The IMAGE PROCESSING Handbook

Fourth Edition

John C. Russ

Materials Science and Engineering Department
North Carolina State University
Raleigh, North Carolina

CRC PRESS

Boca Raton   London   New York   Washington, D.C.

Library of Congress Cataloging-in-Publication Data

Russ, John C.
The image processing handbook / John C. Russ. — 4th ed.
    p. cm.
    Includes bibliographical references and index.
    ISBN 0-8493-1142-X (alk. paper)
    1. Image processing—Handbooks, manuals, etc. I. Title
TA1637 .R87 2002
621.36′7—dc21

2002073595

Visit the CRC Press Web site at www.crcpress.com

Introduction

Image processing is used for two somewhat different purposes:

1. Improving the visual appearance of images to a human viewer
2. Preparing images for measurement of the features and structures present

The techniques that are appropriate for each of these tasks are not always the same, but there is considerable overlap. This book covers methods that are used for both tasks.

To do the best possible job, it helps to know about the uses to which the processed images will be put. For visual enhancement, this means having some familiarity with the human visual process, and an appreciation of what cues the viewer responds to in images. It is also useful to know about the printing or display process, because many images are processed in the context of reproduction or transmission.

The measurement of images generally requires that features be well defined, either by edges or unique brightness, color, texture, or some combination of these factors. The types of measurements that will be performed on entire scenes or individual features are important in determining the appropriate processing steps.

It may help to recall that image processing, similar to food processing or word processing, does not reduce the amount of data present but simply rearranges it. Some arrangements may be more appealing to the senses, and some may convey more meaning, but these two criteria may not be identical nor call for identical methods.

This handbook presents an extensive collection of image processing tools, so that the user of computer-based systems can both understand those methods provided in packaged software, and program those additions that may be needed for particular applications. Comparisons are presented of different algorithms that may be used for similar purposes, using a selection of representative pictures from light and electron microscopes, as well as macroscopic, remote sensing and astronomical images.

In revising the book for this new edition, I tried to respond to some of the comments and requests of readers and reviewers. New chapters on the measurement of images and the subsequent interpretation of the data were added in the second edition, and a section on surface images was added in the third edition. New chapters in this edition discuss in some depth the stereological interpretation of measurements on sections through three-dimensional structures, and the various logical approaches to feature classification. The sections on the ever-advancing hardware for image capture and printing have been expanded and information added on the newest technologies. More examples have been added in every chapter, and the reference list was expanded and brought up to date.

As in past editions, I resisted suggestions to put "more of the math" into the book. Excellent texts are available on image processing, compression, mathematical morphology, etc. that provide as much rigor and as many derivations as may be needed. Many of them are referenced here, but the thrust of this book remains teaching by example. Few people learn the principles of image processing from the equations. Just as we use images to "do science," so most of us use images to learn about many things, including imaging itself. The hope is that, by seeing what various operations do to representative images, you will discover how and why to use them. Then, if you need to look up the mathematical foundations, they will be easier to understand.

The reader is encouraged to use this book in concert with a real source of images and a computer-based system, and to freely experiment with different methods to determine which are most appropriate for his or her particular needs. Selection of image processing tools to explore images when you do not know the contents beforehand is a much more difficult task than using tools to make it easier for another viewer or a measurement program to see the same things you have discovered. It places greater demand on computing speed and the interactive nature of the interface, but it particularly requires that you become a very analytical observer of images. If you can learn to see what the computer sees, you will become a better viewer and obtain the best possible images, suitable for further processing and analysis.

To facilitate this hands-on learning process, I collaborated with my son, Chris Russ, to produce a CD-ROM that can be used as a companion to this book. The Image Processing Tool Kit contains more than 300 images, many of them the examples from the book, plus nearly 200 Photoshop-compatible plug-ins that implement many of the algorithms discussed here. These can be used with Adobe Photoshop® or any of the numerous programs (some of them free), which implement the Photoshop plug-in interface, on either Macintosh or Windows computers. Information about the CD-ROM is available on-line at http://ReindeerGraphics.com/

Acknowledgments

All the image processing and the creation of the resulting figures included in this book were performed on an Apple Macintosh® computer. Many of the images were acquired directly from various microscopes and other sources using color or monochrome video cameras and digitized directly into the computer. Others were digitized using a digital camera (most with a Polaroid DMC), and some were obtained using a 36-bit color scanner (Agfa), often from images supplied by many co-workers and researchers. These are acknowledged wherever the origin of an image could be determined. A few examples, taken from the literature, are individually referenced.

The book was delivered to the publisher in digital form (on a writable CD), without intermediate hard copy, negatives, or prints of the images, etc. Among other things, this means that the author must bear full responsibility for any errors because no traditional typesetting was involved. (It has also forced me to learn more than I ever hoped to know about some aspects of this technology!) However, going directly from disk file to print also shortens the time needed in production and helps to keep costs down, while preserving the full quality of the images. Grateful acknowledgment is made of the efforts by the editors at CRC Press to educate me and to accommodate the unusually large number of illustrations in this book (about 2000 figures and a quarter of a million words).

Special thanks are due to Chris Russ (Reindeer Games Inc., Asheville, NC), who has helped to program many of these algorithms and contributed invaluable comments, and to Helen Adams, who has proofread many pages, endured many discussions, and provided the moral support that make writing projects such as this possible.

John C. Russ
Raleigh, NC

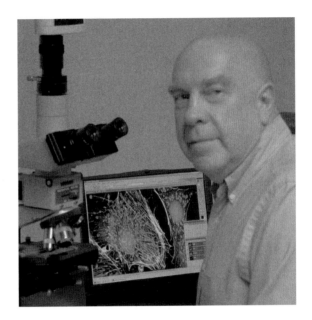

Table of Contents

5 Processing Images in Frequency Space. 277

6 Segmentation and Thresholding 333

Acquiring Images

Human reliance on images for information

Humans are primarily visual creatures. Not all animals depend on their eyes, as we do, for 99% or more of the information received about their surroundings. Bats use high-frequency sound, cats have poor vision but a rich sense of smell, snakes locate prey by their heat emission, and fish have organs that sense (and in some cases generate) electrical fields. Even birds, who are highly visual, do not have our eye configuration. With a few exceptions (e.g., owls), their eyes are on opposite sides of their heads, providing nearly 360-degree coverage but little in the way of stereopsis, and they have four or five different color receptors (we have three, loosely described as red, green, and blue). It is difficult to imagine what the world "looks like" to such animals. Even the word "imagine" contains within it our bias toward images, as does much of our language. People with vision defects wear glasses because of their dependence on this sense. We tolerate considerable hearing loss before resorting to a hearing aid and, practically speaking, no prosthetic devices are available for the other senses of touch, taste, and smell.

This bias in everyday life extends to how we pursue more technical goals as well. Scientific instruments commonly produce images to communicate their results to the operator, rather than generating audible tones or emitting a smell. Space missions to other planets and equally arduous explorations of the ocean depths always include cameras as major components, and we judge the success of those missions by the quality of the images returned. This suggests a few of the ways in which we have extended the range of our natural vision. Simple optical devices such as microscopes and telescopes allow us to see things that are vastly smaller or larger than we could otherwise. Beyond the visible portion of the electromagnetic spectrum (a narrow range of wavelengths between about 400 and 700 nanometers), we now have sensors capable of detecting infrared and ultraviolet light, x-rays, radio waves, and, perhaps soon, even gravity waves. **Figure 1** shows an example of an image presenting radio telescope data in the form of an image in which grey scale brightness represents radio intensity. Such devices and presentations are used to further extend our imaging capability.

Signals other than electromagnetic radiation can be used to produce images as well. Novel new types of microscopes that use atomic-scale probes to "feel" the specimen surface present their data as images. Acoustic waves at low frequency produce sonar images, while at gigahertz frequencies

Figure 1. *Radio astronomy produces images such as this view of NGC 1265. These are often displayed with false colors to emphasize subtle variations in signal brightness.*

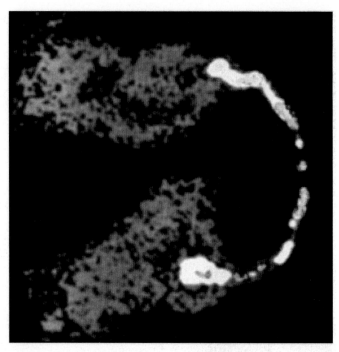

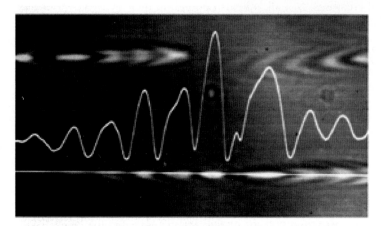

Figure 2. *Scanning acoustic microscope image (with superimposed signal profile along one scan line) of a polished cross section through a composite. The central white feature is a fiber intersecting the surface at an angle. The arcs on either side are interference patterns, which can be used to measure the fiber angle.*

the acoustic microscope produces images with resolution similar to that of the light microscope, but with image contrast that is produced by local variations in the attenuation and refraction of sound waves rather than light. **Figure 2** shows an acoustic microscope image of a composite material, and **Figure 3** shows a sonogram of a baby in the womb.

Some images, such as holograms or electron diffraction patterns, are recorded in terms of brightness as a function of position, but are unfamiliar to the observer. **Figures 4** and **5** show electron diffraction patterns from a transmission electron microscope, in which the atomic structure of the samples is revealed (but only to those who know how to interpret the image). Other kinds of data including weather maps with specialized symbols, graphs of business profit and expenses, and charts with axes representing time, family income, cholesterol level, or even more obscure parameters, have become part of our daily lives. **Figure 6** shows a few examples. The latest developments in computer interfaces and displays make extensive use of graphics, again to take advantage of the large bandwidth of the human visual pathway.

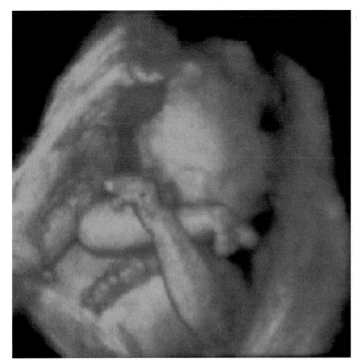

Figure 3. Surface reconstruction of sonogram imaging, showing a 26-week-old fetus in the womb.

Figure 4. An electron diffraction pattern from a thin foil of gold. The ring diameters correspond to diffraction angles, which identify the spacings of planes of atoms in the crystal structure.

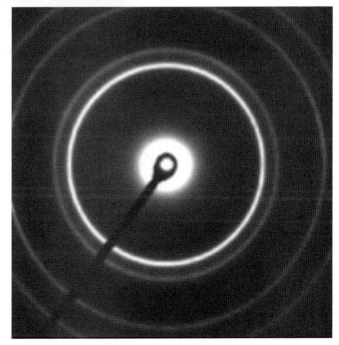

Some important differences exist between human vision, the kind of information it yields from images, and the ways in which it appears to do so, and imaging devices that use computers for technical purposes. Human vision is primarily qualitative and comparative, rather than quantitative. We judge the relative size and shape of objects by mentally rotating them to the same orientation, overlapping them in our minds, and performing a direct comparison. This has been shown by tests in which the time required to recognize features as being the same or different is proportional to the degree of misorientation or intervening distance. **Figure 7** shows an example.

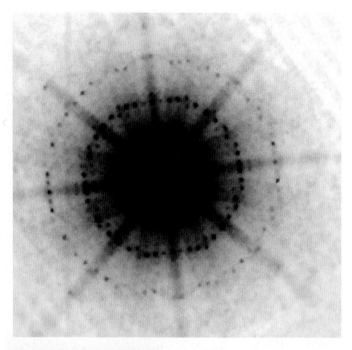

Figure 5. *A convergent beam electron diffraction (CBED) pattern from an oxide microcrystal, which can be indexed and measured to provide high accuracy values for the atomic unit cell dimensions.*

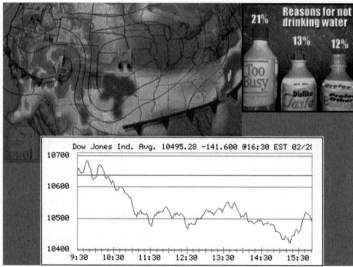

Figure 6. *Typical graphics used to communicate news information include one-dimensional plots such as stock market reports, two-dimensional presentations such as weather maps, and simplified charts using images.*

Humans are especially poor at judging color or brightness of features within images unless they can be exactly compared by making them adjacent. Gradual changes in brightness with position or over time are generally ignored as representing variations in illumination, for which the human visual system compensates automatically. This means that only abrupt changes in brightness are easily seen. Research into human vision indicates that these discontinuities, which usually correspond to physical boundaries or other important structures in the scene being viewed, are extracted from the raw image falling on the retina and sent up to the higher-level processing centers in the cortex.

These characteristics of the visual system are responsible for a variety of visual illusions (**Figure 8**). Some of these illusions enable researchers to study the visual system itself, and others suggest ways that computer-based systems can emulate some of the very efficient (if not always exact) ways that our eyes extract information. Gestalt theory says that this is done by dealing with the

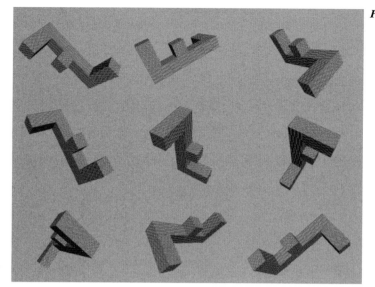

Figure 7. Several views of a complex three dimensional figure. Which of the representations is/are identical and which are mirror images? The time needed to decide is proportional to the misalignment, indicating that we literally "turn the objects over" in our minds to compare them.

Figure 8. A few common illusions:

(***a***) the two horizontal lines are identical in length, but appear different because of grouping with the diagonal lines;

(***b***) the diagonal lines are parallel, but the crossing lines cause them to appear the diverge due to grouping and inhibition;

(***c***) the illusory triangle may appear brighter than the surrounding paper, and is due to grouping and completion;

(***d***) the two inner squares have the same brightness, but the surrounding frames cause us to judge them as different due to brightness inhibition.

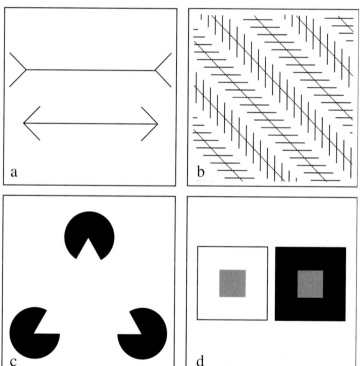

image as a whole, rather than by breaking it down to constituent parts. The idea that grouping of parts within images is done automatically by our vision system, and is central to our understanding of scenes, has been confirmed by many experiments and offers important insights into human physiology and psychology. One of the things it explains is why camouflage works (**Figure 9**).

Our purpose in this book is not to study the human visual pathway, but a brief overview can help us to understand how we see things so that we become better observers. The interested reader may want to explore Frisby, 1980; Marr, 1982; Rock, 1984; and Hubel, 1988. Computer-based image processing and analysis use algorithms based on human vision methods when possible, but also employ other methods that seem not to have direct counterparts in human vision.

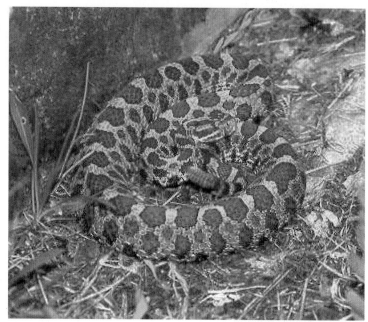

Figure 9. An example of camouflage. Patches of color on this rattlesnake break up the overall shape and make it difficult to recognize.

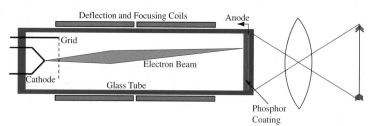

Figure 10. Functional diagram of a vidicon tube. Light striking the phosphor coating changes its local resistance and, thus, the current that flows as the electron beam scans in a raster pattern.

Video cameras

When the first edition of this book was published, in 1990, the most common way of acquiring images for computer processing was with a video camera. Mounted onto a microscope, or using appropriate optics to view an experiment, the camera sent an analog signal to a separate "frame grabber" or analog-to-digital converter (ADC) interface board in the computer, which then stored numeric values in memory.

The basic form of the original type of video camera is the vidicon, illustrated in **Figure 10**. It functions by scanning a focused beam of electrons across a phosphor coating applied to the inside of an evacuated glass tube. The light enters the camera through the front glass surface (and a thin metallic anode layer) and creates free electrons in the phosphor. These vary the local conductivity of the layer, so the amount of current that flows to the anode varies as the beam is scanned, according to the local light intensity. This analog (continuously varying) electrical signal is amplified and, as shown in **Figure 11** conforms to standards of voltage and timing (the standards and timing are slightly different in Europe than the U.S., but the basic principles remain the same).

Digitizing the voltage is accomplished by sampling it and generating a comparison voltage. The child's game of "guess a number" illustrates that it takes only eight guesses to arrive at a value that defines the voltage to one part in 256 (the most widely used type of ADC). The first guess is 128, or half the voltage range. If this is, for example, too large, the second guess subtracts 64. Each successive approximation adds or subtracts a value half as large as the previous. In eight steps, the

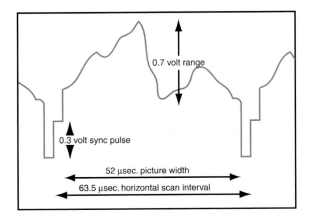

final (smallest) adjustment is made. The result is a number that is conveniently stored in the 8-bit memory of most modern computers.

The tube-type camera has several advantages and quite a few drawbacks. Scanning the beam with electromagnetic or electrostatic fields can produce a distorted scan (pincushion or barrel distortion, or more complicated situations) and is subject to further degradation by stray fields from wiring or instrumentation. **Figure 12** shows an example of pincushion distortion, as well as vignetting and loss of focus. Maintaining focus in the corners of the image takes special circuitry, and the corners may also be darkened by the additional thickness of glass through which the light must pass (vignetting). The sealed vacuum systems tend to deteriorate with time, and the "getter" used to adsorb gas molecules may flake and fall onto the phosphor if the camera is used in a vertical orientation. The response of the camera (voltage vs. brightness) approximates the logarithmic response of film and the human eye, but this varies for bright and dark scenes. Recovery from bright scenes and bright spots is slow, and blooming can occur in which bright light produces spots that spread laterally in the coating and appear larger than the features really are.

The tube-type camera does have some advantages. The spatial resolution is very high, limited only by the grain size of the phosphor and the size of the focused beam spot. Also, the phosphor has a spectral response that can be made quite similar to that of the human eye, which sees color from red (about 0.7 µm wavelength) to blue (about 0.4 µm). Adaptations of the basic camera design with intermediate cathode layers or special coatings for intensification are capable of acquiring images in very dim light (e.g., night scenes, fluorescence microscopy).

Figure 12. *Example of an image showing pincushion distortion, as well as loss of focus and vignetting in the edges and corners.*

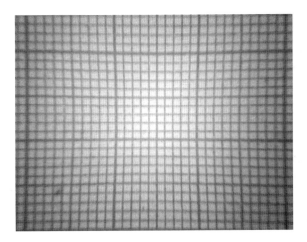

CCD cameras

The tube-type camera has now been largely supplanted by the solid-state chip camera, the simplest form of which is the CCD (charge-coupled device). The camera chip contains an array of diodes that function as light buckets. Light that enters the semiconductor raises electrons from the valence to the conduction band, so the number of electrons is a direct measure of the light intensity. The diodes are formed by photolithography, so they have a perfectly regular pattern with no image distortion, or sensitivity to the presence of stray fields. The devices are also inexpensive and rugged, compared to tube cameras. CCDs were first invented and patented at Bell Labs (in 1969), have been strongly involved in the NASA-JPL space program because they provide a reliable way to acquire images from satellites and space probes, and now are even displacing film in consumer and professional still cameras.

The basic operation of a CCD is illustrated in **Figure 13**. Each bucket represents one "pixel" in the camera (this word has a lot of different meanings in different contexts, as will be explained below, so it must be used with some care). With anywhere from a few hundred thousand to several million detectors on the chip, it is impractical to run wires directly to each one in order to read out the signal. Instead, the electrons that accumulate in each bucket due to incident photons are transferred, one line at a time, to a readout row. On a clock signal, each column of pixels shifts the charge by one location. This places the contents of the buckets into the readout row, and that row is then shifted, one pixel at a time but much more rapidly, to dump the electrons into an amplifier, where it can be sent out as an analog signal from a video camera, or measured immediately to produce a numeric output from a digital camera.

The simplest way of shifting the electrons is shown in **Figure 14**. Every set of three electrodes on the surface of the device constitutes one pixel. By applying a voltage to two of the electrodes, a field is set up in the semiconductor that acts like a bucket. Electrons are trapped in the central region by the high fields on either side. Note that this does not reduce the area sensitive to incoming photons, because electrons generated in the high field regions will quickly migrate to the low field bucket where they are held. By changing the voltage applied to the regions in six steps or phases, as shown in the figure, the electrons are shifted by one pixel. First, one field region is lowered and the electrons spread into the larger volume. Then the field on the other side is raised, and the electrons have been shifted by one-third of the pixel height. Repeating the process acts like a conveyor belt, and is the reason for the name "charge-coupled device."

Figure 13. The basic principle of CCD operation, illustrated as a set of buckets and conveyors (after Janesick, 2001).

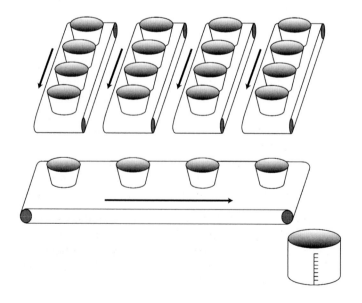

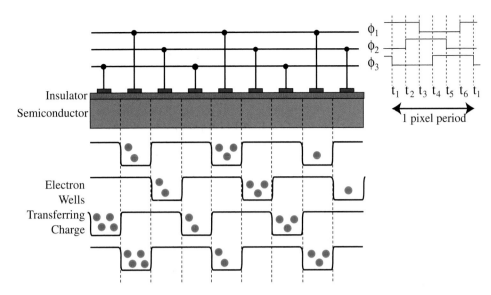

Figure 14. *Varying voltages on a set of three electrodes shifts electrons from one pixel to another.*

One significant problem with the chip camera is its spectral response. Even if the chip is reversed and thinned so that light enters from the side opposite to the electrodes, very little blue light penetrates into the semiconductor to produce electrons. On the other hand, infrared light penetrates easily and these cameras have red and infrared (IR) sensitivity that far exceeds that of human vision, usually requiring the installation of a blocking filter to exclude it (because the IR light is not focused to the same plane as the visible light and would produce blurred or fogged images). **Figure 15** shows this spectral response, which can be further tailored and extended by using materials other than silicon. The chip can reach quite high total efficiency when antireflective coatings are applied, limited primarily by the "fill factor" — the area fraction of the chip that contains active devices between the narrow ditches that maintain electrical separation. Also, the chip camera has an output that is linearly proportional to the incident light intensity, convenient for some measurement purposes but very different from human vision and photographic film, which are logarithmic.

Human vision notices brightness differences of about 2%, that is, a constant ratio of change rather than a constant increment. Film is characterized by a response to light exposure which (after chemical development) produces a density vs. exposure curve such as that shown in **Figure 16**. The low end of this curve represents the fog level of the film, the density that is present even without exposure. At the high end, the film saturates to a maximum optical density, for instance based on the maximum physical density of silver particles. In between, it has a linear relationship whose slope represents the contrast of the film. A steep slope corresponds to a high-contrast film that exhibits a large change in optical density with a small change in exposure. Conversely, a low-contrast film has a broader latitude to record a scene with a greater range of brightnesses. The slope of the curve is usually called "gamma" and some chip cameras, particularly those used for consumer video camcorders, may include circuitry that changes their output from linear to logarithmic so that the image contrast is more familiar to viewers.

When film is exposed directly to electrons, as in the transmission electron micrograph, rather than photons (visible light or x-rays), the response curve is linear rather than logarithmic. Many photons are needed to completely expose a single halide particle for development, but only a single electron. Consequently, electron image films and plates are often very high in density (values greater than 4) which creates difficulties for most scanners.

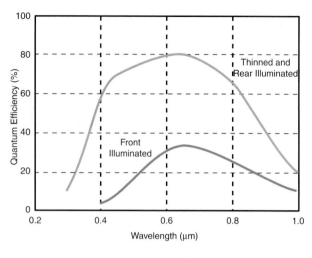

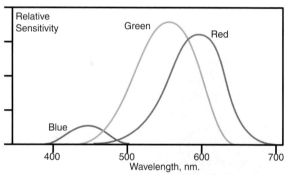

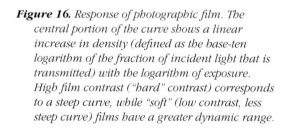

Figure 15. Spectral response of a silicon based chip (***a***), compared with the color sensors in the human eye (***b***), which are commonly identified as red, green, and blue sensitive but actually cover a range of long, medium, and short wavelengths.

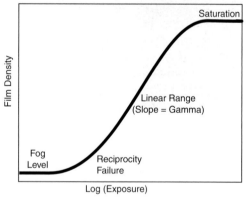

Figure 16. Response of photographic film. The central portion of the curve shows a linear increase in density (defined as the base-ten logarithm of the fraction of incident light that is transmitted) with the logarithm of exposure. High film contrast ("hard" contrast) corresponds to a steep curve, while "soft" (low contrast, less steep curve) films have a greater dynamic range.

The trend in camera chips has been to make them smaller and to increase the number of pixels or diodes present. Some scientific chips, such as those used in the Hubble telescope, occupy an entire wafer. But for consumer devices, making them one-third, one-quarter, or even two-tenths of an inch in overall (diagonal) dimension places many devices on a single wafer and allows greater economic yield. Putting more pixels into this reduced chip area (for more spatial resolution, as discussed below) makes the individual detectors small, but the ditches between then have to remain about the same size to prevent electrons from diffusing laterally. The result is to reduce the total efficiency markedly. Some devices place small lenses over the diodes to capture light that would otherwise fall into the ditches, but these add cost and also are not so uniform as the diodes themselves (which are typically within 1% across the entire chip).

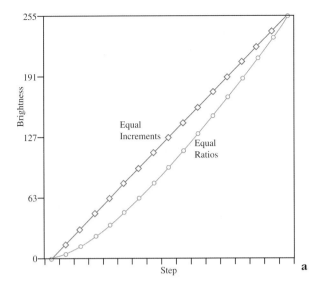

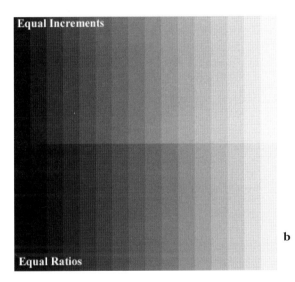

Figure 17. Comparison of visibility of grey level steps from linear (equal steps) and logarithmic (equal ratios) detectors:
*(**a**) plots of intensity;*
*(**b**) display of the values from figure a.*

The other effect of making the detectors small is to reduce their capacity for electrons, called the well capacity. A typical 15 μm pixel in a scientific grade CCD has a capacity of about 500,000 electrons, which with low readout noise (which can be achieved in special situations) of a few electrons gives a dynamic range greater than photographic film. Even larger well capacity and dynamic range can be achieved by combining more detectors in each pixel (binning) by using more steps in the phase shifting. Conversely, reducing the area of the detector also reduces the well size and, with it, the dynamic range. Increasing the noise, for instance by reading out the signal at video rates (each horizontal line in 52 μs for U.S. video), dramatically reduces the dynamic range and a typical consumer grade video camera has no more than about 64 distinguishable brightness levels (studio cameras meet the broadcast video specification of 100 levels). With the chip camera, they are linear with brightness, so they produce even fewer viewable grey levels as shown in **Figure 17**. This performance is much inferior to film, which can distinguish thousands of brightness levels.

Camera artefacts and limitations

Video cameras that use chips have several problems, which contribute to the specific types of defects present in the images which must be dealt with by subsequent processing. One is the fact that video signals are interlaced (**Figure 18**). This clever trick to minimize visual flicker in broadcast television images was accomplished with tube cameras simply by scanning the electron beam in the same interlace pattern as the display television set. With a chip camera, it requires that the array be read out twice for every 30th of a second frame, once to collect the even numbered lines and again for the odd numbered lines. In fact, many cameras combine two lines to get better sensitivity, averaging lines 1 and 2, 3 and 4, 5 and 6, and so on, in one interlace field, and then 2 and 3, 4 and 5, 6 and 7, etc., in the other. This reduces vertical resolution but for casual viewing purposes is not noticeable. Motion can cause the even and odd fields of a full frame to be offset from each other, producing a significant degradation of the image as shown in the figure. A similar effect occurs with stationary images if the horizontal retrace signal is imprecise or difficult for the electronics to lock onto; this is a particular problem with signals played back from consumer video recorders.

During the transfer and readout process, unless the camera is shuttered either mechanically or electrically, photons continue to produce electrons in the chip. This produces a large background signal that further degrades dynamic range and may produce blurring. Electronic shuttering is usually done one line at a time so that moving images are distorted. Some designs avoid shuttering problems by doubling the number of pixels, with half of them opaque to incoming light. A single transfer shifts the electrons from the active detectors to the hidden ones, from which they can be read out. Of course, this reduces the active area (fill factor) of devices on the chip, costing 50% in sensitivity.

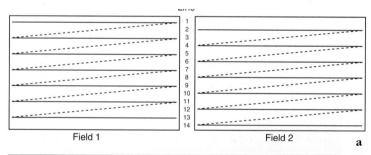

Field 1 Field 2 **a**

*Figure 18. Interlace scan covers even numbered lines in a 1/60th of a second field, and even numbered lines in a second field (**a**). When motion is present, this produces an offset in the complete image (**b**).*

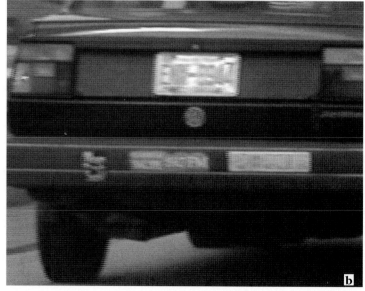

The high speed of horizontal line readout can produce horizontal blurring of the signal, again reducing image resolution. This is partially due to inadequate time for the electrons to diffuse along with the shifting fields and the time needed to recover electrons from traps (impurities in the silicon lattice), and partially to the inadequate frequency response of the amplifier, which is a trade-off with amplifier noise. Even though the individual electron transfers are very efficient, better than 99.99% in most cases, the result of being passed through many such transfers before being collected and amplified increases the noise. This varies from one side of the chip to the other, and from the top to the bottom, and can be visually detected in images if there is not a lot of other detail or motion to obscure it.

Many transfers of electrons from one detector to another occur during readout of a chip, and this accounts for some of the noise in the signal. Purely statistical variations in the production and collection of charge is a relatively smaller effect. The conversion of the tiny charge to a voltage and its subsequent amplification is the greatest source of noise in most systems. Readout and amplifier noise can be reduced by slowing the transfer process so that fewer electrons are lost in the shifting process and the amplifier time constant can integrate out more of the noise, producing a cleaner signal. Cooling the chip to about –40°C also reduces the noise from these sources and from dark current, or thermal electrons. Slow readout and cooling are used only in non-video applications, of course. Janesick (2001) discusses the various sources of noise and their control in scientific CCDs of the type used in astronomical imaging (where they have almost entirely replaced film) and in space probes.

Color cameras

Color cameras can be designed in three principle ways, as shown in **Figures 19**, **20** and **21**. For stationary images (which includes many scientific applications such as microscopy, but excludes "real-time" applications such as video), a single detector array can be used to acquire three sequential exposures through red, green and blue filters, respectively, which are then combined for viewing (**Figure 19**). The advantages of this scheme include low cost and the ability to use different exposure times for the different color bands, which can compensate for the poorer sensitivity of the CCD chip to blue light.

Many high-end consumer and most professional and scientific grade video cameras use three sensors (**Figure 20**). A prism array splits the incoming light into red, green, and blue components

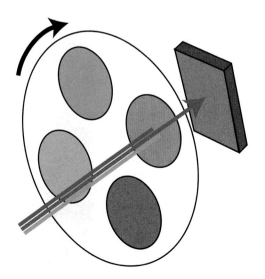

Figure 19. Schematic diagram of a color wheel camera. The fourth filter position is empty, allowing the camera to be used as a monochrome detector with greater sensitivity for dim images (e.g., fluorescence microscopy).

Figure 20. *Schematic diagram of a three-chip color camera.*

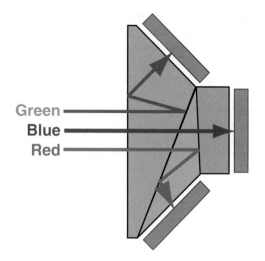

Green ——
Blue ——
Red ——

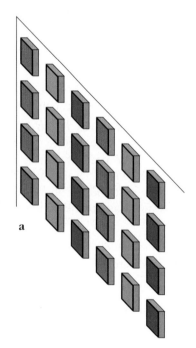

a

Figure 21. *Stripe (**a**) and Bayer (**b**) filter patterns used in single chip cameras.*

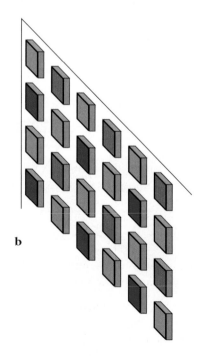

b

which are recorded by three different sensors whose outputs are combined electronically to produce a standard video image. This approach is more costly, because three chips are needed, but for video applications they need not be of particularly high resolution (fewer pixels). The optics and hardware to keep everything in alignment add some cost, and the depth of the prism optics makes it impractical to use short focal length (wide angle) lenses.

Video images are often digitized into a 640×480 array of stored pixels, but this is not the actual resolution of the image. The broadcast bandwidth limits the high frequencies and eliminates any rapid variations in brightness and color. A video image has no more than 330 actual elements of resolution in the horizontal direction for the brightness (luminance) signal, and about half that for the color (chrominance) information. Color information is intentionally reduced in resolution because human vision is not very sensitive to blurring of color beyond boundary lines.

Of course, video signals can be further degraded by poor equipment. Recording video on consumer-grade tape machines can reduce the resolution by another 50% or more, particularly if the record head is dirty or the tape has been used many times before. Video images are just not very high resolution, although some forms of HDTV (high definition television) may improve things in the future. Consequently, video technology is usually a poor choice for scientific imaging unless there is some special need to capture "real-time" images (i.e., 25–30 frames per second) to record changes or motion. Digital cameras have largely replaced them now, as they produce much higher resolution images and at lower cost.

Most digital cameras use a single pixel array, often of very high pixel (detector) count, with a color filter that allows red, green and blue light to reach specific detectors. Different patterns may be used (**Figure 21**), with the Bayer pattern being very common. Notice that it assigns twice as many detectors for green as for red or blue, which mimics to some extent the human eye's greater sensitivity to green. The problem with the single-chip camera, of course, is that the image resolution in each color channel is reduced. The red intensity at some locations must be interpolated from nearby sensors, for example. It is also necessary to design the filters to give the same brightness sensitivity in each channel. If this is not done well, a herringbone pattern will appear in images of a uniform grey test card and color fringes will appear along edges in the picture.

Interpolation techniques for Bayer pattern color filters reduce the image resolution as compared to the number of individual detectors in the camera (which is generally the specification advertised by the manufacturer). The quality of the interpolation, judged by its ability to preserve sharp boundaries in brightness while minimizing the introduction of color artefacts, varies inversely with the computational requirements. A comparison of several patented methods can be found in (Ramanesh, 2000).

Camera resolution

The signal coming from the chip is an analog voltage, of course, even if the digitization takes place in the camera itself, so the interpolation is done in the amplifier stage, by the use of appropriate time constants. This means that the voltage cannot vary rapidly enough to correspond to brightness differences for every pixel. In most cases, because of this interpolation, the actual image resolution with a single chip camera and filter arrangement will be one-half to two-thirds the value that might be expected by the advertised number of pixels in the camera. And some cameras record images with many more stored pixels than the chip resolution would warrant in any case. Such empty magnification contributes no additional information in the image.

Comparing cameras based on actual resolution rather than the stated number of recorded pixels can be quite difficult. It is important to consider the multiple meanings of the word "pixel." In some contexts, it refers to the number of light detectors in the camera (without regard to any color filtering, and sometimes including ones around the edges that do not contribute to the actual image but are used to measure dark current). In other contexts, it describes the number of recorded brightness or color values stored in the computer, although these may represent empty magnification. In other situations, it is used to describe the displayed points of light on the computer monitor, even if the image is shown in a compressed or enlarged size. It makes much more sense to separate these various meanings and to talk about resolution elements when considering real image resolution. This refers to the number of discrete points across the image that can be distinguished from each other, and is sometimes described in terms of the number of line pairs that can be resolved. This is half the number of resolution elements, because one element is needed for the line and one for the space between lines, and it depends on the amount of brightness contrast between the lines and the spaces and, of course, the amount of noise (random variations) present in the image.

The situation is even more complicated with some digital cameras that shift the detector array to capture multiple samples of the image. The most common method is to use a piezo device to offset the array by half the pixel spacing in the horizontal and vertical directions, capturing four images that can be combined to nearly double the resolution of the image as data are acquired from the gaps between the original pixel positions. For an array with colored filters, additional shifts can produce color images with resolution approaching that corresponding to the pixel spacing; and some studio cameras displace the entire sensor array to different regions of the film plane to collect tiles that are subsequently assembled into an image several times as large as the detector array. Of course, the multiple exposures required with these methods means that more time is required to acquire the image.

With either the single-chip or three-chip camera, the blue channel is typically the noisiest due to the low chip sensitivity to blue light and the consequent need for greater amplification. In many cases, processing software that reduces image noise using one of the averaging or median filters discussed in Chapter 3 can be applied separately to each color channel, using different parameters according to the actual noise content, to best improve image appearance.

Because of the longer exposure times, which collect more electrons and so reduce noise due to statistics and amplification, and because of the much slower readout of the data from the chip, which may take several seconds instead of 1/30th of a second, digital cameras using the same chip technology as a video camera can produce much better image quality. Digital still cameras read out the data in one single pass (progressive scan), not with an interlace. By cooling the chip and amplifier circuitry to reduce dark currents, integration (long exposures up to tens of seconds or, for some astronomical applications, many minutes) can be used to advantage because of the high dynamic range of some chip designs. In addition, the ability to use a physical rather than electronic shutter simplifies chip circuitry and increases fill factor. The number of pixels in video cameras need not be any greater than the resolution of the video signal, which, as noted previously, is quite poor. In a digital still camera, very high pixel counts can give rise to extremely high resolution, which is beginning to rival film in some cases.

An interesting crossover is also occurring between high-end consumer and professional scientific-grade cameras. In addition to dedicated cameras for attachment to microscopes or other separate optics, manufacturers are producing consumer cameras with enough resolution (3–6 million pixels at this writing) that it is becoming practical to use them in technical applications, and simple optical attachments are making it easy to connect them to microscopes. **Figure 22** shows two of the cameras in use in the author's laboratory. The large, dedicated camera cost more than six times the small one. The small one is also portable with its own storage, and useful for many other applications. At the same time, professional digital cameras with extremely high resolution detector arrays, interchangeable lenses, etc., are providing capabilities that compete strongly with traditional 35mm and larger film cameras. Every manufacturer of cameras has recognized the shift away from film and toward digital recording, and an incredibly wide variety of cameras is now available with new developments appearing frequently.

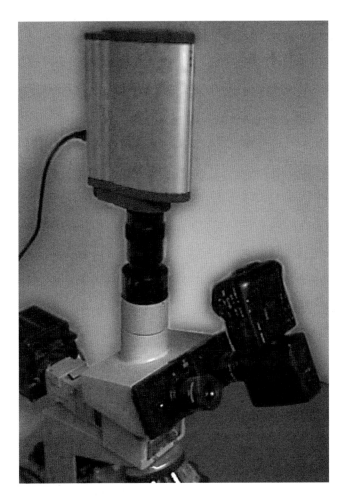

Figure 22. Two digital cameras mounted on the author's microscope. The top camera (Polaroid DMC Ie) provides greater bit depth and compensation for illumination temperature. The one mounted on the eyepiece (Nikon 990) has greater spatial resolution, and can be used without a tethered computer. Both cameras store images as uncompressed TIFF files.

CMOS cameras

A competitor to the CCD design for chips now appearing on the horizon, CMOS (complementary metal oxide semiconductor) uses a different fabrication approach that promises several potential advantages. The most important is cost, because the manufacturing process is similar to that used for other common chips such as computer memory, whereas CCDs require separate fabrication lines. It is also possible to incorporate additional circuitry on the CMOS chip, such as the amplifiers and readout and control electronics, and the digitizer, leading to the possibility of a single-chip camera. This may lead to less expensive systems, but with more costly development procedures. The devices will also be more compact and possibly more rugged. CMOS devices also require lower voltages and have lower power requirements, which can be important for portable devices.

Another potential advantage is windowing, the possibility to read out a portion of the array rather than the entire array, because row–column addressing (just like memory chips) can be used to access any pixel. This can provide rapid updating for focusing, measurement of regions of interest, etc.

On the other hand, CMOS devices have much higher noise than CCDs. Partly, this is due to the fact that the CCD has less on-chip circuitry and uses a common output amplifier for less variability. CMOS has higher dark currents, and thus more noise. Also, there is more capacitance in the output wiring, which degrades amplifier noise characteristics. CMOS uses amplifiers for each pixel, producing a unique nonuniformity for each chip called fixed pattern noise (FPN). FPN can in principle be removed by recording the pattern and post processing with software to remove it, but this further reduces the useful dynamic range. The amplifiers also take up more area on the chip, further reducing fill factor, and with it well capacity and dynamic range. Each pixel requires at least two or three transistors to control the detector, plus the amplifier, and fill factors are often less than 30%. The sensitivity and dynamic range of the CCD is much greater, due to the larger size of the detector, lower noise, etc.

Although CMOS detector production facilities are similar in principle to those used for computer memory and other devices, in fact the quest for lower noise has led to the use of special fabrication processes and techniques to reduce trapping and other defects, which largely eliminates this commonality. Defect control for acceptable yields currently limits CMOS arrays to 1–2 million pixels, whereas CCDs with up to 16 million pixels are currently available.

CMOS is expected to dominate in the low-end consumer market for camcorders and snapshot cameras, toys, and other specialty applications such as surveillance video cameras, but not to challenge CCDs for scientific and technical applications requiring high fidelity, resolution, and dynamic range for some time to come.

Focusing

Regardless of what type of camera is employed to acquire images, it is important to focus the optics correctly to capture the fine details in the image. Usually, the human eye is used to performing this task. In some situations, such as automated microscopy of pathology slides or surveillance tracking of vehicles, automatic focusing is required. This brings computer processing into the initial step of image capture. Sometimes, in the interests of speed, the processing is performed in dedicated hardware circuits attached to the camera; but, in any case, the algorithms are the same as might be applied in the computer. In many cases the focusing is accomplished in software by stepping the optics through a range of settings and choosing the one that gives the "best" picture.

Several different approaches to automatic focus are used. Cameras used for macroscopic scenes may employ methods that use some distance-measuring technology (e.g., using high frequency sound or infrared light to determine the distance to the subject so that the lens position can be adjusted). In microscopy applications, this is impractical and the variation in the image itself with focus adjustment must be used. Various algorithms are used to detect the quality of image sharpness, and all are successful for the majority of images in which there is good contrast and fine detail present. Each approach selects some implementation of a high-pass filter output that can be realized in various ways, using either hardware or software, but must take into account the effect of high frequency noise in the image and the optical transfer function of the optics (Green et al., 1985; Firestone et al., 1991; Boddeke et al., 1994).

Electronics and bandwidth limitations

Video cameras of either the solid-state or tube type produce analog voltage signals corresponding to the brightness at different points in the image. In the standard RS-170 signal convention, the voltage varies over a 0.7-volt range from minimum to maximum brightness, as shown above in Figure 11. The scan is nominally 525 lines per full frame, with two interlaced 1/60th-second fields combining to make an entire image. Only about 480 of the scan lines are actually usable, with the remainder lost during vertical retrace. In a typical broadcast television picture, more of these lines are lost due to overscanning, leaving about 400 lines in the actual viewed area. The time duration of each scan line is 62.5 µs, part of which is used for horizontal retrace. This leaves 52 µs for the image data, which must be subdivided into the horizontal spacing of discernible pixels. For PAL (European) television, these values are slightly different, based on a 1/25th-second frame time and more scan lines, but the resulting resolution is similar.

Broadcast television stations are given only a 4-MHz bandwidth for their signals, which must carry color and sound information as well as the brightness signal we have so far been discussing. This narrow bandwidth limits the number of separate voltage values that can be distinguished along each scan line to a maximum of 330, as mentioned previously, and this value is reduced if the signal is degraded by the electronics or by recording using standard videotape recorders. Consumer-quality videotape recorders reduce the effective resolution substantially; in "freeze frame" playback, they display only one of the two interlaced fields, so that only about 200 lines are resolved vertically. Using such equipment as part of an image analysis system makes choices of cameras or digitizer cards on the basis of resolution quite irrelevant.

Even the best system can be degraded in performance by such simple things as cables, connectors, or incorrect termination impedance. Another practical caution in the use of standard cameras is to avoid automatic gain or brightness compensation circuits. These can change the image contrast or linearity in response to bright or dark regions that do not even lie within the digitized portion of the image, and increase the gain and noise for a dim signal.

Figure 23 shows a micrograph with its brightness histogram. This is an important tool for image analysis, which plots the number of pixels as a function of their brightness values. The histogram as shown is well spread out over the available 256 brightness levels, with peaks corresponding to each of the phases in the metal sample. If a bright light falls on a portion of the detector in the solid-state camera that is not part of the image area of interest (e.g. due to internal reflections in the optics), automatic gain circuits in the camera may alter the brightness–voltage relationship so that the image changes. This same effect occurs when a white or dark mask is used to surround images placed under a camera on a copy stand. The relationship between structure and brightness is changed, making subsequent analysis more difficult.

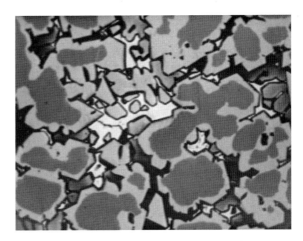

Figure 23. A grey-scale image digitized from a metallographic microscope and its brightness histogram, which plots the number of pixels with each possible brightness value.

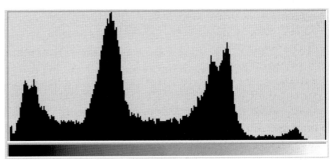

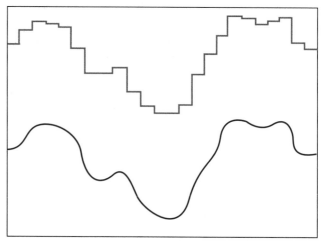

Figure 24. *Digitization of an analog voltage signal such as one line in a video image (blue) produces a series of numbers that represent a series of steps (red) equal in time and rounded to integral multiples of the smallest measurable height increment.*

Issues involving color correction and calibration will be dealt with in the following paragraph, but obtaining absolute color information from video cameras is nearly impossible considering the broad range of wavelengths passed through each filter, the variation in illumination color (e.g., with slight voltage changes on an incandescent bulb) and the way the color information is encoded.

The analog voltage signal is usually digitized with an 8-bit "flash" ADC (analog-to-digital converter). This is a chip using successive approximation techniques to rapidly sample and measure the voltage in less than 100 ns, producing a number value from 0 to 255 that represents the brightness. This number is immediately stored in memory and another reading made, so that a series of brightness values is obtained along each scan line. **Figure 24** illustrates the digitization of a signal into equal steps both in time and value. Additional circuitry is needed to trigger each series of readings on the retrace events so that positions along successive lines are consistent. Digitizing several hundred points along each scan line, repeating the process for each line, and storing the values into memory while adjusting for the interlace of alternate fields produces a digitized image for further processing or analysis.

Pixels

It is most desirable to have the spacing of the pixel values be the same in the horizontal and vertical directions (i.e., square pixels), as this simplifies many processing and measurement operations. Accomplishing this goal requires a well-adjusted clock to control the acquisition. Since the standard video image is not square, but has a width-to-height ratio of 4:3, the digitized image may represent only a portion of the entire field of view. Digitizing boards, also known as frame grabbers, were first designed to record 512 × 512 arrays of values, because the power-of-two dimension simplified design and memory addressing. Most of the current generation of boards acquire a 640 wide by 480 high array, which matches the image proportions and the size of standard VGA display monitors while keeping the pixels square. Because of the variation in clocks between cameras and digitizers, it is common to find distortions of a few percent in pixel squareness. This can be measured and compensated for after acquisition by resampling the pixels in the image as discussed in Chapter 3.

Of course, digitizing 640 values along a scan line that is limited by electronic bandwidth and contains only 300+ meaningfully different values produces an image with unsharp or fuzzy edges and "empty" magnification. Cameras that are capable of resolving more than 600 points along each scan line can sometimes be connected directly to the digitizing electronics to reduce this loss of horizontal resolution. Digital camera designs bypass the analog transmission altogether, sending digital values to the computer, but these are generally slower than standard video systems as discussed previously.

Pixels have a finite area, so those that straddle a boundary effectively average the brightness levels of two regions and have an intermediate brightness that depends on how the pixels lie with respect to the boundary. This means that a high lateral pixel resolution and a large number of distinguishable grey levels are needed to accurately locate boundaries. **Figure 25** shows several examples of an image with varying numbers of pixels across its width, and **Figure 26** shows the same image with varying numbers of grey levels.

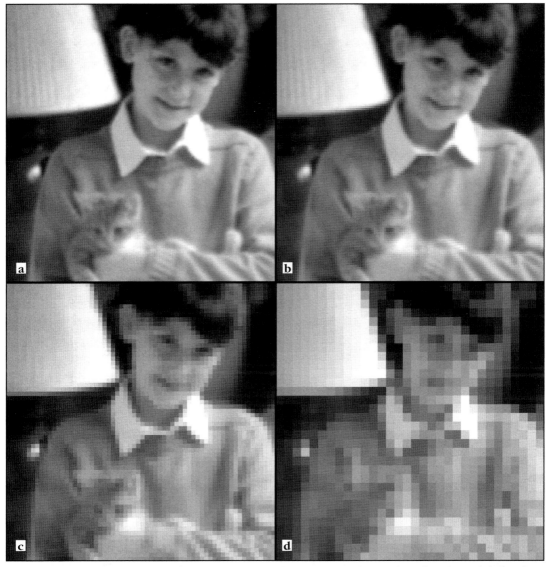

Figure 25. Four representations of the same image, with variation in the number of pixels used: (**a**) 256 × 256; (**b**) 128 × 128; (**c**) 64 × 64, (**d**)32 × 32. In all cases, a full 256 grey values are retained. Each step in coarsening of the image is accomplished by averaging the brightness of the region covered by the larger pixels.

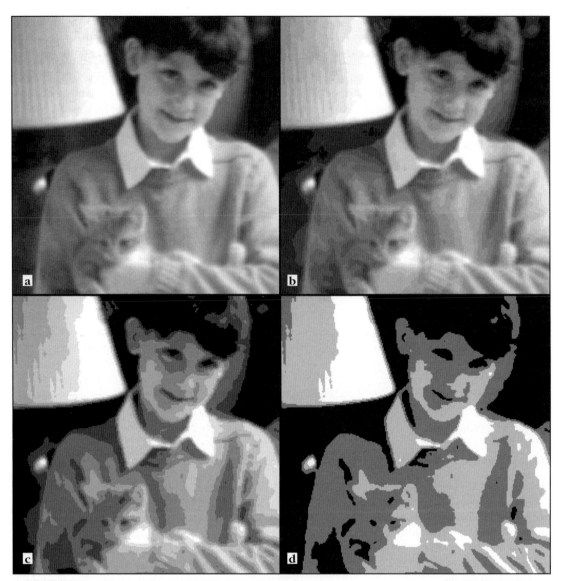

Figure 26. Four representations of the same image, with variation in the number of grey levels used: (a) 32; (b) 16; (c) 8; (d) 4. In all cases, a full 256 × 256 array of pixels are retained. Each step in the coarsening of the image is accomplished by rounding the brightness of the original pixel value.

For the most common types of image acquisition devices, such as video cameras, the pixels represent an averaging of the signal across a finite area of the scene or specimen; however, this is not so in other situations. At low magnification, for example, the scanning electron microscope beam samples a volume of the specimen much smaller than the dimension of a pixel in the image, as does the probe tip in a scanned probe microscope. Range imaging of the moon from the Clementine orbiter read the elevation of points about 10 cm in diameter using a laser range finder, but the points were spaced apart by 100 meters or more.

In these cases, the interpretation of the relationship between adjacent pixels is slightly different. Instead of averaging across boundaries, the pixels sample points that are discrete and well separated. Cases of intermediate or gradually varying values from pixel to pixel are rare, and the problem instead becomes how to locate a boundary between two sampled points on either side. If there are many points along both sides of the boundary, and the boundary can be assumed to have some geometric shape (such as a straight line), fitting methods can be used to locate it to a fraction of the pixel spacing. These methods are discussed further in Chapter 9 on image measurements.

Grey-scale resolution

In addition to defining the number of sampled points along each scan line, and thus the resolution of the image, the design of the ADC also controls the precision of each measurement. Inexpensive commercial flash analog-to-digital converters usually measure each voltage reading to produce an 8-bit number from 0 to 255. This range may not be used entirely for an actual image, which may not vary from full black to white. Also, the quality of most cameras and other associated electronics rarely produces voltages that are free enough from electronic noise to justify full 8-bit digitization anyway. A typical "good" camera specification of 49-dB signal-to-noise ratio implies that only 7 bits of real information are available, and the eighth bit is random noise; but 8 bits corresponds nicely to the most common organization of computer memory into bytes, so that one byte of storage can hold the brightness value from one pixel in the image.

Some cameras and most scanners produce more than 256 distinguishable brightness values, and for these it is common to store the data in two bytes or 16 bits, giving a possible range of 65536:1, which exceeds the capability of any current imaging device (but not some other sources of data that may be displayed as images, such as surface elevation measured with a scanned probe as discussed in Chapter 13). For a camera with a 10- or 12-bit output, the values are simply shifted over to the most significant bits and the low order bits are either zero or random values. For display and printing purposes 8 bits is enough, but the additional depth can be very important for processing and measurement, as discussed in subsequent chapters. In some systems the histogram of values is still expressed as 0–255 for compatibility with the more common 8-bit range, but instead of being restricted to integers, the brightness values can take on real values.

Figure 27 shows an image that appears to be a uniform grey. When the contrast range is expanded we can see the faint lettering present on the back of this photographic print. Also evident is a series of vertical lines which are due to the digitizing circuitry, in this case electronic noise from the high-frequency clock used to control the time base for the digitization. Nonlinearities in the ADC, electronic noise from the camera itself, and degradation in the amplifier circuitry combine to make the lowest two bits of most standard video images useless, so that only about 64 grey levels are actually distinguishable in the data. As noted previously, higher performance cameras and circuits exist, but do not generally offer "real-time" video speed (30 frames per second).

When this stored image is subsequently displayed from memory, the numbers are used in a digital-to-analog converter to produce voltages that control the brightness of a display, often a cathode ray tube (CRT). This process is comparatively noise-free and high resolution, since computer display technology has been developed to a high level for other purposes. A monochrome (black/grey/white) image displayed in this way, with 640 × 480 pixels, each of which can be set to one of 256 brightness levels (or colors using pseudo-color techniques to be discussed below), can be used with many desktop computers.

The human eye cannot distinguish all 256 different levels of brightness in this type of display, nor can they be successfully recorded or printed using inexpensive technology, such as ink-jet or laser printers discussed in Chapter 2. About 20–30 grey levels can be visually distinguished on a CRT or photographic print, suggesting that the performance of the digitizers in this regard is more than adequate, at least for those applications where the performance of the eye was enough to begin with.

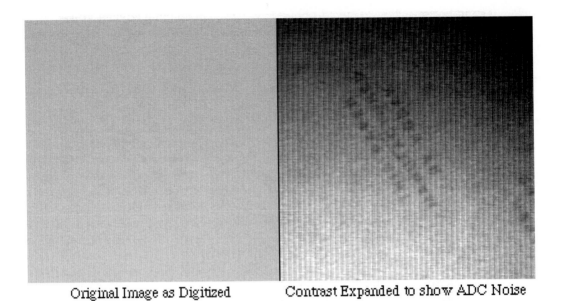

Original Image as Digitized   Contrast Expanded to show ADC Noise

Figure 27. Digitized camera image of the back of a photographic print, showing the periodic noise present in the lowest few bits of the data from the electronics (especially the clock) in the analog to digital converter.

Images acquired in very dim light, or some other imaging modalities such as x-ray mapping in the scanning electron microscope (SEM), impose another limitation of the grey-scale depth of the image. When the number of photons (or other particles) collected for each image pixel is low, statistical fluctuations become important. **Figure 28** shows a fluorescence microscope image in which a single video frame illustrates extreme statistical noise, which would prevent distinguishing or measuring the structures present.

Noise

Images in which the pixel values vary even within regions that are ideally uniform in the original scene can arise either because of limited counting statistics for the photons or other signals, losses introduced in the shifting of electrons within the chip, or due to electronic noise in the amplifiers or cabling. In either case, the variation is generally referred to as noise, and the ratio of the contrast which is actually due to structural differences in the image to the noise level is the signal-to-noise ratio. When this is low, the features present may be invisible to the observer. **Figure 29** shows an example in which several features of different size and shape are superimposed on a noisy background with different signal-to-noise ratios. The ability to discern the presence of the features is generally proportional to their area, and independent of shape.

In the figure, a smoothing operation is performed on the image with the poorest signal-to-noise ratio, which somewhat improves the visibility of the features. The methods available for smoothing noisy images by image processing are discussed in the chapters on spatial and frequency domain methods; however, the best approach to noisy images, when it is available, is simply to collect more signal and improve the statistics.

Adding together more video frames is shown in **Figure 28**. The improvement in quality is proportional to the square root of the number of frames. Because each frame is digitized to 8 bits, adding together up to 256 frames as shown requires a total image storage capability that is 16 bits (2 bytes) deep. Acquiring frames and adding together the pixels at video rates generally requires

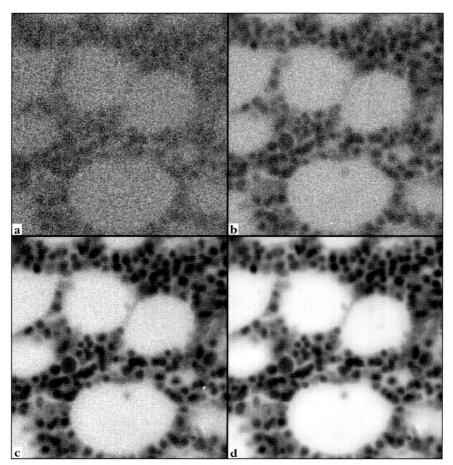

Figure 28. Averaging of a noisy (low photon intensity) image (light microscope image of bone marrow): *one frame (**a**); addition of 4 (**b**), 16 (**c**) and 256 (**d**) frames.*

specialized hardware, and performing the operation in a general-purpose computer limits the practical acquisition to only a few of the video frames per second. This limitation discards a large percentage of the photons that reach the detector. It is more efficient to use a camera capable of integrating the signal directly for the appropriate length of time, and then to read the final image to the computer, which also reduces the noise due to readout and digitization. Digital cameras are available with this capability, and with cooled chips can reduce electronic noise during long acquisitions of many minutes. Most uncooled camera chips will begin to show unacceptable pixel noise due to dark current with integration times of more than a few seconds.

Acquiring images from a video camera is sometimes referred to as "real-time" imaging, but of course this term should properly be reserved for any imaging rate that is adequate to reveal temporal changes in a particular application. For some situations, time-lapse photography may only require one frame to be taken at periods of many minutes. For others, very short exposures and high rates are needed. Special cameras that do not use video frame rates or bandwidths can achieve rates up to ten times that of a standard video camera for full frames, and even higher for small image dimensions. These cameras typically use a single line of detectors and optical deflection (e.g., a rotating mirror or prism) to cover the image.

For many applications, the repetition rate does not need to be that high. Either stroboscopic imaging or simply a fast shutter speed may be enough to stop the important motion to provide a sharp

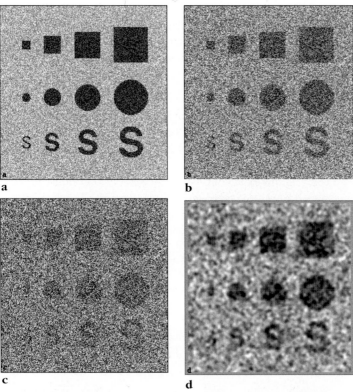

Figure 29. Features on a noisy background:
(a) signal to noise ratio 1:1;
(b) signal to noise ratio 1:3;
(c) signal to noise ratio 1:7;
(d) image c after spatial smoothing.

a

b

c

d

image. Electronic shutters can be used to control solid state imaging devices, instead of a mechanical shutter. Exposure times under 1/1000th of a second can easily be achieved, but of course this short exposure requires plenty of light.

High depth images

Other devices that produce data sets that are often treated as images for viewing and measurement produce data with a much greater range than a camera. For instance, a scanned stylus instrument that measures the elevation of points on a surface may have a vertical resolution of a few nanometers with a maximum vertical travel of hundreds of micrometers, for a range-to-resolution value of 10^5. This would require storing data in a format that preserved the full resolution values, and such instruments typically use 4 bytes per pixel.

In some cases with cameras having a large brightness range, the entire 12- or 14-bit depth of each pixel is stored; however, because this depth exceeds the capabilities of most CRTs to display, or of the user to see, reduction may be appropriate. If the actual brightness range of the image does not cover the entire possible range, scaling (either manual or automatic) to select just the range actually used can significantly reduce storage requirements. In other cases, especially when performing densitometry, a nonlinear conversion table is used. For densitometry, the desired density value varies as the logarithm of the brightness; this is discussed in detail in Chapter 9. A range of 256 brightness steps is not adequate to cover a typical range from 0 to greater than 3 in optical density with useful precision, because at the dark end of the range, 1 part in 256 represents a step of more than 0.1 in optical density. Using a digitization with 12 bits (1 part in 4096) solves this problem, but it is efficient to convert the resulting value with a logarithmic lookup table to store an 8-bit value (occupying a single computer byte) that is the optical density.

Lookup tables (LUTs) may be implemented either in hardware or software. They simply use the original value as an index into a stored or precalculated table, which then provides the derived value. This process is fast enough that acquisition is not affected. The context for LUTs discussed here is for image acquisition, converting a 10-, 12-, or 14-bit digitized value with a nonlinear table to an 8-bit value that can be stored. LUTs are also used for displaying stored images, particularly to substitute colors for grey scale values to create pseudo-color displays. This topic is discussed later in this chapter.

Many images do not have a brightness range that covers the full dynamic range of the digitizer. The result is an image whose histogram covers only a portion of the available values for storage or for display. **Figure 30** shows a histogram of such an image. The flat (empty) regions of the plot indicate brightness values at both the light and dark ends that are not used by any of the pixels in the image. Expanding the brightness scale by spreading the histogram out to the full available range, as shown in the figure, may improve the visibility of features and the perceived contrast in local structures. The same number of brightness values are missing from the image, as shown by the gaps in the histogram, but now they are spread uniformly throughout the range. Other ways to stretch the histogram nonlinearly are discussed in Chapter 3.

Because the contrast range of many astronomical images is too great for photographic printing, special darkroom techniques have been developed. "Unsharp masking" (**Figure 31**) increases the ability to show local contrast by suppressing the overall brightness range of the image. The suppression is done by first printing a "mask" image, slightly out of focus, onto another negative. This negative is developed and then placed on the original to make the final print. This superposition reduces the exposure in the bright areas so that the detail can be shown. The same method can also be used in digital image processing, either by subtracting a smoothed version of the image or by using a Laplacian operator (both are discussed in Chapter 3 on spatial domain processing). When the entire depth of a 12- or 14-bit image is stored, such processing may be needed in order to display the image for viewing on a CRT.

Some perspective on camera performance levels is needed. Although a standard video camera has about 300,000 sensors, and a high performance digital camera may have a few million, the human eye has about 1.5×10^8. Furthermore, these are clustered particularly tightly in the fovea, the central area where we concentrate our attention. It is true that only a few dozen brightness levels can be distinguished in a single field, but the eye adjusts automatically to overall brightness levels covering nine orders of magnitude to select the optimal range (although color sensitivity is lost in the darkest part of this range).

Some cameras use a single-line CCD instead of a two-dimensional array. This gives high resolution but requires physically scanning the line across the film plane, much like a flat-bed scanner. Most of these systems store the image digitally, converting the signal to a full-color image (for instance with 8 to 12 bits each of red, green, and blue data).

Figure 30. *Linear expansion of a histogram to cover the full range of storage and/or display.*

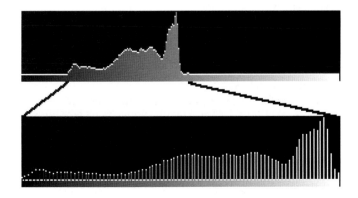

Figure 31. Unsharp masking:
(**a**) *a telescope image originally recorded on film of the Orion nebula;*
(**b**) *the same image using unsharp masking. An out-of-focus photographic print is made onto negative material, which is then placed on the original to reduce the exposure in bright areas when the final print is made (adapted from a 1920s photographic darkroom manual). This reduces the overall contrast so that local variations become visible.*

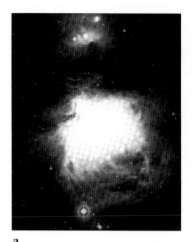

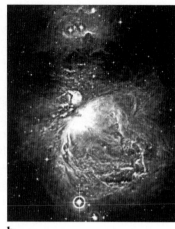

a   b

There is a major difference between the interlace scan used in conventional television and a non-interlaced or "progressive" scan. The latter gives better quality because there are no line-to-line alignment or shift problems. Most high definition television (HDTV) proposals use progressive scan. The format requires a higher rate of repetition of frames to fool the human eye into seeing continuous motion without flicker, but it has many other advantages. These include simpler logic to read data from the camera (which may be incorporated directly on the chip), more opportunity for data compression because of redundancies between successive lines, and simpler display or storage devices. Most scientific imaging systems such as digital cameras, direct-scan microscopes (i.e., the scanning electron microscope (SEM), scanning tunneling microscope (STM), the atomic force microscope (AFM), etc.), flat-bed scanners, film or slide digitizers, and similar devices, use progressive rather than interlaced scan.

HDTV proposals include many more differences from conventional television than the use of progressive scan. The pixel density is much higher, with a wider aspect ratio of 16:9 (instead of the 4:3 used in NTSC television) and the pixels are square. A typical HDTV proposal presents 1920 × 1080 pixel images at the rate of 30 full scans per second, for a total data rate exceeding 1 gigabit per second, which is several hundred times as much data as current broadcast television. One consequence of this high data rate is the interest in data compression techniques, discussed in the next chapter, and the investigation of digital transmission techniques, perhaps using cable or optical fiber instead of broadcast channels. Whatever the details of the outcome in terms of consumer television, the development of HDTV hardware is likely to produce spin-off effects for computer imaging, such as high pixel density cameras with progressive scan output, high bandwidth recording devices, and superior CRT displays. For example, color cameras being designed for HDTV applications output digital rather than analog information by performing the analog-to-digital conversion within the camera, with at least 10 bits each for red, green, and blue.

It is also interesting to compare camera technology to other kinds of image acquisition devices. The scanning electron (SEM) or scanning tunneling microscope (STM) typically use from a few hundred to about 1000 scan lines. Those that digitize the signals use 8 or sometimes 12 bits, and so are similar in image resolution and size to many camera systems. **Figure 32** shows schematically the function of an SEM. The focused beam of electrons is scanned over the sample surface in a raster pattern while various signals generated by the electrons are detected. These include secondary and backscattered electrons, characteristic x-rays, visible light, and electronic effects in the sample.

Other point-scanning microscopes, such as the STM, the confocal scanning light microscope (CSLM), and even contact profilometers, produce very different signals and information. All provide

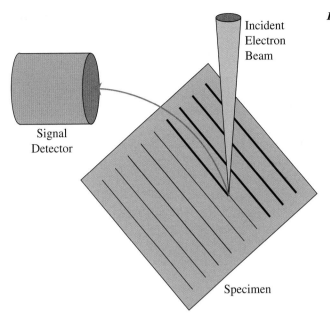

Incident Electron Beam

Signal Detector

Specimen

Figure 32. *The scanning electron microscope (SEM) focuses a fine beam of electrons on the specimen, producing various signals which may be used for imaging as the beam is scanned in a raster pattern.*

a time-varying signal that is related to spatial locations on the sample by knowing the scanning speed and parameters, which allows storing the data as an image.

Significantly larger arrays of pixels are available from flat-bed scanners. These devices use a linear solid-state detector array, and can typically scan areas at least 8 inches by 10 inches, and sometimes up to four times that size. Although primarily intended for the desktop publishing market, they are readily adapted to scan electrophoresis gels used for protein separation, or photographic prints or negatives. A high-quality negative can record more than a thousand distinguishable brightness levels and several thousand points per inch (both values are much better than prints). Scanners are also used for digitizing photographic negatives such as medical x-rays and 35-mm slides. Commercial scanners are used in publishing and to convert films to digital values for storage (for instance in Kodak's Photo-CD format). At the consumer level, scanners with 300 to as many as 1200 pixels per inch are common for large-area reflective originals, and 2500 to 3500 pixels per inch for 35-mm slide film. Most digitize full-color red, green, and blue (RGB) images.

These devices are quite inexpensive, but rather slow, taking tens of seconds to digitize the scan area. Another characteristic problem they exhibit is pattern noise in the sensors: If all of the detectors along the row are not identical in performance, a "striping" effect will appear in the image as the sensor is scanned across the picture. If the scan motion is not perfectly smooth, it can produce striping in the other direction. This latter effect is particularly troublesome with hand-held scanners that rely on the user to move them and sense the motion with a contact roller that can skip, but these devices should not be used for inputting images for measurement anyway (they are marketed for reading text), because of the tendency to skip or twist in motion.

By far the greatest difficulty with such scanners arises from the illumination. There is often a drop-off in intensity near the edges of the scanned field because of the short length of the light source. Even more troublesome is the warm-up time for the light source to become stable. In scanners that digitize color images in a single pass by turning colored lights on and off, stability and consistent color is especially hard to obtain. On the other hand, making three separate passes for red, green, and blue often causes registration difficulties. Even for monochrome scanning, it may take several repeated scans before the light source and other electronics become stable enough for consistent measurements.

Color imaging

Most real-world images are not monochrome, of course, but full color. The light microscope produces color images, and many tissue specimen preparation techniques make use of color to identify structure or localize chemical activity in novel ways. Even for inorganic materials, the use of polarized light or surface oxidation produces color images to delineate structure. The SEM would seem to be a strictly monochromatic imaging tool, but color may be introduced based on x-ray energy or backscattered electron energy. **Figure 33** shows individual grey scale images from the x-ray signals from a mineral sample imaged in the SEM. The x-ray images show the variation in composition of the sample for each of nine elements (Al, Ca, Fe, K, Mg, Na, O, Si, Ti). More individual images are available than just the three red, green, and blue display channels, with no obvious "correct" choice for assigning colors to elements. **Figure 34** shows a few possibilities, but it is important to keep in mind that no single color image can show all of the elements at once. Assigning several of these arbitrarily (e.g., to the red, green, and blue planes of a display), may aid the user in judging the alignment of regions and areas containing two or more elements. Colored x-ray maps are now fairly common with the SEM, as are similar concentration maps based on measured intensities from ion microprobes, but other uses of color such as energy loss in the transmission electron microscope (TEM) are still experimental.

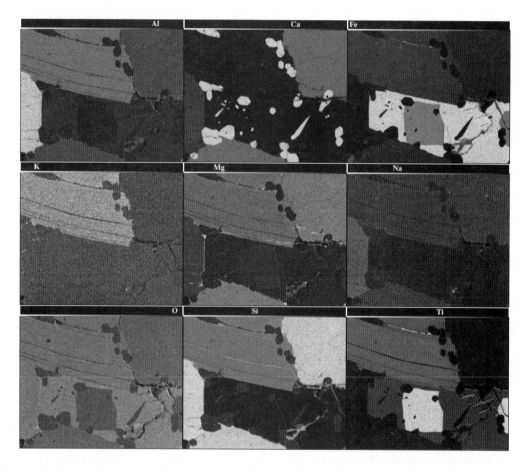

Figure 33. *Scanning electron microscope images of a polished sample of mica. The individual X-ray images or "dot maps" show the localization of the corresponding elements within various minerals in the sample.*

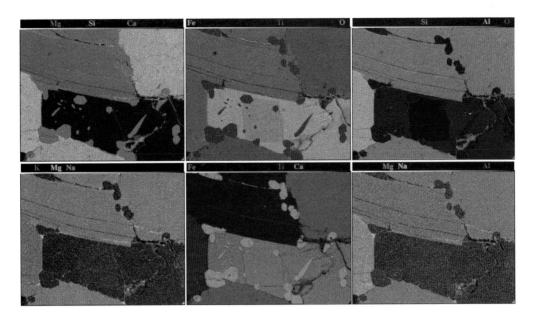

Figure 34. Composite color images made by assigning various images from Figure 33 to the red, green, or blue channels of the display. This assists in the identification and arrangement of the various minerals.

Similar use of color is potentially useful with other kinds of microscopes, although, in many cases, these possibilities have not been exploited in commercial instruments. This is also true for macroscopic imaging tools. A simple example is the use of color to show altitude in air traffic control displays. This use of color increases the bandwidth for communicating multidimensional information to the user, but the effective use of these methods will require some education of users, and would benefit from some standardization.

The use of color to encode richly multidimensional information must be distinguished from the very common use of false-color or pseudo-color to substitute colors for brightness in a monochrome image. Pseudo-color is used because of the limitation mentioned before in our visual ability to distinguish subtle differences in brightness. Although we can only distinguish about 20–30 shades of grey in a monochrome image, we can distinguish hundreds of different colors. Also, it is may aid communication to describe a particular feature of interest as "the dark reddish-blue one" instead of "the medium grey one."

The use of color scales as a substitute for brightness values allows us to show and see small changes locally, and identify the same brightness values globally in an image. This should be a great benefit, since these are among the goals for imaging discussed below. Pseudo-color has been used particularly for many of the images returned from space probes. It would be interesting to know how many people think that the rings around Saturn really are brightly colored, or that Halley's Comet really is surrounded by a rainbow-colored halo. The danger in the use of pseudo-color is that it can obscure the real contents of an image. The colors force us to concentrate on the details of the image, and to lose the gestalt information. Examples of image processing in this book will use pseudo-color selectively to illustrate some of the processing effects and the changes in pixel values that are produced, but often pseudo-color distracts the human eye from seeing the real contents of the enhanced image.

Pseudo-color displays as used in this context simply substitute a color from a stored or precalculated table for each discrete stored brightness value. As shown in **Figure 35**, this should be distinguished from some other uses of color displays to identify structures or indicate feature

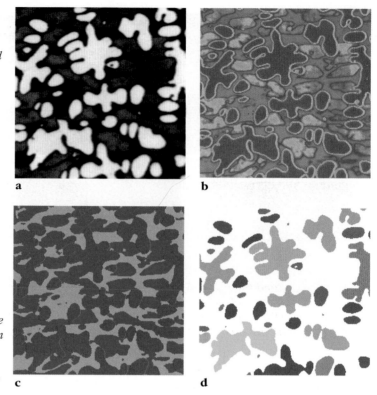

Figure 35. Different uses for pseudo-color displays:
(**a**) portion of a grey-scale microscope image of a polished metallographic specimen with three phases having different average brightnesses;
(**b**) image **a** with pseudo-color palette or LUT which replaces grey values with colors (note the misleading colors along boundaries between light and dark phases);
(**c**) image **a** with colors assigned to phases (this requires segmentation of the image by thresholding and other logic to assign each pixel to a phase based on grey-scale brightness and neighboring pixel classification);
(**d**) lightest features from image **a** with colors assigned based on feature size (this requires the steps to create image **c**, plus collection of all touching pixels into features and the measurement of the features.

properties. These also rely on the use of color to communicate rich information to the viewer, but require considerable processing and measurement of the image before this information becomes available.

Color can be used to encode elevation of surfaces (see Chapter 13). In scientific visualization it is used for velocity, density, temperature, composition, and many less obvious properties. These uses generally have little to do with the properties of the image and simply take advantage of the human ability to distinguish more colors than grey-scale values.

Most computer-based imaging systems make it easy to substitute various lookup tables (LUTs) of colors for the brightness values in a stored image. These work in the same way as input lookup tables, described earlier. The stored grey scale value is used to select a set of red, green, and blue brightnesses in the LUT that control the voltages sent to the display tube. Many systems also provide utilities for creating tables of these colors, but few guidelines exist to assist in constructing useful ones. All we can do here is advise caution. One approach is to systematically and gradually vary color along a path through color space. Examples (**Figure 36**) are a rainbow spectrum of colors or a progression from brown through red and yellow to white, the so-called heat scale. This gradual variation can help to organize the different parts of the scene. Another approach is to rapidly shift colors, for instance by varying the hue sinusoidally. This enhances gradients and makes it easy to see local variations, but may completely hide the overall contents of some images (**Figure 37**).

Some image sources may use color to encode a variety of different kinds of information, such as the intensity and polarization of radio waves in astronomy; however, by far the most common type of color image is that produced by recording the intensity at three different wavelengths of visible light. Video deserves consideration as a suitable medium for this type of image, since standard

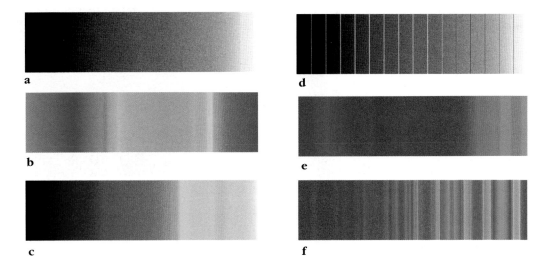

Figure 36. Six examples of display look-up tables (LUTs). *(**a**) monochrome (grey-scale); (**b**) spectrum or rainbow (variation of hue, with maximum saturation and constant intensity); (**c**) heat scale; (**d**) monochrome with contour lines (rainbow colors substituted every 16th value); (**e**) tri-color blend of three primary colors; f) sinusoidal variation of hue with linear variation of saturation and intensity.*

broadcast television uses color in a way that is visually satisfactory. The National Television Systems Committee (NTSC) color encoding scheme used in the U.S. was developed as a compatible add-on to existing monochrome television broadcasts. It adds the color information within the same, already narrow bandwidth limitation. The result is that the color has even less lateral resolution than the brightness information.

Color subsampling reduces the amount of data in an image by representing color data with lower resolution than luminance (brightness) data. This is done in the YUV color space (Y = luminance or brightness, U and V = chrominance or color) described later in this chapter. Uncompressed YUV color is represented as 4:4:4. The common subsampling options are 4:2:2, 4:2:0, 4:1:1, and YUV-9:

4:2:2. — full-bandwidth sampling of Y and 2:1 horizontal sampling of U and V. This is the sampling scheme most commonly used in professional and broadcast video and in tape formats such as D-1 and Digital Betacam. It looks good, but the data compression ratio is only 1.5:1.

4:2:0. — full-bandwidth sampling of Y and 2:1 sampling of U and V in both the horizontal and vertical dimensions. That is, for every four luminance samples, there are two chrominance samples every other line. This yields a 2:1 reduction in data. 4:2:0 is the color space used in MPEG compression.

4:1:1. — full-bandwidth sampling of Y and 4:1 horizontal sampling of U and V. This is the color space of the digital video (DV) formats. It uses U and V samples four pixels wide and one pixel tall, so color bleeding is much worse in the horizontal than in the vertical direction.

YUV-9. — this is the color format used in most of the video compression on the internet. For every 16 luminance Y samples in a 4 × 4-pixel block, there is only one U and one V sample, producing smaller files with correspondingly lower color fidelity. YUV-9 subsampling often results in noticeable color artifacts around the edges of brightly colored objects, especially red.

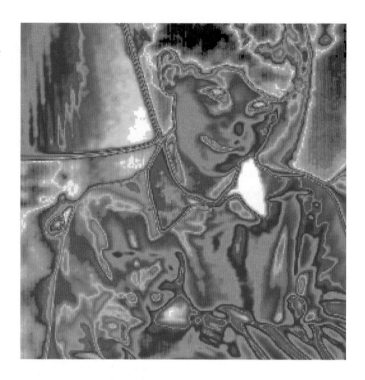

Figure 37. The same image used in Figures 25 and 26 with a pseudocolor display LUT. The gestalt contents of the image are obscured.

Such limitations are acceptable for television pictures because the viewer tolerates colors that are less sharply bounded and uses the edges of features defined by the brightness component of the image where they do not exactly correspond. The same tolerance has been used effectively by painters, and may be familiar to parents whose young children have not yet learned to color "inside the lines." **Figure 38** shows an example in which the bleeding of color across boundaries or variations within regions is not confusing to the eye.

The poor spatial sharpness of NTSC color is matched by its poor consistency in representing the actual color values (a common joke is that NTSC means "Never The Same Color" instead of "National Television Systems Committee"). Videotape recordings of color images are even less

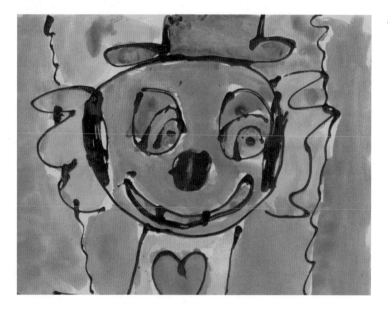

Figure 38. A child's painting of a clown. Notice that the colors are unrealistic, but their relative intensities are correct and the painted areas are not exactly bounded by the lines. The dark lines nevertheless give the dimensions and shape to the features, and we are not confused by the colors which extend beyond their regions.

useful for analysis than monochrome ones, but the limitations imposed by the broadcast channel do not necessarily mean that the cameras and other components may not be useful. An improvement in the sharpness of the color information in these images is afforded by Super-VHS or S-video recording equipment, also called component video, in which the brightness or luminance and color or chrominance information are transmitted and recorded separately.

Some color cameras intended for technical purposes bring out the red, green, and blue signals separately so that they can be individually digitized. Recording the image in computer memory then simply involves treating each signal as a monochrome one, converting it to a set of numbers, and storing it in memory. If the signals have first been combined, the encoding scheme used is likely to be YIQ or YUV (defined in the "color spaces" section), which are closely related to the NTSC broadcasting scheme. Much better fidelity in the image can be preserved by not mixing together the color and brightness information. Instead of the composite signal carried on a single wire, some cameras and recorders separate the chrominance (color) and luminance (brightness) signals onto separate wires. This so-called component, Y-C or S-video format is used for high-end consumer camcorders (Hi-8 and S-VHS formats). Many computer interfaces accept this format, which gives significant improvement in the quality of digitized images, as shown in **Figure 39**.

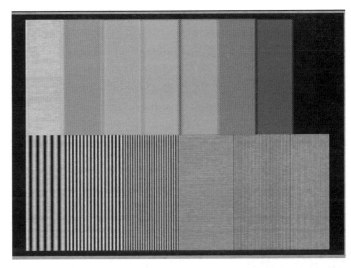

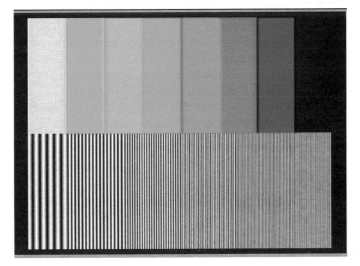

*Figure 39. Comparison of (**a**) composite and (**b**) component video signals from a signal generator, digitized using the same interface board. Note the differences in resolution of the black and white stripes and the boundaries between different colors.*

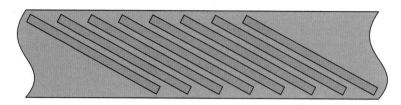

Figure 40. In digital video, each video frame is recorded digitally in ten tracks on metal-coated magnetic tape (12 tracks for the larger PAL format). Each track contains video, audio, and timing information.

Another development in video that is important is digital video (DV) recording. Similar to analog video tape recorders, digital video writes each scan line onto the tape at an angle using a moving head that rotates as the tape moves past it (**Figure 40**); however, the signal is encoded as a series of digital bits that offers several advantages. Just as CD technology replaced analog audio tapes, the digital video signal is not subject to loss of fidelity as images are transmitted or copies are made. More important, the high frequency information that is discarded in analog recording because of the 4 MHz upper frequency limit imposed by conventional broadcast TV is preserved in DV. Digital video records up to 13.5 MHz for the luminance (brightness) information, and up to one-fourth that for the chrominance (color) information. This produces much sharper edge delineation at least for the brightness data in the image, and greatly improves the usefulness of the resulting images. The digital video signal is fully preserved on the tape recording, unlike conventional analog recorders which impose a further bandwidth reduction on the data, and are susceptible to quality loss due to dirty heads, worn tape, or making successive copies from an original.

The result is that DV images have about 500 × 500 pixel resolution and nearly 8 bits of contrast, and can be read into the computer without a separate digitizer board since they are already digital in format. The IEEE 1394 standard protocol for digital video (also known as firewire) establishes a standard serial interface convention that is available on consumer-priced cameras and decks, and is being supported by many computer manufacturers as well. Inexpensive interface boards are available, and the capability is built into the basic circuitry of some personal computers, even laptops. Most of these digital cameras can be controlled by the computer to select individual frames for transfer. They can also be used to record single frames annotated with date and time, turning the digital video tape cartridge into a tiny but high-fidelity storage format for hundreds of single images.

Digital camera limitations

The current development of the digital still-frame cameras for the consumer market involves practically every traditional maker of film cameras and photographic supplies. Many of these are unsuitable for technical applications because of limitations in the optics (fixed focus lenses with geometric distortions), and limited resolution (although even a low-end 320 × 240 pixel camera chip is as good as conventional analog video recording). Some cameras interpolate between the pixels on the chip to create images with empty magnification. In most cases this produces artefacts in the image that are serious impediments to quantitative measurement.

The use of image compression creates the most important problem. In an effort to pack many images into the smallest possible memory, JPEG and other forms of image compression are used. As discussed in Chapter 2, these are lossy techniques that discard information from the image. The discarded data is selected to minimally impact the human interpretation and recognition of familiar images — snapshots of the kids and the summer vacation — but the effect on quantitative image analysis can be severe. Edges are broken up and shifted, color and density values are altered, and

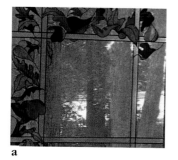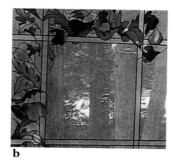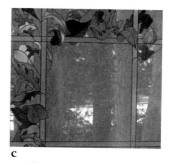

a   b   c

*Figure 41. Images of the same scene (see text) recorded using: (**a**) a 3-chip video camera and analog to digital converter; (**b**) an inexpensive consumer digital camera; and (**c**) a research-grade digital camera.*

fine details can be eliminated or moved. The important advantage of the higher-end consumer and professional cameras is that they offer storage or transfer to the computer without any lossy compression, and this is much preferred for technical applications.

Figure 41 compares images of the same scene using three different cameras. The subject is a difficult view through a stained glass window, with a dark interior and bright daytime exterior. This produces a very high contrast range, regions that are saturated in color and others with low saturation, subtle differences and fine detail. The first image is video from a 3-chip color video camera acquired using a high-quality analog to digital converter producing a 640 × 480 pixel image and averaging eight frames. The second image was acquired with a consumer digital camera, also as a 640 × 480 pixel image, using the highest quality compression setting (least compression). The third image was acquired with a research-grade digital camera as a 1600 × 1200 pixel image.

The original colors are represented with greater fidelity in the third image. In addition to color shifts, the first two images have brightness values that are clipped to eliminate the brightest and darkest values, and the video image does not produce 256 distinct values of red, green, and blue so that the image has missing values within the range. The consumer digital camera apparently applies a hi-pass or sharpening filter that exaggerates contrast at edges producing dark and light borders. Other artefacts are present in the first two images as well: scan line noise in the video image and square blocks resulting from the JPEG compression in the consumer digital camera image. Enlarging the image to see fine details makes apparent the far higher resolution of the research grade digital image. In **Figure 42** a region is expanded to show fine details in each of the images. The research grade digital camera image renders these with greater fidelity in both the high-brightness and high-saturation regions.

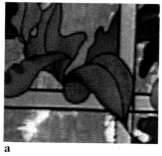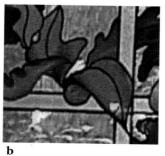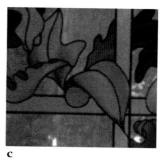

a   b   c

*Figure 42. Enlarged regions of the images in **Figure 41**, showing the greater resolution and fidelity in the high-end digital camera image.*

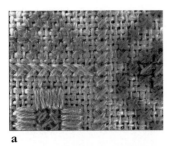
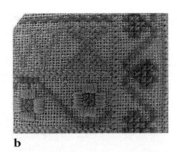
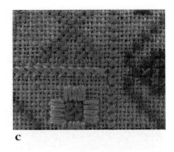

a   b   c

Figure 43. *Macro images using the same three cameras as in* **Figures** *41 and 42. Note the variations in resolution and color rendition.*

The high-resolution digital camera offers the same advantages for recording of images in microscope and other technical applications. **Figure 43** shows three images obtained with the same three cameras using a low power microscope to view an antique cross-stitch fabric specimen. Identification of individual characteristics (and occasional errors) in the formation of the stitches and tension on the threads is of interest to cultural anthropologists to identify individual handiwork. This requires a low enough magnification to see the overall pattern, while identification of the threads and dyes used requires a high enough resolution to see individual fibers, and good color fidelity to represent the dyes. **Figure 44** shows an enlargement of one small region of the three images. The differences in resolution and color fidelity between these images is another demonstration of the importance of using a high-quality camera.

A few words of caution may be useful. The slower readout from digital cameras makes focusing more difficult: the camera produces a preview image that updates a few times a second. This is fine for selecting fields of view, but for convenient focusing it is important to adjust the optics so that the camera is truly parfocal with the eyepiece image. Some digital cameras also put out a live video signal that can be connected to a monitor for previews, albeit with only video resolution. Some digital cameras do not have a useful preview image but instead rely on a viewfinder that is of little practical use. Also the area of the image sensing chip is smaller than film but larger than many video cameras so that standard transfer optics may not provide complete coverage; clipping or vignetting can result.

On the other hand, it is possible in some instances to use very low-end cameras to acquire useful images. For instance, digital cameras intended for video conferencing are available that deliver 64

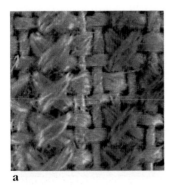
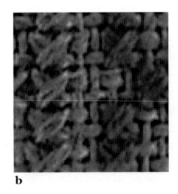
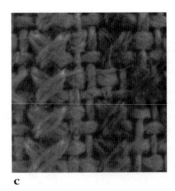

a   b   c

Figure 44. *Enlargement of a portion of the images in* **Figure 43,** *showing the appearance of individual fibers.*

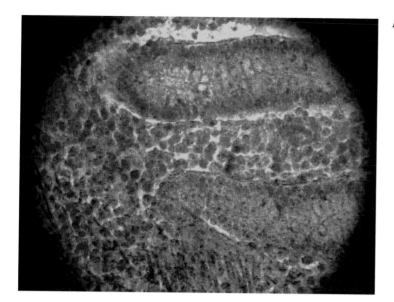

Figure 45. View of a biological thin section using a video conferencing camera placed on the eyepiece of a bench microscope. Despite significant vignetting, the main details of the slide are visible.

Figure 46. Using the same camera as in *Figure 45* with a loupe to record an image for forensic examination.

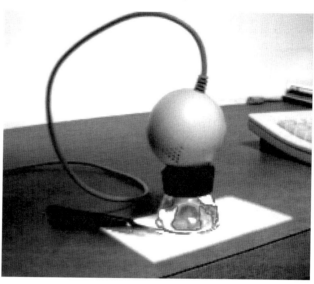

grey levels or 32 levels of red, green, and blue with 320×240 pixel resolution (about as good as many examples of digitized video) at about 10 frames per second via a simple serial or parallel interface to the computer. No digitizer or separate power supply is required, and the digitization is built into the camera chip requiring no hardware to be added to the computer. Such cameras cost well under $100 and can be quite useful for purposes such as capturing an image for videoconferencing.

The illustration in **Figure 45** was obtained by holding one such camera directly onto the eyepiece of a microscope with duct tape. The automatic gain control in the software was turned off because the black area around the image confused the automatic adjustment. **Figure 46** shows another example of the use of the same camera. Placing it on an 8X loupe allows direct capture of images when (as in this forensic case) it was essential to collect images and nothing else except the camera and a laptop computer was available. The biggest flaws with this setup were the difficulty in controlling the specimen illumination and the distortion caused by the very wide angle view from the optics.

Color spaces

Conversion from RGB (the brightness of the individual red, green, and blue signals at defined wavelengths, as captured by the camera and stored in the computer) to YIQ/YUV and to the other color encoding schemes is straightforward and loses no information except for possible round-off errors. Y, the "luminance" signal, is just the brightness of a panchromatic monochrome image that would be displayed by a black-and-white television receiver. It combines the red, green, and blue signals in proportion to the human eye's sensitivity to them. The I and Q (or U and V) components of the color signal are chosen for compatibility with the hardware used in broadcasting; the I signal is essentially red minus cyan, while Q is magenta minus green. The relationship between YIQ and RGB is shown in **Table 1**. An inverse conversion from the encoded YIQ signal to RGB simply requires inverting the matrix of values.

RGB (and the complementary CMY subtractive primary colors used for printing) and YIQ are both hardware-oriented schemes. RGB comes from the way camera sensors and display phosphors work, while YIQ or YUV stem from broadcast considerations. **Figure 47** shows the "space" defined by RGB signals: it is a Cartesian cubic space because the red, green, and blue signals are independent and can be added to produce any color within the cube. Other encoding schemes are available, which are more useful for image processing and are more closely related to human perception.

Table 1. Interconversion of RGB and YIQ color scales

Y = 0.299 R + 0.587 G + 0.114 B	R = 1.000 Y + 0.956 I + 0.621 Q	
I = 0.596 R − 0.274 G − 0.322 B	G = 1.000 Y − 0.272 I − 0.647 Q	
Q = 0.211 R − 0.523 G + 0.312 B	B = 1.000 Y − 1.106 I + 1.703 Q	

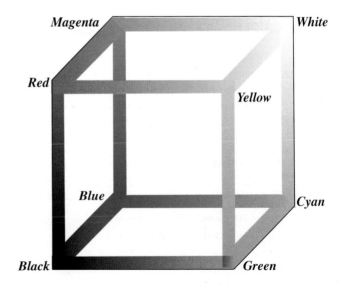

Figure 47. RGB Color Space, showing the additive progression from Black to White. Combining Red and Green produces Yellow, Green plus Blue produces Cyan, and Blue plus Red produces Magenta. Greys lie along the cube diagonal with equal proportions of Red, Green, and Blue. Cyan, Yellow, and Magenta are subtractive primaries used in printing, which, if subtracted from White, leave Red, Blue, and Green, respectively.

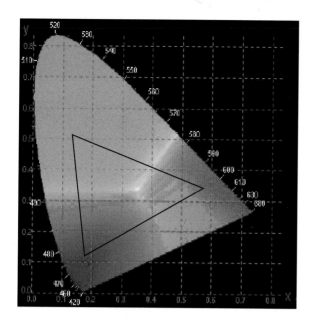

Figure 48. The CIE chromaticity diagram. The colors are fully saturated along the edge. Numbers give the wavelength of light in nanometers. The inscribed triangle shows the colors that typical color CRTs can produce by mixing of red, green and blue light from phosphors.

The oldest of these is the CIE (Commission Internationale de L'Éclairage) chromaticity diagram. This is a two-dimensional plot defining color, shown in **Figure 48**. The third axis is the luminance, which corresponds to the panchromatic brightness which, like the Y value in YUV, would produce a monochrome (grey-scale) image. The other two primaries, called x and y are always positive (unlike the U and V values) and combine to define any color that we can see.

Instruments for color measurement utilize the CIE primaries, which define the dominant wavelength and purity of any color. Mixing any two colors corresponds to selecting a new point in the diagram along a straight line between the two original colors. This means that a triangle on the CIE diagram with its corners at the red, green, and blue locations of emission phosphors used in a cathode ray tube (CRT) defines all of the colors that the tube can display. Some colors cannot be created by mixing these three phosphor colors, shown by the fact that they lie outside the triangle. The range of possible colors for any display or other output device is the gamut; hardcopy printers generally have a much smaller gamut than display tubes as discussed in Chapter 2. The edge of the bounded region in the diagram corresponds to pure colors, and is marked with the wavelength in nanometers.

Complementary colors are shown in the CIE diagram by drawing a line through the central point, which corresponds to white light. Thus, a line from green passes through white to magenta. One of the drawbacks of the CIE diagram is that it does not indicate the variation in color that can be discerned by eye. Sometimes this is shown by plotting a series of ellipses on the diagram. These are much larger in the green area, where small changes are poorly perceived, than elsewhere.

The CIE diagram provides a tool for color definition, but corresponds neither to the operation of hardware nor directly to human vision. An approach that does is embodied in the HSV (hue, saturation, and value), HSI (hue, saturation, and intensity) and HLS (hue, lightness, and saturation) systems. These are closely related to each other and to the artist's concept of tint, shade, and tone. In this system, hue is the color as described by wavelength, for instance the distinction between red and yellow. Saturation is the amount of the color that is present, for instance the distinction between red and pink. The third axis (called lightness, intensity, or value) is the amount of light, the distinction between a dark red and light red, or between dark grey and light grey.

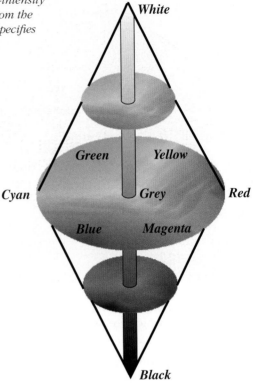

Figure 49. *Bi-conic representation of hue-saturation-intensity space. Greys lie along the central axis. Distance from the axis gives the Saturation, while direction (angle) specifies the hue.*

The space in which these three values is plotted can be shown as a circular or hexagonal cone or double cone, or sometimes as a cylinder. It is useful to imagine the space as a double cone, in which the axis of the cone is the grey scale progression from black to white, distance from the central axis is the saturation, and the direction is the hue. **Figure 49** shows this concept schematically.

This space has many advantages for image processing. For instance, if the algorithms discussed in Chapter 3 such as spatial smoothing or median filtering are used to reduce noise in an image, applying them to the RGB signals separately will cause color shifts in the result, but applying them to the HSI components will not. Also, the use of hue (in particular) for distinguishing features in the process called segmentation (Chapter 6) often corresponds to human perception and ignores shading effects. On the other hand, because the HSI components do not correspond to the way that most hardware works (either for acquisition or display), it requires computation to convert RGB-encoded images to HSI and back.

The HSI spaces are useful for image processing because they separate the color information in ways that correspond to the human visual system's response, and also because the axes correspond to many physical characteristics of specimens. One example of this is the staining of biological tissue. To a useful approximation, hue represents the stain color, saturation represents the amount of stain, and intensity represents the specimen density; however, these spaces are awkward ones mathematically: not only does the hue value cycle through the angles from 0 to 360 degrees and then wrap around, but the conical spaces mean that increasing the intensity or luminance can alter the saturation. A geometrically simpler space that is close enough to the HSI approach for must applications and easier to deal with mathematically is the spherical L·a·b model. L, as usual, is the grey scale axis, or luminance, while **a** and **b** are two orthogonal axes that together define the color and saturation (**Figure 50**). The **a** axis runs from red (+**a**) to green (–**a**) and the **b** axis from yellow (+**b**) to blue (–**b**). Notice that the hues do not have the same angular distribution in this

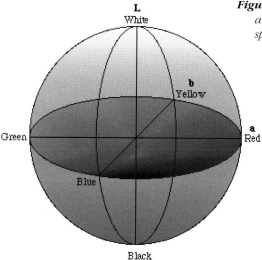

Figure 50. *The L•a•b color space. Grey values lie along a vertical north–south line through the sphere.*

space as in the usual color wheel. These axes offer a practical compromise between the simplicity of the RGB space that corresponds to hardware and the more physiologically based spaces such as CIE and HSI which are used in many color management systems, spectrophotometers and colorimeters.

Conversion between RGB space and hue-saturation-intensity coordinates can be performed in several ways, depending on the shape of the HSI space that is used. The most common choices are a sphere, cylinder, or double cone. In all cases, the intensity axis is aligned along the body diagonal of the cube, but none of the HSI space geometries exactly fits the shape of the RGB cube. This means in order to represent colors in both space the saturation values must be distorted somewhat in the conversion process. This can be seen in the example of **Figure 70** (below) in which a high-resolution panchromatic satellite image is used to replace the intensity channel in an image constructed by merging three lower-resolution R, G, B images.

A spherical color model similar to L·a·b can used as an intermediate step in converting from RGB to HSI. This is simpler than a true HSI space because it uses orthogonal axes instead of representing color as an angle. In this spherical space, the luminance (intensity) value is simply the average of R, G, and B, and the a and b values are coordinates along two orthogonal directions. A typical conversion is

$$\begin{bmatrix} L \\ a \\ b \end{bmatrix} = \begin{bmatrix} 1/3 & 1/3 & 1/3 \\ -\sqrt{2/6} & -\sqrt{2/6} & 2\sqrt{2/6} \\ 1/\sqrt{2} & -1/\sqrt{2} & 0 \end{bmatrix} \bullet \begin{bmatrix} R \\ G \\ B \end{bmatrix} \tag{1}$$

From these values, the hue and saturation can be calculated as

$$H = \tan^{-1}\left(\frac{b}{a}\right) \tag{2}$$

$$S = \sqrt{a^2 + b^2}$$

Alternatively, the conversion can be performed for a conical space:

$$I = \frac{R+G+B}{3}$$

$$S = 1 - \frac{3 \cdot \min(R,G,B)}{R+G+B}$$

$$H = \begin{cases} \cos^{-1}(z) & if (G \geq R) \\ 2\pi - \cos^{-1}(a) & if (G \leq R) \end{cases}$$

$$z = \frac{(2B-G-R)/2}{\sqrt{(B-G)^2 + (B-R)/(G-R)}}$$

(3)

Ledley et al. (1990) showed that the difference between these two RGB-HSI conversions lies principally in the saturation values. A fuller analysis of how this affects combinations of RGB images such as the satellite imagery in **Figure 70** can be found in Tu et al. (2001), where ways to compensate for the saturation changes are proposed.

Hardware for digitizing color images accepts either direct RGB signals from the camera, or the Y-C component signals, or a composite signal (e.g., NTSC) and uses electronic filters to separate the individual components and extract the red, green, and blue signals. As for the monochrome case discussed above, these signals are then digitized to produce values, usually 8-bit ones ranging from 0 to 255 each for R, G, and B. This takes 3 bytes of storage per pixel, so a 640×480 pixel image would require nearly 1 megabyte of storage space in the computer. With most cameras and electronics, the signals do not contain quite this much information, and the lowest 2 or more bits are noise. Consequently, some systems keep only 5 bits each for R, G, and B, which can be fit into two bytes. This reduction is often adequate for internet graphics and some desktop publishing applications, but when packed this way, the color information is hard to get at for any processing or analysis operations.

Color images are typically digitized as 24-bit RGB, meaning that 8 bits or 256 (linear) levels of brightness for red, green, and blue are stored. This is enough to allow display on video or computer screens, or for printing purposes, but, depending on the dynamic range of the data, may not be enough to adequately measure small variations within the image. Since photographic film can capture large dynamic ranges, some scanners intended for transparency or film scanning provide greater range — as much as 12 bits (4096 linear levels) for R, G, and B. These 36-bit images may be reduced to an "optimum" 8 bits when the image is stored. One of the problems with the dynamic range of color or grey scale storage is that the brightness values are linear, whereas the film (and human vision) are fundamentally logarithmic, so that in the dark regions of an image the smallest brightness step that can be stored is quite large and may result in visual artefacts or poor measurement precision for density values.

Further reduction of color images to 256 colors using a lookup table in which the best 256 colors are matched to the contents of the image is commonly used for computer images. This reduces the file size. The lookup table itself requires only 3×256 bytes to specify the R, G, B values for the 256 colors, which are written to the display hardware. Only a single byte per pixel is needed to select from this palette of colors. The most common technique for selecting the optimum palette is the Heckbert or median cut algorithm, which subdivides color space based on the actual RGB values of the pixels in the original image. For visual purposes such a reduction often provides a displayed image that is satisfactory, but for image analysis purposes this should be avoided.

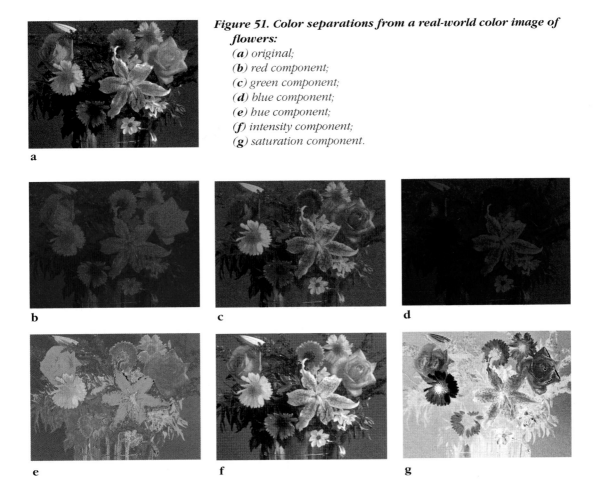

Figure 51. Color separations from a real-world color image of flowers:
(*a*) original;
(*b*) red component;
(*c*) green component;
(*d*) blue component;
(*e*) hue component;
(*f*) intensity component;
(*g*) saturation component.

a

b   c   d

e   f   g

In many situations, although color images are acquired, the "absolute" color information is not useful for image analysis. Instead, it is the relative differences in color from one region to another that can be used to distinguish the structures and features present. In such cases, it may not be necessary to store the entire color image. Various kinds of color separations are available. Calculation of the RGB components (or the complementary CMY values) is commonly used in desktop publishing, but not often useful for image analysis. Separating the image into hue, saturation, and intensity components (also called planes or channels) can also be performed. **Figures 51** and **52** show two examples, one a real-world image of flowers, and the second a microscope image of stained biological tissue. Note that some structures are much more evident in one separation than another (e.g., the pink spots on the white lily petals are not visible in the red image, but are much more evident in the green or saturation images). Also, note that for the stained tissue, the hue image shows where the stains are and the saturation image shows how much of the stain is present. This distinction is also evident in the stained tissue sample shown in **Figure 53**.

It is possible to compute the amount of any particular "color" (hue) in the image. This calculation is equivalent to the physical insertion of a transmission filter in front of a monochrome camera. The filter can be selected to absorb a complementary color (for instance, a blue filter will darken yellow regions by absorbing the yellow light) and transmit light of the same color, so that the resulting image contrast can be based on the color distribution in the image. Photographers have long used yellow filters to darken the blue sky and produce monochrome images with dramatic contrast for clouds, for example. The same color filtering can be used to convert color images to monochrome (grey scale). **Figures 54** and **55** show examples in which the computer is used to

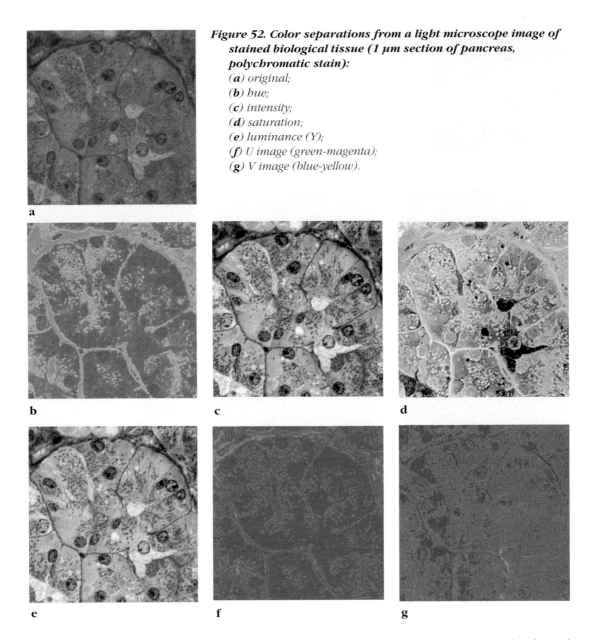

Figure 52. Color separations from a light microscope image of stained biological tissue (1 μm section of pancreas, polychromatic stain):
(**a**) original;
(**b**) hue;
(**c**) intensity;
(**d**) saturation;
(**e**) luminance (Y);
(**f**) U image (green-magenta);
(**g**) V image (blue-yellow).

a

b

c

d

e

f

g

apply the filter. This method offers greater flexibility than physical filters, because the desired wavelength can be specified, the operation can be performed later, using a stored image, and a drawer full of physical filters is not needed.

Reducing a color image to grey scale is useful in many situations and can be accomplished in many ways in addition to the obvious methods of selecting an R, G, B or H, S, I image plane, or applying a selected color filter. If obtaining the maximum grey scale contrast between structures present in the image is desired to facilitate grey scale image thresholding and measurement, then a unique function can be calculated for each image that fits a line through the points representing all of the pixels' color coordinates in color space. This least-square-fit line gives the greatest separation of the various pixel color values and the position of each pixel's coordinates as projected onto the line can be used as a grey scale value that gives the optimum contrast (Russ, 1995e). **Figure 56** shows an example.

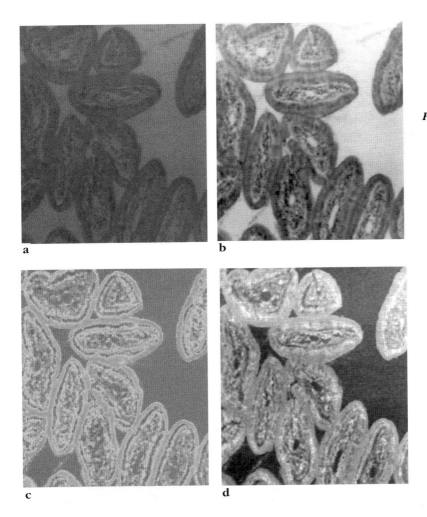

a　　　　b

c　　　　d

Figure 53. Microtomed tissue section of paraffin embedded mouse intestine, Feulgen stained and counter stained with fast green, Bouin's fixative (specimen courtesy of Dr. Barbara Grimes, North Carolina State University): (a) original color image; *(b)* intensity component of image a; *(c)* hue component of image **a**; *(d)* saturation component of image **a**.

Color correction

When images are acquired under different lighting conditions, the color values recorded are affected. Human vision is tolerant of considerable variation in lighting, apparently using the periphery of the viewing field to normalize the color interpretation. Some cameras, especially video cameras, have an automatic white point correction that allows recording an image from a grey card with no color, and using that to adjust subsequent colors. This same correction can be applied in software, by adjusting the relative amount of red, green and blue to set a region that is known to be without any color to pure grey. The method is easy, but does not work well in images that have some regions with highly saturated color and others with little color.

Another approach to color balance is to find a region of known color, or which is to be matched to a region in another image, and to rotate the hues of all colors in the image until they match. This often works well as an adjustment for varying illumination, but only for colors with similar hue values to the point that is matched. **Figure 57** shows an example. It is unrealistic to expect the effect of illumination to shift different colors by the same amount, and to affect only hue and not intensity or saturation.

The most complete approach to color adjustment is tristimulus correction. This requires measuring a test image with areas of pure red, green and blue color, such as the calibration card shown in **Figure 58**. In practical situations, such a card can be included in the scene being digitized. The camera

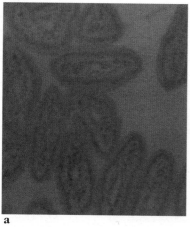

a

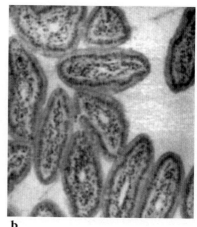

b

Figure 54. Filtering of the image in Figure 53: (**a**) *application of a 480 nm filter to the original color image;* (**b**) *monochrome intensity from image c.*

Figure 55. Cast aluminum alloy containing 7.4% Ca, 0.8%Si, 0.2%Ti, showing two intermetallic phases (Al4Ca in blue, CaSi2 in reddish violet) (*original image from H-E. Bühler, H. P. Hougardy (1980)* Atlas of Interference Layer Metallography, *Deutsche Gesellschaft für Metallkunde, Oberursel):*
(**a**) *original color image;*
(**b**) *the panchromatic intensity component of image* **a** *showing inability to distinguish two of the phases;*
(**c**) *application of a 590 nm filter;*
(**d**) *monochrome intensity from image* **c**;
(**e**) *the hue component of image* **a**.

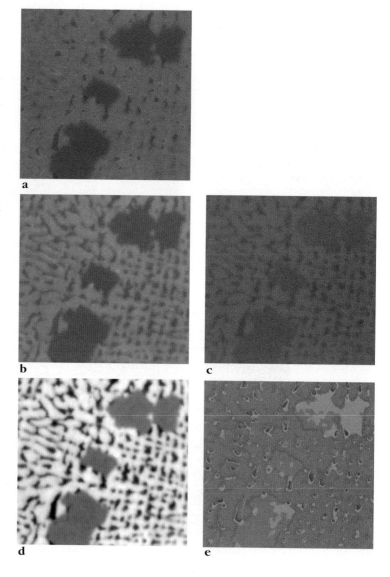

a

b

c

d

e

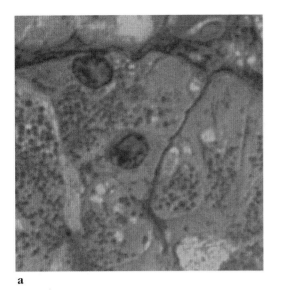 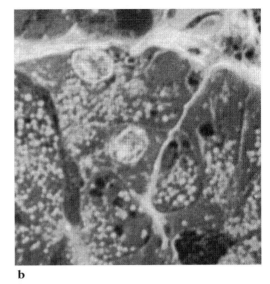

a　　　　　　　　　　　　　　　　　b

Figure 56. *Color image of stained biological tissue (**a**) and the optimal grey scale image produced by fitting a line through the pixel color coordinates as described in the text (**b**).*

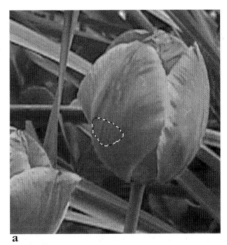

Figure 57. Color matching by shifting hue values:

*(**a**) image of a flower in shade, with an area marked for hue measurement;*

*(**b**) another similar flower imaged in direct sunlight, with an area marked for matching;*

*(**c**) image a with the hue rotated by 12° to match the hue in the two test areas.*

a

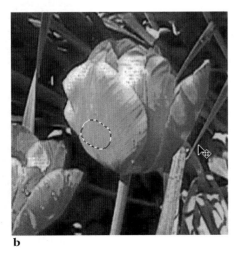 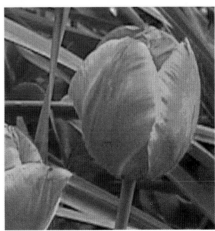

b　　　　　　　　　　　　　　　　　c

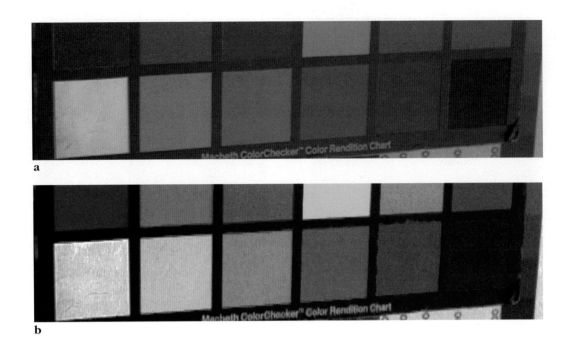

a

b

Figure 58. A portion of a Macbeth color checker chart (GretagMacbeth Corp., New Windsor, NY):
*(a) original image; (b) after tristimulus correction using the values in **Table 2c**.*

(or scanner) will record some intensity for red, green, and blue in each of the areas. This produces a matrix of values as shown in **Table 2**, which can be inverted to generate the tristimulus correction matrix. Calculating new red, green, and blue values by multiplying of this matrix times the measured R, G, B values produces an image in which the calibration areas are adjusted to pure red, green, and blue, and other colors in the image are also corrected, as shown.

Color displays

Of course, color is also important as a vehicle for communicating to the computer user. Most computers use color monitors that have much higher resolution than a television set but operate on essentially the same principle. Smaller phosphor dots, a higher-frequency scan and higher-bandwidth amplifiers, and a single progressive scan (rather than interlace) produce much greater sharpness and color purity.

Besides color video monitors, other kinds of displays may be used with desktop computers. For example, many notebook computers use a liquid crystal display (LCD). The passive type of LCD display has much poorer saturation and is also slower than the somewhat more costly active-matrix type that uses a separate transistor to control each pixel (or actually, each of the RGB cells that together make up a pixel in a color display). Even the best active-matrix color LCDs, however, are inferior to most CRTs because of their lower brightness and narrower viewing angle. They also have an inferior brightness and contrast range for each color, which reduces the number of distinct colors that can be displayed.

These same display devices may be connected to a computer and placed on an overhead projector to show images on a screen. Although very convenient, and acceptable for presentations in a small room, they are inferior to dedicated projection devices. These may either use a very bright (and color corrected) light source with small LCD panels and appropriate optics, or three separate

Table 2. Calculation of tristimulus color correction for Figure 58

Matrix a — measured average R, G, B intensities in red, green, and blue target areas of original image

Area	Measured intensity: Red	Green	Blue
Red	90.223	45.865	35.556
Green	59.933	86.941	40.296
Blue	38.088	36.635	43.028

Matrix b — normalized intensity matrix (values from **a** divided by 255)

0.353826	0.179863	0.139435
0.235031	0.340945	0.158024
0.149365	0.143667	0.168737

Matrix c — inverse of matrix **b**

4.94557	-1.46508	-2.71469
-2.27990	5.52036	-3.28586
-2.43661	-3.40327	11.12704

CRTs with red, green, and blue filters. In the latter case, the resolution is potentially higher because the individual CRTs have continuous phosphor coatings; although, careful alignment of the optics is needed to keep the three images in registration; readjustment may be needed every time the equipment is moved or even as it heats up. Getting enough brightness for viewing large images in rooms with imperfect light control is also a challenge.

A new class of displays uses the digital light modulation principle developed by Texas Instruments. An array of tiny mirrors produced by photolithography on silicon wafers (the same technology used to create electronic devices) is used to reflect light from the illumination source through appropriate optics to a viewing screen. The mirrors can be flipped from the "on" to the "off" position in nanoseconds. Moving each mirror back and forth rapidly to control the fraction of the time that it is in the "on" position controls the brightness of each pixel. A rotating filter wheel allows the array to sequentially project the red, green, and blue channels, which the eye perceives as a color display.

Other kinds of flat-panel computer displays, including electroluminescence and plasma (gas discharge), are fundamentally monochrome. Arrays of red, green, and blue LEDs can in principle be arranged to make a flat-panel display, but the difficulty of generating blue light with these devices and the prohibitive cost of such devices has so far prevented their common use. Arrays of colored light bulbs are used to show images in some sports stadia.

It takes combinations of three color phosphors (RGB) to produce the range of colors displayed on the CRT. The brightness of each phosphor is controlled by modulating the intensity of the electron beam in the CRT that strikes each phosphor. Using a separate electron gun for each color and arranging the colored dots as triads is the most common method for achieving this control. To prevent stray electrons from striking the adjacent phosphor dot, a shadow mask of metal with holes for each triad of dots can be used. Each of the three electron beams passes through the same hole in the shadow mask and strikes the corresponding dot. The shadow mask increases the sharpness and contrast of the image, but reduces the total intensity of light that can be generated by the CRT.

A simpler design that increases the brightness applies the phosphor colors to the CRT in vertical stripes. It uses either a slotted pattern in the shadow mask or no mask at all. The simplicity of the Sony Trinitron design makes a tube with lower cost, no curvature of the glass in the vertical direction, high display brightness, and fewer alignment problems; however, the vertical extent of the phosphor and of the electron beam tends to blur edges in the vertical direction on the screen. Although this design has become fairly common for home television, most high-performance computer CRTs use triads of phosphor dots because of the greater sharpness it affords the image, particularly for lines and edges.

Image types

In traditional images with which we are visually experienced, the brightness of a point is a function of the brightness and location of the light source combined with the orientation and nature of the surface being viewed. These "surface" or "real-world" images are actually rather difficult to interpret using computer algorithms, because of their three-dimensional nature, and the fact that some surfaces may obscure others. Even for relatively flat scenes in which precedence is not a problem and the light source is well controlled, the combination of effects of surface orientation and the color, texture, and other variables make it difficult to quantitatively interpret these parameters independently. Only in the case of a carefully prepared flat and polished surface (as in the typical metallographic microscope) can interpretation of contrast as delineating phases, inclusions, grains, or other structures be successful. For additional background on image formation, and the role of lighting and optics, see (Jahne, 1997).

A second class of images that commonly arises in microscopy shows the intensity of light (or other radiation) that has come through the sample (for additional background on light microscopes and their use for imaging, see texts such as Smith, 1990; Bracegirdle and Bradbury, 1995; Bradbury and Bracegirdle, 1998). These transmission images start with a uniform light source, usually of known intensity and color. The absorption of the light at each point is a measure of the density of the specimen along that path. For some kinds of transmission images, such as those formed with electrons and x-rays, diffraction effects due to the coherent scattering of the radiation by atomic or molecular structures in the sample may also be present. These often complicate analysis, because diffraction is strongly dependent on the exact orientation of the crystalline lattice or other periodic microstructure.

To illustrate the complications that factors other than simple density can cause, **Figure 59** shows a transmission electron microscope (TEM) image of a thin cobalt foil. The evident structure is the magnetic domains in this ferromagnetic material. In each striped domain, the electron spins on the atoms have spontaneously aligned. There is no change in the atomic structure, sample density, or thickness, although the image certainly can fool the eye into thinking such variations may be present.

Likewise, **Figure 60** shows an image of a colloidal gold particle on an amorphous carbon film viewed in a high-resolution TEM. The so-called atomic resolution shows a pattern of dark spots on the substrate that appear more-or-less random, while within the gold particle they are regularly arranged. The arrangement is a result of the crystalline structure of the particle, and the spots are related to the atom positions. The spots are not simply the atoms, however, because the

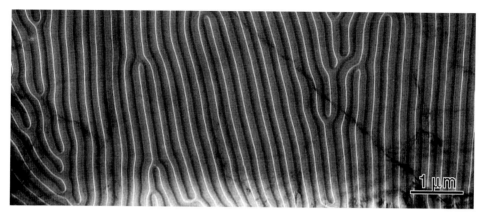

Figure 59. *TEM image of a thin metal foil of cobalt. The striped pattern reveals ferromagnetic domains, in which the electron spins of the atoms are aligned in one of two possible directions (image courtesy Hitachi Scientific Instruments).*

relationship between the structure and the image is very complex, and depends strongly on the microscope parameters and on the amount of defocus in the lens. Calculating the expected image contrast from a predicted structure is possible, and can be done routinely for simple structures. The inverse calculation (structure from image) is more interesting, but can only be accomplished by iteration.

In another subclass of transmission images, some colors (or energies) of radiation may be selectively absorbed by the sample according to its chemical composition or the presence of selective stains and dyes. Sometimes, these dyes also emit light of a different color themselves, which can be imaged to localize particular structures. In principle, this is very similar to the so-called "X-ray maps" made with the scanning electron microscope (SEM), in which electrons excite the atoms of the sample to emit their characteristic x-rays. These are imaged using the time-base of the raster scan of the microscope to form a spatial image of the distribution of each selected element, since the wavelengths of the x-rays from each atom are unique. In many of these emission images,

Figure 60. *TEM image of colloidal gold particle on an amorphous carbon substrate, used to show extremely high microscope resolution (image courtesy Hitachi Scientific Instruments).*

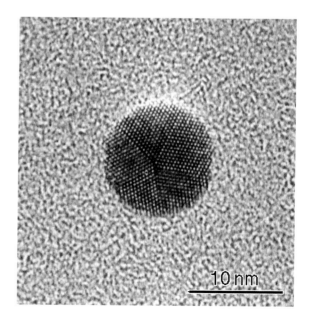

density variations, changes in the thickness of the specimen, or the presence of other elements can cause at least minor difficulties in interpreting the pixel brightness in terms of concentration or amount of the selected target element or compound.

A third class of images uses the pixel brightness to record distances. For example, an atomic force microscope image of a surface shows the elevation of each point on the surface, represented as a grey-scale (or pseudo-color) value. Range images are produced by raster-scan microscopes such as the scanning tunneling microscopes (STM) and atomic force microscopes (AFM), or by physical scanning with a profilometer stylus. They are also produced by interferometric light microscopes, and at larger scales by laser ranging, synthetic aperture radar, side-scan sonar, and other techniques. Additional methods that present an image in which pixel brightness values represent range information obtained indirectly by other means include stereoscopy, shape-from-shading, and motion blur.

Range imaging

Most of the measurement tools available for very flat surfaces provide a single-valued elevation reading at each point in an x,y raster or grid. Chapter 13 discusses the processing and measurement of surface range images in detail. This set of data is blind to any undercuts that may be present. Just as radar and sonar have wavelengths in the range of centimeters to meters (and thus are useful for measurements of large objects such as geologic landforms), so a much shorter measuring scale is needed for high precision, or very flat surfaces. Attempts to use SEM, conventional light microscopy, or confocal scanning light microscopy (CSLM) either on the original surfaces or on vertical sections cut through them, have been only partially satisfactory. The lateral resolution of the SEM is very good, but its depth resolution is not. Stereo pair measurements are both difficult to perform and time consuming to convert to an elevation map or range image of the surface, and the resulting depth resolution is still much poorer than the lateral resolution.

Conventional light microscopy has a lateral resolution of better than one micrometer, but the depth of field is neither great enough to view an entire rough surface nor shallow enough to isolate points along one iso-elevation contour line. The CSLM improves the lateral resolution slightly and greatly reduces the depth of field while at the same time rejecting scattered light from out-of-focus locations. The result is an instrument that can image an entire rough surface by moving the sample vertically and keeping only the brightest light value at each location, or can produce a range image by keeping track of the sample's vertical motion when the brightest reflected light value is obtained for each point in the image. It is the latter mode that is most interesting for surface measurement purposes. The resolution is better than one micrometer in all directions.

Figure 61 shows a reconstructed view of the surface of a fracture in a brittle ceramic. It is formed from 26 planes, separated by 1 µm in the z direction, each of which records a pixel only if that location is brighter than any other plane. The perspective view can be rotated to present a very realistic image of the surface, but plotting the same information in the form of a range image (in which each pixel brightness corresponds to the plane in which the brightest reflection was recorded) is more useful for measurement. **Figure 62** shows this presentation of the same surface along with an elevation profile along an arbitrary line across the surface.

This method is interesting for many macroscopically rough samples, such as fractures and some deposited coatings, but it is not adequate for the really flat surfaces that are currently being produced in many applications. The surface irregularities on a typical polished silicon wafer or precision-machined mirror surface are typically of the order of nanometers.

Three principal methods have been applied to such surfaces. Historically, the profilometer provided a tool that would accurately measure vertical elevation with a resolution approaching a nanometer. Although it has been widely used, the profilometer has two serious disadvantages for many

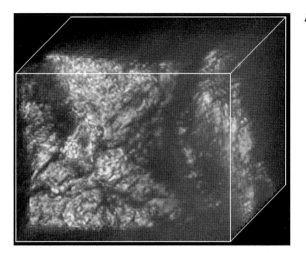

Figure 61. Reconstructed 3D image of a brittle fracture surface in a ceramic, imaged with a confocal scanning light microscope.

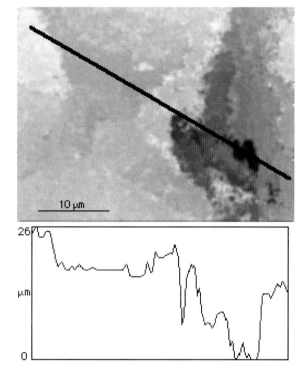

Figure 62. Range image produced from the data in *Figure 61,* with an elevation profile along an arbitrary line.

surface applications. The first is that it determines elevations only along a single profile. Although the analysis of such elevation profiles is straightforward, their relevance to complex surfaces that may have anisotropic properties is questionable. The second limitation is the large tip size, which makes it impossible to follow steep slopes or steps accurately.

This leaves the interferometric light microscope and the AFM as the methods of choice for studying very flat surfaces. Both are somewhat novel instruments. One is a modern implementation of the principles of light interference discovered a century ago, while the other is a technology invented and rapidly commercialized only within the past decade.

The interferometric light microscope (see the review by Robinson et al., 1991) reflects light from the sample surface as one leg in a classic interferometer, which is then combined with light from a reference leg. **Figure 63** shows a schematic diagram. The usual principles of phase-sensitive

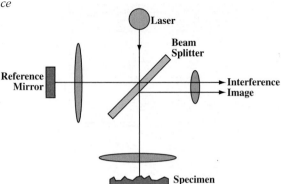

Figure 63. *Schematic diagram of an interference microscope.*

interference occur so that changes in path length (due to different elevations of points on the surface) produce changes in the intensity of the light. This image is then digitized using an appropriate CCD detector array and analog-to-digital conversion, so that a brightness value (and from it a derived elevation value) is recorded for each point on the surface. Although the wavelength of light used is typically about 630 nm, phase differences between the two legs of the interferometer of one-thousandth of the wavelength produce a change in intensity so that the vertical resolution is a few Ångstroms. The lateral resolution, however, is still of the order of one micrometer, limited by the wavelength of the light used and the design of the optics.

The interferometric light microscope suffers if the surface has high slopes or a highly specular finish, since no light will be reflected back to the detector. Such points become drop-outs in the final image. For visual purposes, it is satisfactory to fill in such missing points with a median or smoothing filter (Chapter 3), but, of course, this may bias subsequent measurements.

The vertical resolution of the interferometric microscope is very high, approaching atomic dimensions. Although the lateral resolution is much lower, it should be quite suitable for many purposes. The absolute height difference between widely separated points is not measured precisely, because the overall surface alignment and the shape or "figure" of the part is not known. It is common to deal with the problems of alignment and shape by fitting a function to the data. Determining a best-fit plane or other low-order polynomial function by least squares fitting to all of the elevation data and then subtracting it is called "detrending" the data or "form removal." It is then possible to display the magnitude of deviations of points from this surface; however, the absolute difference between points that are widely separated is affected by the detrending plane, and the ability to distinguish small differences between points that are far apart is reduced.

Figure 64 shows a very flat surface (produced by polishing a silicon wafer) imaged in a commercial interferometric light microscope (Zygo) using both Fizeau and Mirau sets of optics. The field of view is the same in both images, and the total vertical range of elevations is only about 2 nm. The two bright white spots toward the bottom of the image are probably due to dirt somewhere in the optics. These artefacts are much less pronounced with the Mirau optics. In addition, the ringing (oscillation or ripple pattern) around features that can be seen in the Fizeau image is not present with the Mirau optics. These characteristics are usually interpreted as indicating that the Mirau optics are superior for the measurement of very flat surfaces. On the other hand, the Mirau image has less lateral resolution (it appears to be "smoothed"). A pattern of horizontal lines can be discerned that may come from the misalignment of the diffuser plate with the raster scan pattern of the camera.

The AFM is in essence a profilometer that scans a complete raster over the sample surface, but with a very small tip (see the review by Wickramasinghe, 1989). The standard profilometer tip cannot

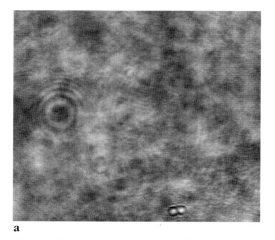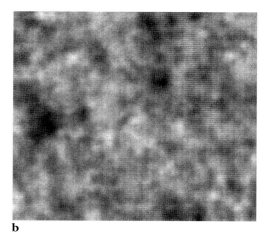

a   b

Figure 64. Comparison of interferometric range images on a flat polished silicon wafer using Fizeau (*a*) and Mirau (*b*) optics.

follow very small or very steep-sided irregularities on the surface because of its dimensions, which are of the order of µm. The AFM tip can be much smaller and sharper, although it is still not usually fine enough to handle the abrupt steps (or even undercuts) present in microelectronic circuits and some other surfaces. The tip can be operated in either an attractive or repulsive mode of interaction between the electrons around the atom(s) in the tip and those in the surface. Usually, repulsive mode (in which the tip is pressed against the surface) does a somewhat better job of following small irregularities, but it may also cause deformation of the surface and the displacement of atoms.

Other modalities of interaction are used for these scanned-tip microscopes. The STM was the original, but it can only be used for conductive specimens and is strongly sensitive to surface electronic states, surface contamination, and oxidation. Lateral force, tapping mode, and other modes of operation developed within the last few years offer the ability to characterize many aspects of surface composition and properties, but the straightforward AFM mode is most often used to determine surface geometry, and presents quite enough complexities for understanding.

As indicated in the schematic diagram of **Figure 65**, the usual mode of operation for the AFM is to move the sample in x, y, and z. The x, y scan covers the region of interest, while the z motion brings the tip back to the same null position as judged by the reflection of a laser beam. The necessary motion is recorded in a computer to produce the resulting image. Modifications that move the tip instead of the sample, or use a linear-array light sensor to measure the deflection of the tip rather than wait for the specimen to be moved in z, do not change the basic principle. The motion is usually accomplished with piezoelectric elements whose dimensions can be sensitively adjusted by varying the applied voltage; however, there is a time lag or creep associated with these motions that appears in the modulation transfer function (MTF) of the microscope as a loss of sensitivity at the largest or smallest dimensions (lowest and highest frequencies). Locating the x, y coordinates of the tip interferometrically instead of based on the piezo driver voltages can overcome some of these problems.

Although the AFM has in principle a lateral resolution of a few Angstroms, as well as vertical sensitivity in this range, it is not always possible to realize that performance. For one thing, the adjustment of scan speeds and amplifier time constants for the visually best picture may eliminate some of the fine-scale roughness and thus bias subsequent analysis. Conversely, it may introduce additional noise from electrical or mechanical sources. Special care must also be taken to eliminate vibration.

Figure 65. Schematic diagram of an atomic force microscope (AFM).

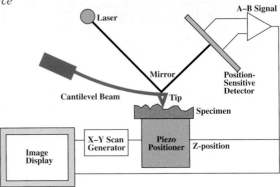

Figure 65. Schematic diagram of an atomic force microscope (AFM).

Most of the attention to the performance of the AFM, STM, and related instruments has been concerned with the high-resolution limit (Denley, 1990a; Denley, 1990b; Grigg et al., 1992). This is generally set by the shape of the tip, which is not easy to characterize. Many authors (Reiss et al., 1990; Pancorbo et al., 1991; Aguilar et al., 1992) have shown that it may be possible to deconvolve the tip shape and improve the image sharpness in exactly the same way that it is done for other imaging systems. This type of deconvolution is discussed in Chapters 5 and 13.

Figure 66 shows a sample of polished silicon (traditional roughness values indicate 0.2–0.3 nm magnitude, near the nominal vertical resolution limit for interferometry and AFM) with a hardness indentation. One limitation of the AFM can be seen by generating a rendered or isotropic display of the indentation, which shows that the left side of the indentation appears to be smoother than the right. This difference is an artefact of the scanning, because the tip response dynamics are different when following a surface down (where it may lag behind the actual surface and fail to record deviations) or up (where contact forces it to follow irregularities). In addition, the measured depth of the indentation is much less than the actual depth, because the tip cannot follow the deepest part of the indentation and because the calibration of the AFM in the vertical direction is less precise than in the x,y directions.

Tools for surface characterization are available with sufficient lateral and vertical resolution for application to a variety of surface range measurements. The interferometer is more convenient to use than the AFM, operates over a wide range of magnifications, and accepts large samples. It also introduces less directional anisotropy due to the instrument characteristics. The AFM, on the

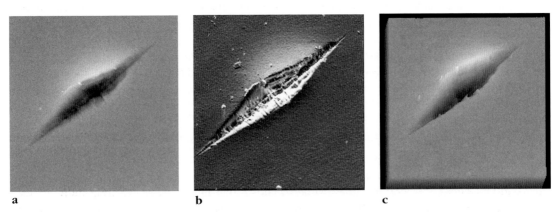

a b c

*Figure 66. AFM image of a Knoop hardness indentation in metal, shown as range (**a**), rendered (**b**) and isometric (**c**) presentations.*

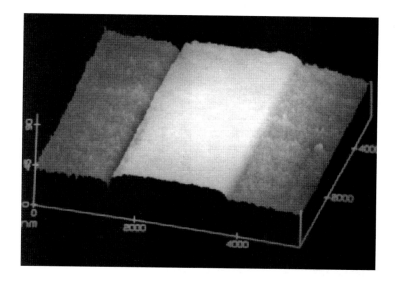

Figure 67. Scanning tunneling microscope (STM) image. The specimen actually is flat-surfaced silicon, with apparent relief showing altered electron levels in a 2μm wide region with implanted phosphorus. (image courtesy of J. Labrasca, North Carolina State University, and R. Chapman, Microelectronics Center of North Carolina).

other hand, has higher lateral resolution which may be required for the metrology of very fine features, now becoming commonplace in integrated circuit fabrication and nanotechnology.

It is important to keep in mind that the signal produced by many microscopes is only indirectly related to the surface elevation. In some cases, it may represent quite different characteristics of the sample such as compositional variations or electronic properties. In **Figure 67**, the apparent step in surface elevation provides an example. The surface is actually flat, but the electronic properties of the sample (a junction in a microelectronic device) produce the variation in signal.

Multiple images

For many applications, a single image is not enough. Multiple images may constitute a series of views of the same area, using different wavelengths of light or other signals. Examples include the images produced by satellites, such as the various visible and infrared wavelengths recorded by the Landsat Thematic Mapper (TM), and images from the SEM in which as many a dozen different elements may be represented by their x-ray intensities. These images may each require processing; for example, x-ray maps are usually very noisy. Then, they are often combined either by using ratios, such as the ratio of different wavelengths used to identify crops in TM images, or Boolean logic, such as locating regions that contain both iron and sulfur in an SEM image of a mineral. **Figure 68** shows an example in which two satellite color photographs of the same region, one covering the usual visual range of wavelengths and one extending into the near infrared, are combined by constructing the ratio of infrared to green intensity as a vegetation index, insensitive to the local inclination of the surface to the sun. Combinations reduce, but only slightly, the amount of data to be stored.

Satellite images are typically acquired in several wavelengths, covering the visible and near infrared bands. Landsat images, for example, can be combined to generate a "true color" image by placing bands 1, 2, and 3 into the blue, green, and red channels of a color image, respectively. Other satellites produce images with higher resolution, although without color sensitivity. **Figure 69** shows three color channels with ground resolution of about 15 meters, and one panchromatic grey scale image with ground resolution of 5 meters. Combining the three low resolution channels to produce a color image, converting this to HSI, and then replacing the intensity channel with the higher resolution image, produces a result shown in **Figure 70** with both color information and high spatial resolution. The fact that the color data are not as sharp as the brightness data does not hinder viewing or interpretation, as discussed previously.

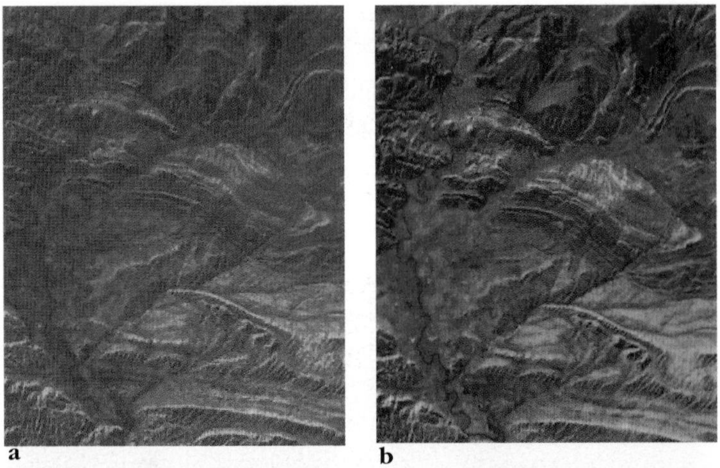

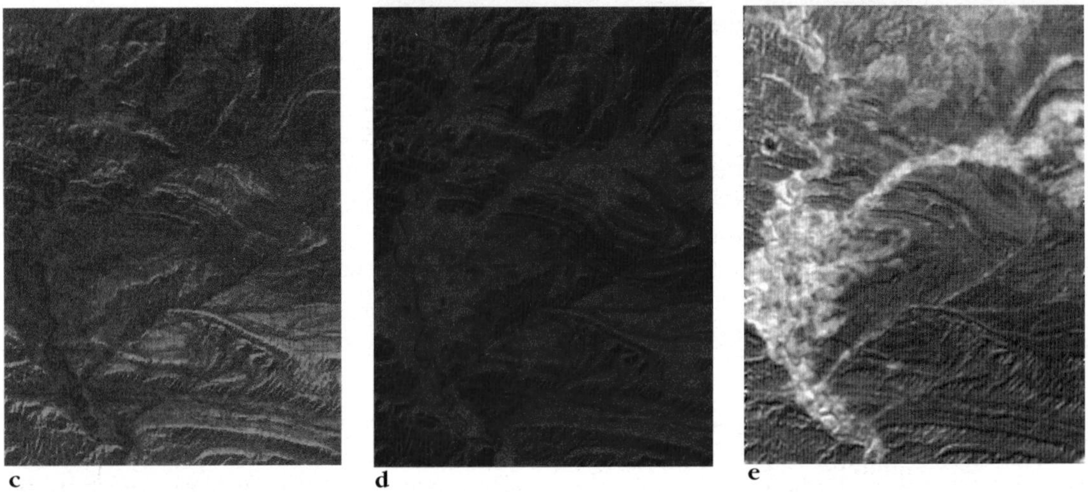

Figure 68. Landsat Thematic Mapper images in visual and infrared color of a 20 km region at Thermopolis, Wyoming (original image from Sabins, 1987):
(a) visible light;
(b) infrared light;
(c) result of filtering the visible image at 520 nm;
(d) filtering the infrared image at 1100 nm;
(e) the ratio of the green (visible) to red (IR) filtered intensities.

Another multiple image situation is a time sequence. This could be a series of satellite images used to track the motion of weather systems or a series of microscope images used to track the motion of cells or beating of cilia. In all of these cases, the need is usually to identify and locate the same features in each of the images, even though there may be some gradual changes in feature appearance from one image to the next. If the images can be reduced to data on the location of only a small number of features, then the storage requirements are greatly reduced.

A technique known as motion flow works at a lower level. With this approach, matching of pixel patterns by a correlation method is used to create a vector field showing the motion between successive images. This method is particularly used in machine vision and robotics work, in which the successive images are very closely spaced in time. Simplifying the vector field can again result in modest amounts of data, and these are usually processed in real time so that storage is not an issue. The principal requirement is that the local texture information needed for matching be present. Thus, the images must be low in random noise and each image should contain simple and distinctive surfaces with consistent illumination. The matching is performed using cross-correlation, in either the spatial or frequency domain (as discussed in Chapter 5).

A set of images can also produce three-dimensional information. They are usually a series of parallel slice images through a solid object (**Figure 71**). Medical imaging methods such as tomography and magnetic resonance images can produce this sort of data. So can some seismic imaging techniques. Even more common are various serial section methods used in microscopy. The classic method for producing such a series of images is to microtome a series of sections from the original sample, image each separately in the light or electron microscope, and then align the images afterwards.

Optical sectioning, especially with the CSLM, which has a very shallow depth of field and can collect images from deep in partially transparent specimens, eliminates the problems of alignment. **Figure 72** shows several focal section planes from a CSLM. Some imaging methods, such as the SIMS (secondary ion mass spectrometer), produce a series of images in depth by physically eroding the

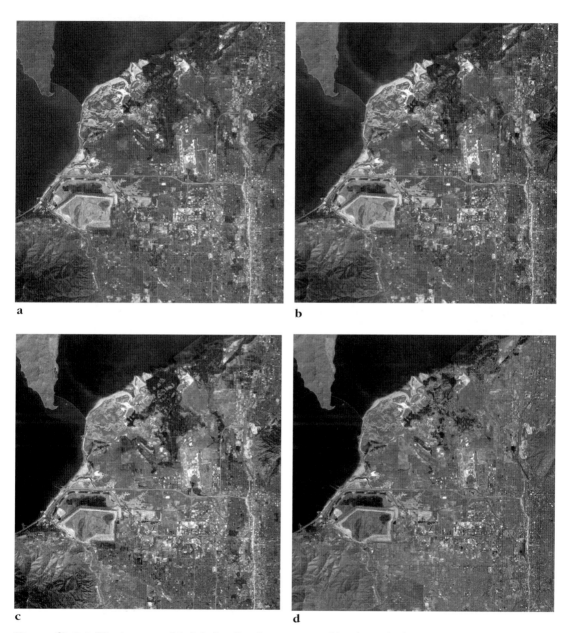

a   b

c   d

Figure 69. Satellite images of Salt Lake City (courtesy Y. Siddiqul, I-Cubed Corp., Ft. Collins, CO):
  (**a**) *Band 1 (blue) 15-m resolution;*
  (**b**) *Band 2 (green) 15-m resolution;*
  (**c**) *Band 3 (red) 15-m resolution;*
  (**d**) *Panchromatic, 5-m resolution.*

Figure 70. Combination of planes :
(a) RGB composite using 20-m resolution images,
Figure 69 a, b, *and* **c;**
(b) replacement of the intensity channel of image **a**
with the higher resolution panchromatic image from
Figure 69d.

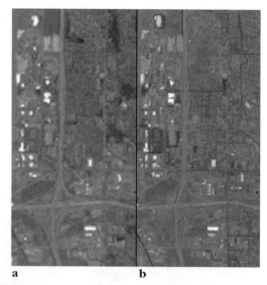

a   b

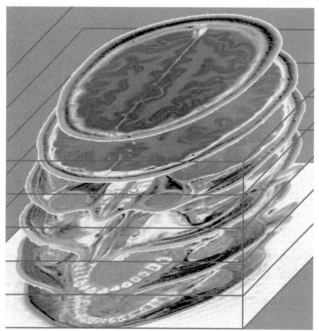

Figure 71. *Multiple planes of pixels
(sections through a human head) fill
three-dimensional space. Voxels (volume
elements) are ideally cubic for
processing and measurement of 3D
images.*

sample, which also preserves alignment. **Figure 73** shows an example of SIMS images. Sequential polishing of harder samples such as metals also produces new surfaces for imaging, but it is generally difficult to control the depth in order to space them uniformly.

The ideal situation for three-dimensional interpretation of structure calls for the lateral resolution of serial section image planes to be equal to the spacing between the planes. This produces cubic "voxels" (volume elements), which have the same advantages for processing and measurement in three dimensions that square pixels have in two; however, it is usually the case that the planes are spaced apart by much more than their lateral resolution, and special attention is given to interpolating between the planes. In the case of the SIMS, the situation is reversed and the plane spacing (as little as a few atom dimensions) is much less than the lateral resolution in each plane (typically about 1 μm).

Some techniques directly produce cubic voxel images, such as three-dimensional tomography. In this case, a series of projection images, generally using x-rays or electrons, are obtained as the sample is rotated to different orientations, and then mathematical reconstruction calculates the density of each voxel. The resulting large, three-dimensional image arrays may be stored as a series of planar slices. When a three-dimensional data set is used, a variety of processing and display modes are available. These are discussed in more detail in Chapter 12. **Figure 74** shows examples of sectioning through a series of x-ray tomographic and magnetic resonance images (MRI) in the x, y, and z planes.

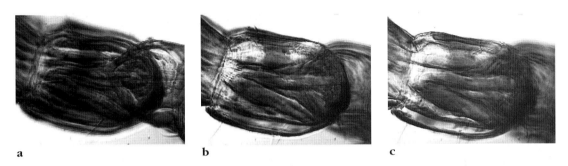

a   b   c

Figure 72. *Serial section images formed by transmission confocal scanning laser microscopy (CSLM). These are selected views from a series of sections through the leg joint of a head louse, with optical section thickness about 0.5 µm.*

Figure 73. *SIMS (secondary ion mass spectrometer) images of Boron implanted in a microelectronic device. The images are selected from a sequence of 29 images covering a total of about 1 µm in depth. Each image is produced by physically removing layers of atoms from the surface, which erodes the sample progressively to reveal structures at greater depth.*

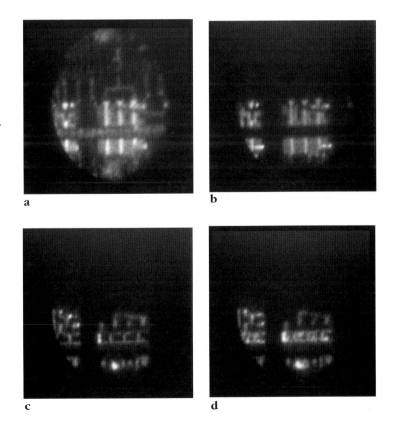

a   b

c   d

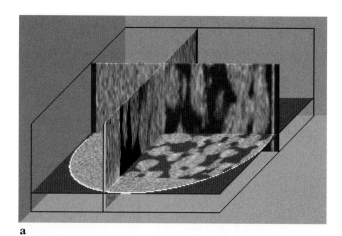

Figure 74. Examples of three-dimensional data sets formed by a series of planar images:
(**a**) A sintered ceramic imaged by x-ray tomography (CAT), with a characteristic dimension of a few μm; the dark regions are voids. The poorer resolution in the vertical direction is due to the spacing of the image planes, which is greater than the lateral pixel resolution within each plane.
(**b**) A human head imaged by magnetic resonance imaging (MRI — the same data set as shown in **Figure 71**), with characteristic dimension of centimeters. The section planes can be positioned arbitrarily and moved to reveal the internal structure.

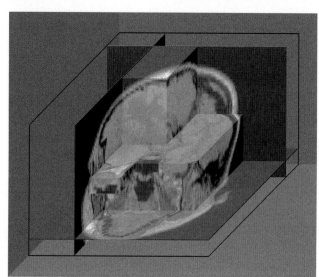

b

Stereoscopy

Three-dimensional information can also be obtained from two images of the same scene, taken from slightly different viewpoints. Human stereoscopy gives us depth perception, although we also get important data from relative size, precedence, perspective, atmospheric haze, and other cues, which were discovered and used very effectively by artists during the Renaissance. Similar to other aspects of human vision, stereoscopy is primarily comparative, with the change of vergence angle of the eyes as we shift attention from one feature to another indicating to the brain which is closer. **Figure 75** shows schematically the principle of stereo fusion, in which the images from each eye are compared to locate the same feature in each view. The eye muscles rotate the eye to bring this feature to the fovea, and the muscles provide the vergence information to the brain. Notice that this implies that stereoscopy is only applied to one feature in the field of view at a time, and not to the entire scene. From the amount of vergence motion needed, the relative distance of the object is ascertained. Only comparative measurements are made, so only the direction or relative amount of motion required to fuse the images of each object is required.

Not all animals use this method. The owl, for instance, has eyes that are not movable in their sockets. Instead, the fovea has an elongated shape along a line that is not vertical, but angled toward

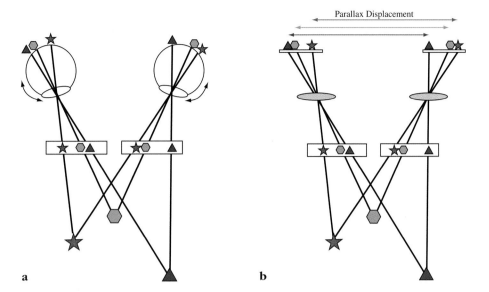

Figure 75. Stereoscopic depth perception:

(a) The relative distance to each feature identified in both the left and right eye views is given by differences in the vergence angles by which the eyes must rotate inward to bring each feature to the central fovea in each eye. This is accomplished one feature at a time. Viewing stereo pair images provides the same visual cues to the eyes and produces the same interpretation.

(b) Measurement of images to obtain actual distances uses the different parallax displacements of the features in two images. The distance between the two view points must be known. Locating the same feature in both images is the hardest part of the task for automated analysis.

the owl's feet. The owl tilts his head to accomplish fusion (bringing the feature of interest to the fovea) and judges the relative distance by the tilt required.

Although the human visual system makes only comparative use of the parallax, or vergence, of images of an object, it is straightforward to measure the relative displacement of two objects in the field of view to calculate their relative distance, or of the angle of vergence of one object to calculate its distance from the viewer. This is routinely done at scales ranging from aerial photography and map making to scanning electron microscopy.

Measurement of range information from two views is quite straightforward in principle. The lateral position of objects in these two views is different depending on their distance. From these parallax displacements, the distance can be computed by a process called stereoscopy, or sometimes photogrammetry. Computer fusion of images is a difficult task, however, that requires locating matching points in the images. Brute-force correlation methods that try to match many points based on local texture are fundamentally similar to the motion flow approach. This produces many false matches, but these are assumed to be removed by subsequent noise filtering. The alternate approach is to locate selected points in the images that are "interesting," based on their representing important boundaries or feature edges, which can then be matched more confidently. The areas between the matched points are then assumed to be simple planes.

No matter how fusion is accomplished, the displacement of the points in the two images, or parallax, gives the range. This method is used for surface elevation mapping, ranging from satellite or aerial pictures used to produce topographic maps (in which the two images are taken a short time

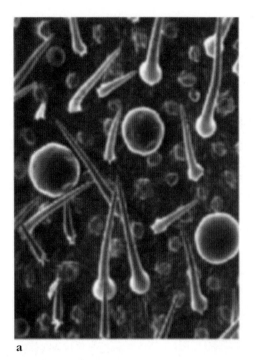 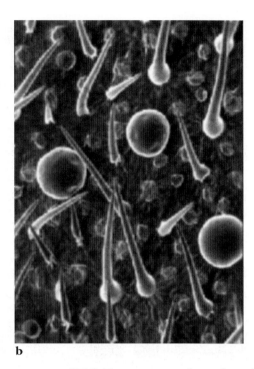

a   b

Figure 76. Stereo pair images from the scanning electron microscope (SEM). The specimen is the surface of a leaf; the two images were obtained by tilting the beam incident on the specimen by 8° to produce two points of view (images courtesy Japan Electron Optics Laboratory, Peabody, MA).

apart as the satellite or airplane position changes) to scanning electron microscope metrology of semiconductor chips (in which the two images are produced by tilting the sample). **Figure 76** shows an example of a stereo pair from an SEM; **Figure 77** shows two aerial photographs and a complete topographic map drawn from them.

The utility of a stereoscopic view of the world to communicate depth information resulted in the use of stereo cameras to produce "stereopticon" slides for viewing, which was very popular more than 50 years ago. Stereo movies (requiring the viewer to wear polarized glasses) have enjoyed brief vogues from time to time. Publication of stereo-pair views to illustrate scientific papers is now relatively common. The most common formats are two side-by-side images about 7.5 cm apart (the distance between human eyes), which an experienced viewer can see without optical aids by looking straight ahead and allowing the brain to fuse the two images, and the use of different colors for each image. Overprinting the same image in red and green (or red and blue) allows the viewer with colored glasses to see the correct image in each eye, and again the brain can sort out the depth information (**Figure 78**). Some SEMs display true stereo views of surfaces using this method. Of course, this only works for grey scale images. Computer displays using polarized light and glasses are also used to display three-dimensional data, usually synthesized from calculations or simulations rather than direct imaging.

Several different measurement geometries are used (Boyde, 1973). In all cases, the same scene is viewed from two different locations, and the distance between those locations is precisely known. Sometimes this is accomplished by moving the viewpoint, for instance, the airplane carrying the camera. In aerial photography, the plane's speed and direction are known, and the time of each picture is recorded with it to give the distance traveled.

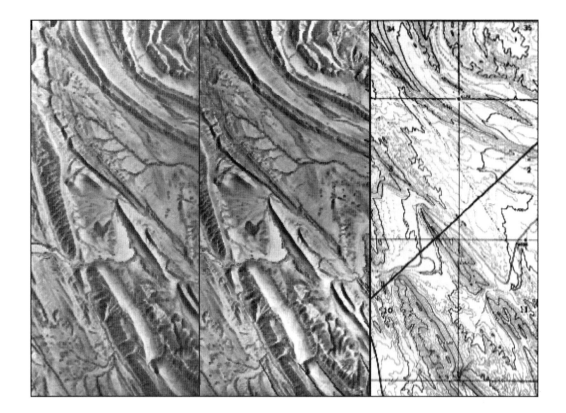

Figure 77. *Stereo pair images from aerial photography, and the topographic map showing iso-elevation contour lines derived from the parallax in the images. The scene is a portion of the Wind River in Wyoming. (From Sabins, Jr. F.F. [1987]. Remote Sensing: Principles and Interpretation, 2nd ed., W.H. Freeman, NewYork. With permission.)*

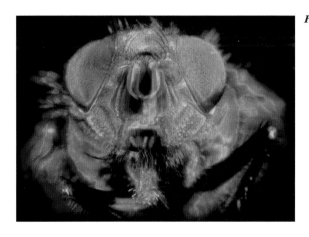

Figure 78. *Red/cyan stereo image of a fly's head. This image was captured as two separate SEM images, which were then superimposing as different color planes. To view the image, use glasses with a red filter in front of the left eye, and either a green or blue filter in front of the right eye.*

In **Figure 79**, *S* is the shift distance (either the distance the plane has traveled or the distance the SEM stage was translated) and *WD* is the working distance or altitude. The parallax $(d_1 - d_2)$ from the distances between two points as they appear in the two different images (measured in a direction parallel to the shift) is proportional to the elevation difference between the two points.

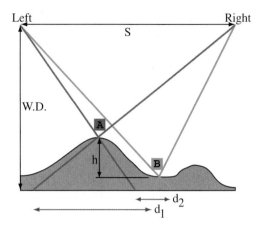

Figure 79. *Geometry used to measure the vertical height difference between objects viewed in two different images obtained by shifting the sample or viewpoint (typically used for aerial photography).*

$$h = WD \cdot \frac{(d_1 - d_2)}{S} \qquad (4)$$

If the vertical relief of the surface being measured is a significant fraction of *WD*, then foreshortening of lateral distances as a function of elevation will also be present in the images. The x and y coordinates of points in the images can be corrected with the following equations. This means that rubber-sheeting to correct the foreshortening is needed to allow fitting or "tiling" together a mosaic of pictures into a seamless whole.

$$X' = X \cdot (WD - h) / WD$$

$$Y' = Y \cdot (WD - h) / WD \qquad (5)$$

Much greater displacement between the two eyepoints can be achieved if the two views are not in parallel directions, but are instead directed inward toward the same central point in each scene. This is rarely done in aerial photography, because it is impractical when trying to cover a large region with a mosaic of pictures and is not usually necessary to obtain sufficient parallax for measurement. When examining samples in the SEM, however, it is very easy to accomplish this by tilting the sample between two views. In **Figure 80**, the two images represent two views obtained by tilting the specimen about a vertical axis. The points A and B are separated by a horizontal distance d_1 or d_2 that is different in the two images. From this parallax value and the known tilt angle δ applied between the two images, the height difference h and the angle θ of a line joining the points (usually a surface defined by the points) can be calculated (Boyde, 1973) as:

$$\theta = \tan^{-1} \left\{ \frac{\cos\delta - d_2 / d_1)}{\sin\delta} \right\} \qquad (6)$$

$$h_1 = \frac{(d_1 \cdot \cos\delta - d_2)}{\sin\delta}$$

Notice that the angle θ is independent of the magnification, since the distances enter as a ratio.

When two angled views of the same region of the surface are available, the relative displacement or parallax of features can be made quite large relative to their lateral magnification. This makes it

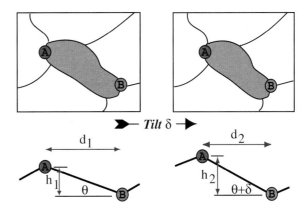

Figure 80. Geometry used to measure the vertical height difference between points viewed in two different images obtained by tilting the sample (typically used for microscopy).

possible to measure relatively small amounts of surface relief. Angles of 5 to 10° are commonly used; for very flat surfaces, tilt angles as great as 20° can sometimes be useful. When large angles are used with rough surfaces, the images contain shadow areas where features are not visible in both images and fusion becomes very difficult. Also, when the parallax becomes too great in a pair of images, it can be difficult for the human observer to fuse the two images visually if this step is used in the measurement operation.

Many of the measurements made with stereo-pair photographs from both SEM and aerial photography are made using extensive human interaction. The algorithms that have been developed for automatic fusion require many of the image processing operations that will be described in later chapters to make possible the identification of the same features in each image. For the moment, it is enough to understand the principle that identifying the same points in left and right images, and measuring the parallax, gives the elevation. With data for many different pairs of points, it is possible to construct a complete map of the surface. The elevation data can then be presented in a variety of formats, including a range image encoding elevation as the brightness or color of each pixel in the array. Other display modes, such as contour maps, isometric views, or shaded renderings can be generated to assist the viewer in interpreting these images, which are not common to our everyday experience. The range image data are in a suitable form for many types of image processing and for the measurement of the surface area or the volume above or below the surface.

The majority of elevation maps of the earth's surface being made today are determined by the stereoscopic measurement of images, either taken from aerial photography or satellite remote imaging. Of course, two-thirds of the earth is covered by water and cannot be measured this way. Portions of the sea bottom have been mapped stereoscopically by side-scanned sonar. The technology is very similar to that used for the radar mapping of Venus, except that sonar uses sound waves (which can propagate through water) and radar uses high-frequency (millimeter length) electromagnetic radiation that can penetrate the opaque clouds covering Venus.

The synthetic aperture radar (SAR) used by the Magellan probe to map Venus does not directly give elevation data to produce a range image. The principle of SAR is neither new, nor is it restricted to satellites and space probes. Aerial mapping of desert regions has been used to penetrate through the dry sand and map the underlying land to find ancient watercourses, for instance. The principle of SAR is that the moving satellite (or other platform) emits a series of short pulses directed downwards and to one side of the track along which it is moving. Direction parallel to the track is called the azimuth and the direction perpendicular to it is called the range (not to be confused with the range image that encodes the elevation information). The name "synthetic aperture" refers to the fact that the moving antenna effectively acts as a much larger antenna (equal in size to the distance the antenna moves during the pulse) that can more accurately resolve directions in azimuth.

The radar records the intensity of the returning pulse, the travel time, and the Doppler shift. The intensity is a measure of the surface characteristics, although the radar (or sonar) reflectivity is not always easy to interpret in terms of the surface structure and is not directly related to the albedo (or reflectivity) for visible light. The travel time for the pulse gives the range. For a perfectly flat surface, there would be an arc of locations on the surface that would have the same range from the antenna. Because of the motion of the satellite or airplane, each point along this arc produces a different Doppler shift in the signal frequency. Measuring the Doppler shift of each returned pulse provides resolution along the arc. Each point on the ground contributes to the return pulse with a unique range and Doppler shift, which allows a range map of the ground to be reconstructed.

The surface is not flat, therefore multiple combinations of location and elevation are possible, which could produce the same return signal. Combining the measurements from several overlapping sweeps (for Magellan, several sequential orbits) allows the elevation data to be refined. The database for Venus resolves points on the ground with about 120-m spacing and has elevation data with resolutions that vary from 120 to 300 m (depending on where along the track, and how far from the center of the track, they were located). For each point, the elevation and the reflectivity are stored (**Figure 81**). In many of the published renderings of these data, the elevation values are used to construct the surface shape and the reflectivity values are used to color the surface (**Figure 82**). Of course, the colors do not reflect the actual visual appearance of the surface.

Synthetic aperture ranging with either radar or sonar is not the only way these signals can be used to construct a range map. Directing a beam straight down and measuring the echo, or return time, gives the range at a single point. Many such measurements can be used to construct a map or image. The simple "fish-finder" type of sonar can be used to construct a map of a lake bottom in this way, if the boat is steered back and forth in a raster pattern to cover the whole surface. Other signals can be used, as well. The Clementine mission to the moon used a laser beam from the orbiting space craft in a similar fashion. By pulsing the laser and waiting for the echo, points were measured every few hundred meters across the entire lunar surface with a vertical resolution of about 40 m.

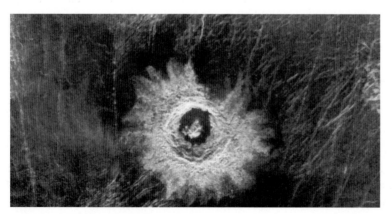

Figure 81. Range image of Venus obtained from synthetic aperture radar (courtesy Jet Propulsion Laboratory, Pasadena, CA).

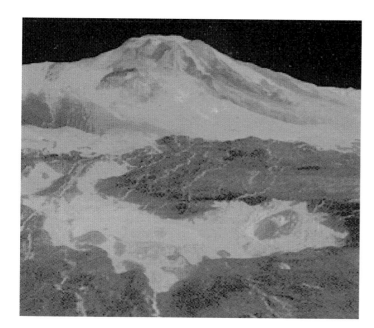

Figure 82. Rendered surface of Venus from SAR data (courtesy Jet Propulsion Laboratory, Pasadena, CA).

Imaging requirements

Given the diversity of image types and sources described earlier, several general criteria can be prescribed for images intended for computer processing and analysis. The first criteria is the need for global uniformity. The same type of feature should look the same wherever it appears in the image. This implies that brightness and color values should be the same and, consequently, that illumination must be uniform and stable for images acquired at different times. When surfaces are nonplanar, such as the earth as viewed from a satellite or a fracture surface in the microscope, corrections for the changing local orientation may be possible, but this usually requires extensive calculation and/or prior knowledge of the surface and source of illumination.

Figure 83 shows an example of a microscope image with nonuniform illumination. Storing a "background" image with no specimen present (by moving to a clear space on the slide) allows this nonuniformity to be leveled. The background image is either subtracted from or divided into the original (depending on whether the camera has a logarithmic or linear response). This type of leveling is discussed in Chapter 3 on correcting image defects, along with other ways to obtain the background image when it cannot be acquired directly.

The requirement for uniformity limits the kinds of surfaces that are normally imaged. Planar surfaces, or at least simple and known ones, are much easier to deal with than complex surfaces. Simply connected surfaces are much easier to interpret than ones with arches, bridges, caves and loops that hide some of the structure. Features that have precedence problems, in which some features hide entirely or in part behind others, present difficulties for interpretation or measurement. Illumination that casts strong shadows, especially to one side, is also undesirable in most cases. The exception occurs when well-spaced features cast shadows that do not interfere with each other. The shadow lengths can be used with the known lighting geometry to calculate feature heights. **Figure 84** shows an example in aerial photography. One form of sample preparation for the TEM deposits a thin film of metal or carbon from a point source, which also leaves shadow areas behind particles or other protrusions that can be used in the same way (**Figure 85**).

In addition to global uniformity, we generally want local sensitivity to variations. This means that edges and boundaries must be well delineated and accurately located. The resolution of the camera sensor was discussed earlier. Generally, anything that degrades high frequencies in the signal

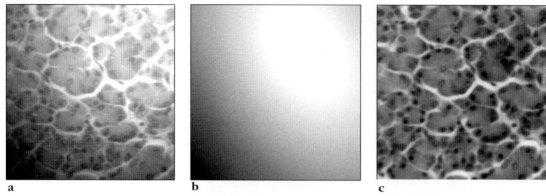

a   b   c

Figure 83. *A microscope image obtained with nonuniform illumination (due to a misaligned condenser lens). The "background" image was collected under the same conditions, with no sample present (by moving to an adjacent region on the slide). Subtracting the background image and expanding the contrast of the difference produces a "leveled" image with uniform brightness values for similar structures.*

chain will disturb the subsequent ability to identify feature boundaries or locate edges for measurement. On the other hand, such simple problems as dust on the optics can introduce local variations that may be mistaken for image features, causing serious errors.

Measurement of dimensions requires that the geometry of the imaging system be well known. Knowing the magnification of a microscope or the altitude of a satellite is usually straightforward. Calibrating the lateral scale can be accomplished either by knowledge of the optics or by using an image of a known scale or standard. When the viewing geometry is more complicated, either because the surface is not planar or the viewing angle is not perpendicular, measurement is more difficult and requires determination of the geometry first, or the inclusion of a scale or fiducial marks on the object being viewed.

Figure 84. *Aerial photograph in which length of shadows and knowledge of the sun position permit calculation of the heights of trees and the height of the piles of logs in the lumberyard, from which the amount of wood can be estimated.*

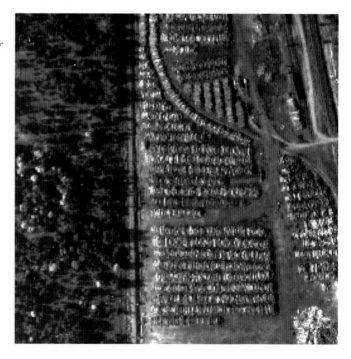

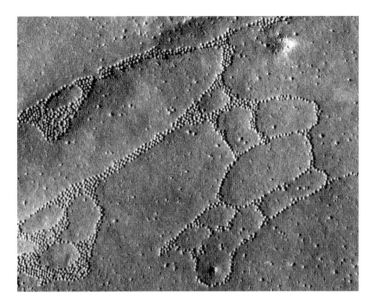

Figure 85. *Electron microscope image showing shadowed particles delineating the gap junctions between cells, revealed by freeze-fracturing the tissue.*

Figure 86 shows the simplest kind of distortion when a planar surface is viewed at an angle. Different portions of the image have different magnification scales, which makes subsequent analysis difficult. It also prevents combining multiple images of a complex surface into a mosaic. This problem is evident in two applications at very different scales. Satellite images of the surface of planets are assembled into mosaics covering large areas only with elaborate image warping to bring the edges into registration. This type of warping is discussed in Chapter 3. SEM images of rough surfaces are more difficult to assemble in this way, because the overall specimen geometry is not so well known, and the required computer processing is more difficult to justify.

Measuring brightness information, such as density or color values, requires a very stable illumination source and sensor. Color measurements are easily affected by changes in the color temperature of an incandescent bulb due to minor voltage fluctuations or as the bulb warms up or ages. Fluorescent lighting, especially when used in light boxes with x-ray films or densitometry gels, may be unstable or may introduce interference in solid-state cameras due to the high-frequency flickering of the fluorescent tube. Bright specular reflections may cause saturation, blooming, or shifts in the camera gain.

It helps to bear in mind the purpose if digitizing an image into a computer. Some of the possibilities are listed in the following paragraphs, and these place different restrictions and demands on the hardware and software used. Subsequent chapters discuss these topics in greater detail. The emphasis throughout this book is on the results produced by various processing and measurement techniques, with plain English descriptions of the methods and illustrations comparing different approaches. Numerous books provide computer codes that implement various algorithms, such as (Parker, 1997; Ritter and Wilson, 2001; Pavlidis, 1982; Myler and Weeks, 1993; Umbaugh, 1998; Seul et al., 2000; Lichtenbelt et al., 1998), with more books rolling off the presses every month.

A great many books on digital image processing are also available, some of which delve deeply into the mathematical underpinnings of the science, and others which concentrate on applications in a particular field. A representative selection includes (Gonzalez and Woods, 1993; Pratt, 1991; Rosenfeld and Kak, 1982; Weeks, 1996; Pitas, 2000; Nikolaidis and Pitas, 2001; Costa & Cesar, 2001; Sonka et al., 1999; Kriete, 1992; Hader, 1992; Sanchez and Canton, 1999; Russ, 2001). The emphasis in this text is on the generality of the methods, showing that the same techniques apply to a broad range of types of images, and trying to educate the user in the performance and results instead of the theory.

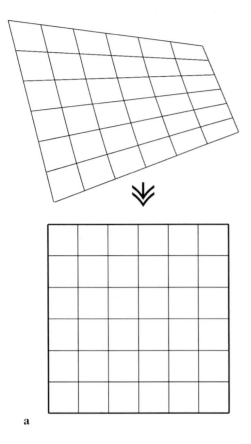

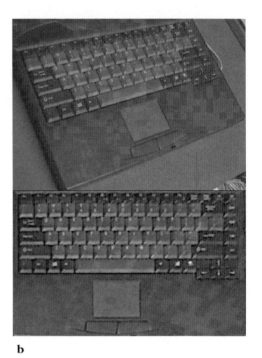

Figure 86. Geometric distortion occurs when a surface is viewed from a position away from the surface normal. Correcting this distortion to obtain a rectilinear image that can be properly processed and measured, or fitted together with adjoining images, requires knowing the viewing geometry and/or including some known fiducial marks in the scene which can be used to determine it.

a

b

Storing and filing of images becomes more attractive as massive storage devices (such as writable DVD disks) drop in price or where multiple master copies of images may be needed in more than one location. In many cases, this application also involves hardcopy printing of the stored images and transmission of images to other locations. If further processing or measurement is not required, then compression of the images is worthwhile. The advantage of electronic storage is that the images do not degrade with time and can be accessed by appropriate filing and cross-indexing routines. On the other hand, film storage is far cheaper and offers much higher storage density as well as higher image resolution, and it is likely that devices for examining film will still be available in 100 years, which may not be the case for DVD disks.

Enhancement of images for visual examination requires a large number of pixels and adequate pixel depth so that the image can be acquired with enough information to perform the filtering or other operations with fidelity and then display the result with enough detail for the viewer. Uniformity of illumination and control of geometry are not of great importance. When large images are used, and especially for some of the more time-consuming processing operations, or when interactive experimentation with many different operations is intended, this application may benefit from very fast computers or specialized hardware.

Measurement of dimensions and density values can often be performed with modest image resolution if the magnification or illumination can be adjusted beforehand to make the best use of the image sensor. Processing may be required before measurement (for instance, derivatives are often used to delineate edges for measurement), but this can usually be handled completely in software. The most important constraints are tight control over the imaging geometry, and the uniformity and constancy of illumination.

Quality control applications usually do not involve absolute measurements so much as watching for variations. In many cases, this is handled simply by subtracting a reference image from each acquired image, point by point, to detect gross changes. This can be done with analog electronics at real-time speeds. Preventing variation due to accidental changes in the position of camera or targets, or in illumination, is a central concern.

Microstructural research in either two or three dimensions usually starts with image measurement and has the same requirements as noted previously, plus the ability to subject the measurement values to appropriate stereological and statistical analysis. Interpretation of images in terms of structure is different for images of planar cross sections or projections (**Figure 87**). The latter are familiar to human vision, while the former are not; however, section images, such as the one in **Figure 88**, contain rich information for measurement in three dimensions that can be revealed by statistical analysis. Projection images, such as the one in **Figure 89**, may present greater difficulties for interpretation.

Three-dimensional imaging utilizes large data sets, and in most cases the alignment of two-dimensional images is of critical importance. Some three-dimensional structural parameters can be inferred from two-dimensional images. Others, principally topological information, can only be determined from the three-dimensional data set. Processing and measurement operations in three dimensions place extreme demands on computer storage and speed. Displays of three-dimensional information in ways interpretable by, if not familiar to, human users are improving, but need further development of algorithms. They also place considerable demands on processor and display speed.

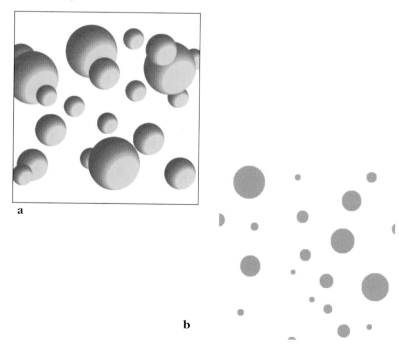

Figure 87. *Projection images, such as the spheres shown in (a), are familiar, showing the external surfaces of features; however, some features are partially or entirely obscured and it is not easy to determine the number or size distribution. Cross-section images, as shown in (b), are unfamiliar and do not show the maximum extent of features, but statistically it is possible to predict the size distribution and number of the spheres.*

a

b

Figure 88. *Light microscope image of section through a colored enamel coating applied to steel (courtesy V. Benes, Research Institute for Metals, Panenské Brezany, Czechoslovakia). The spherical bubbles arise during the firing of the enamel. They are sectioned to show circles whose diameters are smaller than the maximum diameter of the spheres, but since the shape of the bubbles is known it is possible to infer the number and size distribution of the spheres from the data measured on the circles.*

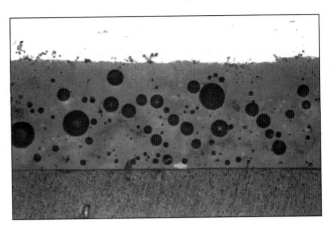

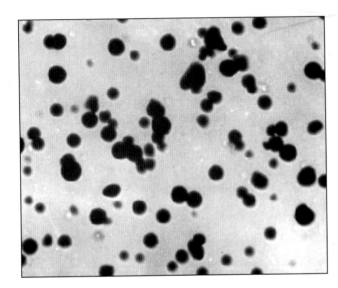

Figure 89. *Transmission electron microscope image of latex spheres in a thick, transparent section. Some of the spheres are partially hidden by others. If the section thickness is known, the size distribution and volume fraction occupied by the spheres can be estimated, but some small features may be entirely obscured and cannot be determined.*

Classification and recognition is generally considered to be the high-end task for computer-based image analysis. It ranges in complexity from locating and recognizing isolated objects belonging to a few well-established classes to much more open-ended problems. Examples of the former are locating objects for robotic manipulation or recognizing targets in surveillance photos. An example of the latter is medical diagnosis, in which much of the important information comes from sources other than the image itself. Fuzzy logic, expert systems, and neural nets are all being applied to these tasks with some success. Extracting the correct information from the image to feed the decision-making process is more complicated than simple processing or measurement, because the best algorithms for a specific application must be determined as part of the logic process.

These tasks all require the computer-based image processing and analysis system, and by inference the image acquisition hardware, to duplicate some operations of the human visual system. In many cases they do so in ways that copy the algorithms we believe are used in vision, but in others quite different approaches are used. Although no computer-based image system can come close to duplicating the overall performance of human vision in its flexibility or speed, there are specific tasks at which the computer surpasses any human. It can detect many more imaging signals than just visible light; is unaffected by outside influences, fatigue or distraction; performs absolute measurements rather than relative comparisons; can transform images into other spaces that are beyond normal human experience (e.g., Fourier, Wavelet, or Hough space) to extract hidden data; and can apply statistical techniques to see through the chaotic and noisy data that may be present to identify underlying trends and similarities.

These attributes have made computer-based image analysis an important tool in many diverse fields. The image scale may vary from the microscopic to the astronomical, with substantially the same operations used. For the use of images at these scales, see especially Inoue (1986) and Sabins (1987). Familiarity with computer methods also makes most users better observers of images, able to interpret unusual imaging modes (such as cross sections) that are not encountered in normal scenes, and conscious of both the gestalt and details of images and their visual response to them.

2

Printing and Storage

Printing and storage

Creating hardcopy representations of images, for example, to use as illustrations in reports, is important to many users of image processing equipment. It is also usually important to store the images so that they can be retrieved later, for instance to compare with new ones or to transmit to another worker. Both of these activities are necessary because it is rarely possible to reduce an image to a compact verbal description or a series of measurements that will communicate to someone else what we see or believe to be important in the image. In fact, it is often difficult to draw someone else's attention to the particular details or general structure that may be present in an image that we may feel are the significant characteristics present, based on our examination of that image and many more. Faced with the inability to find descriptive words or numbers, we resort to passing a representation of the image on, perhaps with some annotation. Arlo Guthrie describes this procedure in his song, "Alice's Restaurant," as "twenty-seven 8 by 10 color glossy pictures with circles and arrows and a paragraph on the back of each one."

Printing

This book is printed in color, using high-end printing technology not normally available to a single image processing user. But many everyday jobs can be handled quite well using quite inexpensive machines; the quality, speed, and cost of both monochrome and color printers are improving rapidly. A typical monochrome (black on white) laser printer costs about a thousand dollars and has become a common accessory to desktop computer systems. These printers are designed primarily to print text, and simple graphics such as line drawings. Most can, however, be used to print images as well. We have come a very long way since computer graphics consisted of printing Christmas posters using Xs and Os on a teletype to represent different grey levels (**Figure 1**). In this chapter, we will examine the technology for printing images that can be used in desktop computer-based image processing systems.

For this purpose, it does not matter whether or not the printers use a high level page description language such as PostScript®, which is used to produce smooth characters and lines at the maximum printer resolution, so long as they allow the computer to transmit to the printer an array of individual pixel brightness values. Most printers that can create any graphics output in addition to

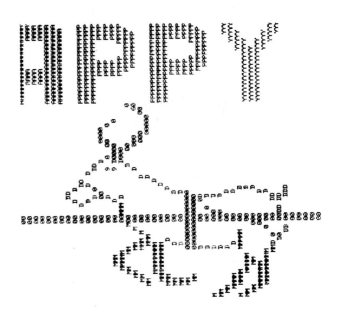

Figure 1. Portion of a 1960s-era teletype printout of a Christmas calendar poster.

simply printing text can be controlled in this way. This means that "daisy wheel" or other formed-character printers (now virtually obsolete) are not useful for imaging. That is how the Snoopy posters were made, by creatively arranging to overprint groups of characters to produce different levels of darkness. But dot-matrix printers using inked ribbons, ink jet printers, thermal printers, and other devices that form their output as an array of dots on paper *can* be used to print images. The quality of the result is primarily a function of the size and spacing of the dots.

A basic level of confusion that often arises in interpreting the specifications of a printer in terms of image quality has to do with "dots per inch" (dpi) and "lines per inch" (lpi) (sometimes also called pixels per inch for even more confusion). For any of the printers mentioned previously, but particularly for laser printers, the specification of dpi resolution is the number of tiny black dots (or whatever color ink is used) that the printer can deposit on paper. Usually, it is the same in both the line (horizontal) and page (vertical) directions on the paper, although some printers have different dpi resolution in the two directions. Normally, the dots are used to form characters and lines. A low number of dpi will cause the characters to look rough and the lines to appear stair-stepped or "aliased." Resolution of 300 to 600 dpi or more for laser printers is now very common. It is capable of producing quite acceptable output for text and line drawings used in reports and correspondence.

However, the dots placed on the paper by these printers are black, and do not have an adjustable grey scale needed to print images. To create a grey scale for images, it is necessary to use groups of these dots, a technique generally known as halftoning. It is commonly used in newspapers, magazines, and books (including this one), and as we will see can be used for color as well as monochrome images. The differences in halftone quality between (for instance) a newspaper and a book lie fundamentally in the number of dots per inch that can be placed on the paper and the way they are organized to produce a grey scale (or color) result.

The basis of halftoning lies in the grouping of the individual black dots produced by the printer. A group of (for instance) 16 dots in a 4 × 4 array may be called a halftone cell. Within the cell, some or all of the dots may actually be printed. Where no dot is printed, the white paper shows through. If the cell is reasonably small, the observer will not see the individual dots but will instead

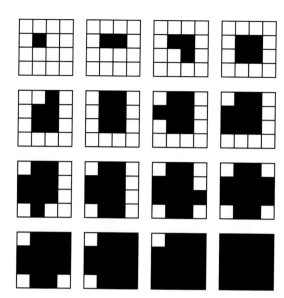

Figure 2. Halftone grey scale produced with a 4 × 4 dot cell. Printing dots in all, some or none of the locations generates 17 different grey values.

Figure 3. Representation of a grey scale image by halftoning.

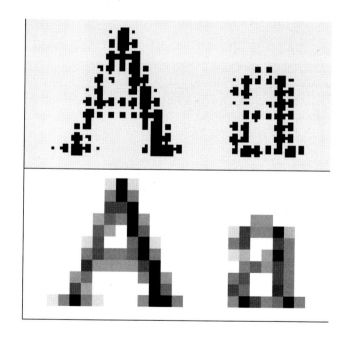

visually average the amount of dark ink and light paper, to form a grey scale. In this example, shown in **Figure 2**, 17 possible levels of grey are available, ranging from solid black (all dots printed) to solid white (no dots printed).

In a 300 dpi printer, the individual black dots can be placed on the paper with a spacing of 1/300th of an inch in each direction. Grouping these into 4 × 4 halftone cells would produce 300 ÷ 4 = 75 cells per inch. This is close to the resolution of pixels on a typical video display used with an image-processing computer. If each pixel corresponds to a halftone cell, then an image can be printed with about the same dimension as it appears on the screen. Each halftone cell uses one of its 17 possible grey levels to represent the grey scale of the pixel. **Figure 3** illustrates how these printed cells represent the grey levels in typical anti-aliased text.

Of course, because an original image might typically have 256 grey levels, this appears to be a rather poor representation of the brightness information; however, that is not the only nor even the most serious limitation. Instant prints from Polaroid® film show only about the same number of distinct grey levels (the film is quite a bit better than the print) and are considered quite useful for many scientific as well as casual purposes (for instance, the recording of scanning electron microscope images).

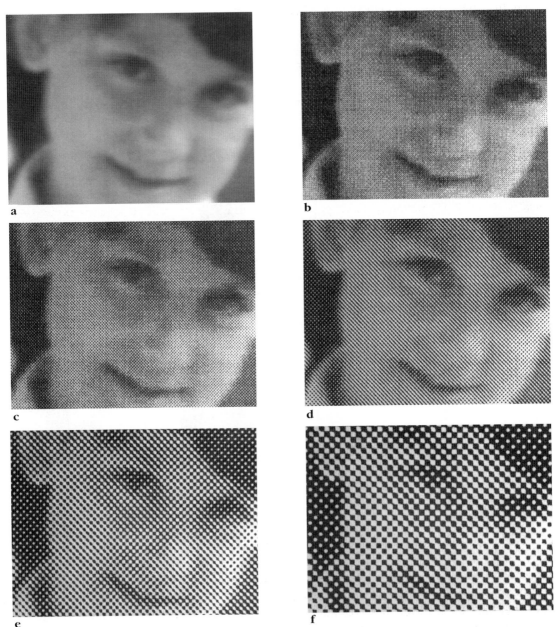

Figure 4. Printed halftone images of the same image using a 300-dpi Postscript laser printer: (a) original image; (b) 100 lines per inch; (c) 75 lines per inch; (d) 50 lines per inch; (e) 32 lines per inch; (f) 25 lines per inch. Increasing the number of halftone cells improves the lateral resolution at the expense of the number of grey levels that can be shown.

One problem with the halftoning method illustrated in **Figure 4** is that the dots and cells are large enough to be visually distinguished by the observer. In a magazine or book, the size of the cells is smaller. The cell size is usually described as a halftone screen or grid: the spacing of the screen in number of lines per inch corresponds to twice the number of cells per inch discussed above. A screen with well over 100 lines per inch (often 115 or 133 lines per inch) is used to produce high quality printed illustrations. Even in a newspaper illustration, a screen of at least 85 lines per inch is typically used. **Figure 4** shows several examples of halftone output from a typical laser printer, in which the number of halftone cells is varied to trade off grey scale versus lateral resolution. The output from the current generation of desktop laser printers is adequate for some reports, but not for publication.

Not only are more lines per inch of resolution desired to preserve the sharpness of features in the image, at the same time more grey levels must be represented by these more finely spaced cells. That means that the printer (or imagesetter, as these higher-quality devices are generally called) must be capable of placing a much larger number of very much smaller dots. A grey scale of 65 levels can be formed with an 8×8 array of dots in a cell. With a 125-line screen, this would correspond to $8 \times 125 = 1000$ dpi. This is about the starting point for typeset quality used to print images for commercial purposes. Color (introduced below) imposes additional restrictions that require even higher resolution (smaller dots).

An additional difficulty with the halftoning method outlined above arises from the dots themselves. Each of the various printing methods produces dots in a different way. Dot-matrix printers use small pins to press an inked ribbon against the paper. Ink-jet printers produce tiny ink droplets. Some of these printers deposit the ink in a liquid form that penetrates into the paper making slightly fuzzy dots, while in others the ink has solidified and adheres to the paper without penetration. The better grades of paper have surface coatings that prevent the ink from spreading or penetrating. Thermal printers use a pin to pass an electrical current through the coating on a paper. One kind of paper is coated with a white oxide of zinc that is reduced by the current to deposit a dark spot of metal at the location; other thermal papers are based on the chemistry of silver. Laser printers work essentially like a xerographic copier. The light from the laser (or in some versions from a photodiode) falls on a selenium-coated drum and by the photoelectric effect produces a localized electrostatic charge. This in turn picks up carbon particles (the toner or "ink"), which are then transferred to the paper and subsequently heated to remain permanently.

Dots on paper

All of these technologies are limited by the ability to make a small, dark spot on the paper. The size of the carbon particles used as the toner in copier or laser printer cartridges limits the spatial resolution, and special finely ground toner is needed for resolutions of 600 dpi and higher values. The limitation in making higher resolution laser printers is not primarily in the additional memory needed in the printer, nor by the need to focus the light to a smaller spot on the drum, but in the toner particle size. Some systems disperse the toner using liquid carriers to improve the control of toner placement.

Similar restrictions limit the other printing methods. The difficulty of depositing a small but dark ink spot by the impact of a pin onto a ribbon, or the fuzziness of the dot written by thermal printing, have prevented those techniques from advancing to higher resolutions. Ink-jet printers can generate small drops and hence deposit small dots, but the inks tend to spread on the paper. Indeed, the roughness of the paper surface, and the need for special coatings to prevent the inks from soaking into the paper fibers or spreading across the surface or the toner particles from falling off, become critical issues. It is not enough to purchase a high quality printer; the use of special paper

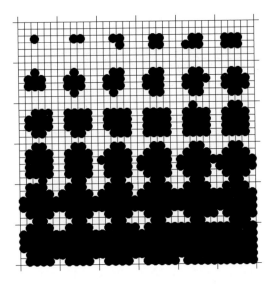

Figure 5. *A 6 × 6 dot halftone that can produce 37 grey levels. The use of approximately round dots large enough to touch diagonally causes them to overlap and produce darker cells than ideal.*

with a proper surface finish for the particular printer is needed to achieve the quality of image printing that the printer technology makes available (Lee and Winslow, 1993).

Because the dots produced by printers are generally imperfect and rough-edged, it is hard to control them so that the grey scale produced by the array of dots within the cell is uniform. Most dots are larger than their spacing so that solid black areas can be printed. This is good for printing text characters, which are intended to be solid black, although it means that the dots overlap some of the white areas in the cell, which darkens the halftone grey scale. **Figure 5** shows this for the case of a 6 × 6 dot halftone cell. At the dark end of the scale, adjacent grey levels may be indistinguishable, while at the light end the difference between the first few levels may be very great.

For the case of a 4 × 4 dot cell illustrated above using a 300 dpi printer, 17 nominal grey levels, and 75 cells per inch, the darkening or "gain" of the grey scale will produce images of marginal quality. If the printer resolution is much higher so that finer halftone cells with more steps can be created, it is possible to correct for this tendency to darken the images by constructing a mapping that translates the pixel grey value to a printed grey value that compensates for this effect. These "gamma" curves are applied within the software so that more-or-less equal steps of brightness can be printed on the page.

However, the human eye does not respond linearly to grey scale, but logarithmically. This means that to produce a printed image in which the visual impression of brightness varies linearly with pixel value, a further adjustment of the gamma curve is needed (as shown in **Figure 6**) to compress the dark values even more and expand the light ones. Because of these limitations, a printing scale with 65 grey values defined by an 8 × 8 dot halftone cell may be able to show only about half that many shades in the actual printed image.

Halftone grids in a typesetter or imagesetter are not limited by the size or perfection of the dots. Instead of coarse toner particles or contact with an inked ribbon, typesetters use light to expose a photographic emulsion, which is then developed to produce either a film or a print. The size of the silver grains in the film emulsion is far smaller than the effective dot size and the dots can be controlled in both size and shape with great precision. There is still a need for a gamma curve to compensate for the nonlinear response of human vision, however.

If the variation of brightness across an image is gradual and the total number of grey levels is small, it is possible to generate a visual effect known as banding or posterization. This is illustrated

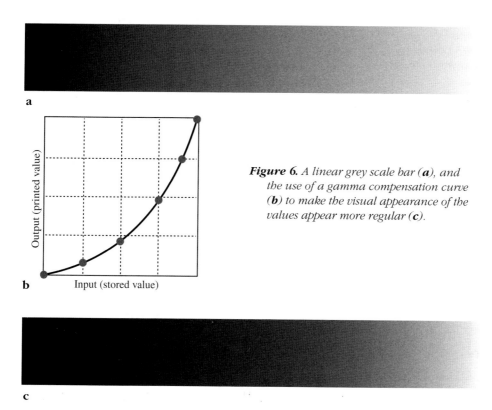

a

b

Figure 6. A linear grey scale bar (**a**), and
the use of a gamma compensation curve
(**b**) to make the visual appearance of the
values appear more regular (**c**).

c

in **Figure 7**. The step from one brightness level to the next appears as a contour line in the printed image and is visually recognized as a feature in the picture, when in fact it is purely an artefact of the printing process. Banding can be avoided by increasing the number of grey levels used, or in some cases by modifying the way in which the dots within the halftone cell are used to generate the grey scale. Generally, the rule for the maximum number of grey shades available is 1 + $(dpi/lpi)^2$, where dpi is the printer resolution in dots per inch (e.g., 300 or 600 for a typical laser printer) and lpi is the lines per inch of the halftone screen (e.g., 75 lines per inch for the example discussed above). This assumes that all of the grey levels can actually be used, subject to the darkening ("dot gain") and gamma effects mentioned above.

In the examples shown in **Figures 2** and **3**, an arrangement of dots was used that produced more-or-less round regions of black within a white frame. With a larger dot array in each cell, an even more regular circular pattern can be constructed. The round dot pattern is one of the more

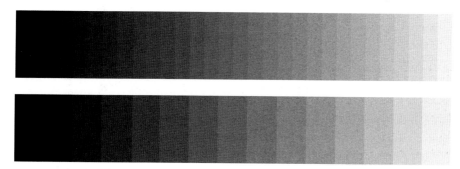

Figure 7. A grey scale bar showing banding when printed with only 32 or 16 grey steps.

Figure 8. Printouts of a portion of an image of Saturn (shown in entirety in Figure 20) using different dot patterns within the same size halftone cells:
(a) round;
(b) horizontal line;
(c) diagonal line;
(d) plus;
(e) cross.

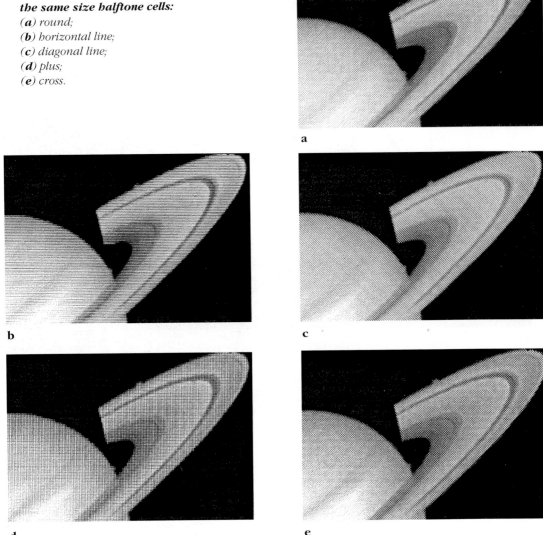

a

b

c

d

e

commonly used arrangements; however, many others are possible, including lines and crosses (**Figure 8**). Each of these produces some visual artefacts that may be useful for artistic effects but generally interfere with viewing the actual image contents. For instance, the diamond pattern used by most Postscript printers as an approximation to round dots causes dot densities less than 50% black to appear quite different from ones that are 50% or more black. The reason for this is that at the 50% point the dots touch from one cell to the next so that the eye perceives a sudden transition from dark dots on a white background to the reverse, even if the individual dots are not visually evident. Of course, all such artefacts degrade the representation of the original grey scale image.

If the dots within each halftone cell are randomly distributed, fewer visual artefacts are likely. However, this requires additional computer processing within the printer and is not a commonly available feature. Other printers use programs that analyze the neighbor cells (pixels). If cells on one side are dark and on the other side are light, the program may use a pattern of dots that is shifted toward the dark neighbors to produce a smoother edge. This works quite well for generating smooth boundaries for printed text characters and minimizing jagged edges on lines, but it is not clear that it provides any consistent benefit for grey scale image printing.

Printers of modest dpi resolution cannot produce halftone cells that are small and still represent many grey levels, and visually distracting patterns may appear in images if regular patterns of dots are used within the cells. Hence, another approach used with these printers is to use "dithering" to represent the image. In a simple random dither, each possible position where the printer can place a black dot corresponds to a point in the image whose grey scale value is examined. If the point is very dark, there

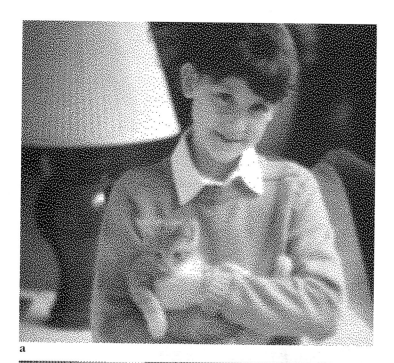

a

Figure 9. Two different dither patterns for the "girl" image (shown in Chapter 1, Figure 25):
(a) random dots;
(b) patterned dots.

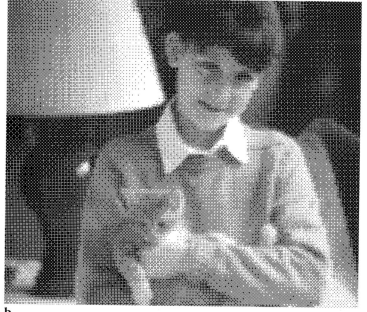

b

is a high probability that the dot should be printed (and vice versa). A random number is generated and compared to the grey scale; if the number is below the grey scale value for that point (both properly scaled), then the dot is printed on the page.

As shown in **Figure 9**, even coarse dithering can produce a viewable representation of an image. Many different types of dithering patterns are used, some of them random or pseudo-random and others with various patterned arrangements of the dots. Usually, the particular dither pattern used is determined either by the printer itself or the interface software provided for it. There is a rich literature on the design of dither patterns, but the user of the image analysis system may not have much control or choice of them. Dithered images are generally good at showing gradually varying brightness gradients, since human vision responds to an average dot density or spacing. But sharp edges will be blurred, broken up, or displaced because there is no continuous line or boundary printed, and it is difficult to compare the brightness of regions within the image. Dithered printing is usually considered to be a "low-end" method for producing crude hard copy and not suitable for use in reports or publications.

Despite the limitations discussed previously, monochrome image printing using a halftoning method and a printer with 300–600 dpi capability is adequate for many kinds of image processing applications and the resulting images are suitable in quality for reports. For higher quality work, photographic recording can be used. This process may seem like a step backward, especially when the image may have started out on film in the first place before it was digitized into the computer. But because facilities for handling photographic images, duplicating them, and making halftone screens photographically for printing are well developed, fully understood, and comparatively inexpensive, this is often the most effective solution. Forcing a "high-tech" solution in which images are directly merged into a report within the computer may not be worthwhile in terms of time or cost if only a small number of copies are needed. Mounting photographs on a few pages or inserting them as separate pages is still a quite suitable presentation method. No doubt as printing technology continues to advance, the balance will continue to shift toward direct printing from the computer.

Color printing

Printing color images is much more complicated and difficult. The usual method, which you can see by looking at the color images in this book with a magnifier, is to create halftones for each of several different color inks and superimpose them to produce the printed color image. Many complexities are involved in this process. The following section discusses the complexities that are important for most networked or desktop color printers.

Displaying a color image on a computer monitor or television set is accomplished by illuminating red, green, and blue phosphors with the electron beam in the cathode ray tube (CRT). There are exceptions, of course, the most important being the flat-panel liquid crystal (LCD) displays used for projectors and notebook computers. There are also large-screen displays (such as used at sporting events) that consist of arrays of discrete lights. Each of these methods generate the colors in different ways, but it is still the visual mixing together of red, green, and blue that produces the full range of colors that can be shown.

This range is called the "gamut" of the device (Stone et al., 1988). In a display that emits red, green, and blue light (RGB), it is possible to generate a large fraction of the total range of colors that the human eye can see. **Figure 10** shows the CIE color diagram that was introduced in Chapter 1, adding the typical color gamut for an RGB display and an ink-jet color printer superimposed on the diagram. One of the features of the CIE diagram is that colors add together along straight lines, so the three phosphor colors define the corners of a triangle that enclose all of the possible

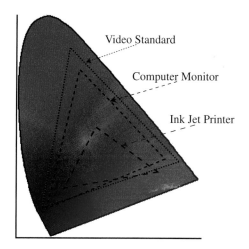

Figure 10. The CIE color diagram discussed in Chapter 1 with gamuts shown for broadcast television, a typical computer monitor, and a typical ink-jet printer.

Figure 11. Comparison of RGB (additive) and CMY (subtractive) color spaces. The additive color space adds red, green, and blue emissive colors to a black background, while subtractive color space removes cyan, magenta, and yellow colors from a white background.

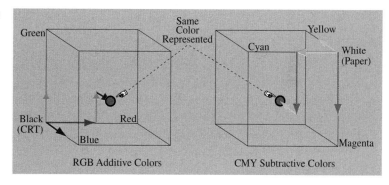

color combinations. The missing colors that cannot be generated using these particular phosphors include points near the outside of the diagram, which are the most saturated colors.

The concept of the color gamut applies equally well to other color display and recording devices. However, the gamut is not always as simple in shape as the triangle shown in the figure. For one thing, printing uses subtractive rather than additive color. In terms of the color cube (also introduced in Chapter 1 and shown in **Figure 11**) the blank paper starts off as white and the addition of cyan, magenta, and yellow inks removes the complementary colors (red, green, and blue,

Figure 12. Combinations of RGB additive colors on a black background, and CMY subtractive colors on a white background.

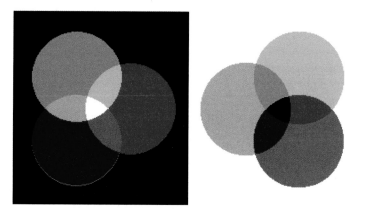

respectively) from the reflected light to produce the possible range of colors. It is common to call these colors CMY to distinguish them from the additive RGB colors.

The theory of subtractive printing, summarized in **Figure 12**, suggests that the mixture of all three colors will produce black (just as with additive RGB color, the summation of all three colors produces white); however, actual printing with CMY inks generally cannot produce a very good black, but instead gives a muddy greyish brown because of impurities in the inks, reflection of light from the surface of the ink (so that it does not pass through all of the ink layers to be absorbed), and difficulty in getting complete coverage of the white paper.

The most common solution is to add a separate, black ink to the printing process. This reduces the need for large amounts of the colored inks, reduces the thickness of ink buildup on the page, and reduces cost. But from the standpoint of image quality, the most important factor is that it allows dark colors to be printed without appearing muddy. The four-color, cyan-magenta-yellow-black system (CMYK) uses four halftone screens, one for each ink, but although converting from RGB colors (or CIE, HSI, or any other equivalent color space coordinate system) to CMY (often called process color) is straightforward, converting to CMYK is not. Rules to calculate how much black to put into various color representations depend on visual response to colors, the kind of paper to be printed, the illumination the print will be viewed with, and even the contents of the images.

Algorithms for converting from CMY to CMYK involve specifying levels of undercolor removal (UCR) and grey component replacement (GCR) which are essentially arbitrary, are little documented, and vary considerably from one software program to another (Agfa, 1992). The general approach is to use the value of whichever of the three components (CMY) is darkest to determine an amount of black to be added. For instance, for a color containing 80% cyan, 50% magenta, and 30% yellow, the 30% value would be taken as an index into a built-in calibration curve or lookup table. This might indicate that a 15% value for the black ink should be chosen for grey component replacement. Then, the amount of the principal color (in this example cyan), or, according to some algorithms, the amounts of all of the colors, would be reduced (grey component replacement). It is difficult to design algorithms for these substitutions that do not cause color shifts. Also, the substitutions do not work equally well for printing with different combinations of ink, paper finish, etc.

Color prints are generally not as vivid or saturated as the image appears on the CRT. In addition, the colors depend critically on the paper finish and viewing conditions. Changing the room light will slightly alter the visual appearance of colors on an RGB monitor, but because the monitor is generating its own illumination this is a secondary effect. Since a print is viewed by reflected light, changing the amount of light or the color temperature of room light with a print can completely alter the appearance of the image. The color temperature (a handy way of describing the spectrum of intensity vs. color) of incandescent bulbs, fluorescent bulbs, direct sunlight, or open sky are all quite different.

Human vision can be tricked by combinations of illumination and shadow, inks or other colored coatings, surface finish (smooth, or textured in various ways), and even the presence of other adjacent colors in the field of view to change the way we judge colors in an image. These other colors may even lie outside the image itself; consider how a colored mat can change the appearance of an art print. When "true" color prints of an image are required, it is necessary to perform extensive calibrations of a specific printer and monitor so that acceptable fidelity is obtained. This is of great concern in advertising; if you purchase clothing from a mail order catalog, you expect the colors of the cloth to match the printed photograph, which is no easy task. The process usually works by adjusting the monitor output (with lookup tables in the display hardware) so that the appearance of colors there is tailored to match the ability of a specific printer/paper/ink combination to reproduce them.

For most (but certainly not all) applications of image processing, the purpose of printing in color is to distinguish the variously colored regions present; some inaccuracy in the fidelity of the colors is acceptable. If exact color matching is not necessary in a particular application then the task becomes much easier, although you will still need to be concerned about the color gamut of the printer, the consistency of colors (to allow comparison of different images or regions), and of course the resolution of the printer. The color gamut is important because colors of increasing saturation in the original image, which can be distinguished on the video display, may become similar in the print image if the saturation exceeds the range of the printer.

Producing CMYK halftones (so-called color separations) and superimposing them to produce color prints sounds simple enough, but it harbors many problems that commercial printers must deal with routinely. One is how to superimpose the halftone screens so that they do not produce visual

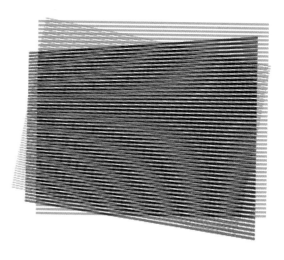

Figure 13. *Moiré pattern produced by overlaying arrays of color dots.*

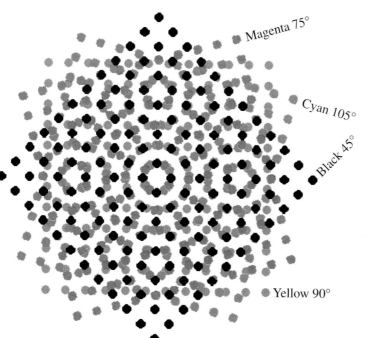

Figure 14. *Ideal screen angles for CMYK color printing place the halftone screens at angles of 45° (black), 75° (magenta), 90° (yellow), and 105° (cyan).*

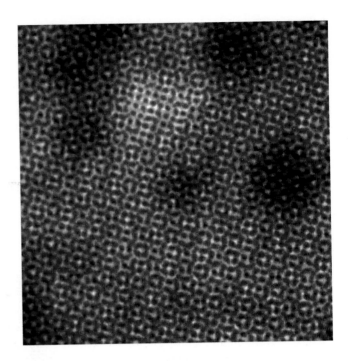

Figure 15. *Example of color halftone image printed in an earlier edition of this textbook.*

moiré patterns in the image. **Figure 13** shows an example of a moiré effect produced by different color patterns. The lines that appear are an artefact of the spacing and alignment of the individual patterns. Traditional offset printing defines "ideal" screen angles for the four CMYK screens as 45, 70, 90 and 105° respectively, as shown in **Figure 14**. This aligns the colored dots to form small rosettes that together make up the color. **Figure 15** shows an example; note that the dots vary in size to control the amount of each color, and that some of the halftone spots may be partly superimposed on each other. Because some inks are partially transparent, this can produce various color biases depending on the order of printing.

In most printing, the colors are not intended to be superimposed on each other, but printed adjacent to each other, and to allow some white paper to show. Most color printing methods suffer from the fact that as more color is added, the white paper is covered and the appearance becomes darker. This is another reason that high-resolution halftone screens and very small printing dots must be used. Generally, when four halftone grids or color separations are used, the dpi of the printer must be doubled for each color to get an equivalent printing resolution to monochrome printing. In other words, each pixel now requires four interleaved halftone cells, one for each color. Because the dot size for each of the four colors is only one-fourth of the area, printing a solid expanse of one color is not possible, which further reduces the maximum saturation that can be achieved and hence the gamut of the printer.

Most desktop printers do not provide control over the screen angles, and many printers simply use a zero angle for all four screens due to the way the printing mechanism works (for instance, a typical color ink-jet printer). Some page description languages (e.g., PostScript Level 2) include provision for such control, but only high-end typesetters and imagesetters generally respond to those commands.

All of the problems present in printing monochrome or grey scale images, such as banding, posterization, limited numbers of intensity levels, and so forth, are also present in producing the color separations. In addition, color printing introduces the additional problems of screen angles and moiré patterns. Finally, alignment and registration of the colors must be considered, since in many printers they are printed one at a time and the paper must be handled in several passes. Some alternative printing methods exist that deposit multiple colors in a single pass, but these have their own problems of allowing inks to dry without mixing.

The printing and registration of colors presents one additional problem in some cases. Consider a region of a uniform color that is a mixture of two or more of the primary printed colors and is adjacent to a region of a different color. At the boundary, the colors must change abruptly from one color to the other; however, the two-color screens are not aligned dot for dot, and along the boundary there will be cases in which one of the two left-side color dots may be present close to one of the two right-side color dots. This can give rise to false color lines along boundaries. In graphic arts, such artefacts are usually avoided by trapping to remove the colors at the boundaries in a particular order, or covering up the boundary with a black line. Obviously, such tricks are not available in printing real images where every pixel may be different.

Printing hardware

The discussion so far of converting the image to CMY or CMYK values and superimposing them as separate halftone screens on the printed page has ignored the physical ways that such color printing is performed (Kang, 1997, 1999). Few computer users will have ready access to imagesetters and offset printing presses that have high enough resolution to produce such high quality results. There is a considerable variation in the quality, cost, and performance of different types of desktop printers. Some of the more common currently available methods include ink jet, thermal wax, dye sublimation, and color laser printers. This section will offer some comparison of these technologies, recognizing that continuous progress in print quality is being made as many vendors compete for their slice of a rapidly growing market. In all of these comparisons it is important to keep cost in mind. Many of the printers themselves have dropped significantly in price, but the cost of consumables — paper, ink, etc. — keep the overall cost of each copy quite high for most of these devices.

To assist in comparing the various printer types, **Figure 16** shows a portion of an image printed using several of the technologies discussed in the following section.

Figure 16. Magnified (30x) views of the same image printed using different devices:
(a) photograph;
(b) Xerox copy;
(c) black and white laser printer;
(d) dye-sublimation printer;
(e) phase change solid ink printer;
(f) color laser printer;
(g) ink jet printer in low-resolution mode;
(h) ink jet printer in high-resolution mode;
(i) ink jet printer using uncoated bond paper (images from M. Jurgens, Queens University).

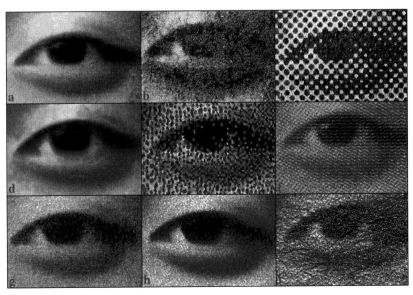

Color laser printers are the most economical for many applications, because they use plain paper and have relatively high speeds. The high initial cost of the printer is offset by very low cost per copy. They work by separating the image into CMY or CMYK colors and using each to control the illumination of a separate charged drum that picks up the corresponding color toner and deposits it on the paper. One major problem with these printers is the difficulty of keeping everything in alignment, so that the paper does not shrink or shift as it goes from one drum through a heater to bake the toner and on to the next drum. The use of a relatively thick paper with a smooth finish helps. In addition, the order in which the toners must be applied is critical, because with most models presently available the dots are not really laid down as a set of halftone screens at different angles (as discussed previously). Instead, they tend to overlay each other, which makes it difficult to achieve good color saturation or accurate color blending.

Figure 17 shows an enlarged example of a color laser printer output. Note that the saturated colors such as red are formed by combining two toner colors (red = blue + magenta) and give good coverage of the white paper, but more subtle colors are not so clear and may appear muddy. In fact, a plot of the gamut (maximum saturation limits for colors) of this type of printer is not too meaningful because the most saturated colors are rather well defined but the less saturated ones are not, and are more difficult to distinguish from each other. Color laser prints are generally a marginal choice for image reproduction, although they may be satisfactory for reports, or for computer graphics consisting primarily of saturated colors.

Dye-sublimation (or dye-diffusion) printers continue to represent the high end of image quality available in desktop printers. They require special coated paper (or transparency material). The inks or dyes are transferred one at a time from a master color sheet or ribbon to the paper, with a typical resolution of about 300 dpi. A portion of the color ribbon as large as the paper is consumed in making each print, even if only a small amount of the color is needed.

The low resolution value of 300 dpi, as compared with 1200+ dpi for most of the other types of color printers described here, does not indicate the actual print quality because the print is formed

Figure 17. *Enlarged view of color laser printer output, with areas of fully saturated and unsaturated colors.*

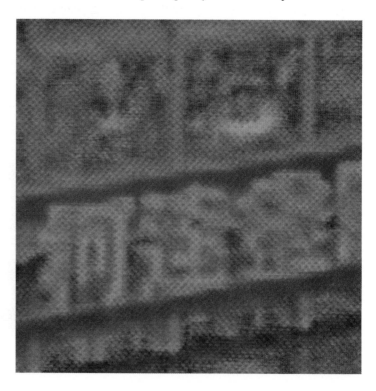

in a different way. Rather than assembling tiny printer dots to build up the color, these printers can control the amount of each color more directly. The amount of dye that is transferred from the ribbon to each pixel on the hardcopy is controlled by heating the print head to sublime or vaporize varying amounts of dye. A control to one part in 256 is typical, although the use of a corrective gamma function for each color to balance the colors so that the print appears similar to the screen image (so-called "color-matching") may reduce the effective dynamic range for each color to about 1 part in 100. Still, that means that about 1 million (100^3) different color combinations can be deposited at each point in the recorded image.

Dye-sublimation printers do not use a halftone or dither pattern. The dyes diffuse into the polyester coating on the paper and blend to produce continuous color scales. Each of the 300 printed regions per inch on the paper contains a uniform proportioned blend of the three or four dye colors. The lack of any halftone or dither pattern and the blending and spreading of the color dyes within the coating (instead of lying on the surface as inks do) produces an image that is very smooth and pleasing in its appearance. Magnification (**Figure 16d**) reveals the continuous tone and the just-visible pixelation pattern.

It is sometimes claimed that these printers are "near photographic" in output quality, but in several important respects that is not true. The saturation is less than a good photographic print, so that the color gamut is lower, and the 300 dpi resolution compounded by the spreading of the dye in the coating, produces much poorer sharpness than a photographic print (which can easily resolve several thousand points per inch). This spreading is somewhat worse along the direction of paper movement than across it, which can cause some distortion in images or make some edges less sharp than others. On the dye-sublimation print, large areas of uniform or gradually varying color will appear quite smooth because there is no dither or halftone to break them up, but edges and lines will appear fuzzy.

In addition to these technical limitations, the relatively high cost of dye-sublimation printers and of their materials has limited their use as dedicated printers for individual imaging systems. At the same time, their rather slow speed (because each print requires three or four separate passes with a different color ribbon or a ribbon with alternating color panels) has made them of limited use on networks or for making multiple copies. Still, they have been the preferred choice for making direct, hardcopy printouts of images. They are even finding use in commercial outlets, where consumers can insert their slides or color negatives into a scanner, select the image and mask it if desired, and then directly print out a hard copy to take home. The glossy finish of the coated paper probably causes many customers to think they have a traditional photographic print, although the effects of temperature, ozone, and humidity on useful life are much worse.

Some ***dry ink*** printers (also called phase change printers since the ink is melted and transferred to the paper) and thermal-wax printers are used for printing images, although they are best suited to computer graphics because of their bright colors and glossy results. They work well on overhead transparencies, which are fine for producing business graphics presentations, but are not usually an acceptable medium for image-processing output. The print head in a thermal-wax printer contains heating elements that melt the wax and transfer the color to the paper. This process is repeated for each color, which may cause alignment problems. In many cases, the dots are too large and the resulting number of shades for each color too small, and the resolution too poor, to show details well in images. The image appears as flat, shiny plates of ink pressed onto but not into the paper surface (**Figure 16e**).

Ink-jet printers are certainly at this time the most widely used devices for producing hard copies of images. The printers are quite inexpensive (although the consumable supplies are not), and the resolution is quite high (many current models offer 1200–1440 dpi). Ink jet printers are by far the most sensitive to paper quality among all of the technologies discussed here. Quality prints

Figure 18. Wicking of ink on an uncoated paper.

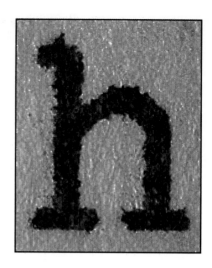

require a paper with both internal sizing and surface coatings to prevent the ink from wicking into the cellulose fibers (**Figure 18**), while promoting adhesion and providing a bright white background. Pigments such as $CaCO_3$ or TiO_2 also serve to whiten the paper. Surface coatings such as gelatin or starch are hydrophobic to prevent the ink from spreading, are smoother than the raw cellulose fibers, and may additionally be rolled (calendered) to provide an even more uniform surface. Inks must be carefully formulated with very tiny pigment particles (if these are used instead of dyes) to allow small droplets (the current state of the art is 4 picoliter drops for each tiny printer dot) to be uniformly and consistently transferred to the paper.

Longevity of the prints is strongly affected by exposure to ultraviolet light, humidity, temperature, ozone, acidity of the paper, etc. Some manufacturers now offer "archival" quality inks and papers, meaning that the paper has a high pH (usually due to added alkaline buffers to reduce acidity that causes discoloration or physical deterioration of the paper) and a high rag content (fibers other than cellulose), and the ink contains pigments that do not break down with exposure to UV radiation; however, it should not be expected that even these prints will survive well for long periods unless storage conditions are carefully controlled. Achieving acceptable lifetimes for computer-printed hardcopy continues to present challenges to equipment manufacturers.

Two types of ink are used in these printers, some containing pigment particles and others containing dyes. The inks containing pigment particles are less affected by paper variables (flatness, surface coatings, etc.) and suffer less environmental degradation by light, moisture, or ozone, or other airborne contaminants. Thus, they are often called "archival" inks, although the actual life of prints and the resistance to color shifts during storage still depend upon storage conditions. The pigment particles are not absorbed into the paper or its surface coatings, which makes them more sensitive to smearing or scratching. Dye-based inks, which are more common, dry quickly, and because they are more reflective than pigment-based inks (which produce color mainly by absorbing light) produce brighter colors and a broader range of colors.

In order to expand the gamut of the printers, and to improve the ability to render subtle shades such as skin tones, many ink jet printers now use more than the four CMYK inks. In a typical six-color system called CcMmYK, two less saturated cyan and magenta inks are available as well. Eight-color systems introduce less saturated yellow and black inks, and others may be used in addition. Algorithms for converting the stored RGB values for each pixel to appropriate blends of multiple inks are complex, proprietary, and highly ad hoc. Many ink-jet printers offer multiple quality levels. The faster settings also consume less ink, producing acceptable draft images with less saturated colors, while the slower settings are used for final copies.

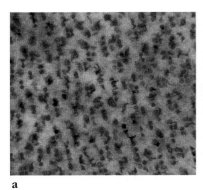
a

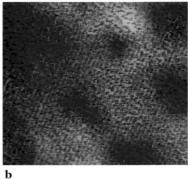
b

Figure 19. Ink-jet printer output (six-color CcMmYK inks): (**a**) light area with well-defined separate dots; (**b**) superposition of more colors produces greater saturation but covers more white paper for a darker result.

In light areas of printouts, the individual droplets can be seen (**Figure 19a**). Ideally these would all be perfectly round, identical size, well spaced color dots. In practice, they often deteriorate rapidly as printers age, are affected by temperature, and of course by the paper being used. When more color is present and more different ink colors are used, they superimpose on each other and cover the paper, producing a darker image (**Figure 19b**). As noted previously, this is the opposite behavior to the appearance of the image on the CRT display, where more color produces a brighter pixel.

As noted earlier, the gamut of a printer is usually described by an outline on a color wheel or CIE diagram of the maximum color saturations achievable, as shown again in **Figure 20**. The actual situation is much more complicated because saturation varies with brightness as mentioned above. By printing out swatches covering the entire three-dimensional color space, it is possible to construct a more complete representation of a printer's gamut. **Figure 21** shows an example, for an Epson six-color ink-jet printer, using the L·a·b representation of color space described previously. Printers with multiple inks can produce thousands of different hues, and modulate colorant density to produce high tonal resolution and subtle difference in color; however, notice that, as with all such gamut plots, certain colors cannot be represented on the hard copy.

Ink jet printers can also be equipped with a selection of grey inks, which when controlled by appropriate software can do an extremely good job of printing grey scale images. By selecting

Figure 20. *Color wheel comparing typical gamuts for ink-jet and dye sublimation printers.*

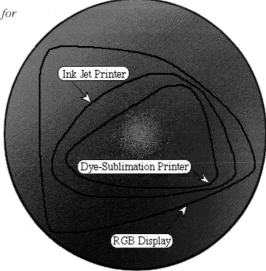

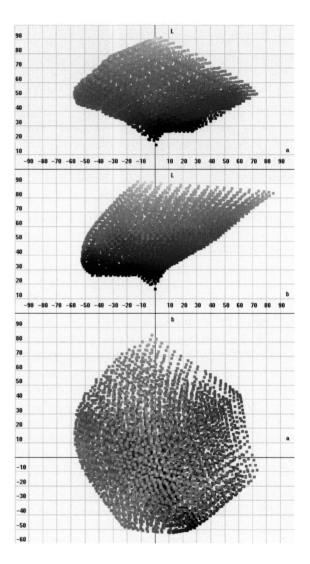

Figure 21. *Three-dimensional gamut for a six-color CcMmYK ink jet printer, displayed as cross sections through L·a·b color space (From Rezanaka, I. and Eschbach, R., Eds. (1996).* Recent Progress in Ink-Jet Technologies. *Soc. Imaging Science and Tech., Springfield, VA. With permission.)*

different ink densities as well as controlling the placement of tiny drops, a grey scale can be constructed that is very similar to photographic prints, and with a very acceptable spatial resolution. Selection of paper with good surface finish is still important.

Film recorders

In many cases, especially for color images, printing directly from the computer to paper is expensive and the quality limited. But the image looks good on the computer screen and it is tempting just to photograph it from there to create slides or prints using conventional film methods. Certainly, this is convenient. I have hundreds of slides that I once used in lectures (before the advent of affordable compact projectors that connected directly to my laptop computer allowed for more convenient and higher quality presentations) that were produced in exactly this way. I kept a 35-mm camera loaded with slide film on a tripod near my desk. When there was something on the screen that might be useful as a slide, I just moved the camera into position and, with a permanent exposure setting of f8 at 1/2 second (for ASA 100 slide film), snapped the picture. You do need to make sure that there are no reflections of windows or room lights on the monitor. When the roll was finished, I sent it off and got back a box of quite useful slides. I have done this enough times to know that there is no need even to bracket the exposures. The exposure setting of f8 is about optimal for lens sharpness and gives plenty of depth of field for the slight curvature of the computer monitor, while 1/2 second is long enough to capture enough full raster scans so that no visible line shows where the scan was when the shutter opened or closed.

Although these pictures are fine for lecture slides, they are not useful for many other purposes. It is always obvious that they are photographs of the computer screen and not the actual images that have been captured or processed. This is due partly to the fact that they usually include the menu bars, cursor, and other open windows on the screen. It is possible to eliminate those, and many image-processing programs have a "photo mode" that displays just the image with the rest of the screen dark.

Unfortunately, other clues reveal how such an image is recorded. It is difficult to align the camera so that it is exactly perpendicular to the center of the screen. This misalignment produces a distortion of the image. In addition, the curvature of the screen causes a pincushion distortion of the image that is hard to overcome, and even with flat screen displays there tends to be vignetting. Special cameras intended for recording images from computer monitors have hoods to shield against stray light and align the camera lens, and may incorporate corrective optics to correct some of the distortions and minimize these problems. Still, other more serious difficulties remain.

Most color displays use an array of red, green, and blue phosphors arranged as triads of round dots. The electron beams are focused onto the phosphors and further restricted by an aperture screen (shadow mask) that prevents the electrons from straying from one dot to another. The other approach to monitor design, used in the Sony Trinitron, has a single electron gun, no shadow mask and the color phosphor arranged in vertical stripes. This design provides brighter images, since more of the screen is covered with phosphor and there is no shadow mask. On the other hand, the colors are less pure and lines or edges less sharp depending on their orientation. Varying the intensity of the electron beam controls the relative brightness of the phosphors and the resulting color that is perceived by the human observer, who blends the individual dots together. Modern computer displays have color triads with a spacing of about 0.25 mm. Human vision does not resolve these at normal viewing distances, so the colors are visually blended.

The image is made up of a regular pattern of color dots that the film records, perhaps with some systematic distortion due to the screen curvature and camera position. This pattern may be visible when a slide is projected onto a large screen. There is a temptation to use these films to prepare prints for publication, which reveals their major flaw. When the prints are subsequently converted to halftones, the array of dots photographed from the screen will interact with the screen of the halftone to produce a moiré pattern that can be quite objectionable.

Film has high resolution, good color saturation and dynamic range, and inexpensive processing, which make it an excellent recording medium. But photographing a color monitor is not the right way to record the image. Dedicated film recorders solve the problems mentioned above by using a monochrome CRT with a continuous phosphor and a flat face. The continuous phosphor gives a very high resolution with no structure to cause moiré patterns, while the flat face eliminates distortions. With only a single electron beam, sharp focus and uniform intensity can be maintained from center to edges much better than with video displays; the fixed optics also provide sharp focus across the image with no vignetting or distortion.

A motorized filter wheel containing red, green, and blue filters is placed between the CRT and the camera. Software much like that used to drive a printer is used to separate the image into red, green, and blue components and these are displayed one at a time on the CRT with the appropriate filter in place. The much higher display resolution allows entire images to be displayed with full pixel resolution, which is not usually possible on the computer monitor (unless you have a very large one). The filter densities are adjusted to balance the film sensitivity. All three color components are recorded on the same frame of the film. With most recorders, the entire process is automatic, including film transport and compensation for different film speeds and sensitivities (for instance, slide or print film).

The only drawbacks are the exposure time of several seconds and the delay until the film is developed, and of course the cost of the entire unit. The cost varies as a function of resolution (from 2000 dots horizontally up to as much as 16,000 dots), and the flexibility to handle different sizes and types of film. High-end recorders are used to expose movie film frame by frame to produce movies containing "virtual reality" and rendered computer images (e.g., *Toy Story*), or to restore old classics by removing dirt and making color corrections (e.g., *Snow White*). Recorders that are price-competitive with color printers can be used for routine production of 35-mm slides. Nevertheless, the use of such recorders has not become widespread, and there is still a general preference for printing images directly onto paper.

File storage

When working on a computer-based, image-analysis system, images can be saved as disk files. There seems to be no reason to consider these files as being any different from other disk files, which may contain text, drawings, or programs. In one sense this is true: files contain a collection of bytes that can represent any of those things as well as images. But from a practical point of view, there are several reasons for treating image files as distinct, because they may require somewhat different storage considerations:

1. Image files are usually large. In terms of computer storage, the old adage that a picture is worth one thousand words is clearly a vast understatement. A single video frame (typically 640 × 480 pixels) in monochrome occupies about 300 kilobytes (KB), while one in full color requires about 1 megabyte (MB). A series of images forming a time sequence, or a three-dimensional array of voxel data (which can be considered as a series of planes) can be far larger. A 500 × 500 × 500 voxel tomographic reconstruction requires 125 MB, or twice that if the density values for the voxels have a dynamic range that exceeds 256 levels. This means that the storage capacity used must be large, preferably open-ended by allowing some kind of removable media, and reasonably fast. It also increases the interest in storage methods that utilize compression to reduce file size.
2. Imaging usually requires saving a large number of files. This reinforces the requirement for large amounts of fast storage, but it also means that access to the stored images will be needed. Constructing a database that can access images in a variety of ways, including showing the user small thumbnail representations, using keywords, and other indexing tools, is an important need that has been recognized by many software producers. Automatically extracting classification data from the image to assist in searching is a more difficult problem.
3. Data management in the era of computers has not yet fully exploited the possibilities of coping with relatively straightforward records that contain text and numbers. The "file cabinet" metaphor is a poor and limited one. Search engines on the internet compile lists of the words used on trillions of sites so they can produce fast results, but everyone who has used them knows that the process finds many extraneous sites and misses many of interest. The real issue for computerized file storage is access to files and finding documents. Adding a field to a database primarily constructed to hold text entries does not make it into an imaging database. For instance, keeping a picture of each employee in a personnel file may be worthwhile, but it would hardly allow a user to locate employees by knowing what they looked like. That would require looking at every image.

One type of database that involves images works in essentially the opposite direction. A geographical information system (GIS) stores multiple images and maps. These record different kinds of information, which is keyed to locations. There may also be text records keyed to those locations. By overlaying and correlating the multiple map representations, it becomes possible to compare the locations of features on one map (e.g., roads or buildings) with those on others (types of soil or vegetation, underground aquifers, etc.). There are important issues to resolve in constructing a GIS, since the various maps and images (including aerial and satellite photos) must be aligned and registered, taking into account their different resolutions. In addition, displaying such rich multidimensional data presents challenges beyond those faced in most image databases.

There may be some other factors to consider in designing an optimum system for image storage. For instance, in forensic, medical and some other applications, it may be important to keep a record of all accesses to the image and of any processing or editing steps that may be applied. Also, some standardization of storage formats is important if images are to be shared between users or between different systems. Some users may want to archive images essentially forever but rarely access any particular image, while others may make continued and repeated accesses but be willing to discard images after a certain time (or when a project is completed). The data may be intended for access by many users, over a network, or be restricted to a single user. If a set of images is to be distributed widely as a permanent and unalterable resource, the requirements change again.

There are some beginnings of solutions to most of these problems and indications that many more will be forthcoming. The introduction of the Photo-CD format by Kodak indicates their expectation of considerable consumer usage of this type of storage. It is easy to imagine someone trying to find an old picture of "Aunt Sarah," for example. If the photo is stored as a faded print in an old shoe box, the searcher may have a rough idea of where to look in the attic for the box and then be willing to sort through the contents looking for the picture. But in the era of computer technology, it will seem natural that somehow the computer can find the picture just by being asked for it. Obviously, that is not a trivial task, but many companies are trying to respond to the challenge.

Storage media

Kodak's Photo-CD is an example of one kind of media that is being used for image storage. Actually, we will see in the following paragraphs that Photo-CD also defines a storage format, not just the use of CD disks; it is possible to store images on CDs in other formats as well. Projects as diverse as archaeological digs and remote sensing (satellite imagery) have found it convenient and inexpensive to distribute collections of images on CDs as a reference resource. The CD (Compact Disk) is just a plastic platter with reflective dots imprinted onto it, physically identical to audio CDs. The format of the dots, which mark changes from 1s to 0s rather than the actual bit values, is shown in **Figure 22**.

The reflective dots on a CD duplicated in quantity are physically imprinted in a pressing operation and covered by a hard plastic that is quite resistant to damage. This technique lends itself to

Figure 22. Storage format for CD data. Pits and lands in the aluminum layer reflect laser light, with the pits scattering the light and producing a darker reflection. Transitions from bright to dark indicate ones and places where no transition occurs indicate zeroes.

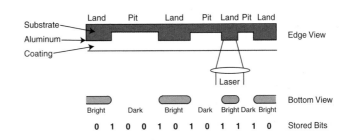

creating many copies of a disk inexpensively. Current prices for making duplicates from a master are less than a dollar per copy and continue to decline. Distributing a library of images in this way makes sense, as does distributing software, etc., because practically every modern computer has a reader for these disks.

Data on CDs are written on one single continuous spiral track, in blocks of 2048 bytes (plus the block address and some error detection sums). The entire track is written at one time, which requires the data to be continuously supplied to the write head as the disk spins. The CD format is much more difficult to use as a random-access device for either writing or reading than a conventional disk with its multiple circular tracks and fixed sectors, which make locating particular blocks of data much easier.

Pressing CDs from a master creates pits in the plastic substrate that are coated with aluminum and then sealed with a protective plastic layer. The plastic layer not only prevents physical damage, but also prevents oxidation of the aluminum that would reduce its reflectivity. In a CD-R (recordable) disk, the writing is done by a laser whose light is absorbed in a dye layer. The dye decomposes and is deposited on the metal layer, darkens it, and produces the same pattern of reflective and dark regions that the physical lands and pits do in the pressed CD.

CD-R disks are widely used as "write-once" storage devices for archiving files. CD-R drives are inexpensive and can be connected to a computer just like any other disk drive (for instance, using a standard SCSI or USB interface); they are standard equipment on many models. Files are written to a blank disk (which cost less than 50 cents at this time and continue to become less expensive). The writing process is not very fast; with the 4X drive in the laptop on which I am writing this, it takes 15 minutes to write a full disk. But that disk provides storage of more than 600 megabytes, enough to hold this entire book. After it has been written, the CD-R disk can be read in exactly the same drive as a pressed CD-ROM, or used as a master to duplicate the more durable pressed disks in quantity. CD-R disks have become so reliable and inexpensive that many people, myself included, use them instead of floppy disks to transmit even small amounts of data, when a physical disk is more suitable than transmission over the internet. The entire text and all of the nearly 2000 illustrations in this book were written onto a CD-R for backup and for transmission to the publisher.

One of the limitations of the CD is that in most cases, this writing operation must be performed in a single session. All of the files to be placed on the disk must be available on the host computer and written at the same time, so that the disk directory can be created for subsequent reading. In creating the Photo-CD format, Kodak introduced the idea of multiple directories (or multiple sessions) so that a disk could be taken in to the photo finisher to add more images (e.g., another roll of film) to an existing disk; however, not all drives or software that can read CDs are able to access the additional directories, and there is considerable overhead (about 9 MB) associated with the directories for each additional session.

At present, the most practical use of CDs is to produce entire disks of images or other data for storage or distribution. The images are archival in nature, since users are not able to modify them on the original disk. Reading from CD drives is generally rather slow. Even the newer drives that operate at 12 to 20 times or more the speed of the platter from that used for audio disks have reading speeds an order of magnitude less than a standard magnetic hard disk used in the computer. However, for accessing archival images that speed may be quite acceptable.

Higher-density formats such as those used in digital video disks (DVD) offer an order of magnitude more storage on the same size disk, with the same advantages and drawbacks as CDs, but as yet user-writable drives or media are less common. Re-writable CDs (CD RW) that use disks of the same size that can be erased and rewritten are slightly more expensive, but share the same problems of slow speed and lose the advantage of being tamper-proof. Writable but not alterable disks are especially useful in situations (medical and forensic imaging are the most oft-cited examples) in which images must be stored permanently. Such drives are also used for financial records and other applications in which assurances are needed that data cannot be tampered with, either intentionally or accidentally.

Magnetic recording

The most common type of hard disks in computers use magnetic storage. The disk platter (of glass or metal) is coated with a thin layer of magnetic material much like that used in audio tapes. Reading and writing are done using a magnetic head that "flies" just above the disk surface, riding on a cushion of air pressure produced by the spinning disk surface. This method has exceptions: some drives use a flexible polymer substrate more like simple floppy disks, with the magnetic head in physical contact with the disk coating. Such differences affect the long-term durability of the media, the reading and writing speed, the physical density of storage and the amount of information that can be written onto a single disk. But from the user's point of view the details of the design technology are secondary considerations.

Removable magnetic storage disks with capacities of several hundred megabytes are commonly available (e.g., the popular "Zip" disk). Removable types of storage are desirable, because any conventional hard disk, even one with tens or hundreds of gigabytes of storage, will sooner or later fill up with images (usually sooner). Any system that is intended for serious image analysis work is going to require some form of removable and hence unlimited storage.

The speed of access of a conventional hard disk is somewhat faster than the removable types, and quite a bit faster than slow methods such as CDs. This speed makes it attractive to copy files onto a hard disk for access, and to write them to the removable media only when work is at least temporarily complete. With that approach, the hard disk serves as a short-term storage location for work in progress, but the removable media are still used to store images for long-term purposes. The hard disk is also the place where the computer operating system, and all of the various programs including those used for image analysis, are stored.

No consideration needs to be given to floppy disks because of their inability to hold large amounts of data. The typical diskette size of 1.4 MB can usually only hold one or a few images, and sometimes not even that. A single color image obtained from a color scanner with 600 dpi resolution (a widely available level of performance), taken from an original 8 × 10-inch photograph, would require about 81 MB of storage. Such files are not conveniently stored on floppy disks. Even a typical video image, requiring about 900 KB, takes up most of one floppy disk. That may be acceptable for sending one image to a colleague but is hardly useful for storage of many images, even ignoring the rather slow reading and writing speeds of these drives and the comparative fragility of the disks.

Tape drives are even slower. A single 4-mm tape, the same type of cassette used for digital audio recording, can hold several gigabytes of files, with a drive costing a few hundred dollars. But because access to any particular location on the tape requires rewinding and searching, these devices are really only useful for backing up a random access hard disk. Saving a collection of images on a tape for archival storage might make sense, however, as it is less expensive than any other form of digital storage except CD-R. Generally, tapes are less robust than disks because they are subject to stretching even in normal use and can easily be damaged by mishandling.

Likewise, magnetic storage is generally less "archival" than optical storage because stray fields or high temperatures can cause accidental erasure. The CD has the best claim to be archival, but this claim applies to the pressed disks; the CD-R recordable disks claim only a 5–10 year life with good storage conditions. Instead of using magnetic tapes and drives simply to back up a large disk drive, it is possible with existing software to treat the tape as though it is a large (and rather slow) disk, that is, to access files randomly. This requires loading a directory into memory identifying where each file is on the tape, which takes memory space. Also, the reading times are not suitable if the files must be accessed very often. But such a medium might be used as a large and inexpensive data storage medium over a network.

One of the most recent developments in storage is network servers with arrays of redundant hard disks (RAID storage) that work in parallel for extremely high speed with error protection. The transmission of large images over ethernet still takes more time than local storage, but the advantages of shifting the responsibilities for maintaining and backing up storage to the information technology (IT) experts in your organization and the availability of images to all computers on the network makes this an attractive option in many situations.

If your purpose is archival storage of images, then regardless of what medium you select, you should prepare to invest in extra drives and interfaces. It is not likely that any of the current media will be readable by common storage devices in 10 years, so you will need to keep your own spare parts and working systems. And even then it may be difficult to transfer the images to the next generation of computers through different interfaces and networks. If you doubt this, consider the storage media in common use 10 years ago (8-inch floppy disks, mag-optical disks, Bernoulli, hard disk cartridges, etc.), none of which can be read with any ease today. Storage such as punched cards and DECtape, from 20 years ago, are unreadable except in a few very unusual circumstances because the machines are simply gone or in museums.

Another cost of archival storage is maintaining backup copies at some remote site, with appropriate security and fire protection, and having a routine method of storing regular backups there. It is really not enough simply to back up your hard disk to a tape or CD every Friday and drop the backup off in your safety deposit box on the way home, if your data are really worth keeping for many years. This is certainly the case for remote sensing tapes (a good example, by the way, of the changing face of storage — most of the early tapes can be read only on a handful of carefully preserved drives), medical records, and so on. For many kinds of records, and particularly images, photographic film is still the method of choice; it offers decades of storage, takes very little space, and can be accessed with standard equipment.

But for most people, the purpose of storing large numbers of images (certainly hundreds, perhaps thousands, probably not tens of thousands) is not so much for archival preservation as for access. The ability to find a previous image, to compare it to a current one, and to find and measure similarities and differences, is an obvious need in many imaging tasks. Choosing a storage technology is not the really difficult part of filling this need. A selection between any of the technologies mentioned above can be based on the tradeoffs among cost, frequency and speed of access, and the size of the storage required. The technical challenge lies in finding a particular image after it has been stored.

Databases for images

Saving a large number of images raises the question of how to locate and retrieve any particular image. If the storage uses removable media, the problem is compounded. These problems exist for any large database, for instance one containing personnel or sales records. But some unique problems are involved in searching for images. Database management programs are being introduced with some features intended specifically for images, but much remains to be done in this area.

Most database management routines offer the ability to search for entries based on some logical combination of criteria based on keywords or the contents of search fields. For images, it might be useful to search, for example, for images recorded between October 1 and 15, from a camera attached to a particular microscope, using transmitted light through a 500 nm color filter, obtained from slide #12345 corresponding to patient ABCDE, etc. It might also be nice to find the images that contain a particular type of feature, for example satellite images of lakes in a certain range of sizes, whose infrared signature indicates that they have a heavy crop of algae.

The first of these tasks can be handled by many existing database searching routines, provided that the classification data have been entered into the appropriate fields for each image. The second task calls for much more intensive computer processing to extract the desired information from each image. It requires close coupling of the image analysis software with the database management routine. Such a system can be implemented for a specific application, but general and flexible solutions are not yet widely available in spite of considerable effort.

Searching through multiple fields or lists of keywords is typically specified by using Boolean logic, for instance that the creation date must lie before a certain value and that either one or another particular keyword must be present (and that multiple keywords must occur close together in the text), but that the image must not be in color. These types of searches are similar to those used in other kinds of database managers and internet search engines. A potentially more useful type of search would use fuzzy logic. For instance looking for features that were "round" and "yellow" does not specify just what criterion is used to judge roundness, nor what range of numeric values are required, nor what combination of color components or range of hue values is sufficiently yellow.

Sometimes described as "query by image content" (QBIC), this approach seeks to include visually important criteria such as color, texture, and shape of image objects and regions (Pentland et al., 1994; Yoshitaka and Ichikawa, 1999; Rui et al., 1999). Depending on the field of use, quite different criteria may be important for searching. For instance in a medical application the user might want to find "other images that contain a tumor with a texture like this one" (which implies the concept of the object named *tumor*, as well as the description of the texture), while in surveillance the target might be "other images that contain objects of similar shape to this airplane." Key issues for such a search include derivation and computation of the attributes of images and objects that provide useful query functionality, and retrieval methods based on similarity as opposed to exact match. Queries may be initiated with one or a few example images ("query by example"), perhaps with subsequent refinement. Effective human interfaces for such query systems are also in development.

Implementing a search for the example of "round" and "yellow" features would require first measuring a representative sample of features in the images in the database to obtain measures for roundness (perhaps the ratio of shortest to longest dimension, but other shape criteria are discussed in Chapter 9) and hue. Some systems also use spatial frequency data to characterize texture. Histograms of frequency versus value for these parameters would then allow conversion of the adjectives to numbers. For instance, "round" might be taken to mean objects falling within the uppermost 5–10% of the range of actual values, and "yellow" the range of hues values bracketing true yellow and enclosing a similar fraction of the observations.

A program that might potentially be shown an example image and then told to search the internet for similar ones is still very far away. Part of the problem is that it is difficult to know beforehand what aspects of an image may later prove to be important. When we search through pictures in a shoebox, they vary widely. This usually allows them to be visually distinguished at a glance, but how will a search program know who is Aunt Sarah? And the meaning of the image content is also obscure except to a human with much additional background knowledge.

For example, **Figure 23** shows several images found on the internet (each from a different web site) in a fraction of one second using a search engine with the target "ACC + basketball + tournament + photo." Notice that several of the pictures show several players and the ball, but the uniform colors vary (and one image is not in color). Some do not show the ball, while one shows only the ball and net. Three show neither players nor the ball, but other things that are recognizably

Figure 23. *Basketball images as discussed in the text.*

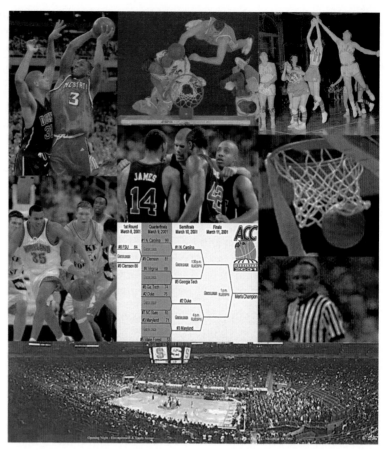

connected to basketball (a referee, a tournament bracket chart, and a basketball court). At the present and foreseeable state of the art, showing any one picture to a query-by-example program would not find the others.

An even more difficult scenario is present in many scientific imaging situations. There may be a very large number of quite similar images, such as liver tissue sections with the same colored stain from many patients, or satellite images of populated areas with many buildings, in which visual and machine methods of locating a particular image are hardly useful at all. A very experienced operator may be able to recognize some key features of interest, but not to describe them to the software in a meaningful or exclusive way. In such cases a search based on keywords, dates, patient records, location, etc. may be more appropriate. On the other hand, query by content systems have been used successfully for locating paintings and other artwork (Holt and Hartwick, 1994).

Several commercial programs claim to offer some degree of search capabilities for images. By far the best known and most fully documented is the IBM QBIC system, a prototype development kit from IBM Almaden Research with more than 10 years of experience and development (Niblack et al., 1993; Faloutsos et al., 1994; Flickner et al., 1995). It allows a user to query a collection of images based on colors, textures, shapes, locations and layout. For example, "find an image with a green background and a round red object in the upper left." This and other similar systems first process the images in the files to extract information such as the histogram (for mean and standard deviation of brightness and hue), and to segment the image into homogenous regions for measurement of size and shape, and then search through these signatures for specific numeric values (De Marsicoi et al., 1997).

An even more powerful approach to resolving fuzzy criteria into numeric values ranks all of the observations according to dimension, hue or some other objective criterion and then uses the rank numbers to decide how well a particular object conforms to the adjective used. If a feature was ranked 10th in roundness and 27th in yellowness out of a few hundred features, it would be considered round and yellow. On the other hand, if it was ranked 79th in one or the other attribute, it would not be. Both of these methods ultimately use numeric values, but judge the results in terms of the actual range of observations encountered in the particular type of application. And they do not use traditional "parametric" statistics that try to characterize a population by mean and standard deviation, or other narrow descriptors.

Fuzzy logic offers some powerful tools for classification without requiring the user to decide on numerical limits; however, although fuzzy logic has been enthusiastically applied to control circuits and consumer products, its use in database searching is still rather limited. That, combined with the time needed to measure large numbers of representative images to give meaning to the users' definition within a particular context, seems to have delayed the use of this approach in image database management. Consequently, most searching is done using specific values (e.g., a creation date after December 1, 2001, instead of "recent") and Boolean matching with user-specified criteria.

Typically, it is up to the user to establish the criteria that may be interesting for future searches before the database is established and the images are stored away. If the proper fields have not been set up, there is no place to save the values. It is impossible to overstate the importance of designing the proper search fields and lists of keywords ahead of time, and the difficulty of adding more fields retrospectively. No simple guidelines are used for setting up fields, because each imaging application has unique requirements. Establishing dozens or even hundreds of search fields with large numbers of keywords is a minimum requirement for any image database management routine.

Of course, it is still necessary to fill the search fields with appropriate values and keywords when the image is saved. Some of the fields may be filled automatically, with things like date and time, operator name, perhaps some instrument parameters such as magnification or wavelength, location (this could either be latitude and longitude, or coordinates on a microscope slide), and so forth. Even patient or sample ID numbers can in principle be logged in automatically; some laboratories are using bar code labeling and readers to automate this function. Doing this at the time the image is acquired and saved is not too burdensome, but obviously supplying such information retrospectively for a set of images is difficult and error-prone.

But the really interesting keywords and descriptors require the human observer to fill in the fields. Recognition and identification of the contents of the image, selection of important characteristics or features while ignoring others, and then choosing the most useful keywords or values to enter in the database is highly dependent on the level of operator skill and familiarity, both with the images and with the program.

Not surprisingly, the entries can vary greatly. Different operators, or the same operator on different days, may produce different classifications. One method that is often helpful in constraining operators' choice of keywords is setting up a glossary of words that the operator can select from a menu, as opposed to free-format entry of descriptive text. The same glossary is later used in selecting logical combinations of search terms.

Values for measurement parameters that are included in the database can usually be obtained from an image analysis program. In later chapters on image measurement, we will see that automatic counting of features, measurement of their sizes, location, densities, and so forth, can be performed by computer software. But in general this requires a human to determine what it is in the image that should be measured. These programs may or may not be able to pass values directly to the database; in many practical situations manual retyping of the values into the database is required, offering further opportunities for omissions and errors to creep in.

Even in cases in which the target is pretty well known, such as examining blood smear slides, or scanning the surface of metal for cracks containing a fluorescent dye, there is enough variation in sample preparation, illumination conditions, etc., to require a modest amount of human oversight to prevent errors. And often in those cases the images themselves do not need to be saved, only the numeric measurement results. Saving entire images in a database is most common when the images are *not* all nearly the same, but vary enough to be difficult to describe by a few numbers or keywords.

A very different type of database uses the image as the organizing principle, rather than words or numbers. Numerical or text data in the database is keyed to locations on the images. This approach, mentioned previously, is generally called a geographical information system (GIS) and is used particularly when the images are basically maps. Imagine a situation in which a number of aerial and satellite photographs of the same region have been acquired. Some of the images may show visible light information, but perhaps with different resolutions or at different times of day or seasons of the year. Other images may show the region in infrared bands or consist of range images showing elevation. There may also be maps showing roads and buildings, land use patterns, and the locations of particular kinds of objects (fire hydrants, electrical transformers). Tied to all of this may be other kinds of data including mail addresses, telephone numbers, and the names of people, for example. Other kinds of information may include temperatures, traffic patterns, crop yields, mineral resources, and so forth.

Organizing this information by location is not a simple task. For one thing, the various images and maps must somehow be brought into registration so that they can be superimposed. The resolution and scales are typically different, and the "depth" of the information is quite variable as well (and certainly consists of much more than a grey scale value for each pixel). Finding ways to access and present this data so that comparisons between quite disparate kinds of information can be made presents real challenges. Even searching the database is less straightforward that might be imagined. For instance, selecting coordinates (e.g., latitude and longitude) and then asking for various kinds of information at that location is comparatively straightforward. Computerized maps (distributed on CD) are presently available that can be accessed by a laptop computer connected to a GPS (Global Positioning System) receiver that picks up timing signals from the network of satellites to figure out location anywhere on the earth with an accuracy of a few meters. That can obviously be used to bring up the right portion of the map. But if you are driving a car using such a system to navigate, your question may be "show me the routes to follow to the nearest gas station, or hospital, or to avoid the 5:00 p.m. traffic jam and reach the main highway." Clearly, these questions require access to additional information on streets, traffic lights and timing, and many other things. And that same database can also be accessed by entering a telephone number or zip code. This is current technology; the promise is for much richer databases and more flexible ways to access and display the information.

Browsing and thumbnails

This section started out with the idea that saving images so that they can later be compared to other images is necessary precisely because there is no compact way to describe all of the contents of the image, nor to predict just what characteristics or features of the image may be important later. That suggests that using brief descriptors in a database may not provide a tool to locate particular images later. Consequently, most image databases also provide a way for the user to see the image, or at least a low-resolution "thumbnail" representation of it, in addition to whatever logical search criteria are employed.

Some approaches to image databases write the full image and one or more reduced resolution copies of the image onto the disk so that they can be quickly loaded when needed. This may include, in addition to the full original copy of the image, a very small version to use as a display thumbnail for browsing, a version with a resolution and color gamut appropriate for the system printer, and perhaps others. Since most of the auxiliary versions of the image are much smaller in storage requirements than the original, keeping the lower resolution copies does not significantly increase the total space required, and it can greatly speed up the process of accessing the images. Kodak's Photo-CD is an example of a storage format that maintains multiple resolution versions of each image. In some cases it is practical to use a lossy compression technique to save the lower resolution versions of the images, to further reduce their storage requirements or to facilitate internet transmission.

The reason for thumbnails, or some kind of reduced size representation of the images in the database, is that allowing the user to "browse" through the images by showing many of them on the screen at the same time is often an essential part of the strategy of looking for a particular image. The difficulties with keywords and multiple data fields noted previously mean that they can rarely be used in a Boolean search to find one particular or unique image. At best, they may isolate a small percentage of the stored images, which can then be presented to the user to make a visual selection. Even highly successful and widely reported search systems, such as the Automated Fingerprint Identification System (AFIS), rely on skilled human operators to review the 10–20 best matches found by the system based on measured values (the minutiae in each fingerprint) to perform conclusive identification.

Browsing through images is very different than the search strategies that are used for most other kinds of data. It is common on most computer systems, either as part of the system software itself, or as basic utility routines, or as part of applications, to incorporate intelligent search capabilities that can locate files based not only on the values of data fields (e.g., a creation date for the file) or keywords, but also by examining the actual contents of the files. For instance, the word processor being used to write this chapter can search through all of the files on my hard disk for any document containing the phrases "image" and "database" in close proximity to each other, and then show me those files by name and with the phrases displayed in context.

But that approach is possible because the files are stored as text. There may be special formatting characters present (and indeed, it is possible to search for those as well: "Find documents containing the word 'large' in Times New Roman italics") but the bulk of the file content is a straightforward ASCII representation of the letters that make up the words and phrases. Searching strategies for text, including ignoring capitalization or requiring an exact match, and allowing for "wild card" characters (e.g., "find documents containing the phrase 'fluorescen# dye'" would find both fluorescent and fluorescence), are widely used. Much effort has gone into the development of efficient search algorithms for locating matches.

A relatively new development in text searches uses natural language rules to interpret the text. This search technique distinguishes among nouns, verbs, and adjectives to extract some meaning from the text. That, combined with the use of a thesaurus and dictionary so that words can be substituted, allows specifying target text by entering a few topical sentences, and then having the search engine look for and rank matches.

How can this technique be used for images? Certainly there is no way to simply match a specific series of bytes. The image data are typically stored on disk as a sequence of pixel values. For many monochrome images, storage requires one byte per pixel, and the values from 0 to 255 represent the grey scale of the data. For images that have greater dynamic range, two bytes per pixel may be needed; some computers store the high byte and then the low byte, and some the reverse. For color, at least three bytes per pixel are needed. These may be stored with all three values in some fixed order for each pixel, or the entire row (or even the entire image) may be stored separately for the red, green and blue values (or other color space representation).

Dozens of different storage formats are available for images. Few image database management routines support more than a handful of formats, expecting that most users will select a format according to specific needs, or as used by a few particular programs. When images must be imported from some "foreign" format, it is usually possible to translate them using a dedicated program. This is particularly needed when different dedicated computers and programs acquire images from various instruments, and then transmit them to a single database for later analysis.

A few relatively "standard" formats, such as TIFF ("tagged image file format") files, are used on several different computer platforms, while others may be unique to a particular type of computer (e.g., PICT on the Macintosh, BMP on the PC) or even proprietary to a particular program (e.g., the PSD format used by Adobe Photoshop®). In the latter case, the widespread use of the program can make the format a kind of standard in its own right. Some of these "standards" (TIFF is an excellent example) have so many different options that many programs do not implement all of them. The result is that a TIFF file written by one program may not be correctly read by another program that uses a different subset of the 100 or so options.

Some storage formats include various kinds of header information that describes formats, color tables and other important data more or less equivalent to the formatting of a text document. Some compress the original data in various ways, and some of the methods do so in a "lossless" manner that allows the image to be reconstructed exactly, while others accept some losses and approximate some pixel values in order to reduce the storage requirement.

For instance, the Macintosh PICT format is a lossless method that represents a line of pixels with the same value by listing the value once, and then the number of times it is repeated. For computer graphics, animation, and rendered drawings from drafting programs, this "run-length encoding" (RLE) method is very efficient. It is also used to transmit faxes over telephone lines. But it does not offer much compression for typical real-world images because groups of pixels are not usually uniform.

If compression of the data is present, the computer must read the entire image file and reconstruct the image in memory before anything can be done with it. But even if the data can be scanned directly within the disk file, how can it be searched to locate a particular image based on the contents? There is not generally a specific sequence of pixel values along one line of the image (most images are stored in a raster format, as a series of lines) that is the target. There is not even usually a specific two-dimensional pattern of pixel values. Features in images are more irregular than that, and may occur in unexpected locations, sizes and orientations.

Statistical averages of the image, as may be summarized in its brightness histogram, most predominant color, etc., may sometimes be useful, but they are rarely computed while searching for a particular image in the database. Instead, if such parameters are considered important, they are determined beforehand, when the image is stored, and written into specific fields so that they can be searched using standard logical tests.

There is one approach to data matching that is sometimes applied to this kind of searching. Cross-correlation of a target image with each image in a database is a way to look for images that are similar to the target, in a very particular sense. The use of cross-correlation is discussed and illustrated in Chapter 5, because it is usually implemented using Fourier transforms. These can be speeded up by using dedicated hardware, but even so it can be quite time consuming to search through a large database for a best match.

One application of this approach is matching surveillance photos to identify targets of possible military interest. For example, cross-correlation of an aerial image of an airport against a database of images of airplanes, each type viewed in many different orientations, will match the type of airplanes and their locations in the image. For more diverse images, or ones containing features that are more variable in their shape, contrast or color, this method is less suitable.

When images are stored in a database that extends over several physical disks, particularly when removable media are used, many of the images may not be accessible or online when the search is made. The usual solution to this problem is to keep the descriptive keywords and other search fields, plus at least a thumbnail representation of the image, in a file with the main program. This allows rapid searching to find a subset of the images that may be examined visually by the user. The program has the location of each image stored in its file, so it can then request the user to insert the particular disks to load the actual images. Even with this approach, the search file can be quite large when hundreds or thousands of images are included in the database. The search file can itself require a large (and fast) disk for storage.

On the other hand, for several reasons, the search fields, keywords, thumbnails, and other ancillary information should be stored with the image instead of in a central data file. Such storage makes the file containing the image self-contained, so that it can be copied with all its information intact. It is also possible to maintain a record of who has accessed the image and when, or to keep a detailed record of whatever changes have been made to an image. Such information may be very important in reconstructing the history of processing an image.

Image database programs may also be required to limit access to images, for instance with passwords. A networked file server may allow one group of users to read images from the files, another group to add images to the database, and a third group to process or modify images. Since images are large, moving them across local area networks from a central location to many workstations is a far from trivial consideration. This is particularly a concern in medical imaging and remote sensing applications, where a large number of images are to be accessed by a moderate number of users.

Finally, the question for any image searching routine is just how it is to be used. Finding one or several images according to some criteria is usually not the end result but the beginning. How can the image(s) now be loaded into whatever program is to be used for processing or measurement? Some database management programs can act as a filter that is used by any program opening a file. This is convenient for loading images but may not lend itself to adding images to the database. Other management programs can simply locate the images and copy them onto a local disk (and perhaps convert their format or decompress them), so that the user may more easily open them into the desired application.

Lossless coding

Image compression was mentioned previously. This is desired for storage or transmission in order to reduce the rather large size of most image files, and is quite an active area of study. We will not review all of the techniques for compression described in the literature, since most of them are not implemented in standard software packages available for dedicated image processing. Most of the methods fall into just a few categories, and representative examples of each are discussed in the following paragraphs.

Image compression methods can be judged by two criteria. One is the time needed to accomplish the compression and decompression and the degree of compression achieved. This is particularly important when images are being compressed for "real-time" transmission, as in video conferencing, or perhaps when transmitting large images via the internet. The second criterion is the degree of preservation of the image. It is this latter area of concern that will be primarily discussed here.

The first and most important distinction between compression methods is whether they are lossless or lossy techniques. A lossless method is one that allows exact reconstruction of all of the individual pixel values, while a lossy method does not. Lossless methods, often referred to as image coding rather than compression, have been around for some time, with much of the original development being directed toward the transmission of images from the space probes. The communication bandwidth provided by these low-power transmitters did not allow sending many images from the remote cameras unless some method was used to reduce the number of bits per pixel.

A simple, early approach was to send just the difference between each pixel and the previous one (sometimes called "delta compression"). Because most areas of the image had little change, this reduced the average magnitude of the numbers, so that instead of requiring (for instance) 8 bits per pixel, fewer bits were needed. This is another way of saying that images are highly correlated. A histogram of the differences between adjacent pixels has a peak near zero and few large values, as shown in **Figures 24** and **25** for images that have different histograms of pixel brightness values.

Further approaches to compression used algorithms that examined several preceding pixels, predicted the next value based on some kind of fitting algorithm, and then just stored the difference from that. Advances on those methods use pixels on preceding lines as well, for further improvement in the predicted value and hence reduction in the difference values (Daut et al., 1993). Obviously, a method that looks at preceding lines is suitable for so-called progressive scan imaging rather than an interlaced scan as used in broadcast television. Most of these compression algorithms were originally designed and utilized with live image sources. If the image has already been stored in memory, then the full array of pixels is available.

An additional refinement codes the differences between a pixel and either its predicted value or its predecessor more efficiently. For instance, in recording each wavelength band in Landsat images a 4-bit number is used for most differences, with two values of the 16 possible numbers reserved

Figure 24. Example image ("Girl") with its histogram, and the results of compression by calculating differences between each pixel and its left-hand neighbor. The original image has a broad range of pixel brightness values. The histograms of the original and compressed image show that the latter has most values near zero. Contrast of the displayed compression image has been expanded to show pixel differences.

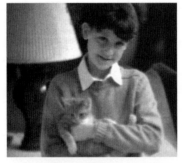
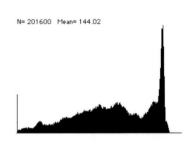

N= 201600 Mean= 144.02

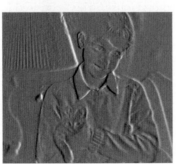
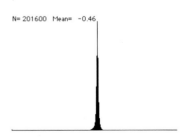

N= 201600 Mean= -0.46

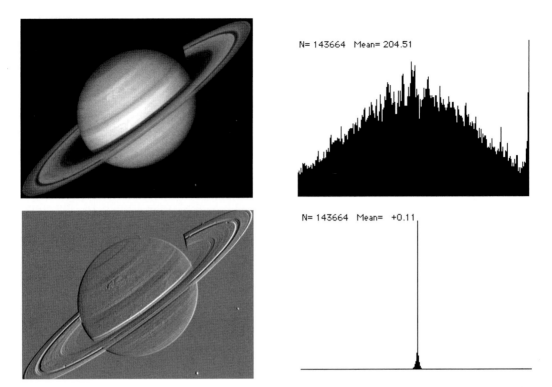

N= 143664 Mean= 204.51

N= 143664 Mean= +0.11

Figure 25. *Example image ("Saturn") with its histogram, and the results of compression by calculating differences between each pixel and its left-hand neighbor. The original image contains many black pixels. The histograms of the original and compressed image show that the latter has most values near zero. Contrast of the displayed compression image has been expanded to show pixel differences.*

as flags indicating that a (rare) larger difference value follows, either positive or negative. An average of about 4.3 bits per pixel is needed to store the images, instead of the full 8 bits.

If further optimization is made to allow variable length codes to be used to represent differences, storage requirements can be further reduced to about 3.5 bits per pixel for the Landsat data. One of the most widely used variable-length coding schemes is Huffman coding. This uses the frequency with which different grey values occur in the image in order to assign a code to each value. Shorter codes are used for the more frequently occurring values, and vice versa. This can be done either for the original grey values, or for the pixel difference values. Huffman coding is also used for other types of data, including text files. Because some letters are used more than others in English, it is possible to assign shorter codes to some letters (in English, the most frequently used letter is E, followed by TAOINSHRDLU). Morse code for letters represents an example of such a variable length coding for letters (not an optimal one).

As a simple example of the use of Huffman codes for images, consider an image in which the pixels (or the difference values) can have one of 8 brightness values. This would require 3 bits per pixel (2^3 = 8) for conventional representation. From a histogram of the image, the frequency of occurrence of each value can be determined and as an example might show the following results (**Table 1**), in which the various brightness values have been ranked in order of frequency. Huffman coding provides a straightforward way to assign codes from this frequency table, and the code values for this example are shown. Note that each code is unique and no sequence of codes can be mistaken for any other value, which is a characteristic of this type of coding.

Table 1. Example of Huffman codes assigned to brightness values

Brightness Value	Frequency	Huffman code
4	0.45	1
5	0.21	01
3	0.12	0011
6	0.09	0010
2	0.06	0001
7	0.04	00001
1	0.02	000000
0	0.01	000001

Notice that the most commonly found pixel brightness value requires only a single bit, but some of the less common values require 5 or 6 bits, more than the three that a simple representation would need. Multiplying the frequency of occurrence of each value times the length of the code gives an overall average of:

$$(0.45 \cdot 1) + (0.21 \cdot 2) + (0.12 \cdot 4) + (0.09 \cdot 4) + (0.06 \cdot 4) + (0.04 \cdot 5) + (0.02 \cdot 6) + (0.01 \cdot 6) = 2.33 \text{ bits/pixel}$$

Using software to perform coding and decoding takes some time, particularly for the more "exotic" methods, but this is more than made up in the decreased transmission time or storage requirements. This is true of all of the coding and compression methods discussed here, and is the justification for their use. Information theory sets a lower limit to the size to which an image (or any other file of data) can be reduced, based on the distribution of actual values present. If, for example, an image consists of 256 possible grey levels with actual frequencies of occurrence (taken from a brightness histogram of the image) of $p_0, p_1, \ldots, p_{255}$, then the entropy of the image is

$$H = -\sum_{i=0}^{255} p_i \cdot \log_2 p_i \tag{1}$$

Information theory establishes this as a theoretical limit to the number of bits per pixel needed to represent the image, and provides a performance criterion for actual coding methods. If this calculation is applied to the same example with eight grey levels as used above to illustrate Huffman coding, it calculates H = 2.28 bits per pixel as a minimum. Huffman coding is not optimal except in the unique case in which the frequencies of occurrence of the various values to be represented are exactly integral powers of $1/2$ ($1/4$, $1/8$, . . .). But this example indicates that it does offer a useful degree of compression with modest computational needs. Other coding techniques are available that can approach the theoretical limit, but simple methods like Huffman coding are often good enough to be widely used.

Table 2. Entropy values (bits per pixel) for representative grey-scale images shown in Figures 24, 25, and 26

Image	H (original)	H (difference-coded)
Girl (**Figure 24**)	7.538	3.059
Saturn (**Figure 25**)	4.114	2.019
Bone marrow (**Figure 26a**)	7.780	4.690
Dendrites (**Figure 26e**)	7.415	4.262
Bug (**Figure 26i**)	6.929	3.151
Chromosomes (**Figure 26m**)	5.836	2.968

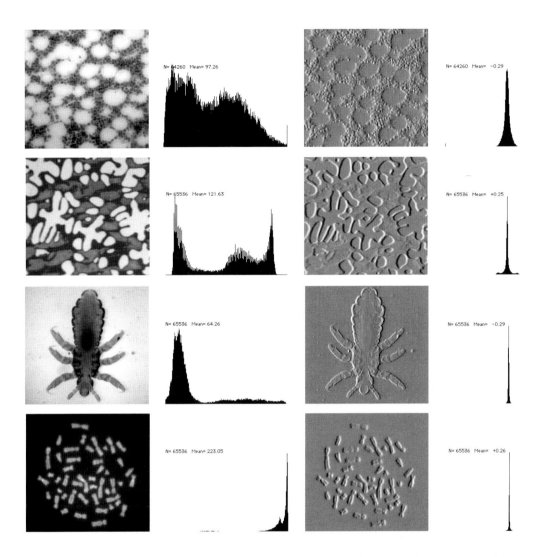

*Figure 26. Application of difference compression (autocorrelation) to various test images, with histograms of pixel values. The entropy values are listed in **Table 2**.*

Table 2 lists the entropy values for a few typical images, which are shown in **Figure 26** along with their original brightness histograms and the histograms of difference values between horizontally adjacent pixels. Some of these images have large peaks in their original histograms that indicate there are many pixels with similar brightness values. This affects both the entropy value and as discussed above the generation of an optimal Huffman code. Notice the reduction in information density (H) as the visual appearance of images becomes simpler and larger areas of uniform brightness are present. Calculating the H values for the difference coding of these images reveals a considerable reduction as shown in the table, averaging about a factor of 2 in additional compression.

The entropy definition can be expanded to cover neighbor pairs by summing the joint probabilities of all pairs of two (or more) grey values for neighbors in the same way. This would apply if a coding scheme was used for pairs or larger combinations of pixels, which in theory could compress the image even further.

Although it is unusual to apply coding methods to all possible pairs of grey values present, a related coding scheme can be used with images just as it is with text files. This approach scans through the file once looking for any repeating patterns of byte values. In a text file, the letter patterns present in English (or any other human language) are far from random. Some sequences of letters such as "ing," "tion," "the," and so forth occur quite often, and can be replaced by a single character. In particular cases, common words or even entire phrases may occur often enough to allow such representation.

A dictionary of such terms can be constructed for each document, with segments selected by size and frequency to obtain maximum compression. Both the dictionary itself and the coded document must be stored or transmitted, but for a large document the combination requires much less space than the original. Compression of typical text documents to half of their original size is commonly achieved in this way. For small documents, using a standard dictionary based on other samples of the language may be more economical than constructing a unique dictionary for each file. Dictionary-based methods, known as a "Lempel-Ziv" technique (or one of its variants, such as Lempel-Ziv-Welch, or LZW), is commonly used to compress text to reduce file sizes.

Applying the same compression algorithm to images, treating the sequence of bytes just as though they represented ASCII characters is not so successful (Storer, 1992). Few exactly repeating patterns exist in most images; even small amounts of random noise cause changes in the pixel values. These noise fluctuations may not be important, and in fact it is easy to argue that much of this "noise" arises in the camera, electronics and digitization and is not part of the scene itself. But our goal in coding the image is to preserve everything so that it can be reconstructed exactly, and there is no *a priori* reason to discard small fluctuations. Deciding that some variations in pixel values represent noise while others represent information is very difficult. Because of these fluctuations, whatever their source, few repeating patterns are found, and the compressed image is usually not significantly smaller than the original.

A close cousin of these coding methods is run-length encoding. This was mentioned before as being used in some of the standard file formats, such as the Macintosh PICT format and the compressed TIFF format used on most computer platforms. Run-length encoding (RLE) looks for any row of pixel brightness values that repeats exactly, and replaces it with the value and the number of pixels. For natural grey scale images, such rows do not occur very often and little compression is achieved; however, for computer graphics, drawings and animation images, this method can achieve very high compression ratios.

Run-length encoding is particularly appropriate for binary (black and white) images. Fax machines use RLE to send images of pages containing text or images via telephone lines. Thresholding is often used as discussed in a subsequent chapter to reduce images to black and white representations of features and background. Such binary images can be efficiently represented by run-length encoding, and in addition the encoded image is directly useful for performing some measurements on images.

Most of the common image formats used in desktop computers and workstations are lossless representations of images. Some simply record all of the pixel values in some regular order, perhaps with header information that gives the dimensions of the image in pixels, the colors represented by the various values, or other similar information. Some use modest coding schemes such as run-length encoding to speed up the reading and writing process and reduce file size. Some, such as TIFF or HDF, are actually a collection of possible formats that may or may nor include coding and compression, and have within the header a flag that specifies the details of the format in the particular file.

Fortunately, program users rarely need to know the details of the format in use. Either the images have been stored by the same program that will later read them back in, or several programs share one of the more-or-less standard formats, or there is a translation facility from one format to another within the programs or provided by a separate program. Quite a few such translation programs have been developed specifically to cope with the problems of translating image files from one computer platform to another.

Reduced color palettes

As part of the storage format for images, many systems try to reduce the number of colors represented within each image. One reason that color images occupy so much storage space is that three color components, usually RGB, are stored for each pixel. In most cases, these occupy one byte each, giving 256 possible values for each component. In a few cases, reduction to 32 grey levels ($2^5 = 32$) is used to allow reducing the storage requirements to 2 bytes, but the visual artefacts in these images due to the magnitude of the changes between colors on smoothly varying surfaces may be distracting. In some other cases, more than 8 bits per color component are used, sometimes as many as the 12 bits ($2^{12} = 4096$) which are generally considered to be required to capture all of the dynamic range of color slide film, and this of course represents a further increase in storage requirements.

Some images can be reduced for storage, depending on their ultimate use, by constructing a unique color coding table. This allows each pixel to have a stored value from 0 to 255 and occupy one byte, while the stored value represents an entry in a table of 256 possible colors to be used to display that image. This method may seem to reduce the amount of information in the image drastically, but it corresponds nicely to the way that many computer screens actually work. Instead of a 24-bit display with 8 bits (256 intensity values) for R, G, and B, many low cost displays use an 8-bit display memory in which each of the possible 256 pixel values is used to select one of 16 million colors (2^{24}). The palette of colors corresponding to each pixel value is stored with the image (it occupies only $3 \times 256 = 768$ bytes), and written to the hardware of the display to control the signals that are output to the cathode ray tube (CRT) or other device. This is sometimes called a lookup table (LUT) since each pixel value is used to "look up" the corresponding display color. Manipulation of the same LUT to produce pseudocolor displays was described in Chapter 1.

If the LUT or palette of color values is properly selected, it can produce quite acceptable display quality. Since the selection of which 256 colors are to be used to show an entire image (typically containing from 1/4 million to 1 million pixels) is critical to the success of this method, various algorithms have been devised to meet the need. The color triplet can be considered (as discussed in Chapter 1) as a vector in a three-dimensional space, which may be RGB, HSI, etc. The process of selecting the best palette for the image consists of examining the points in this space that represent the colors of all the pixels in the image, and then finding the clusters of points in a consistent way to allow breaking the space up into boxes. Each box of points of similar color are then represented by a single color in the palette. This process is usually called vector quantization; there are several iterative algorithms that search for optimal results and are all rather computer intensive (Heckbert, 1982; Braudaway, 1987; Gentile et al., 1990).

Improvements in both visual quality and speed are obtained by using the YCC (broadcast video, also called YIQ and YUV) space with the Y (luminance, or brightness) axis given more precision than the two chrominance signals (yellow-blue and red-green), because human vision is more sensitive to changes in brightness than in color. This is the same argument used for reducing the bandwidth used to transmit the color information in television. The scaling of the values is also nonlinear (Balasubramanian et al., 1994), corresponding to the response of the display CRT to changes in signal intensity. In other words, the goal of the color palette compression is to reproduce the image so that visual observation of the image on a television screen will not show objectionable artefacts such as color banding. And for that goal these methods work well. But if any further quantitative use of the image is intended, the loss of true color information may create obstacles. It may even produce difficulties for printing the images, since the gamut of colors available and the response of the color intensities is different than for CRT displays.

JPEG compression

Much higher compression ratios can often be achieved for images if some loss of the exact pixel values can be tolerated. There is a rich literature discussing the relative merits of different approaches. For instance, the encoding of differences between neighboring pixels can be made lossy and gain more compression simply by placing an upper limit on the values. Since most differences are small, one might represent the small differences exactly but only allow a maximum change of ±7 grey levels. This restriction would reduce the number of bits per pixel from 8 to 4, without any other coding tricks. Larger differences, if they occur, would be spread out over several pixels. Of course, this might distort important edges or boundaries.

Three approaches have become common enough to be implemented in many desktop computers and are fairly representative of the others. The popular JPEG (Joint Photographers Expert Group) standard is widely used in digital cameras and Web-based image delivery. The wavelet transform is newer but will become part of the JPEG standard soon, and claims to minimize some of the visually distracting artefacts that can appear in JPEG images. Fractal compression has also shown promise, and claims to be able to enlarge images by inserting "realistic" detail beyond the resolution limit of the original. Each method will be discussed and examples shown.

The JPEG technique is fairly representative of many of these transform-based compression methods. It uses a discrete cosine transform (DCT) that is quite similar to the Fourier transform method discussed in Chapter 5. The JPEG standard is a collaborative effort of the CCITT (International Telegraph and Telephone Consultative Committee) and the ISO (International Standards Organization), and actually comprises a variety of methods that are not explicitly intended for computer storage; the algorithm deals with a stream of bytes as might be encountered in image transmission.

The JPEG discrete cosine transform consists of several steps:

1. The image is separated into HSI channels and subdivided into 8 × 8 pixel blocks. If the image is not an exact multiple of 8 pixels in width or height, it is temporarily padded out to that size.
2. Each 8 × 8 pixel block is processed using the discrete cosine transform. This is closely related to the more familiar Fourier transform, except that all of the values are real instead of complex. The transform produces another 8 × 8 block of values for the frequency components. Although the original pixel values are 1 byte = 8 bits (0 ... 255), the transformed data are stored temporarily in 12 bits, giving 11 bits of precision plus a sign bit. Except for the possibility of round-off errors due to this finite representation, the DCT portion of the algorithm does not introduce any loss of data (i.e., the original image can be exactly reconstructed from the transform by an inverse DCT).
3. The 64 coefficients for each block are quantized to a lower precision by dividing by a fixed table of values that gives the least precision for high frequency terms. Adjusting the "quality" factor in most implementations increases the factors and reduces more terms to low precision or erases them altogether. This is the "lossy" step in the compression. In most cases, more precision is retained for the intensity or luminance than for the color data. This is because in the intended use of the compression method for human viewing of images, it is generally accepted that more fidelity is needed in image brightness than is needed in color, as mentioned before.
4. The first of the 64 coefficients for each block is the average brightness or "DC" term. It is represented as a difference from the same term for the preceding block in the image. The blocks are listed in raster-scan order through the image.

5. The remaining 63 coefficients for each block are scanned in a zig-zag diagonal order that starts with the lowest frequencies and progresses to the highest. The entire data stream is further compacted by using a Huffman coding as discussed earlier. This step is loss-free.

The decompression or image reconstruction procedure reverses these steps to produce an image that is similar to the original image. Compression and decompression for the DCT are symmetric (same computational complexity and time). Some other compression methods, such as fractal compression of images and Moving Pictures Experts Group (MPEG) compression of movies, are asymmetric and take much longer to achieve the compression than is needed for decompression during playback.

The loss of high-frequency terms results in some image defects and distortions. Since the loss of precision depends on the magnitude of the values, results are different in the various 8 × 8 pixel blocks in the original image, and the exact nature of the defects will vary from place to place. In general, sharp boundaries, edges, corners, and lines require the highest frequencies to accurately reproduce, and it is these that will show the greatest degradation. The results will depend on exactly where the line or corner lies with respect to the 8 × 8 block boundaries. An 8 × 8 block of pixels with a uniform grey value would be compressed to a single coefficient that would be accurately encoded, and all of the remaining coefficients would actually be zero so that no loss would occur. Small deviations from this uniform grey might or might not be preserved.

JPEG, or any similar other approach based on transforms, can be improved in several ways. One is to choose the best possible color space in which to represent the image before starting. For instance, Photo-CD (discussed in the following paragraphs) uses the CIE color space while JPEG uses HSI. Second, instead of dividing the image into non-overlapping tiles, a system using blocks that overlap in both the horizontal and vertical directions can suppress some of the artefacts that appear at block boundaries (Young and Kingsbury, 1993). Third, and perhaps most important, the quantization of terms can be made more flexible. Different scaling factors can be used for each color plane or for different colors, for different frequencies, and perhaps different directions, depending on the intended use of the image (for viewing, printing, etc.). These methods can improve the reconstructed image quality at a given level of compression, with no change in reconstruction time.

The use of JPEG compression or indeed any "lossy" compression technique for images should be restricted to images intended for visual examination and printing, and should not be used for images intended for measurement and analysis. This is true even for relatively high "quality" settings which result in only modest compression. At high-compression settings, even visual examination of images may be affected due to aliasing of edges and lines, loss of resolution, and suppression of contrast.

Figure 27 shows a real-world image that has been JPEG compressed by about 30:1 and then reconstructed. The major features are still quite recognizable, but upon closer inspection there are many artefacts present. Besides the blocky appearance, fine details are missing or altered. There has also been a slight shift in the colors present. For measurement purposes, the image fidelity has been seriously compromised. **Figure 28** shows a much simpler test image and the results of compression. As the degree of compression is increased, the artefacts become more and more serious until the figure is entirely unrecognizable.

All of the commonly used compression methods take advantage of the fact that human vision tolerates (and detects) less spatial resolution in the color information than in the brightness. This provides a useful way to detect that compression have been applied. **Figure 29** shows the hue channel from the images from **Figure 27**; the uncompressed image has values of hue that vary from pixel to pixel, while the compressed version shows the loss of spatial resolution in the color data.

Figure 27. Example image ("Flowers") and the reconstruction after JPEG compression by a factor of 29:1. Note the differences in highly textured areas at the center of each flower, artefacts along edges of petals, and the discontinuity in the stem at the left.

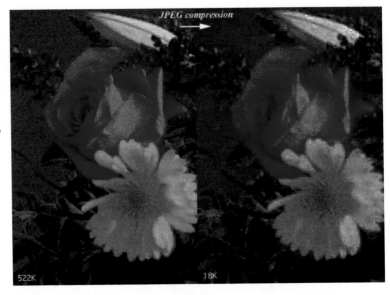

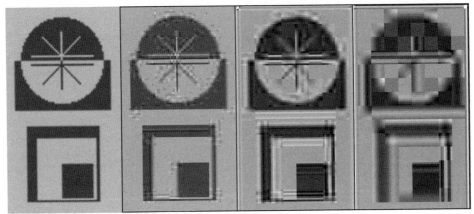

Figure 28. *A test pattern and the result of JPEG compression by factors of 3.5:1, 5.8:1, and 7.9:1 (from left to right).*

JPEG compression has been accepted for use in consumer applications and for transmission of images on the Web primarily because most images contain a wealth of redundant information, and human vision and understanding can recognize familiar objects in familiar settings based on only a few clues. For scientific imaging purposes the artefacts introduced by lossy compression are unacceptable. **Figure 30** shows an example. The image of the film has been compressed by less than 17:1 and visually appears little changed, but a plot of the average intensity across the film shows that minor peaks have been completely eliminated.

The proprietary Kodak Photo-CD algorithm is also a transform method, and shares many of the same advantages and drawbacks as the JPEG method. Because it is intended to work from traditional photographic materials, which have a wide latitude, Photo-CD makes some provision for the extended range that may be present in such images. Whereas JPEG separates the image first into HSI components, as discussed in Chapter 1, Photo-CD uses a modification of the YCC format used for broadcast television, which has one luminance (Y) and two chrominance (C_1 and C_2 or U and V) components (one the red-green balance and the other the yellow-blue balance),

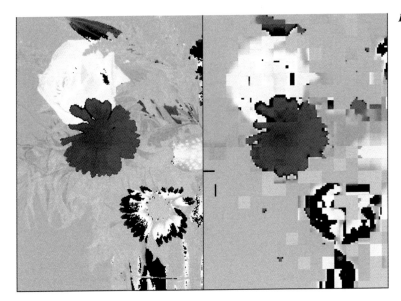

Figure 29. Hue channels from the images in Figure 27. The original image (left) has hue values that vary from pixel to pixel, while in the compressed image the hue values are uniform over larger regions.

Although they cover an extended range in which $Y' = 1.36 \cdot Y$, and the modified C' components are related to RGB by

$$R = Y' + C_2'$$
$$G = Y' - (0.194 \cdot C_1') - 0.509 \cdot C_2' \qquad (3)$$
$$B = Y' + C_1'$$

When each of these is mapped to a 256-level (one-byte) value, a nonlinear relationship is used as shown in **Figure 31**. In addition to mapping the film density to the output of a typical CRT display for viewing of the stored image, this method allows recording information beyond the nominal 100% white, which gives visually important highlights to reflections and other features that can be recorded by film, but not by most charge-coupled device (CCD) cameras. These differences, however, do not alter the basic similarity of approach, fidelity, and efficiency that Photo-CD shares with JPEG.

Judging the quality of compressed and restored images is not a simple matter. Calculating the statistical differences between the original pixel values and the reconstructed values is often used, but does not provide a measure that agrees very well with human judgment, nor with the needs of image measurement and analysis. Human vision responds differently to the same absolute variation between pixels depending on whether they lie in light or dark areas of the image. Differences are usually more objectionable in the dark areas, because of the logarithmic response of human vision. Differences are also judged as more important in regions that are smooth, or strongly and regularly patterned, than in areas that are perceived as random. Displacing an edge or boundary because of pixel differences is usually considered more detrimental than a similar brightness change in the interior of a feature.

Ranking of image quality by humans is often employed to compare different methods, but even with careful comparisons the results are dependent on lighting conditions, the context of the image and others that have been seen recently, and fatigue. It was the result of extensive human comparisons that led to the selection of the JPEG standard that is now widely implemented. The JPEG method is one of many that rely on first transforming the image from the familiar spatial domain to another one that separates the information present according to a set of basis functions.

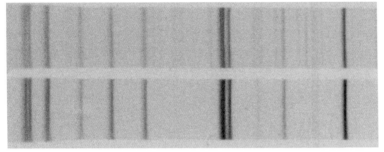

a

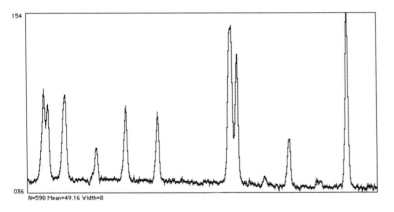

b

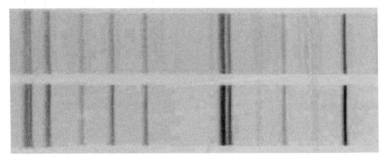

c

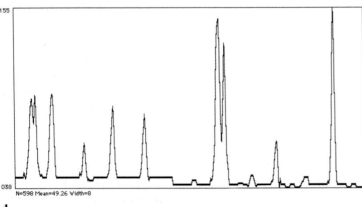

d

*Figure 30. Image of a Debye–Scherer x-ray film before (**a**) and after (**c**) JPEG compression (from 136.3K to 8.1K bytes). The position and density of the vertical lines provide information about crystallographic structure. A plot of the density profile across the images (**b** and **d**, respectively) shows that statistical noise in the spectrum has been removed along with some small peaks, and a new artefact peak introduced, by the compression.*

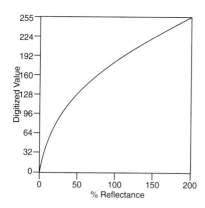

Figure 31. Nonlinear encoding of brightness and extended luminance range used in Kodak's Photo-CD format.

Wavelet compression

The virtue of transforming the image into another space is that it collects the information together in a different way. The Fourier method (and its close cousin the DCT used in JPEG compression) separates the information present according to frequency and orientation. If a complete set of these functions is used, it can exactly and completely reconstruct the original image. Therefore, using the transform by itself is not a lossy method; but if the complete set of functions is used, the numbers required to specify the magnitude and phase take up just as much storage space as the original image. In fact, usually they take up more because the magnitude and phase values are real numbers, and the original pixel values are likely to have been integers that require less storage space.

Of course, many other sets of basis functions besides the sinusoid functions are used in the Fourier approach. Some provide a more efficient representation of the image, in which more of the terms are very small, while some are simply easier to compute. One of the more recently popular methods is the wavelet transform, which offers some computational advantages and can even be obtained optically with lenses and masks (McAulay et al., 1993), or electronically with a filter bank.

The wavelet transform provides a progressive or "pyramidal" encoding of the image at various scales, which is more flexible than conventional windowed approaches like the Fourier transform. The wavelets comprise a normalized set of orthogonal functions on which the image is projected (Chui, 1992). The wavelet functions are localized rather than extending indefinitely beyond the image as sinusoids do, so the wavelet transform tends to deal better with the edges of regions and of the image, and its use for compression avoids the "blockiness" or "quilting" sometimes seen in JPEG compression, where the image is subdivided into 8 × 8 pixel blocks before performing a discrete cosine transform.

Several different wavelet functions are commonly used. The simplest is the Haar, which is just a square step as shown in **Figure 32**, that can be shifted across the image and expanded horizontally. Other wavelet functions, such as the Daubechies order-4 wavelet shown, are less obvious but work the same way and may reduce visual artefacts when compression is performed as described below (Welstead, 1999). Just as the Fourier summation of sinusoids can be used to reconstruct any arbitrary function, so can the summation of wavelet functions (Daubechies, 1992, 1996; Mallat, 1989).

To understand the process of the wavelet transform using the Haar functions, consider the following process. First, find the average intensity for the entire image, and put this value into a single pixel in the upper left corner of the transform (which will be the same size as the original). Now subdivide the image into quadrants, and find the difference between the average values of

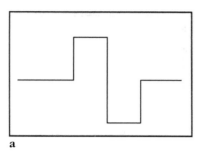
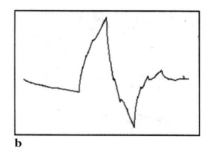

Figure 32. Two wavelets: (a) Haar; (b) Daubechies D4.

each quadrant and the global mean. Place these values into a 2 × 2 block of pixels. Similarly place the difference between each of the two left hand quadrants and the corresponding right hand quadrants into one pixel, and the similar vertical differences into one pixel each, as shown in **Figure 33**. Repeat this process by subdividing the quadrants, and continue until the individual pixels have been reached.

It is clear that the squares and rectangles in the transform that contain the higher frequency differences (which lie downwards and to the right) are much larger and represent much more data

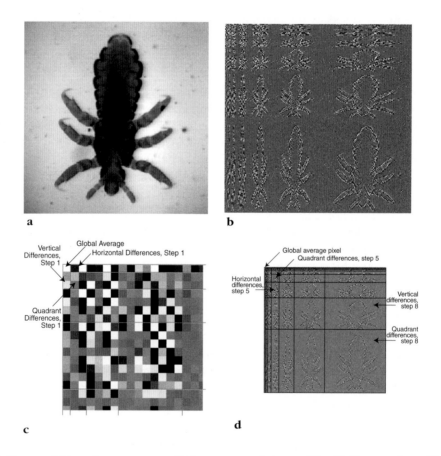

Figure 33. The wavelet transform process applied to an example image ("Bug"). The transform (b) consists of the differences between average values at different scales. These are marked and labeled for the upper left corner of the transform (c) and for the entire transform (d).

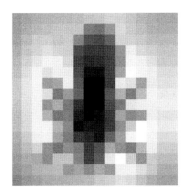 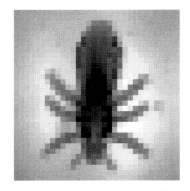 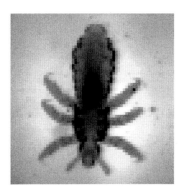

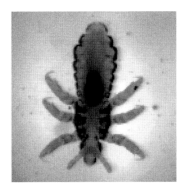

Figure 34. Reconstruction (inverse wavelet transform) adds in each higher frequency term successively. In the example, steps 4, 5, 6, and 7 are shown. Step 8 gives back the original image in this case (the dimension, 256 pixels, equals 2^8).

than those corresponding to low frequency information. The subdividing process amounts to working with higher and higher frequencies in the original image, and the reconstruction of the original image can be carried out using selected frequencies. **Figure 34** shows the process of reconstruction of the image in **Figure 33**, by adding back the differences between pixels at progressively smaller steps. The process reconstructs the original image exactly, without loss. Applications of this approach to a wide variety of time- and space-dependent signals are taking advantage of its efficiency and compactness. In some cases, analysis of the coefficients can provide information about the image content, just as is commonly done with the Fourier transform.

In principle, all these transforms take up just as much space as the original and are loss-free. To achieve compression, the coefficients in the transform are quantized, just as for the JPEG cosine transform. Lossy compression of the image is accomplished by quantizing the magnitudes of the various terms in the transform so they can be represented with fewer bits, and eliminating those that are very small. This can reduce the amount of space required, but also produces loss in the quality of the reconstructed image and introduces various artefacts.

Figure 35 shows the flowers image from **Figure 27** after wavelet compression. Although the artefacts are not visually objectionable in the reconstructed image, examining the difference between the original and the compressed image reveals many differences in detail such as color variations and shifts in the location of edges, which would seriously impact quantitative measurements.

The justification for compression is that the loss of particular terms from the transform may not be visible or at least objectionable to a human viewer, because the information each term represented was spread throughout the entire image and may have contributed little to any particular feature. This is not always the case. The selection of terms with a small amplitude often means the elimination of high frequency information from the image, and this may be important to define edges and boundaries in particular. Just as the most visually objectionable defect in the JPEG cosine

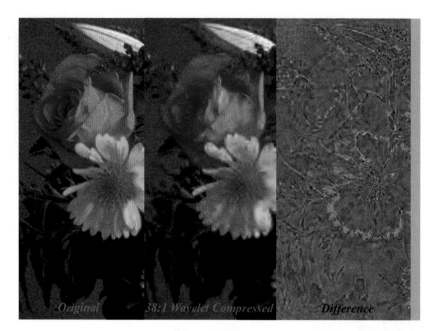

Figure 35. *Wavelet transform applied to the "flowers" image from* **Figure 27**. *Subtracting the original from the reconstructed image shows the differences, which are greatest in those areas of the image with more detail.*

transform is "blocky" artefacts, so the most annoying aspect of the wavelet transform is that details are suppressed more in "busy" parts of the image, so that it is difficult to predict which details will survive and which will not.

Compression using lossy methods is often suitable for images to be used in particular applications such as printing in which the printing device itself may set an upper limit to the fidelity that can be reproduced. It has already been suggested that one use of compression may be to store multiple copies of an image in a database, each with appropriate quality for a specific purpose such as printing or viewing as a thumbnail for searching and recognition. It is also important to determine just how much loss of quality is produced by varying degrees of image compression, so that artefacts capable of altering the analysis of reconstructed images are avoided.

Another application in which compression is normally used (wavelet compression, in fact) is fingerprint files, used by law enforcement agencies for identification. The spacing of the friction ridges on fingertips varies only slightly from one individual to another, so the corresponding set of frequencies is preserved while lower frequencies (e.g., due to shading in the image) and higher frequencies (e.g., due to noise or dust) are discarded.

Fractal compression

Barnsley (Barnsley and Hurd, 1993) has shown another way to transform an image, using what are often referred to as self-affine distortions of the image (shrinking and displacing copies of the original) as the basis functions. In principle, a complete set of these operations would give a set of parameters as large as the original image. Yet, for many images, a small number of functions are required to reconstruct the original image with acceptable fidelity, providing significant compression. The best-known example of this self-affine image generation is the fern produced by iteratively combining smaller copies of the same basic shape.

The four rules in **Table 3** are able to generate a realistic image of a fern. Each rule corresponds to one rotation, displacement and shrinkage of a sub-element of the structure. The rules are applied by starting at any point, selecting one of the rules (with the frequency shown by the probability values, from 1% to 84%), and then moving from the current point to the next point according to the rule. This point is plotted and the procedure iterated to produce the entire figure. The more points, the better the definition of the result as shown in **Figure 36**. The entire fern with 20,000 points shows the self-similarity of the overall shape. As a portion of the image is blown up for examination, more points are required. Finally, the limit of magnification is set by the numerical precision of the values in the computer, as indicated in the figure.

Table 3. Transformations (basis functions) for the Fern image (Figure 36)

1 ($p = 0.840$)	$x' = +0.821 \cdot x + 0.845 \cdot y + 0.088$
	$y' = +0.030 \cdot x - 0.028 \cdot y - 0.176$
2 ($p = 0.075$)	$x' = -0.024 \cdot x + 0.074 \cdot y + 0.470$
	$y' = -0.323 \cdot x - 0.356 \cdot y - 0.260$
3 ($p = 0.075$)	$x' = +0.076 \cdot x + 0.204 \cdot y + 0.494$
	$y' = -0.257 \cdot x + 0.312 \cdot y - 0.133$
4 ($p = 0.010$)	$x' = +0.000 \cdot x + 0.000 \cdot y + 0.496$
	$y' = +0.000 \cdot x + 0.172 \cdot y - 0.091$

From a mathematical point of view, the four transformations are basis functions or mappings which can be added together in proportion (the p, or probability values) to produce the overall object. The same principle has been applied to the compression of photographic images with grey scale or color pixels, where it is known as the Collage Theorem. That there must be such basis functions, or rules for the self-affine distortions, and that they are in principle discoverable, is known (Barnsley et al., 1986; Barnsley, 1988; Khadivi, 1990; Barnsley and Sloan, 1992; Barnsley and Hurd, 1993). The problem of finding the correct mappings is, however, far from trivial. Knowing that such functions must exist gives few leads to discovering them. Each mapping consists of a combination of translation, scaling, rotation, and warping. One proprietary method for finding them has been patented (U.S. Patent #5065447). There are formal procedures for performing fractal compression (Fisher et al., 1992), although the results are not necessarily optimal. It has been shown that nonlinear self-affine transforms can also be used, and may be more efficient.

This technique is described as "fractal compression" because the reconstruction is carried out iteratively (as shown for the fern), and because it provides ever finer levels of detail. In fact, the method can be continued to produce reconstructed images with detail at a much finer scale than the original used to find the basis functions. Such detail looks very impressive, because the enlarged image never shows flat or smooth areas that indicate loss of resolution. Of course, the detail is not real. It is generated under the assumption that whatever patterns are present at large scale in the image are also present with progressively less amplitude at all finer scales. Unlike the JPEG and wavelet methods, fractal compression is not symmetrical. The time needed to compress the image is typically much greater than that needed to reconstruct it.

Fractal compression also has characteristic artefacts. **Figure 37** shows the "Flower" image again, after a 40:1 compression. Subtracting the original from the reconstructed image shows that the colors have been significantly altered, features have been shifted in position, and details inserted that were not present in the original.

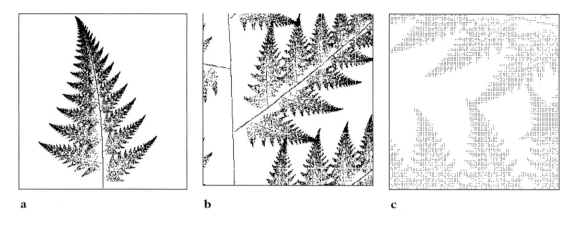

a   b   c

Figure 36. Image of a fern generated with the four transformation rules shown in the text. The structure remains self-similar when expanded, except for the limitation of finite numerical precision in the computer, which rounds off the values in the 100 times expanded image: (a) *fern image with 20,000 points; (**b**) 5× expansion; (**c**) 100× expansion.*

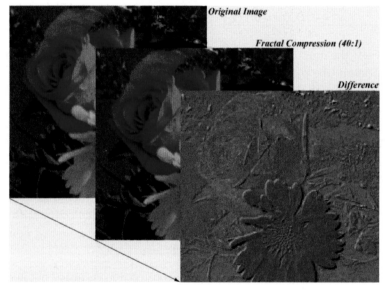

Figure 37. *Fractal compression of the "flowers" image from* **Figure 27**. *Color changes, shifts in position of features, and insertion of detail are all evident in the difference image.*

Digital movies

There is growing interest in using small computers to produce, edit and display digital moving pictures. Two emerging standards (or sets of standards) are Apple's Quicktime and Microsoft's Video for Windows. Both of these methods allow the use of various compression techniques, usually called CODECs (**CO**mpressor-**DEC**ompressors). A CODEC is a program implementation of one of the compression algorithms such as those described earlier. In fact, JPEG is one of the methods provided by currently existing codecs available for both Quicktime and Video for Windows. Some of the codecs run in software only, and others use additional hardware. For JPEG, this can be either a digital signal processor chip programmed to execute the discrete cosine transform, or a dedicated chip designed specifically for the JPEG algorithm.

The JPEG method, however, does not provide as much compression for digital movies as is needed to compress an entire movie onto a single CD-ROM, to broadcast high-definition television (HDTV) images, or to allow digital video conferencing with images transmitted over relatively low bandwidth networks because it does not take into account the considerable redundancy of sequential images. In most cases, a series of images on movie film or videotape has large areas of pixels that are not changing at all with time, or are doing so in relatively smooth and continuous ways. It should be possible to compress these, and in fact quite high compression ratios can be tolerated because for such areas the needed quality of the reconstructed image is not high. Human vision tends to ignore portions of images in which nothing interesting is happening, and no changes are occurring.

The MPEG standards follow the same approach as JPEG. They are based primarily on the need to compress images in order to transmit "consumer" video and the forthcoming HDTV, in order to compress the images enough to permit transmission within the narrow bandwidth used by present television stations, and to fit entire movies onto DVD disks. Of course, for more technical purposes such as tracking features in a sequence of images, or measuring density or color changes as a function of time, different requirements may place different limits on the acceptable quality of reconstruction.

For sequences of images, an additional compression based on similarity between successive frames is employed. MPEG adds several additional steps to reduce the amount of data that must be transmitted. It looks for blocks of similar pixels in successive images, even if they have moved slightly. Only an average of 2 frames per second are normally sent in their entirety. The rest are either encoded as differences from preceding frames, or as interpolations between frames. This approach allows overall compression to approach 200:1 with "acceptable" visual appearance.

A typical HDTV proposal presents 1920 × 1080 pixel images at the rate of 30 per second, for a total data rate exceeding 1 gigabit per second. The images use progressive scan (not interlaced), square pixels, and a wider image aspect ratio of 16:9 instead of the 4:3 used in NTSC video (and most computer display screens). A typical broadcast TV station has a bandwidth that is 250 times too small. Without examining the debate over HDTV, whose standards are still evolving, we can consider if and how application of these methods may be useful for technical images.

It is important to remember that the criterion for these compression methods is the visual acceptance of the reconstructed image, as it is displayed on a television screen. For instance, the MPEG standard, similar to today's broadcast television, encodes the chrominance (color) information with less precision than it does the luminance (brightness) information. This is because tests indicate that human vision of images displayed on a CRT is more tolerant of variations in color than in brightness. The use of images for technical purposes, or even their presentation in other forms such as printed hardcopy viewed by reflected light, may not be so forgiving.

The audio compression used in MPEG is used by itself for music recording (the popular MP3 format). The requirement for fidelity is that high frequencies must be well enough preserved so that (for example) overtone sequences allow the listener to distinguish an oboe from a muted trumpet.

Most of the moving-picture compression methods use key frames, which are compressed using the same method as a still picture. Then, for every image in the sequence that follows the key frame, the differences from the previous image are determined and compressed. For these difference images, as we have seen previously, the magnitude of the values is reduced. Consequently, in performing a further compression of this image by keeping only the "most important" basis functions, the number of terms eliminated can be increased significantly and much higher levels of compression achieved.

Similar to JPEG, MPEG consists of several options, some of which require more computation but deliver more compression. For instance, motion compensation provides a higher degree of compression because it identifies an overall translation in successive images (for instance, when the camera is slowly panned across a scene), and adjusts for that before comparing locations in one image with the previous frame. The MPEG approach is asymmetric: it requires more computation to compress the original data than to decompress it to reconstruct the images.

One of the consequences of this approach to compression is that it is intended only to go forward in time. From a key frame and then successive differences, you can reconstruct each following image, but you cannot easily go back to reconstruct a previous image, except by returning to the nearest preceding key frame and working forward from there. In principle, one key frame at the beginning of each scene in a movie should be enough. In practice, key frames are inserted periodically.

Other compression methods are being developed for sequential images. One is predictive vector quantization that attempts to locate boundaries in each image, track the motion of those boundaries, and use prediction to generate successive images. Sequences of 8-bit grey scale images compressed to an average data rate of less than 0.5 bits per pixel have been reported (Nicoulin et al., 1993; Wu and Gersho, 1993; Wen and Lu, 1993; Hwang et al., 1993). Fractal compression has also been extended to deal with image sequences (Li et al., 1993).

High compression ratios for moving images are appropriate for video conferencing, where the image quality only has to show who is speaking and perhaps what they are holding. For many consumer applications, in which the final image will be viewed on a television screen of only modest resolution, adequate image quality can be achieved at high compression ratios. Tests with human television viewers have long suggested that it is the quality of the sound that is most important, and significant noise and other defects in the individual images are not objectionable.

For most technical applications, however, the types of artefacts produced by still image compression are not acceptable, and the additional ones introduced as a result of temporal compression make matters worse. The user intending to perform analysis of images from a sequence should certainly begin with no compression at all, and only accept specific compression methods if tests indicate they are acceptable for the particular purposes for which the images are to be used.

3

Correcting Imaging Defects

The first class of image processing operations, which is considered in this chapter, is those procedures applied to correct some of the defects in as-acquired images that may be present due to imperfect detectors, limitations of the optics, inadequate or nonuniform illumination, or an undesirable viewpoint. It is important to emphasize that these are corrections that are applied after the image has been digitized and stored, and therefore will be unable to deliver the highest quality result that could have been achieved by optimizing or correcting the acquisition process in the first place.

Of course, acquiring an optimum-quality image is sometimes impractical. If the camera can collect only a small number of photons in a practical time or before the scene changes, then the noise present in the image cannot be averaged out by acquiring and adding more photons or video frames, and other noise reduction means are needed. If the source of illumination cannot be controlled to be perfectly centered and normal to the viewed surface (for instance the sun), or if the surface is curved instead of planar, then the image will have nonuniform illumination that must be corrected afterwards. If the viewpoint cannot realistically be adjusted (for instance the path of a space probe or satellite), or if the surface is irregular (as in the case of a metal fracture), then some parts of the scene will be foreshortened; this must be taken into account in comparing sizes or measuring distances.

Even in typical laboratory setups such as light microscopy, keeping the instrument in ideal alignment may be very time-consuming, and achieving adequate stability to collect dim fluorescence images for a long time very difficult, so that it becomes more practical to trade off some of the ultimately achievable image quality for convenience and speed, and to utilize image processing methods to perform these corrections. When the first space probe pictures were obtained and the need for this type of correction was first appreciated, it required lengthy computations on moderate sized computers to apply them. It is now possible to implement such corrections on desktop machines in times measured in seconds, so that they can be practically applied to routine imaging needs.

Contrast expansion

In Chapter 1, it was noted that the typical digitization process for images produces values from 0 (black) to 255 (white), producing one-byte (8-bit) values, or for color images one byte each for red, green and blue. If the camera and digitizer have more precision, the values may have 10, 12, or

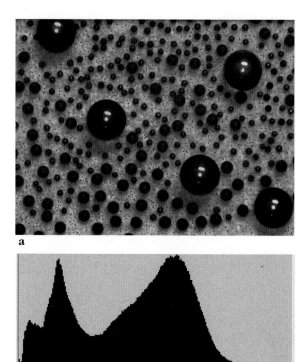

Figure 1. *Image of ball bearings and lead shot from a macro camera. The histogram (**b**) covers the full range from white to black. The small number of white pixels correspond to the specular light reflections from the larger balls.*

a

b

even more bits of precision and typically occupy two bytes each. Although this is the full dynamic range available to the output of the camera sensors, there is no reason that the actual image data will cover the full range. In many situations, the recorded image will have a much smaller range of brightness values, which may either lie toward the middle of the range (intermediate grey values), or toward either the bright or dark end of the range.

The image histogram, a plot of the number of pixels with each possible brightness level, is a valuable tool for examining the contrast in the image. **Figure 1** shows an example image in which the histogram covers the full dynamic range and indicates good contrast. The small number of very bright pixels corresponds to the specular highlights where light is reflected from the largest polished metal balls.

If the inherent range of variation in brightness of the image is much smaller than the dynamic range of the camera, subsequent electronics, and digitizer, then the actual range of numbers will be much less than the full range of 0 through 255. **Figure 2a** shows an example. The specimen is a thin section through tissue, with a blood vessel shown in cross section in a bright field microscope. Illumination in the microscope and light staining of the section produce very little total contrast. The histogram shown next to the image is a plot of the number of pixels at each of the 256 possible brightness levels. The narrow peak indicates that only a few of the levels are represented.

Visibility of the structures present can be improved by stretching the contrast so that the values of pixels are reassigned to cover the entire available range. **Figure 2b** shows this. The mapping is linear and one-to-one. This means that the darkest pixels in the original image are assigned to black, the lightest images are assigned to white, and intermediate grey values in the original image are given new values which are linearly interpolated between black and white. All of the pixels in the original image that had one particular grey value will be assigned the same grey value in the resulting image, but it will be a different one than in the original.

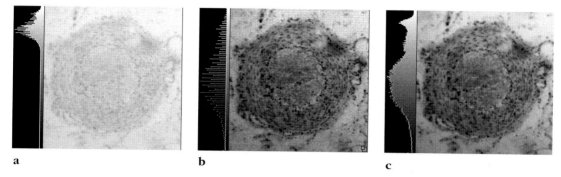

a   **b**   **c**

Figure 2. Light microscope image of a blood vessel:
(a) *has very low initial contrast, as shown by its brightness histogram;*
(b) *Linear expansion of the brightness range by manipulating the display shows a full range of black to white values but causes gaps in the histogram;*
(c) *Acquiring the image with optimum illumination and camera exposure produces similar contrast but without gaps in the histogram, and with less noise.*

This histogram plotted with the image in the figure now shows counts of pixels for grey levels that are spread out across the available brightness scale, but notice that most of the grey values still show zero values in the histogram, indicating that no pixels have those values. The reassignment of grey values has increased the visual contrast for the pixels present, but has not increased the ability to discriminate subtle variations in grey scale that were not recorded in the original image. It has also magnified the brightness difference associated with noise in the original image.

Figure 2c shows the same field of view recorded to utilize the entire range of the camera and digitizer. This may require adjusting the illumination, camera gain or exposure time, etc., and generally requires a lot of trial and error in the settings. The mean brightness of various structures is similar to that shown in **Figure 31b**; however, all of the 256 possible grey values are now present in the image, and very small variations in sample density can now be distinguished or measured in the specimen.

This problem is not restricted to bright images. **Figure 3a** shows a dark image from a scanning electron microscope, with its histogram. The structures on the integrated circuit are revealed when the contrast is stretched out (**Figure 3c**), but this also increases the visibility of the noise, or random "speckle" variations for pixels that represent the same structure and ideally should be uniform in brightness. The problem of image noise will be dealt with as the next topic in this chapter.

These cases are rather extreme. It is often not practical to adjust the illumination, camera gain, etc., to exactly fill the available pixel depth (number of grey levels that can be digitized or stored). Furthermore, increasing the brightness range too much can cause pixel values at the dark and/or light ends of the range to exceed the digitization and storage capacity and to be clipped to the limiting values, which also causes loss of information. **Figure 4** shows an example, a micrograph of a cross section through an enamel coating in which the grey scale range of the bubbles is fine but the polished flat surfaces were brighter than the white limit of the camera and consequently were clipped to a value of 255, losing any detail that might have been present. To avoid such problems, it is common for images to be acquired that do not completely cover the available brightness range.

When contrast expansion is applied to color images, the correct procedure is to convert the image from its stored RGB (red, green, blue) format to HSI (hue, saturation, intensity), and expand the intensity scale while leaving the color information unchanged, as shown in **Figure 5.** This prevents color shifts that would occur if the individual red, green, and blue histograms were linearly expanded to full scale, as shown in **Figure 6**. Such shifts are especially prevalent if the original image consists primarily of just a few colors, or is predominantly of one color.

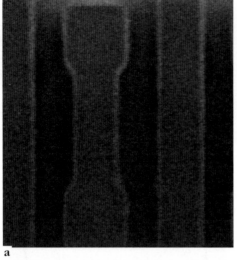

a

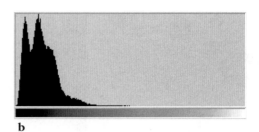

b

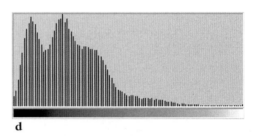

d

Figure 3. A rather dark scanning electron
microscope (SEM) image of lines on an
integrated circuit
(**a**) with its histogram
(**b**) After linear contrast expansion
(**c**) the features and noise are both more
visible, and the histogram
(**d**) shows gaps between values.

c

If these images still have enough different grey levels to reveal the important features in the specimen, then linear contrast expansion may be a useful and acceptable method to increase the
viewer's visual discrimination. More important, this expansion may make it possible to more directly compare images acquired with slightly different brightness ranges by adjusting them all to the
same expanded contrast scale. Of course, this only works if the brightest and darkest class of features are present in all of the images and fields of view.

Other manipulations of the pixel brightness values can also be performed. These are described as
point operations, meaning that the new values assigned depend only on the original pixel value
and not on any of its neighbors, and one-to-one, meaning that all pixels which originally had a
single grey scale value are assigned to another single value, although the process may not be linear. An example would be one which converted brightness to density, which involves a logarithmic relationship. For color images, a transfer function can be used to correct colors for distortion due to the color temperature of the light source, or for atmospheric scattering and
absorption in satellite images. These functions may be implemented with either a mathematical
function or a lookup table.

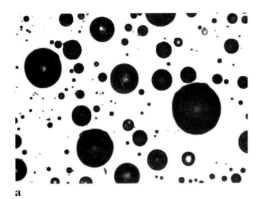

a

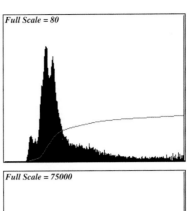

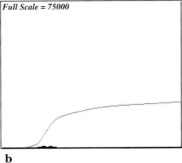

b

Figure 4. Light micrograph of polished section through an enamel coating (**a**). The histogram (**b**) shows that the majority of the pixels are full white, indicating that they were brighter than the dynamic range and were clipped to 255. It is necessary to expand the vertical scale of the histogram to see the peaks for the pixels with grey values corresponding to the bubbles in the coating.

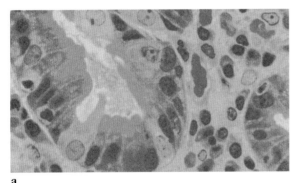

a

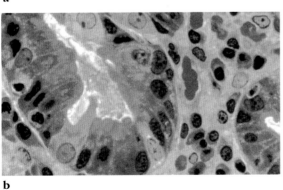

b

Figure 5. Light microscope image of stained tissue (**a**), and the result of expanding contrast by converting to HSI space and linearly expanding the intensity only (**b**).

Chapter 4 illustrates many of these contrast manipulations to enhance the visibility of structures present in the image.

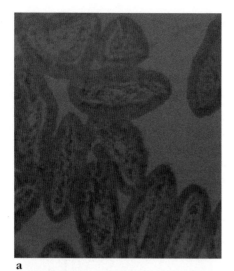

a

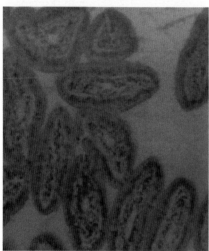

c

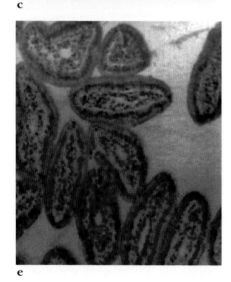

e

Figure 6. Light microscope image of stained tissue *(a)* with histograms of the red, green and blue values *(b)*. Expanding the intensity while leaving hue and saturation unchanged *(c)* expands the range of RGB values but they do not cover the full range *(d)*. Expanding the RGB values individually to full range *(f)* produces color shifts in the image *(e)*.

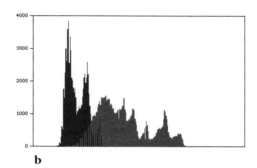

b

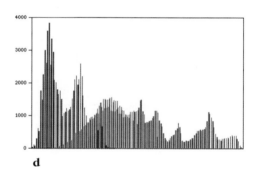

d

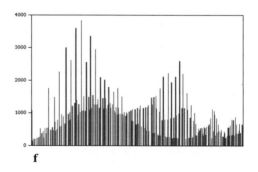

f

Noisy images

The linear expansion of contrast shown in the examples described earlier is often accompanied by an increased visibility for noise (random fluctuations in pixel values) that may be present. Noise is an important defect in images that can take many different forms and arise from various sources.

In Chapter 1, improvement in image quality (technically, signal-to-noise ratio) by averaging a number of frames was demonstrated. One unavoidable source of noise is counting statistics in the image detector due to a small number of incident particles (photons, electrons, etc.). This is particularly the case for x-ray images from the scanning electron microscope (SEM), in which the ratio of incident electrons to detected x-rays may be from 10^5 to 10^6. In fluorescence light microscopy, the fluoresced-light photons in a narrow wavelength range from a dye or activity probe may also produce very dim images, compounded by the necessity of acquiring a series of very-short-duration images to measure activity as a function of time.

Noisy images may also occur due to instability in the light source or detector during the time required to scan or digitize an image. The pattern of this noise may be quite different from the essentially Gaussian noise due to counting statistics, but it still shows up as a variation in brightness in uniform regions of the scene. One common example is the noise in field emission SEM images due to the variation in field emission current at the tip. With a typical time constant of seconds, the electron emission may shift from one atom to another, producing a change of several percent in the beam current. The usual approach to minimize the effects of this fluctuation in the viewed image is to use scan times that are either much shorter or longer than the fluctuation time.

Similar effects can be seen in images acquired using fluorescent lighting, particularly in light boxes used to illuminate film negatives, resulting from an interference or beat frequency between the camera scan and flickering of the fluorescent tube. This flickering is much greater than that of an incandescent bulb, whose thermal inertia smooths out the variation in light emission due to the alternating current. When the noise has a characteristic that is not random in time and does not exhibit "normal" statistical behavior, it is more difficult to place numeric descriptors on the amount of noise. However, many of the same techniques can be used, usually with somewhat less efficacy, to reduce the noise. Periodic noise sources, resulting typically from electrical interference or vibration, may be removed using Fourier transform representation of the image, discussed in Chapter 5.

Assuming that an image represents the best quality that can practically be obtained, this section will deal with ways to suppress noise to improve the ability to visualize and demarcate for measurement the features which are present. The underlying assumptions in all of these methods are that the pixels in the image are much smaller than any of the important details, and that for most of the pixels present, their neighbors represent the same structure. Various averaging and comparison methods can be applied based on these assumptions.

These assumptions are very much the same as those inherent in classical image averaging, in which the assumption is that pixel readings at each location at different times represent the same structure in the viewed scene. This directly justifies averaging or integrating pixel readings over time to reduce random noise. When the signal varies in other ways described previously, other methods such as median filtering (discussed in the following paragraphs) can be used. These methods are directly analogous to the spatial comparisons discussed here except that they utilize the time sequence of measurements at each location.

Important differences exist between noise reduction by the use of frame averaging to combine many sequential readouts from a camera, and the use of a camera that can integrate the charge internally before it is read out. The latter mode is employed in astronomy, fluorescence microscopy, and other applications to very faint images, and is sometimes called "staring" mode since the camera is simply open to the incident light. The two methods might seem to be equivalent, since both add together the incoming signal over some period of time. It is important, however, to understand that there are two quite different sources of noise to be considered.

In a camera used in staring mode, the electrons collected in each transistor on the charge coupled device (CCD) array include those produced by incoming photons and some from the dark current in the device itself. This current is strongly influenced by thermal noise, which can move electrons around at room temperature. Cooling the chip, either by a few tens of degrees with a Peltier cooler or by hundreds of degrees with liquid nitrogen or even liquid helium, can reduce this thermal noise dramatically. An infrared camera must be cooled more than a visible light camera, because the light photons themselves have less energy and so the production of a signal electron takes less energy, so that more dark current would be present at room temperature.

Cameras intended for staring application or long time exposures often specify the operating time needed to half-fill the dynamic range of the chip with dark current. For an inexpensive Peltier-cooled camera, the useful operating time may be several minutes. For a high quality device used for professional astronomy and cooled to much lower temperatures, it may be tens of hours. Collecting an image in staring mode for that length of time would raise the dark level to a medium grey, and any real signal would be superimposed on that background. The production of thermal electrons is a statistical process, therefore, not all pixels will have the same background level. Fluctuations in the background thus represent one type of noise in the image that may be dominant for these types of applications to very dim images. In most cases, this source of noise is small compared to the readout noise.

All cameras have some readout noise. In the typical CCD camera, the electrons from each transistor must be transferred across each line in order to be read out as a voltage to the computer. In a CCD camera, more transfers are needed to shift the electrons from one side of the image to the amplifier and so the resulting noise is greater on one side of the image than on the other. In an interline transfer camera, a separate row of transistors adjacent to each detector is used instead, somewhat reducing the readout noise. Of course, additional sources of noise from the other associated electronics (clock signals, wiring from the camera to the digitizer, pickup of electrical signals from the computer itself, and so forth) may degrade the signal even more. But even if those other sources of noise are minimized by careful design and proper wiring, there is an irreducible amount of noise superimposed on the signal each time the camera image is read out, amplified and digitized.

This noise is generally random, and hence is as likely to reduce as to increase the brightness of any particular pixel. **Figure 7** shows an example of two successive video frames acquired using a good quality digital camera and normal lighting. The images look essentially identical except for the motion of the clock pendulum. However, subtracting one frame from the other (and expanding the contrast) shows the pixel noise present in the images. With digital cameras, as discussed in Chapter 1, the normal procedure is to acquire a single image using an appropriate exposure time, and then transfer the digitized values to the computer. However, some camera designs that are not cooled may acquire several shorter exposures and average the results in the computer.

With video cameras, averaging many frames together causes the random noise from readout to partially cancel while the signal continues to add up. The small well size of the transistors on the very tiny chip make long exposures impractical The consequence is that frame averaging can reduce the relative magnitude of this source of noise in the image, but cannot eliminate it. **Figure 8** shows two video frames of the clock, acquired in dim light with high amplifier gain. The individual images show visible noise, which is even more apparent in the difference image.

For a very dim image, the optimum situation would be to integrate the signal within the camera chip, but without allowing any single pixel to reach saturation. Then reading the data out once will

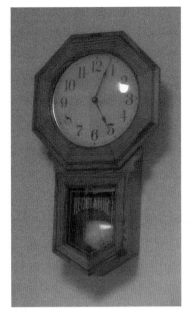
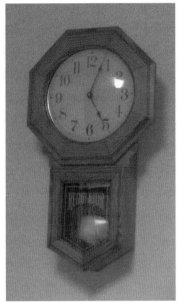
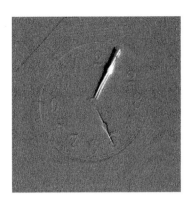

Figure 7. *Two images of the same view, acquired from a digital camera, and the difference between them (pixels enlarged and contrast expanded to show detail).*

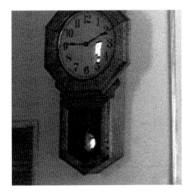
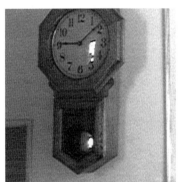
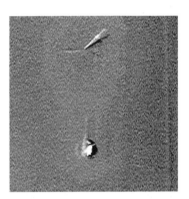

Figure 8. *Two images of the same view, acquired as sequential video frames, and the difference between them (contrast expanded to show detail).*

produce the minimum readout noise and the best image. For a brighter image, or for a camera than can only function at video rates, it may be acceptable to average together a sufficient number of frames to reduce the pixel variations due to random readout noise. This integration may be done in the frame grabber or in the computer program. The frame grabber is generally restricted by the amount of on-board memory, but can often collect every frame with no loss of data. The computer program is more flexible, but the time required to add the frames together may result in discarding some of the video frames, so that the total acquisition takes longer (which may not be a problem if the image does not vary with time). Of course, in fluorescence microscopy bleaching may occur and it may be desirable to collect all of the photons as rapidly as possible, either by frame averaging, or, for a very dim image, by using staring mode if the camera is capable of this.

Figure 9 shows a comparison of two SEM images taken at different scan rates. The fast scan image collects few electrons per pixel and so has a high noise level that obscures details in the

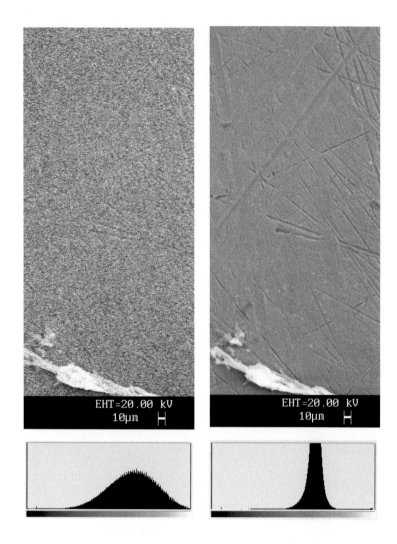

Figure 9. SEM images of a scratched metal surface:
(a) 1-second scan;
(b) histogram of *(a)*;
(c) 20 second scan;
(d) histogram of *(c)*.

image. Slowing the scan rate down from one second to 20 seconds increases the amount of signal and reduces the noise. The histograms show that the variation of brightness within the uniform region is reduced, which is why the visibility of detail is improved.

Neighborhood averaging

The simplest form of spatial averaging is simply to add together the pixel brightness values in each small region of the image, divide by the number of pixels in the neighborhood, and use the resulting value to construct a new image. **Figure 10** shows that this essentially produces an image with a smaller number of pixels. The block size in **Figure 3b** is 4×4, so that sixteen pixel values are added. The noise in this image is random due to the counting statistics of the small number of photons, so the improvement in image quality or signal-to-noise ratio is just the square root of 16, or a factor of 4; however, the image lateral resolution is seriously impacted and the small structures in the image can no longer be separately discerned.

The more common way to accomplish neighborhood averaging is to replace each pixel with the average of itself and its neighbors. This is often described as a "kernel" operation, since implementation can be generalized as the sum of the pixel values in the region multiplied by a set of

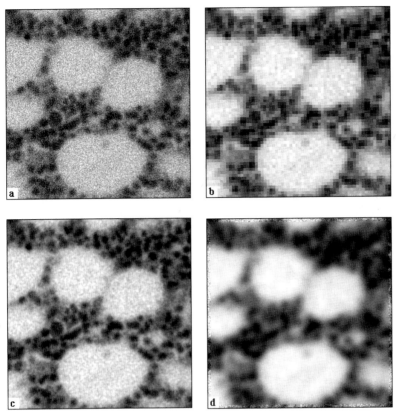

Figure 10. Smoothing by averaging:
(a) *noisy original image (fluorescence light microscopy of bone marrow);*
(b) *each 4 × 4 block of pixels averaged;*
(c) *each pixel replaced by the average of itself and its eight neighbors in a 3 × 3 square block;*
(d) *each pixel replaced by the average of itself and its 120 neighbors in an 11 × 11 square.*

integer weights. The process is also called a "convolution" because it corresponds to a procedure performed in Fourier space (discussed in Chapter 5).

$$P^*_{x,y} \frac{\sum\limits_{i,j=-m}^{+m} W_{i,j} \cdot P_{x+i,y+j}}{\sum\limits_{i,j=-m}^{+m} W_{i,j}} \tag{1}$$

Equation 1 shows the calculation performed over a square of dimension $2m + 1$, which is odd. The neighborhood sizes thus range from 3×3, upward to 5×5, 7×7, etc. It is possible to use non-square regions; for larger neighborhoods an approximation of a circle is preferable to a square but somewhat more difficult to implement. The array of weights W for a simple neighbor averaging contains only 1s, and for a 3×3 region could be written as:

1	1	1
1	1	1
1	1	1

where we understand the convention that these coefficients are to be multiplied by pixels that surround the central pixel, the total normalized by dividing by the sum of weights, and the value written to the location of the central pixel to form a new image.

As a matter of practicality, because storage space is never unlimited, it is common to write the new image back into the same memory as the original; however, when this is done it is important to use the original pixel values for the summation, and not those new ones which have already been calculated for some of the neighbors. This requires keeping a copy of a few lines of the image during the process.

Neighborhood operations including kernel multiplication are usually applied symmetrically around each pixel. This creates a problem for pixels nearer to the edge of the image than the half-width of the neighborhood. Various approaches are used to deal with this problem, including designing special asymmetrical kernels or rules along edges or in corners, assuming that the image edges are mirrors, so that each line of pixels within the image is duplicated beyond it, or assuming that the image wraps around so that the left edge and right edge, and the top and bottom edges, are continuous. In the examples shown here, an even simpler approach has been used: the processing is restricted to that portion of the image where no edge conflicts arise. This leaves lines of unprocessed pixels along the edges of the images, equal in width to half the dimension of the neighborhood. None of these approaches is entirely satisfactory, and in general most processing operations sacrifice some pixels from the image edges.

Figure 10 shows the effect of smoothing using a 3×3 neighborhood average and also an 11×11 neighborhood size. The noise reduction is much greater with the larger region, but is accompanied by a significant blurring of the feature edges.

The amount of blurring can be reduced and more control exerted over the neighborhood averaging procedure by using weight values that are not 1. For example, the values

1	2	1
2	4	2
1	2	1

have several attractive characteristics. First, the central 4 which multiplies the original pixel contents is the largest factor, causing the central pixel to dominate the average and reducing blurring. The values of 2 for the four orthogonally touching neighbors and 1 for the four diagonally touching neighbors acknowledge the fact that the diagonal pixels are in fact farther away from the center of the neighborhood (actually by the factor $\sqrt{2}$). Finally, these weights have a total value of 16, which is a power of two and consequently very easy to divide in a computer implementation of this averaging procedure.

Similar sets of ad hoc weight values can be devised in various sizes. Integers are commonly used to speed implementation, and storage requirements are modest. We will see in Chapter 5, in the context of processing images in frequency space, that these kernels can be analyzed quite efficiently in that domain to understand their smoothing properties. It turns out from that analysis that one of the very useful "shapes" for a weight kernel is that of a Gaussian. This is a set of integers that approximate the profile of a Gaussian function along any row, column or diagonal through the center. It is characterized by a standard deviation, expressed in terms of pixel dimensions. The size of the kernel is generally made large enough that adding another row of terms would insert negligibly small numbers, ideally zeroes into the array, but of course some zero values will be present anyway in the corners since they are farther from the central pixel.

Choosing the actual integers is something of an art, at least for the larger kernels, since the goal is to approximate the smooth analytical curve of the Gaussian, although the total of the weights must usually be kept smaller than some practical limit to facilitate the computer arithmetic (Russ, 1995d). Several Gaussian kernels are shown below, with standard deviations that increase in geometric proportions from less than one pixel to many pixels. The standard deviation for these kernels is the radius (in pixels) containing 68% of the integrated magnitude of the coefficients, or the volume under the surface if the kernel is pictured as a 3D plot of the integer values. This is a two-dimensional generalization of the usual definition of standard deviation; for a one-dimensional Gaussian distribution, 68% of the area under the curve lies within ± one standard deviation.

Of course, the kernel size increases with the standard deviation as well; the total width of the kernel is at least six times the standard deviation. For the largest examples illustrated below, only the upper left quadrant of the symmetrical array is shown. Repeated application of a small kernel, or the sequential application of two or more kernels, is equivalent to the single application of a larger one, which can be constructed as the convolution of the two kernels (applying the weighting factors from one kernel to those in the other as if they were pixel values, and summing and adding to generate a new, larger array of weights).

$\sigma = 0.391$ pixels (3×3)

```
 1   4   1
 4  12   4
 1   4   1
```

$\sigma = 0.625$ pixels (5×5)

```
 1   2   3   2   1
 2   7  11   7   2
 3  11  17  11   3
 2   7  11   7   2
 1   2   3   2   1
```

$\sigma = 1.0$ pixels (9×9)

```
 0   0   1   1   1   1   1   0   0
 0   1   2   3   3   3   2   1   0
 1   2   3   6   7   6   3   2   1
 1   3   6   9  11   9   6   3   1
 1   3   7  11  12  11   7   3   1
 1   3   6   9  11   9   6   3   1
 1   2   3   6   7   6   3   2   1
 0   1   2   3   3   3   2   1   0
 0   0   1   1   1   1   1   0   0
```

$\sigma = 1.6$ pixels (11×11)

```
 1   1   1   2   2   2   2   2   1   1   1
 1   2   2   3   4   4   4   3   2   2   1
 1   2   4   5   6   7   6   5   4   2   1
 2   3   5   7   8   9   8   7   5   3   2
 2   4   6   8  10  11  10   8   6   4   2
 2   4   7   9  11  12  11   9   7   4   2
 2   4   6   8  10  11  10   8   6   4   2
 2   3   5   7   8   9   8   7   5   3   2
 1   2   4   5   6   7   6   5   4   2   1
 1   2   2   3   4   4   4   3   2   2   1
 1   1   1   2   2   2   2   2   1   1   1
```

σ = 2.56 pixels (15 × 15)

```
2  2  3  4  5  5  6  6  6  5  5  4  3  2  2
2  3  4  5  7  7  8  8  8  7  7  5  4  3  2
3  4  6  7  9 10 10 11 10 10  9  7  6  4  3
4  5  7  9 10 12 13 13 13 12 10  9  7  5  4
5  7  9 11 13 14 15 16 15 14 13 11  9  7  5
5  7 10 12 14 16 17 18 17 16 14 12 10  7  5
6  8 10 13 15 17 19 19 19 17 15 13 10  8  6
6  8 11 13 16 18 19 20 19 18 16 13 11  8  6
6  8 10 13 15 17 19 19 19 17 15 13 10  8  6
5  7 10 12 14 16 17 18 17 16 14 12 10  7  5
5  7  9 11 13 14 15 16 15 14 13 11  9  7  5
4  5  7  9 10 12 13 13 13 12 10  9  7  5  4
3  4  6  7  9 10 10 11 10 10  9  7  6  4  3
2  3  4  5  7  7  8  8  8  7  7  5  4  3  2
2  2  3  4  5  5  6  6  6  5  5  4  3  2  2
```

σ =4.096 pixels (21 × 21)

```
5  6  7  8  9 10 11 12 13 13 13 13 13 12 11 10  9  8  7  6  5
6  7  9 10 11 12 14 15 15 16 16 16 15 15 14 12 11 10  9  7  6
7  9 10 12 13 15 16 17 18 18 19 18 18 17 16 15 13 12 10  9  7
8 10 12 13 15 17 18 20 21 21 21 21 21 20 18 17 15 13 12 10  8
9 11 13 15 17 19 21 22 23 24 24 24 23 22 21 19 17 15 13 11  9
10 12 15 17 19 21 23 25 26 27 27 27 26 25 23 21 19 17 15 12 10
11 14 16 18 21 23 25 27 28 29 29 29 28 27 25 23 21 18 16 14 11
12 15 17 20 22 25 27 29 30 31 31 31 30 29 27 25 22 20 17 15 12
13 15 18 21 23 26 28 30 32 33 33 33 32 30 28 26 23 21 18 15 13
13 16 18 21 24 27 29 31 33 34 34 34 33 31 29 27 24 21 18 16 13
13 16 19 21 24 27 29 31 33 34 34 34 33 31 29 27 24 21 19 16 13
13 16 18 21 24 27 29 31 33 34 34 34 33 31 29 27 24 21 18 16 13
13 15 18 21 23 26 28 30 32 33 33 33 32 30 28 26 23 21 18 15 13
12 15 17 20 22 25 27 29 30 31 31 31 30 29 27 25 22 20 17 15 12
11 14 16 18 21 23 25 27 28 29 29 29 28 27 25 23 21 18 16 14 11
10 12 15 17 19 21 23 25 26 27 27 27 26 25 23 21 19 17 15 12 10
9 11 13 15 17 19 21 22 23 24 24 24 23 22 21 19 17 15 13 11  9
8 10 12 13 15 17 18 20 21 21 21 21 21 20 18 17 15 13 12 10  8
7  9 10 12 13 15 16 17 18 18 19 18 18 17 16 15 13 12 10  9  7
6  7  9 10 11 12 14 15 15 16 16 16 15 15 14 12 11 10  9  7  6
5  6  7  8  9 10 11 12 13 13 13 13 13 12 11 10  9  8  7  6  5
```

σ = 6.536 pixels (29 × 29, upper left corner)

```
 7  8  9 10 10 11 12 13 13 14 14 15 15 15 15 ...
 8  9 10 11 11 12 13 14 15 15 16 16 16 17 17 ...
 9 10 11 12 13 13 14 15 16 17 17 18 18 18 18 ...
10 11 12 13 14 15 16 17 17 18 19 19 20 20 20 ...
10 11 13 14 15 16 17 18 19 20 20 21 21 21 21 ...
11 12 13 15 16 17 18 19 20 21 22 22 23 23 23 ...
12 13 14 16 17 18 19 20 21 22 23 24 24 24 24 ...
13 14 15 17 18 19 20 22 23 24 24 25 25 26 26 ...
13 15 16 17 19 20 21 23 24 25 26 26 27 27 27 ...
14 15 17 18 20 21 22 24 25 26 27 27 28 28 28 ...
14 16 17 19 20 22 23 24 26 27 28 28 29 29 29 ...
15 16 18 19 21 22 24 25 26 27 28 29 30 30 30 ...
15 16 18 20 21 23 24 25 27 28 29 30 30 30 31 ...
15 17 18 20 21 23 24 26 27 28 29 30 30 31 31 ...
15 17 18 20 21 23 24 26 27 28 29 30 31 31 31 ...
...
```

σ = 10.486 pixels (43 × 43, upper left corner)

```
 6  6  6  7  7  7  8  8  8  9  9  9  9 10 10 10 10 10 10 10 11 11 ...
 6  6  7  7  7  8  8  8  9  9  9 10 10 10 10 11 11 11 11 11 11 11 ...
 6  7  7  7  8  8  9  9  9 10 10 10 11 11 11 11 11 12 12 12 12 12 ...
 7  7  7  8  8  9  9  9 10 10 10 11 11 11 12 12 12 12 12 12 12 13 ...
 7  7  8  8  9  9  9 10 10 11 11 11 12 12 12 12 13 13 13 13 13 13 ...
 7  8  8  9  9 10 10 10 11 11 12 12 12 13 13 13 13 13 14 14 14 14 ...
 8  8  9  9  9 10 10 11 11 12 12 12 13 13 13 14 14 14 14 14 14 14 ...
 8  8  9  9 10 10 11 11 12 12 13 13 13 14 14 15 15 15 15 15 15 ...
 8  9  9 10 10 11 11 12 12 13 13 14 14 15 15 15 15 15 16 16 16 ...
 9  9 10 10 11 11 12 12 13 13 14 14 15 15 15 16 16 16 16 16 16 ...
 9  9 10 10 11 12 12 13 13 14 14 15 15 15 16 16 16 16 17 17 17 17 ...
 9 10 10 11 11 12 12 13 14 14 15 15 15 16 16 16 17 17 17 17 17 ...
 9 10 11 11 12 12 13 13 14 14 15 15 16 16 17 17 17 18 18 18 18 ...
10 10 11 11 12 13 13 14 14 15 15 16 16 17 17 17 18 18 18 18 18 ...
10 10 11 12 12 13 13 14 15 15 16 16 17 17 17 18 18 18 19 19 19 ...
10 11 11 12 12 13 14 14 15 15 16 16 17 17 18 18 18 19 19 19 19 ...
10 11 11 12 13 13 14 15 15 16 16 17 17 18 18 19 19 19 19 19 ...
10 11 12 12 13 13 14 15 15 16 16 17 17 18 18 19 19 19 19 20 20 ...
10 11 12 12 13 14 14 15 15 16 17 17 18 18 19 19 19 19 20 20 20 ...
10 11 12 12 13 14 14 15 16 16 17 17 18 18 19 19 19 19 20 20 20 20 ...
11 11 12 12 13 14 14 15 16 16 17 17 18 18 19 19 20 20 20 20 20 ...
11 11 12 13 13 14 14 15 16 16 17 17 18 18 19 19 20 20 20 20 20 ...
...
```

```
5  5  5  5  5  5  5  6  6  6  6  6  6  6  6  7  7  7  7  7  7  7  7 7 7 7 7  7  7  ...
5  5  5  5  5  6  6  6  6  6  6  6  6  6  7  7  7  7  7  7  7  7  7  7  7  7  7  7  7 ...
5  5  5  5  6  6  6  6  6  6  6  6  6  7  7  7  7  7  7  7  7  7  7  7  7  7  7  7  7 ...
5  5  5  6  6  6  6  6  6  6  7  7  7  7  7  7  7  7  7  7  7  7  7  8  8  8  8  8  8 ...
5  5  6  6  6  6  6  6  6  7  7  7  7  7  7  7  7  7  8  8  8  8  8  8  8  8  8  8  8 ...
5  6  6  6  6  6  6  6  7  7  7  7  7  7  7  7  8  8  8  8  8  8  8  8  8  8  8  8  8 ...
5  6  6  6  6  6  6  7  7  7  7  7  7  7  7  8  8  8  8  8  8  8  8  8  8  8  8  8  8 ...
6  6  6  6  6  6  7  7  7  7  7  7  7  8  8  8  8  8  8  8  8  8  8  8  8  8  8  8  8 ...
6  6  6  6  6  7  7  7  7  7  7  7  8  8  8  8  8  8  8  8  8  8  8  9  9  9  9  9  9 ...
6  6  6  6  7  7  7  7  7  7  7  8  8  8  8  8  8  8  8  8  8  9  9  9  9  9  9  9  9 ...
6  6  6  7  7  7  7  7  7  7  8  8  8  8  8  8  8  8  8  9  9  9  9  9  9  9  9  9  9 ...
6  6  6  7  7  7  7  7  8  8  8  8  8  8  8  8  8  9  9  9  9  9  9  9  9  9  9  9  9 ...
6  6  7  7  7  7  7  8  8  8  8  8  8  8  9  9  9  9  9  9  9  9  9  9  9  9  9  9  9 ...
6  7  7  7  7  7  7  8  8  8  8  8  8  9  9  9  9  9  9  9  9  9  9  9  9  9  10 10 10 ...
6  7  7  7  7  7  8  8  8  8  8  8  8  9  9  9  9  9  9  9  9  9  9  9 10 10 10 10 10 10 ...
7  7  7  7  7  7  8  8  8  8  8  8  8  9  9  9  9  9  9  9  9  9 10 10 10 10 10 10 10 10 ...
7  7  7  7  7  8  8  8  8  8  8  8  9  9  9  9  9  9  9  9 10 10 10 10 10 10 10 10 10 10 ...
7  7  7  7  7  8  8  8  8  8  8  9  9  9  9  9  9  9  9 10 10 10 10 10 10 10 10 10 10 10 ...
7  7  7  7  8  8  8  8  8  8  9  9  9  9  9  9  9  9 10 10 10 10 10 10 10 10 10 10 10 10 ...
7  7  7  7  8  8  8  8  8  8  9  9  9  9  9  9  9  9 10 10 10 10 10 10 10 10 10 10 10 10 ...
7  7  7  7  8  8  8  8  8  8  9  9  9  9  9  9  9  9 10 10 10 10 10 10 10 10 10 10 10 10 ...
7  7  7  8  8  8  8  8  9  9  9  9  9  9  9  9 10 10 10 10 10 10 10 10 10 10 10 10 10 10 ...
7  7  7  8  8  8  8  8  9  9  9  9  9  9  9 10 10 10 10 10 10 10 10 10 10 10 10 10 10 11 ...
7  7  7  8  8  8  8  8  9  9  9  9  9  9  9 10 10 10 10 10 10 10 10 10 10 11 11 11 11 11 ...
7  7  7  8  8  8  8  8  9  9  9  9  9  9  9 10 10 10 10 10 10 10 10 10 10 11 11 11 11 11 ...
7  7  7  8  8  8  8  8  9  9  9  9  9  9 10 10 10 10 10 10 10 10 10 10 11 11 11 11 11 ...
7  7  7  8  8  8  8  8  9  9  9  9  9  9 10 10 10 10 10 10 10 10 10 10 11 11 11 11 11 ...
7  7  7  8  8  8  8  8  9  9  9  9  9  9 10 10 10 10 10 10 10 10 10 10 11 11 11 11 11 11 ...
```

Figure 11 shows several Gaussian weight kernels plotted as isometric views. Notice that the quantization of the weights using integers produces some distortion. Some systems allow entering kernel weights as real numbers as shown in **Figure 12a**. Many systems generate Gaussian kernels as needed, when the user enters the standard deviation value (**Figure 12b**). The actual smoothing operation can be speeded up considerably in the case of Gaussian filters by separating the operation into two simpler ones. Instead of using the entire square array of weights, which for a 15 × 15 kernel would require 225 multiplications and additions, the filter can be separated into a vertical Gaussian blur with a linear array of weights (15 multiplications and additions) followed by a horizontal Gaussian blur (another 15 for a total of 30). The implementation of many convolution kernels can be separated in this way, but for purposes of understanding the algorithms it is probably better to consider the entire array of weights.

In subsequent sections on image processing, we will see other uses for kernels in which the weights are not symmetrical in magnitude and not all positive. The implementation of the kernel will remain the same, except that when negative weights are present the normalization is usually performed by division by the sum of the positive values only (because in these cases the sum of all the weights is usually zero). For the present our interest is restricted to smoothing of noise in images.

Figure 13 shows the same noisy image as **Figure 10**, along with an image of the same region using image averaging to reduce the statistical noise, as described in Chapter 1. The figure also shows an enlargement of a portion of the image in which the individual pixels can be discerned, as an aid to judging the pixel-to-pixel noise variations in uniform regions and the sharpness of boundaries

Figure 11. Isometric plots of the weight values in Gaussian smoothing kernels:
(a) 5 × 5, σ = 0.625 pixels;
(b) 13 × 13, σ = 2.5 pixels;
(c) 43 × 43, σ = 10.486 pixels (note the stair-stepping produced by integer weight values)

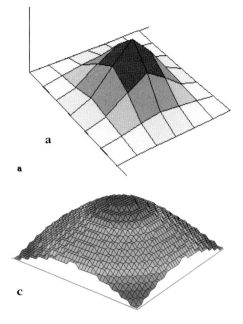

a

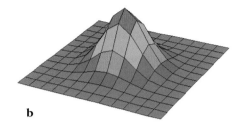

b

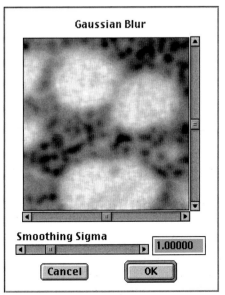

c

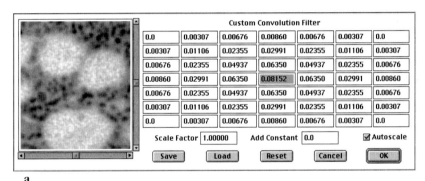

a

b

Figure 12. Gaussian smoothing to reduce noise:
(a) entering real values for a Gaussian filter with standard deviation = 1.0 pixels;
(b) specifying the standard deviation for automatic generation of the weights. The preview displays also expand the image contrast.

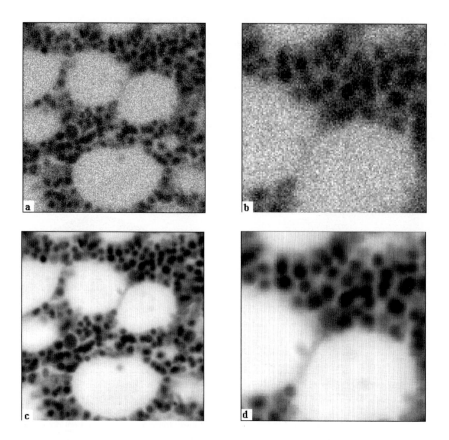

Figure 13. Reduction of noise by temporal averaging:
   (a) *original image (same as Figure 10);*
   (b) *enlarged to show individual pixel detail;*
   (c) *averaging of 256 frames;*
   (d) *enlarged to show individual pixel detail.*

between different structures. Applying smoothing with a Gaussian kernel with a standard deviation of 1.0 pixels produces the improvement in quality shown in **Figure 14**.

This type of averaging can reduce visible noise in the image, but it also blurs edges, displaces boundaries, and reduces contrast. It can even introduce artefacts when two nearby structures are averaged together in a way that creates an apparent feature between them. **Figure 15** shows an example in which the lines of the test pattern are blurred by the 11×11 averaging window causing false lines to appear between them.

In Chapter 4 on image enhancement, the use of kernels in which a ring of negative weight values surrounds a positive central peak will be shown. The purpose of this modification is to sharpen edges and avoid some of the blurring that is produced by smoothing out noise. The same method has long been used for the smoothing of one-dimensional signal profiles, such as x-ray diffraction patterns, spectra, or time-varying electronic signals. This is often performed using a Savitsky and Golay (1964) fitting procedure. Tables of coefficients published for this purpose (and intended for efficient application in dedicated computers) are designed to be used just as the weighting coefficients discussed previously, except that they operate in only one dimension. The process is equivalent to performing a least-squares fit of the data points to a polynomial. The smoothed profiles preserve the magnitude of steps while smoothing out noise. **Table 1** lists these coefficients for

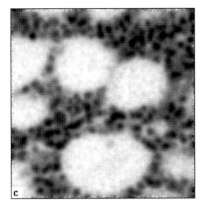

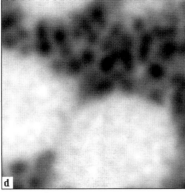

Figure 14. Reduction of noise by Gaussian smoothing (compare with Figure 13a, b): **(a)** *application of a Gaussian filter with standard deviation of 1 pixel;* **(b)** *enlarged to show individual pixel detail.*

*Figure 15. Artefacts due to smoothing. Applying an 11 × 11 smoothing kernel to the test pattern in image **a** produces apparent lines between the original ones, as shown in image **b**.*

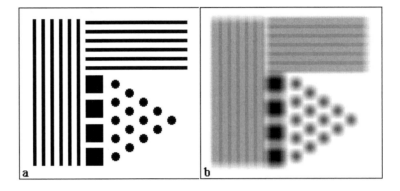

second (quadratic) and fourth (quartic) power polynomials, for fits extending over neighborhoods ranging from 5 to 19 points. These profiles are plotted in **Figure 16**.

This same method can be extended to two dimensions, of course (Edwards, 1982). This can be done either by first applying the coefficients in the horizontal direction and then in the vertical direction, or by constructing a full 2D kernel. **Figure 17** shows the application of a 7 × 7 Savitsky and Golay quadratic polynomial to smooth the image from **Figure 13**.

It is interesting to compare the results of this spatial-domain smoothing to that which can be accomplished in the frequency domain. As discussed in Chapter 5, multiplication of the frequency transform by a convolution function is equivalent to application of a kernel in the spatial domain. The most common noise-filtering method is to remove high frequency information, which represents pixel-to-pixel variations associated with noise. Such removal may be done by setting an aperture on the two-dimensional transform, eliminating higher frequencies, and retransforming. **Figure 18** shows the result of applying this technique to the same image as in **Figure 13**. A circular low-pass filter with radius of 35 pixels and a 10-pixel-wide cosine edge shape (the importance of these parameters is discussed in Chapter 5) was applied. The smoothing is similar to that accomplished in the spatial domain.

As a practical matter, for kernel sizes that are small, or ones that are separable into vertical and horizontal passes like the Gaussian, multiplication and addition of the pixel values in the spatial domain is a faster operation. For kernels that are larger than about 15 × 15 (the limit depends to some extent on the particulars of the individual computer, whether the image can be held entirely in memory or must be accessed from disk, whether multiple processors can be used, etc.) the frequency domain method will be faster; however, because both procedures are mathematically identical, it is generally easier to understand the process based on spatial domain kernels of weights.

Table 1. Savitsky and Golay fitting coefficients

Quadratic polynomial fit

5	7	9	11	13	15	17	19
0	0	0	0	0	0	0	-.0602
0	0	0	0	0	0	-.065	-.0226
0	0	0	0	0	-.0706	-.0186	.0106
0	0	0	0	-.0769	-.0118	.0217	.0394
0	0	0	-.0839	0	.038	.0557	.0637
0	0	-.0909	.021	.0629	.0787	.0836	.0836
0	-.0952	.0606	.1026	.1119	.1104	.1053	.0991
-.0857	.1429	.1688	.1608	.1469	.133	.1207	.1101
.3429	.2857	.2338	.1958	.1678	.1466	.13	.1168
.4857	.3333	.2554	.2075	.1748	.1511	.1331	.119
.3429	.2857	.2338	.1958	.1678	.1466	.13	.1168
-.0857	.1429	.1688	.1608	.1469	.133	.1207	.1101
0	-.0952	.0606	.1026	.1119	.1104	.1053	.0991
0	0	-.0909	.021	.0629	.0787	.0836	.0836
0	0	0	-.0839	0	.038	.0557	.0637
0	0	0	0	-.0769	-.0118	.0217	.0394
0	0	0	0	0	-.0706	-.0186	.0106
0	0	0	0	0	0	-.065	-.0226
0	0	0	0	0	0	0	-.0602

Quartic polynomial fit

5	7	9	11	13	15	17	19
0	0	0	0	0	0	.0464	-.0343
0	0	0	0	0	.0464	-.0464	-.0565
0	0	0	0	.0452	-.0619	-.0619	-.039
0	0	0	.042	-.0814	-.0636	-.0279	.0024
0	0	.035	-.1049	-.0658	-.0036	.0322	.0545
0	.0216	-.1282	-.0233	.0452	.0813	.0988	.1063
.25	-.1299	.0699	.1399	.1604	.1624	.1572	.1494
-.5	.3247	.3147	.2797	.2468	.2192	.1965	.1777
1.5	.5671	.4172	.3333	.2785	.2395	.2103	.1875
-.5	.3247	.3147	.2797	.2468	.2192	.1965	.1777
.25	-.1299	.0699	.1399	.1604	.1624	.1572	.1494
0	.0216	-.1282	-.0233	.0452	.0813	.0988	.1063
0	0	.035	-.1049	-.0658	-.0036	.0322	.0545
0	0	0	.042	-.0814	-.0636	-.0279	.0024
0	0	0	0	.0452	-.0619	-.0619	-.039
0	0	0	0	0	.0464	-.0464	-.0565
0	0	0	0	0	0	.0464	-.0343
0	0	0	0	0	0	0	.0458

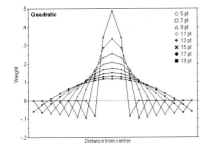 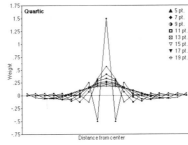

Figure 16. *Savitsky and Golay linear smoothing weights for least squares fitting to quadratic and quartic polynomials.*

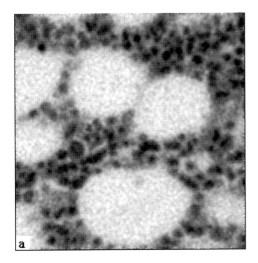 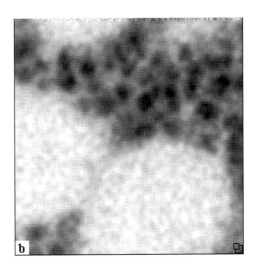

Figure 17. Smoothing with a 7-point wide, quadratic Savitsky and Golay fit:
  (a) same image as **Figure 13**, smoothed;
  (b) enlarged to show pixel detail.

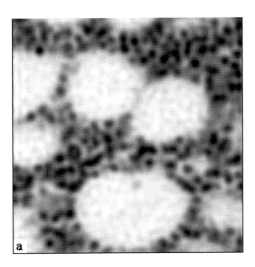 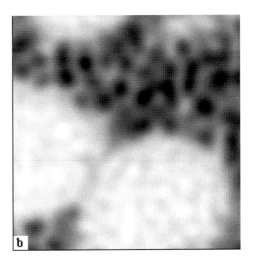

Figure 18. Smoothing in frequency space, using a circular low-pass filter with radius of 35 pixels and a 10-pixel wide cosine edge shape:
  (a) application to image in **Figure 13**;
  (b) enlargement to show pixel detail.

Neighborhood ranking

Smoothing filters do reduce noise, but the underlying assumption is that all of the pixels in the neighborhood represent multiple samples of the same value, in other words, that they all belong to the same feature. Clearly, at edges and boundaries this is not true, and all of the smoothing filters shown above produce some blurring of edges, which is undesirable. The Gaussian filters produce the least edge blurring for a given amount of noise reduction, but cannot eliminate the blurring altogether.

The use of weighting kernels to average together pixels in a neighborhood is a convolution operation, which has a direct counterpart in frequency space image processing. It is a linear operation that uses all of the pixels in the neighborhood, and in which no information is lost from the original image. Other processing operations can be performed in neighborhoods in the spatial domain that also provide noise smoothing. These are not linear and do not utilize or preserve all of the original data.

The most widely used of these methods is based on ranking of the pixels in a neighborhood according to brightness. Then, for example, the median value in this ordered list can be used as the brightness value for the central pixel. As in the case of the kernel operations, this is used to produce a new image and only the original pixel values are used in the ranking for the neighborhood around each pixel.

The median filter is an excellent rejecter of certain kinds of noise, for instance "shot" or impulse noise in which individual pixels are corrupted or missing from the image. If a pixel is accidentally changed to an extreme value, it will be eliminated from the image and replaced by a "reasonable" value, the median value in the neighborhood. This type of noise occurs in CMOS cameras with "dead" transistors that have no output or always put out maximum signals, and in interference microscopes for points on a surface with a locally high slope that returns no light, for example.

Figure 19 shows an example of this type of noise. Ten percent of the pixels in the original image, selected randomly, are set to black, and another ten percent to white. This is a rather extreme amount of noise, but a median filter is able to remove the noise and replace the bad pixels with reasonable values while causing a minimal distortion or degradation of the image. Two different neighborhoods are used: a 3 × 3 square containing a total of nine pixels, and a 5 × 5 octagonal (approximately circular) region containing a total of 21 pixels. **Figure 20** shows several of the neighborhood regions often used for ranking. Of course, the computational effort required rises quickly with the number of values to be sorted, even using specialized methods which keep partial sets of the pixels ranked separately so that as the neighborhood is moved across the image, only a few additional pixel comparisons are needed.

Application of a median filter can also be used to reduce the type of random or speckle noise shown before in the context of averaging. **Figure 21** shows the same image as in **Figure 5**, with a 5 × 5 octagonal median filter applied. There are two principal advantages to the median filter as compared with multiplication by weights. First, the method does not reduce the brightness difference across steps, because the values available are only those present in the neighborhood region, not an average between those values. Second, median filtering does not shift boundaries as averaging may, depending on the relative magnitude of values present in the neighborhood. Overcoming these problems makes the median filter preferred both for visual examination and measurement of images (Huang, 1979, Yang and Huang, 1981).

Figure 22 shows a comparison of uniform averaging, Gaussian filtering, and median filtering applied to a noisy SEM image. The better preservation of edge sharpness by the median filter is apparent. Even with a very large neighborhood (**Figure 22e**) the edges do not shift position, but when the neighborhood radius is larger than the size of any features present, they are eliminated

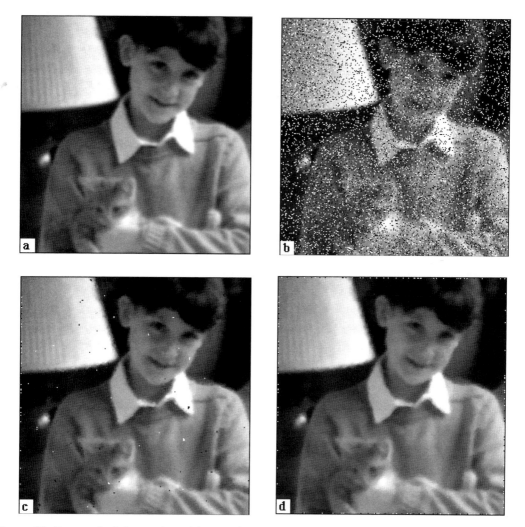

Figure 19. Removal of shot noise with a median filter:
    (a) original image;
    (b) image *a* with 10% of the pixels randomly selected and set to black, and another 10% randomly selected and set to white;
    (c) application of median filtering to image *b* using a 3 × 3 square region;
    (d) application of median filtering to image *b* using a 5 × 5 octagonal region.

and replaced by values from the surrounding background. This is an essential feature of the median filter, which can sometimes be used to advantage to remove dirt or other small, unwanted features from images. For noise reduction purposes, however, it is better to repeat the application of a small median than to use a large one.

Because of the minimal degradation to edges from median filtering, it is possible to apply the method repeatedly. **Figure 23** shows an example in which a 5 × 5 octagonal median filter was applied 12 times to an image. The fine detail is erased in this process, and large regions take on the same brightness values, although the edges remain in place and well defined. This type of leveling of brightness due to repetition of median filtering is sometimes described as contouring or posterization (but those terms also have other meanings that will be presented elsewhere).

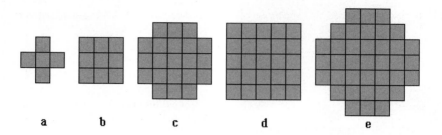

a   b   c   d   e

Figure 20. Neighborhood patterns used for median filtering: (a) *four nearest-neighbor cross;* **(b)** *3 × 3 square containing nine pixels;* **(c)** *5 × 5 octagonal region with 21 pixels;* **(d)** *5 × 5 square containing 25 pixels;* **(e)** *7 × 7 octagonal region containing 37 pixels.*

The concept of a median filter requires a ranking order for the pixels in the neighborhood, which for grey scale images is simply provided by the pixel value. Color images present a challenge to this idea (Sartor and Weeks, 2001; Comer and Delp 1999; Heijmans, 1994). Simple application of the ranking operations to the red, green and blue channels is rarely useful and does not generalize to HSI because hue is an angle that wraps around modulo 360°.

A color median filter can be devised by using as the definition of the median value that pixel whose color coordinates give the smallest sum-of-squares of distances to the other pixels in the neighborhood (Astolo et al., 1990; Oistämö and Neuvo, 1990; Russ, 1995b). The choice of the color space in which these coordinate distances are measured can also present a problem. As discussed earlier, HSI space is generally preferred for processing to RGB space, but there is no unique answer to the question of the relative scaling factors of these different spaces, or how to deal with the angular measure of hue values. **Figure 24** shows an example of an HSI color median filter.

The extension of median filtering (or rank-order filtering in general) from a simple ranking of scalar numbers (the grey scale pixel values) to vectors representing color space values opens the

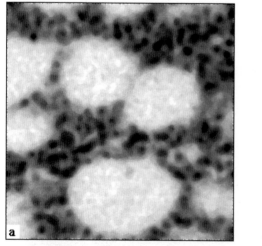

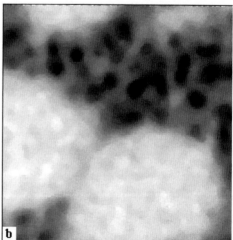

Figure 21. Smoothing with a median filter:
    (a) *the same image as in* **Figure 13** *after application of a 5 × 5 octagonal median filter;*
    (b) *enlargement of image* **a** *to show individual pixels.*

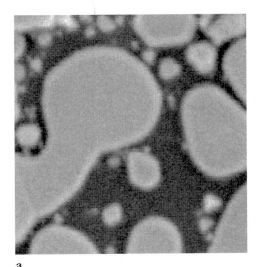

a

Figure 22. Comparison of noise reduction techniques (SEM image enlarged to show pixel detail):
(a) original;
(b) 5 × 5 uniform averaging;
(c) Gaussian filter, standard deviation = 1 pixel;
(d) median filter, 5× 5 octagonal region;
(e) median filter, radius = 15 pixels.

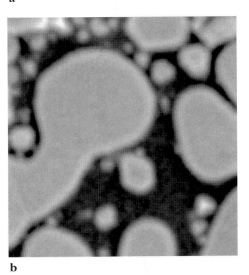

b

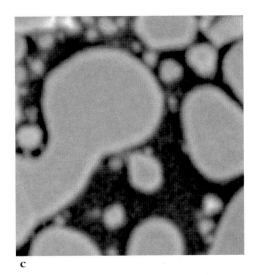

c

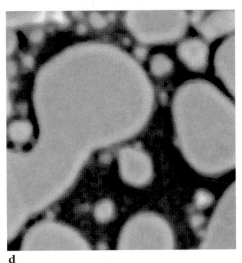

d

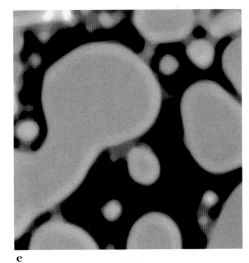

e

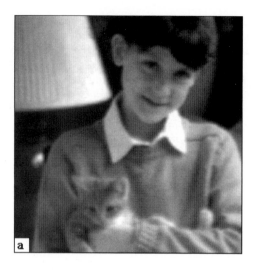

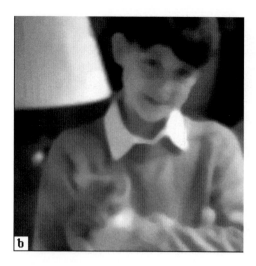

Figure 23. Repeated application of a 5 × 5 octagonal median filter: (a) *original image;* **(b)** *after 12 applications — the fine details have been erased and textured regions leveled to a uniform shade of grey, but boundaries have not shifted.*

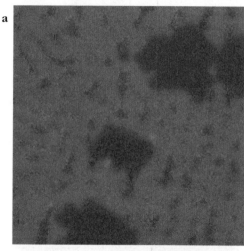

Figure 24. Color image (light micrograph of a metal alloy) with speckle noise, enlarged to show pixel detail:
(a) *original;*
(b) *3 × 3 color median filter applied;*
(c) *median repeated five times.*

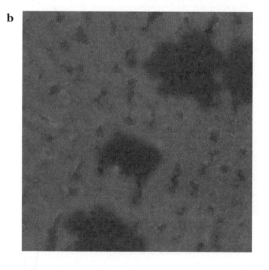

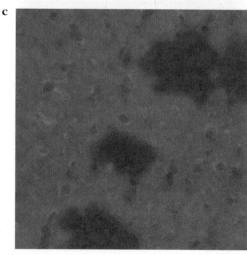

door to more complex uses of vector ranking. Instead of the vector length, it is possible to construct rankings based on vector angles to remove vectors (colors) that point in atypical directions, or hybrid methods that combine direction and distance (Smolka et al., 2001). Vectors need not be restricted to three dimensions, so it is possible to combine many criteria into a total measure of pixel similarity. The performance of these methods is bought at the price of computational complexity, but it is possible in some cases to reconstruct images corrupted by up to 70% noise pixels with quite good accuracy.

Sharpening of edges can be accomplished even better with a mode filter (Davies, 1988). The mode of the distribution of brightness values in each neighborhood is, by definition, the most likely value; however, for a small neighborhood, the mode is poorly defined. An approximation to this value can be obtained with a truncated median filter. For any asymmetric distribution, such as would be obtained at most locations near but not precisely straddling an edge, the mode is the highest point, and the median lies closer to the mode than the mean value. This is illustrated in **Figure 25**. The truncated median technique consists of discarding a few values from the neighborhood so that the median value of the remaining pixels is shifted toward the mode. In the example shown in **Figure 26**, this is done for a 3 × 3 neighborhood by skipping the two pixels whose brightness values are most different from the mean, ranking the remaining seven values, and assigning the median to the central pixel.

Another modification to the median filter is used to overcome its tendency to erase lines which are narrower than the half-width of the neighborhood, and to round corners. The so-called hybrid median, or corner-preserving median, is actually a three-step ranking operation (Nieminen et al., 1987). In a 5 × 5 pixel neighborhood, pixels may be ranked in two different groups as shown in **Figure 27**. The median values of the 45-degree neighbors forming an "X" and the 90-degree neighbors forming a "+" (both groups include the central pixel) are compared to the central pixel and the median value of that set is then saved as the new pixel value. As shown in **Figure 28**, this method preserves lines and corners which are erased or rounded off by the conventional median. In a larger neighborhood, more orientations can be employed; four directions can be used in a 5 × 5 region, producing four values that can be ranked along with the original central pixel.

If the hybrid median filter is applied repeatedly, it can also produce posterization. Because the details of lines and corners are preserved by the hybrid median, the shapes of regions are not smoothed as they are with the conventional median, although the brightness values across steps are still sharpened and posterized, as illustrated in **Figure 29**.

The fact that the hybrid median involves multiple ranking operations, first within each of the groups of pixels and then to compare those medians to the central pixel, does not impose a computational penalty. Each of the ranking operations is for a much smaller number of values than used in a square or octagonal region of the same size. For example, the 5-pixel wide neighborhood

Figure 25. Schematic diagram of an asymmetric histogram distribution of brightness values, showing the relationship between the mode, median and mean. The truncated median filter works by discarding the values in the distribution which are farthest from the mean, and then using the median of the remainder as an estimate for the mode. For a symmetrical distribution values are discarded from both ends and the median value does not change (it is already equal to the mode).

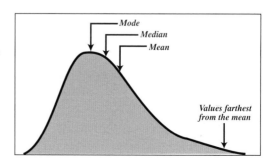

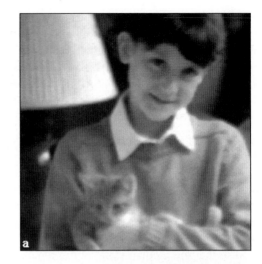

Figure 26. Application of the truncated median filter to posterize the image from Figure 23a:
(a) one application of the 3 × 3 truncated median;
(b) difference between **Figure 26a** and a conventional 3 × 3 median filter, showing the difference in values along edges;
(c) 12 applications of the truncated median filter.

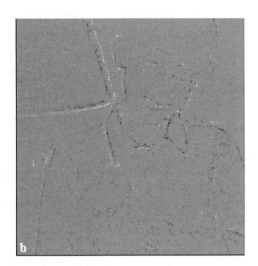

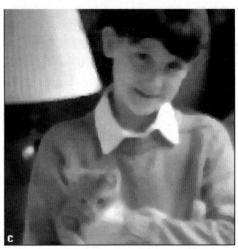

used in the examples contains either 25 (in the square neighborhood) or 21 pixels (in the octagonal neighborhood) which must be ranked in the traditional method. In the hybrid method, each of the groups contains only 9 pixels, and the final comparison involves only three or five values. Even with the additional logic and manipulation of values, the hybrid method is about as fast as the conventional median.

Posterizing an image, or reducing the number of grey levels so that regions become uniform in grey value and edges between regions become abrupt, falls more into the category of enhancement than correcting defects, but is included here as a side effect of median filtering. Other methods can produce this effect. One that is related to the median is the extremum filter, which replaces each pixel value with either the minimum or maximum value in the neighborhood, whichever is closer to the mean value. **Figure 30** shows this operator applied to the image from **Figure 19**. This filter is not edge-preserving and may shift boundaries. When the extremum filter is iterated, it is sometimes called a "toggle" filter (Arce et al., 2000).

Sometimes it is useful to construct a neighborhood that is not round, but has a specific shape based on independent knowledge about the nature of the image. A common defect in video images is the appearance of horizontal lines that indicate variations in signal between the two interlaced fields. A similar defect occurs in atomic force microscope images due to DC signal offsets.

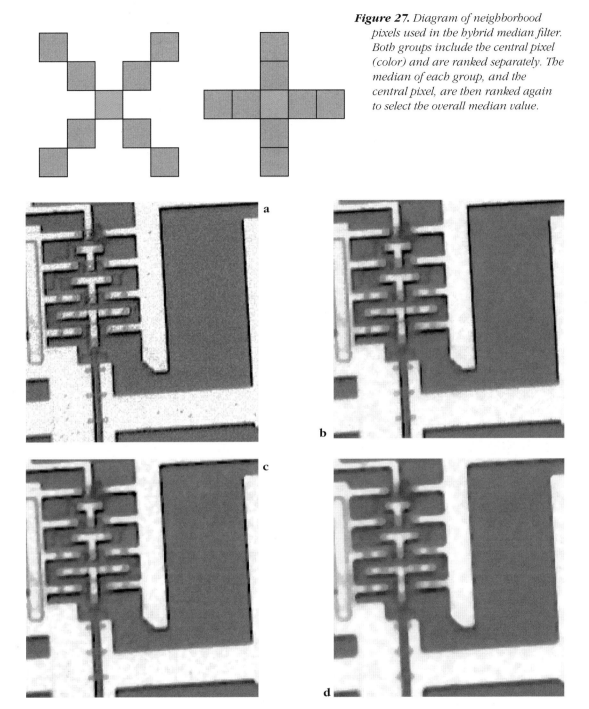

Figure 27. Diagram of neighborhood pixels used in the hybrid median filter. Both groups include the central pixel (color) and are ranked separately. The median of each group, and the central pixel, are then ranked again to select the overall median value.

Figure 28. Application of the hybrid median filter to a light microscope image of an integrated circuit, showing the improved retention of lines and corners:

(a) original image with noise;

(b) application of the 5 × 5 hybrid median filter;

(c) application of a conventional 3 ×3 median, which does not remove all of the noise but still degrades corners and edges somewhat;

(d) application of a conventional 5 × 5 octagonal median filter, showing its greater rounding of corners and elimination of edges.

Figure 29. Repeated application of the hybrid median filter to the noisy image in Figure 10:
(a) original image;
(b) zoomed portion of **Figure 29a** showing individual pixels;
(c) repeated application of a conventional 5-pixel wide median filter;
(d) zoomed portion of **Figure 29c** showing individual pixels;
(e) repeated application of the hybrid 5-pixel wide median filter;
(f) zoomed portion of **Figure 29e** showing individual pixels.
Notice that the brightness values are posterized and smoothed and edge contrast is sharpened, but the shapes of features and edges are not smoothed.

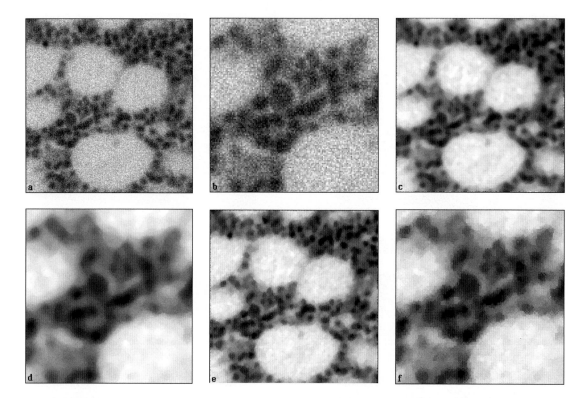

Movie film often exhibits vertical scratches resulting from wear and tear and rubbing against transport devices. If the direction of the lines or scratches is known, a neighborhood may be constructed to remove it.

Figure 31 shows an example of video line noise in a poor quality surveillance tape. This is a common defect that can arise from dirty recording heads, for example. A median neighborhood that is vertical but only one pixel wide can eliminate much of the line noise. Similarly, **Figure 32** shows horizontal streaks in a low voltage SEM image in which the scan rate was too high for the amplifier time constant, which blurs information along the scan line direction. Again, a median filter applied in a vertical stripe corrects the problem.

In most simple cases the neighborhood used in a ranking operation such as a median filter is circular with a radius selected on the basis of the size of the smallest features to be retained. For computational simplicity, a square neighborhood is sometimes used, which can introduce some directional bias into the results. It is also possible to use an adaptive neighborhood, one that includes

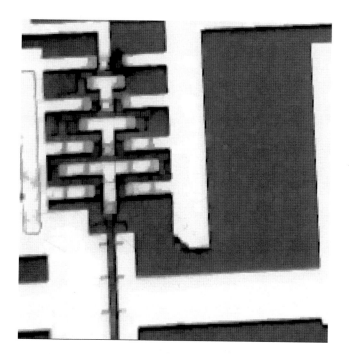

Figure 30. Posterization of the image from *Figure 28*, produced by applying a 3 × 3 extremum filter which replaces each pixel value with either the minimum or maximum value in the neighborhood, whichever is closer to the mean value.

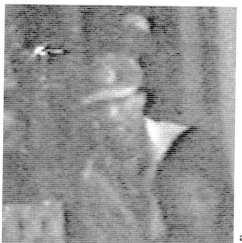

a

Figure 31. Surveillance video image with horizontal scan line noise *(a)*, a custom neighborhood to perform median filtering only in a vertical direction *(b)*, and the result *(c)*.

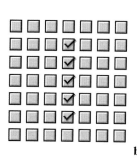

b

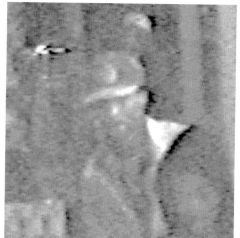

c

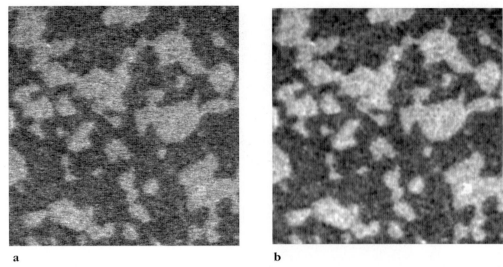

a   b

Figure 32. Low-voltage SEM image of a thin film, with horizontal streaking (a), and the result of applying a vertical median filter (b).

pixels based on their value and position. In general, the goal is to select for ranking a set of N (a small odd number) pixel values. There are several possible methods, all of which start with a larger neighborhood of candidate pixels which are then included in the ranking if they meet additional criteria, which may be used in combination:

1. Pixels where the difference from the central pixel is less than some adjustable threshold
2. The N pixels within the larger neighborhood that are closest in value to the central pixel
3. The N pixels within the larger neighborhood that are closest in value to the central pixel and are contiguous with it and with each other (Kober et al., 2001)

It is also possible to weight the pixels according to their distance from the central pixel, by entering nearby pixel values more than once into the list to be ranked. Generally, at the expense of computational complexity, these methods produce good rejection of impulsive noise (as does the conventional median) and improved rejection of additive random noise.

Other neighborhood noise-reduction methods

A modification to the simple averaging of neighborhood values that attempts to achieve some of the advantages of the median filter is the so-called Olympic filter. The name comes from the system of scoring used in some events in the Olympic games, in which the highest and lowest scores are discarded and the remainder averaged. The same thing is done with the pixel values in the neighborhood. By discarding the extreme values, shot noise is rejected. Then the average of the remaining pixel values is used as the new brightness.

Figure 33 shows an application of this method to the image from **Figure 13**, containing Gaussian noise (random intensity variations or speckle). Because it still causes blurring of edges and still requires sorting of the brightness values, this method is generally inferior to the others discussed and is not often used. **Figure 34** shows an application to the shot noise introduced in **Figure 19**. The performance is quite poor: the features are blurred and yet the noise is not all removed.

Other versions of modified or conditional smoothing omit some of the pixel values in the moving neighborhood from the smoothing operation. The justification is always based on the omitted pixels being different from those that are used, so that they presumably belong to a different region.

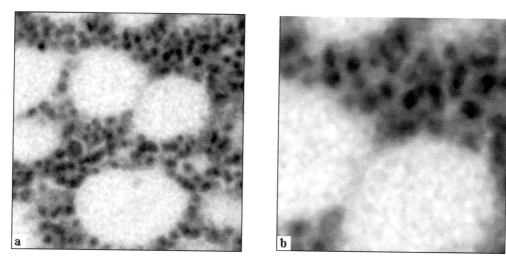

Figure 33. Application of an Olympic filter to Gaussian noise. The four brightest and four darkest pixels in each 5 × 5 neighborhood are ignored and the remaining 17 averaged to produce a new image: (a) application to the image in Figure 10; (b) enlargement to show pixel detail.

Most of the techniques take into account both the location of the pixel in the region and the difference in the value from the original central pixel. For example, fitting a function to the pixels may be used to detect a sharp change in the slope and to omit pixels that lie beyond the edge ("kriging"). **Figure 35** shows one example of such a conditional smoothing process. It does reduce noise, but is not obviously superior to a simple median. All of these methods make some assumptions about the nature of the image and of the noise present, and the better the assumptions fit the actual image, the better the result.

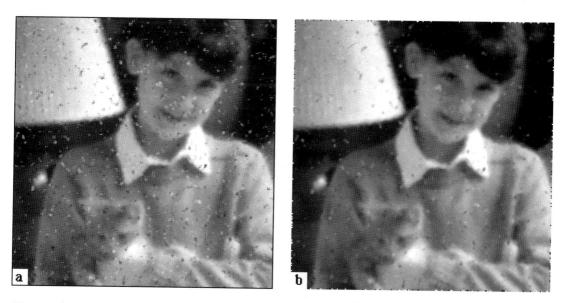

Figure 34. Application of Olympic filter to shot noise. The original image is the same as in Figure 13: (a) the two brightest and two darkest pixels in each 3 × 3 neighborhood are ignored and the remaining five averaged; (b) the four brightest and four darkest pixels in each 5 × 5 neighborhood are ignored and the remaining 17 averaged.

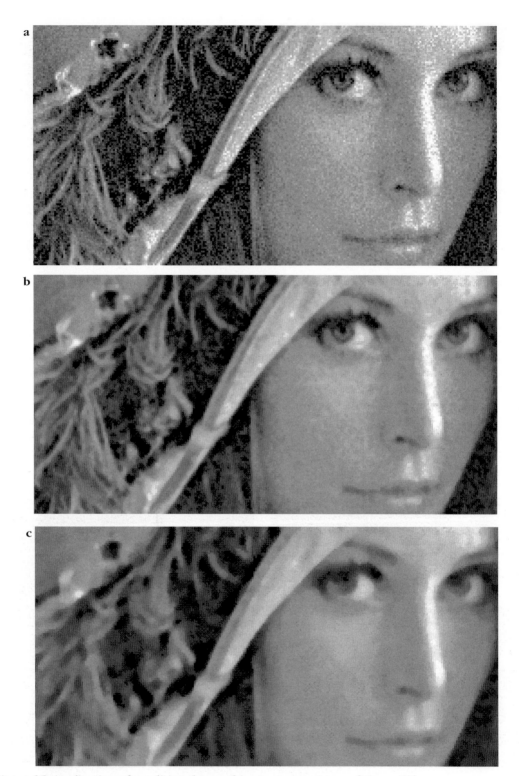

Figure 35. Application of conditional smoothing to a noisy image (Figure 19):
   (a) original;
   (b) conditional smoothing that estimates boundary locations and performs smoothing only using pixels within each region;
   (c) median filter (5-pixel wide octagonal neighborhood).

Other, more complicated combinations of operations are used for very specific types of images. For instance, synthetic aperture radar (SAR) images contain speckle noise which varies in a known way with the image brightness. To remove the noise, the brightness of each pixel is compared to the average value of a local neighborhood. If it exceeds it by an amount calculated from the average and the standard deviation, then it is replaced by a weighted average value. Using some coefficients determined by experiment, the method is reported (Nathan and Curlander, 1990) to perform better at improving signal-to-noise than a simple median filter. This is a good example of an ad hoc processing method based on knowledge of the characteristics of the signal and the noise in a particular situation. In general, any filtering method that chooses between several algorithms or modifies its algorithm based on the actual contents of the image or the neighborhood is called an adaptive filter (Mastin, 1985).

Noise is often modeled as a Gaussian additive function, and noise reduction methods are often tested by adding Gaussian noise to an image, but in fact various noise sources have very widely differing characteristics. Noise that arises from photon or particle counting is generally Poisson, which becomes Gaussian for large numbers. The distribution of exposed grains in film is also approximately Gaussian. The effect of electronic circuitry in cameras and amplifiers can be either additive or multiplicative, and generally affects dark areas differently from bright ones. Noise resulting from light scattering in the atmosphere or from surfaces is generally multiplicative rather than additive. Speckle interferometry encountered in radar imaging is more complex, since it interacts through shifts in phase and polarization. It also tends to have a spatial correlation, which makes it more difficult to model. The removal of speckle by acquiring many short duration images is beyond the scope of this text.

Another way of filtering by ranking is to use the maximum and minimum brightness rather than the median. **Figure 36** shows the results of a two-step operation. First, the brightest pixel value in each region (a 5 × 5 octagonal neighborhood) was used to replace the original pixel values. Then in a second transformation, the darkest pixel value in each region was selected. This type of combined operation requires two full passes through the image, and during each pass only the previous pixel brightness values are used to derive the new ones.

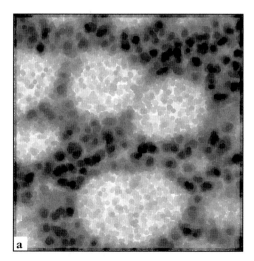 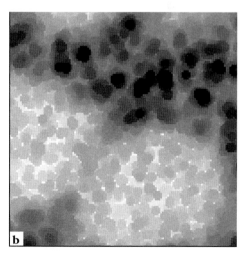

Figure 36. *Grey-scale opening, or erosion and dilation. Two separate ranking operations are performed on the original image from **Figure 5**. First each pixel value is replaced with the brightest value in the neighborhood (5 × 5 octagonal); then using this image, each pixel value is replaced by the darkest value in the same size neighborhood: **(a)** result; **(b)** enlarged to show pixel detail.*

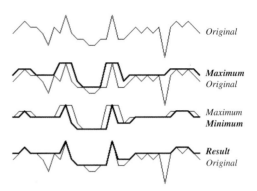

Figure 37. Schematic diagram of the operation of grey-scale erosion and dilation in one dimension, showing (starting from the top): *the original profile with result of first (maximum) pass, producing a new profile through brightest points; the second step in which a new profile passes through the darkest (minimum) points in the result from step 1; comparison of the final result to the original profile, showing rejection of noise and dark spikes but retention of bright features.*

For reasons that will be discussed in more detail in Chapter 7, this type of operation is often described as a grey-scale erosion and dilation, by analogy to the erosion and dilation steps which are performed on binary images. The sequence is also called an opening, again by analogy to operations on binary images. By adjusting the sizes of the neighborhoods (which need not be the same) used in the two separate passes, to locate the brightest and then the darkest values, other processing effects are obtained. These are described in Chapter 4.

As a method for removing noise, this technique would seem to be the antithesis of a median filter, which discards extreme values. It may be helpful to visualize the image as a surface for which the brightness represents an elevation. **Figure 37** shows a one-dimensional representation of such a situation. In the first pass, the brightest values in each region are used to construct a new profile which follows the "tops of the trees." In the second pass, the darkest values in each region are used to bring the profile back down to those points which were large enough to survive the first one, giving a new profile that ignores the dark noise spikes in the original while retaining the bright features. Applying the same operations in the other order (erosion followed by dilation) would have removed bright noise while retaining dark features.

Another method that uses ranking, but in two different size neighborhoods, is useful for locating and removing noise. It is often called a "top hat" or "rolling ball" filter. Imagine the brightness values of the pixels to represent the elevation of a surface. A top hat filter consists of a flat disk that rests on the surface, and a central crown of a smaller diameter, as shown in **Figure 38**. This filter is centered on each pixel in the image, with the brim "resting" on the surface. Any pixels that "stick up" through the crown of the hat are considered to be noise, and replaced. The replacement value may be either the mean or the median value of the pixels covered by the brim of the hat.

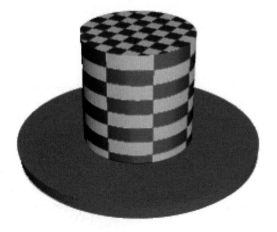

Figure 38. *Diagram of a top hat filter. The brim (red) rests on the "surface" that corresponds to the brightness of pixels in the image. Any pixel with a brightness value able to rise through the crown of the hat is detected and can be replaced with the mean or median of the outer neighborhood. The inner and outer radius of the brim and the height of the crown are all adjustable parameters.*

The implementation of this filter uses two neighborhoods, one a round (or approximately round) region corresponding to the inside or crown of the hat, and a second annular neighborhood surrounding it that corresponds to the brim. In each, the maximum (brightest) value is found. If the difference between the brightest pixel in the interior region and the outside exceeds a threshold (the height of the hat) then the pixel value is replaced with the mean or median of the outside region.

An adaptation of this same logic to a trench-shaped neighborhood (a line of pixels forming the inner region, with parallel lines on both sides forming the outer region) can be used to effectively find and remove scratches, provided they have a known direction. This technique is sometimes used to remove scratches when digitizing film.

If the sense of the brightness values is reversed and darkest pixels are the target of the filter, it is usually called a rolling ball filter. The symbolism is that a sphere rolling on the surface will be unable to touch the bottom of the pit represented by the dark noise pixel. **Figure 39** shows an example. The dust particles on the slide are all smaller than 9 pixels across, so a filter consisting of an inner circle with a radius of 4 pixels and an outer one with a radius of 6 pixels forms the top hat. The dust particles are removed, but because the bug itself is too large to fit inside the inner circle, there is no large difference between the darkest values in the two neighborhoods and the pixels are not altered.

In the next chapter, we will consider the use of this same filter for a different purpose. Instead of removing extreme points as noise, the same operation can be used to find points of interest that are smaller than the crown of the hat and brighter or darker than the local neighborhood. In that case, the points that do *not* protrude through the crown are suppressed, and only those that do are kept. **Figure 39c** also illustrates this property of the top hat. Using the same settings for neighborhood size, but keeping the extreme values and suppressing those that do not have a difference greater than the top hat threshold reveals just the dust particles on the slide.

Defect removal, maximum entropy, and maximum likelihood

As shown, the rolling ball/top hat filter can be used to remove small defects by replacing the pixels with a value taken from the surrounding neighborhood. A more general approach to this type of replacement is to interpolate the replacement values. Real images often contain discrete localized defects, either originating in the specimen itself or in the camera (e.g., dirt on the lens). If the defect is large and irregular in shape, smoothing may leave some of the pixel values from the defect remaining in the resulting image, and it may be impractical to use a neighborhood for rank-based filtering that is large enough to encompass it. In many cases, better results can be obtained by filling in the region of the defect using the adjacent values. In the example shown in **Figure 40**, a hole in a leaf has been manually circled and the pixels replaced by linear interpolation between the edge pixels. The algorithm is similar in effect to stretching a membrane across an irregular opening with an edge of variable height. The elastic membrane forms a lowest-energy surface. Calculating the pixel values within the region is accomplished in the same way.

Instead of manual outlining, regions may be selected by any of the thresholding techniques discussed in Chapter 6. These include specifying a range of brightness or color values that discriminate the defects from their surroundings, or using a region-growing method in which selecting one point in the defect allows the software to include all touching similar pixels. In **Figure 41**, this method was used to select the yellow flower. Then the region was enlarged by two pixels (using dilation, a method discussed in Chapter 7), and the background interpolated from the edge pixels of the region. This approach can be quite useful for removing manually selected features from images. Subtracting the modified image from the original produces an image of just the removed feature, as shown.

Figure 39. Operation of the rolling ball/top hat filter:
(a) original image showing dust particles on the slide next to the insect;
(b) removal of the dust particles by the filter;
(c) image of just the dust particles obtained by keeping only those pixels that are found by the filter.

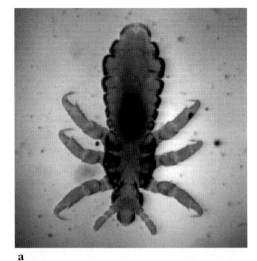

a

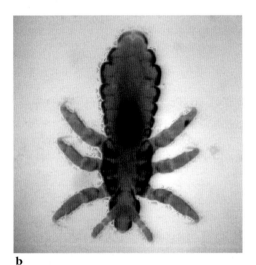

b

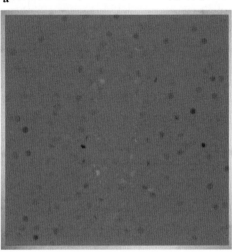

c

Images may contain other defects, such as blur due to motion or out-of-focus optics, in addition to noise. The "inverse filtering" methods described in Chapter 5 under the topic of deconvolution are quite noise sensitive. When the noise that is present can itself be characterized, it may be possible to use a maximum entropy approach to remove the artefacts.

Maximum entropy methods represent a computer-intensive approach to removing artefacts such as noise or blur from images, based on some foreknowledge about the image contents and some assumptions about the nature of the degradation that is to be removed and the image restored (Skilling, 1986; Frieden, 1988). The conventional description of the method is to imagine an image containing N pixels, that has been formed by a total of M photons (where usually $M \gg N$). The number of photons in any single pixel (i.e., the pixel's brightness value) is P_i where i is the pixel brightness value.

The measured image has normalized pixel brightness values $p_i = \sum P_i / M$ that only approximate the "true" image that would be collected if there were no artefacts. The p_i values are just the image histogram. The method used to approach this ideal image is to alter pixel brightness values to maximize the entropy in the image, subject to some constraints. The justification for this method is given in terms of statistical probability and Bayes' theorem, and will not be derived here. In some cases this method produces dramatic improvements in image quality.

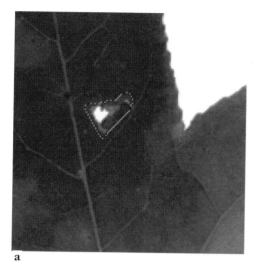
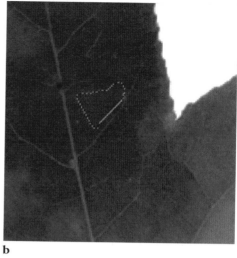

Figure 40. Defect removal by interpolating from the edges of a region:
(a) image of a maple leaf (enlarged) showing a manually drawn region around a hole;
(b) interpolation of values from the edge.

Figure 41. Removing a large feature from a complex image:
(a) selection of a region around a yellow flower (enlarged) by region growing as described in the text;
(b) interpolated background;
(c) difference between **a** and **b**, showing just the removed feature on a varying background.

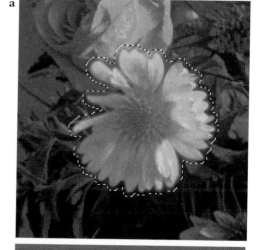
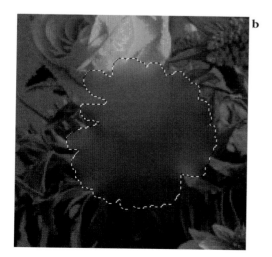
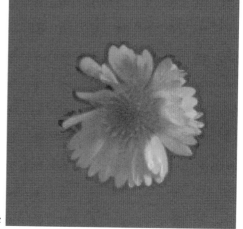

The "entropy" of the brightness pattern is given in a formal sense by calculating the number of ways that the pattern could have been formed by rearrangement, or $S = M!/p_1! \, p_2!, \ldots p_N!$ where ! indicates factorial. For large values of M, this reduces by Stirling's approximation to the more familiar $S = -\sum p_i \log p_i$. This is the same calculation of entropy used in statistical mechanics. In the particular case of taking the log to the base 2, the entropy of the image is the number of bits per pixel needed to represent the image, according to information theory.

The entropy in the image would be maximized in an absolute sense simply by setting the brightness of each pixel to the average brightness. Clearly, this is not the "right" solution. It is the application of constraints that produce usable results. The most common constraint for images containing noise is based on a chi-squared statistic, calculated as $\chi^2 = 1/\sigma^2 \sum (p_i - p_i')^2$. In this expression the p_i values are the original pixel values and the p_i' are the altered brightness values, and σ is the standard deviation of the values. An upper limit can be set on the value of χ^2 allowed in the calculation of a new set of p_i' values to maximize the entropy. A typical (but essentially arbitrary) limit for χ^2 is N, the number of pixels in the array.

This constraint is not the only possible choice. A sum of the absolute value of differences, or some other weighting rule, could also be chosen. This is not quite enough information to produce an optimal image, and so other constraints may be added. One is that the totals of the p_i and p_i' values must be equal. Bryan and Skilling (1980) also require, for instance, that the distribution of the p_i – p_i' values corresponds to the expected noise characteristics of the imaging source (e.g., a Poisson or Gaussian distribution for simple counting statistics). And, of course, we must be careful to include such seemingly "obvious" constraints as non-negativity (no pixel can collect fewer than zero photons). Jaynes (1985) makes the point that there is practically always a significant amount of real knowledge about the image which can be used as constraints, but which is assumed to be so obvious that it is ignored.

An iterative solution for the values of p_i' produces a new image with the desired smoothness and noise characteristics which are often improved from the original image. Other formulations of the maximum entropy approach may compare one iteration of the image to the next, by calculating not the total entropy but the cross entropy, $-\sum p_i \log (p_i/q_i)$ where q_i is the previous image brightness value for the same pixel, or the modeled brightness for a theoretical image. In this formulation, the cross entropy is to be minimized. The basic principle remains the same.

Maximum likelihood reconstruction of an image is another related approach in which the assumption is made that the boundaries between regions should be sharp. In most real images, pixels that straddle any boundary average values from both sides according the exact placement of the edge with respect to the finite size of the pixel. This leads to intermediate brightness or color values that appear to blur the boundary. Reclassifying the pixels to the brightness of one region or the other sharpens the boundaries.

One of the most common statistical approaches to the classification measures the variance of pixels in many subregions of a neighborhood around each pixel as shown in **Figure 42**. Whichever region has the lowest variance is taken to represent the region to which the central pixel should belong, and it is assigned the mean value from that subregion (Kuwahara et al., 1976). **Figure 43** shows an application of the method.

When applied to halftoned images that have been digitized with a scanner, this filter can eliminate the halftone patterns as shown in **Figure 44**. Also note that for real objects such as the flowers and leaves shown, in which the edges of objects are naturally shaded, the filter converts the appearance to that of a painting or cartoon.

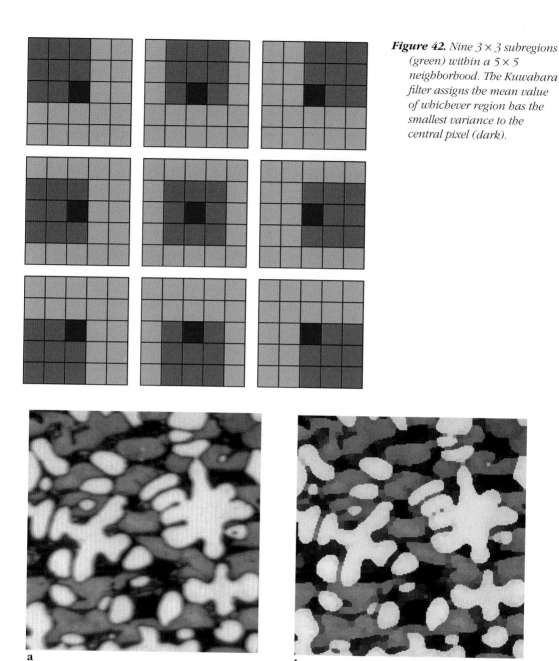

Figure 42. Nine 3 × 3 subregions (green) within a 5 × 5 neighborhood. The Kuwahara filter assigns the mean value of whichever region has the smallest variance to the central pixel (dark).

Figure 43. Application of a maximum likelihood filter:
(a) original image (enlarged to show pixel detail);
(b) filter applied, resulting in sharp region boundaries.

Nonuniform illumination

The most straightforward strategy for image analysis uses the brightness of regions in the image as a means of identification: it is assumed that the same type of feature will have the same brightness (or color, in a color image) wherever it appears in the field of view. If this brightness is different from that of other features, or can be made so by appropriate image processing as discussed in Chapter 4, then it can be used to discriminate the features for counting,

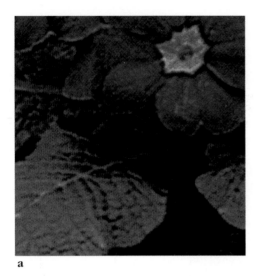 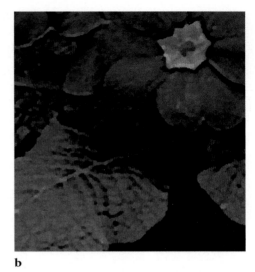

a

b

Figure 44. Application of the maximum likelihood filter to a scanned image with halftone:
  (a) original;
  (b) filter applied.

measurement or identification. Even if there are a few other types of objects that cannot be distinguished on the basis of brightness or color alone, subsequent measurements may suffice to select the ones of interest.

This approach is not without pitfalls, which are discussed further in Chapter 7 in conjunction with converting grey scale images to binary (black-and-white) images. Other approaches are available such as region growing or split-and-merge that do not have such stringent requirements for uniformity of illumination. Simple brightness thresholding, when it can be used, is by far the simplest and fastest method to isolate features in an image, and it is important to consider the problems of shading of images.

When irregular surfaces are viewed, the amount of light scattered to the viewer or camera from each region is a function of the orientation of the surface with respect to the source of light and the viewer, even if the surface material and finish is uniform. In fact, this principle can be used to estimate the surface orientation, using a technique known as shape-from-shading. Human vision seems to apply these rules very easily and rapidly because we are not generally confused by images of real-world objects. We will not pursue those methods here, however.

Most of the images we really want to process are essentially two-dimensional. Whether they come from light or electron microscopes, or satellite images, the variation in surface elevation is usually small compared to the lateral dimensions, giving rise to what is often called "two-and-one-half D." This is not always the case of course (consider a woven fabric examined in the SEM), but we will treat such problems as exceptions to the general rule and recognize that more elaborate processing may be needed.

Even surfaces of low relief need not be flat, a simple example being the curvature of the earth as viewed from a weather satellite. This will produce a shading across the field of view, as will illumination of a macroscopic or microscopic surface from one side. Even elaborate collections of lights, or ring lights, can only approximate uniform illumination of the scene.

For transmission imaging, the uniformity of the light source with a condenser lens system can be made quite good, but it is easy for these systems to get out of perfect alignment and produce shading as well. Finally, it was mentioned in Chapter 1 that lenses or the cameras themselves may cause vignetting, in which the corners of the image are darker than the center because the light is partially absorbed.

Most of these defects can be minimized by careful setup of the imaging conditions, or if they cannot be eliminated altogether, can be assumed to be constant over some period of time. This assumption allows correction by image processing. In many instances, it is possible to acquire a "background" image in which a uniform reference surface or specimen is inserted in place of the actual samples to be viewed, and the light intensity recorded. This image can then be used to "level" the subsequent images. The process is often called "background subtraction" but, in many cases, this is a misnomer. If the image acquisition device is logarithmic with a gamma of 1.0, then subtraction of the background image point-by-point from each acquired image is correct. If the camera or sensor is linear, then the correct procedure is to divide the acquired image by the background. For other sensor response functions, there is no simple correct arithmetic method, and the calibrated response must first be determined and applied to convert the measured signal to a linear or logarithmic space.

In the process of subtracting (or dividing) one image by another, some of the dynamic range of the original data will be lost. The greater the variation in background brightness, the less the remaining variation from that level can be recorded in the image and will be left after the leveling process. This loss and the inevitable increase in statistical noise that results from subtracting one signal from another argue that all practical steps should be taken first to make illumination uniform before acquiring the images, before resorting to processing methods.

Figure 83 in Chapter 1 showed an example of leveling in which the background illumination function could be acquired separately. This acquisition is most commonly done by removing the specimen from the light path, for instance a slide, and storing an image representing the variation. This image can then be used for leveling, although in many cases, it is not practical to remove the specimen, or its presence is a contributor to the brightness variation. This includes situations in which the specimen thickness varies and so the overall absorption of light is affected. Another case is that in which the surface being examined is not perfectly flat, which causes incident light or SEM images to show a varying background.

Figure 45 shows an example of the latter type. The SEM image shows particles on a substrate, which because of the geometry of the surface and of the SEM chamber causes a portion of the image to appear darker than the rest. The human eye is quite tolerant of this kind of gradual brightness variation, and so it is sometimes helpful to apply pseudo-color lookup tables to reveal the shading present in the image. Moving the specimen or changing the magnification alters the pattern of light and dark, in which case it is necessary to perform the correction using the image itself. Fortunately, in many of these situations the variation of background brightness is a smooth and well behaved function of location and can be approximated by simple functions such as polynomials. The leveling in the figure was performed using this method.

Figure 46 shows a situation in which the brightness variation can be extracted directly from the original image. By separating the red, green, and blue planes from the image it is seen that the green image contains the important detail: the blood vessels in the retina of the eye, which are difficult to view because of the overall brightness variation. The red image has nearly the same variation so the ratio of the green to red levels the varying background and makes the vessels more uniform in contrast.

Another situation in which direct measurement of two images allows dividing to correct for nonuniform brightness arises in the transmission electron microscope. It is common, particularly for inorganic samples in materials science, for the specimens to vary in thickness. Computing the ratio of the conventional brightfield image to the zero-loss electrons isolated by a spectrometer attached to the microscope gives a direct measure of the variation in specimen thickness, which can subsequently be used to quantify concentration and structural measurements.

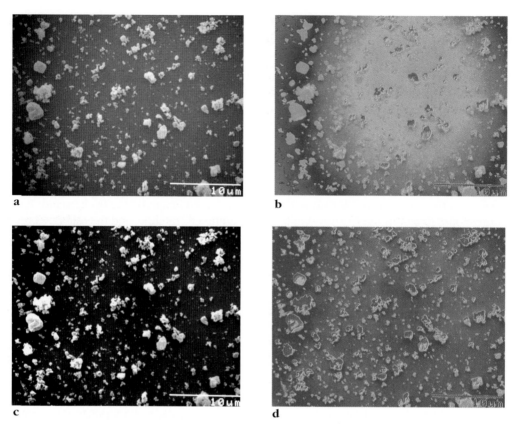

Figure 45. Leveling image contrast:
  (**a**) *SEM image of particulates on a substrate;*
  (**b**) *pseudo-color applied to a to make the shading more visually evident;*
  (**c**) *image leveled by polynomial fitting;*
  (**d**) *pseudo-color applied to **c**.*

Fitting a background function

By selecting a number of points in the image, a list of brightness values and locations can be acquired. These can then used to perform least-squares fitting of a function B(x, y) that approximates the background, and can be subtracted (or divided) just as a physically acquired background image would be. When the user marks these points, for instance by using a pointing device such as a mouse, trackball or light pen, it is important to select locations that should all have the same brightness and are well distributed across the image. Locating many points in one small region and few or none in other parts of the image requires the function to extrapolate the polynomial, and can introduce significant errors. For a second-order polynomial, the functional form of the fitted background is

$$B(x,y) = a0 + a_1 \cdot x + a_2 \cdot y + a_3 \cdot x^2 + a_4 \cdot y^2 + a_5 \cdot xy \qquad (2)$$

This polynomial has six fitted constants, and so in principle could be fitted with only that number of marked points. Likewise, a third-order polynomial would have ten coefficients; however, in order to get a good fit and diminish sensitivity to minor fluctuations in individual pixels, and to have

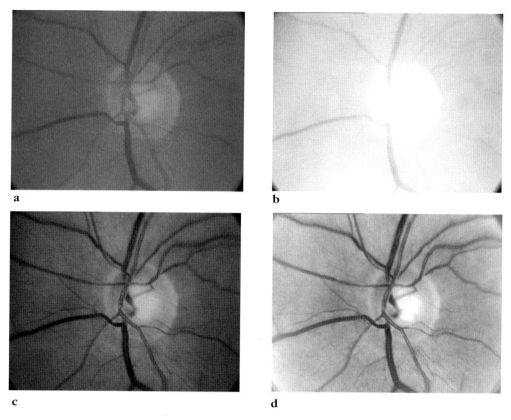

a   b

c   d

Figure 46. Leveling with a measured background:
   (a) retina image from an opthalmoscope, showing shading that makes the capillaries difficult to discern;
   (b) red channel contains no detail but does show the shading;
   (c) green channel has most of the contrast in the image;
   (d) ratio of green to red shows more uniform contrast (original image courtesy George Mansoor, University of Connecticut Health Care).

enough points to sample the entire image area properly, it is usual to require several times this minimum number of points.

Figure 47 shows an example in which a background region can be selected in this way. Points around the periphery of the stamp should all be the same in brightness but vary because of nonuniform illumination. Selecting that region, fitting a polynomial function to it, and subtracting it (because this is a digitized photograph, subtraction is appropriate), levels the resulting image of the background and also the stamp. Notice that one effect of leveling is to make the peaks in the image histogram much narrower, since all of the pixels in the same region have more nearly the same value. Comparison of this result with **Figure 41c** shows that the edge interpolation method is somewhat inferior (note the color shift in the flower) because it provides only linear interpolation and uses fewer pixel values to define the background brightness.

In some cases, it is practical to automatically locate the points for background fitting. Automatic leveling is easiest when there is a distinct structure or phase present that is well distributed throughout the image area and contains the darkest (or lightest) pixels present. In that case, the image can be subdivided into a grid of smaller squares or rectangles, the darkest (or lightest) pixels in each subregion located, and these points used for the fitting.

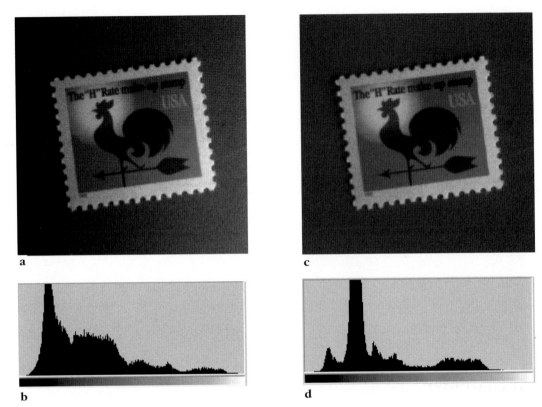

Figure 47. Correction of nonuniform lighting by selecting a background region:
 (a) original image;
 (b) histogram of *a*;
 (c) result of subtracting a polynomial fit to the pixel values in the periphery of the stamp;
 (d) histogram of *c*.

Figure 48 shows an example in which the specimen (a polished ceramic) has an overall variation in brightness due to curvature of the surface. The brightest pixels in each region of the specimen represent the matrix, and so should all be the same. Subdividing the image into a 9×9 grid and locating the brightest pixel in each square gives a total of 81 points, which are then used to calculate a second-order polynomial (six coefficients) by least-squares. The fitting routine in this case reported a fitting error (rms value) of less than two brightness values out of the total 0–255 range for pixels in the image.

Figure 48b shows the calculated brightness using the B(x,y) function, and **Figure 48c** shows the result after subtracting the background from the original, pixel by pixel, to level the image. This leveling removes the variation in background brightness and permits setting brightness thresholds to delineate the pores for measurement, as discussed in Chapter 6.

This approach to automatic leveling can of course be applied to either a light or a dark background. By simultaneously applying it to both the lightest and darkest pixels in each region of the image, it is possible to stretch the contrast of the image as a function of location, as shown schematically in **Figure 49** using a line profile of brightness as an example. This autocontrast method works particularly well when the image loses contrast due to nonuniform illumination or varying sample thickness. **Figure 50** shows an example.

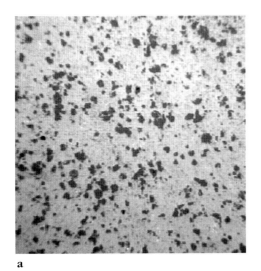

a

b

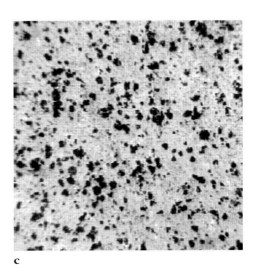

c

Figure 48. Automatic leveling of nonuniform illumination:
(**a**) Reflection light microscope image of ceramic specimen, with nonuniform background brightness due to a non-planar surface;
(**b**) background function calculated as a polynomial fit to the brightest point in each of 81 squares (a 9 × 9 grid);
(**c**) leveled image after subtracting **b** from **a**.

Another approach sometimes used to remove gradual variation in overall brightness employs the frequency transforms discussed in Chapter 5. It assumes that the background variation in the image is a low-frequency signal, and can be separated in frequency space from the higher frequencies that define the features present. If this assumption is justified, and the frequencies corresponding to the background can be identified, then they can be removed by a simple filter in the frequency space representation.

Figure 51 shows an example of this approach. The brightness variation in the original image is due to off-centered illumination in the microscope. Transforming the image into frequency space with a 2D FFT (as discussed in Chapter 5), reducing the magnitude of the first four frequency components by filtering the frequency space image, and retransforming, produces the image shown in the figure.

This method is not entirely successful for this image. The edges of the image show significant variations present because the frequency transform attempts to match the left and right edges and the top and bottom edges. In addition, the brightness of dark and light regions throughout the image which have the same appearance and would be expected to properly have the same brightness show considerable local variations because the brightness variation is a function of the local details, including the actual brightness values and the shapes of the features. There are few practical situations in which leveling can be satisfactorily performed by this method.

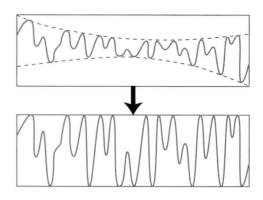

Figure 49. *Schematic diagram of automatic contrast adjustment by fitting polynomials to both the brightest and darkest values across an image and stretching the brightness values between those limits.*

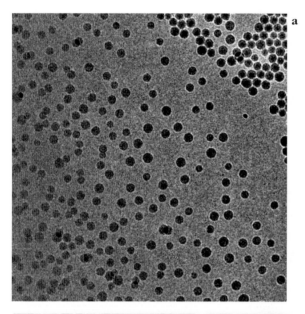

a

Figure 50. TEM image of latex particles:
(a) original, with varying contrast due to changing sample thickness;
(b) after application of automatic contrast by fitting polynomial functions to light and dark pixel values (and applying a median filter to reduce random pixel noise).

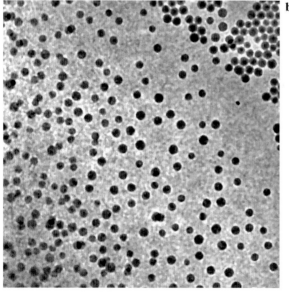

b

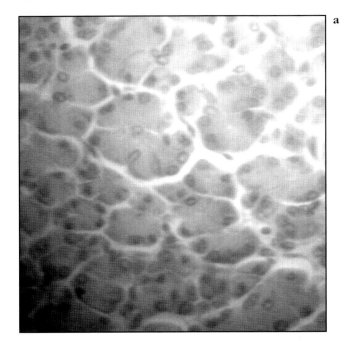

a

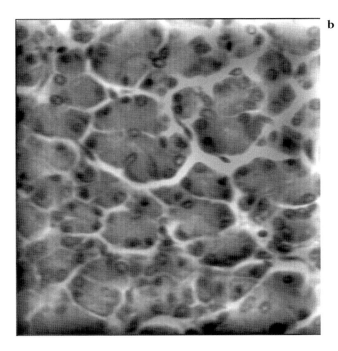

b

Figure 51. Leveling of image brightness and contrast by removal of low-frequency terms in 2D FFT:
(a) original image, showing nonuniform illumination;
(b) attempt to level the brightness by reducing the magnitude to zero of the lowest four frequency components. Notice that in addition to the variations near the edge, the brightness of similar structures is not constant throughout the image.

Rank leveling

When the background varies more abruptly than can be fit to simple functions, another approach can be used. This method is especially useful when the surface is irregular, such as details on a fracture surface examined in the SEM, or a thin section with a fold viewed in the TEM. The assumption behind this method is that features of interest are limited in size and smaller than the scale of background variations, and that the background is everywhere either lighter than or darker than the features. Both requirements are often met in practical situations.

Rank neighborhood operations (such as the median filter) were discussed previously in this chapter, and are also used in Chapter 4. The basic idea behind neighborhood ranking operations is to compare each pixel to its neighbors or combine the pixel values in some small region, minimally the eight touching pixels in a 3 × 3 square. This operation is performed for each pixel in the image, and a new image is produced as a result. In many practical implementations, the new image replaces the original image with only a temporary requirement for additional storage; these implementation considerations are discussed in Chapter 4.

For our present purposes, the neighborhood comparison works as follows: for each pixel, examine the pixels in a 3 × 3 square, a 5 × 5 octagon, or other similar small region. If the background is known to be darker than the features, find the darkest pixel in each neighborhood and replace the value of the original pixel with that darker brightness value. For the case of a background lighter than the features, the brightest pixel in the neighborhood is used instead. These operations are sometimes called grey-scale erosion and dilation, by analogy to the morphological processing discussed in Chapter 7. The result of applying this operation to the entire image is to shrink the features by the radius of the neighborhood region, and to extend the local background brightness values into the area previously covered by features.

Figure 52 illustrates this procedure for an image of rice grains on a dark and uneven background. A neighborhood is used here which consists of 21 pixels in an octagonal 5 × 5 pattern centered on each pixel in the image. The darkest pixel value in that region replaces the original central pixel. This operation is repeated for every pixel in the image, always using the original image pixels and not the new ones from application of the procedure to other pixels. After this procedure is complete, the rice grains are reduced in size as shown in **Figure 52b**. Repeating the operation continues to shrink the grains and to extend the background based on the local background brightness.

After four repetitions (**Figure 52d**), the rice grains have been removed. This removal is possible because the maximum width of any grain is not larger than four times the width of the 5-pixel-wide neighborhood used for the ranking. Knowing how many times to apply this operation depends upon knowing the width (smallest dimension) of the largest features present, or simply watching the progress of the operation and repeating until the features are removed. In some cases, this can be judged from the disappearance of a peak from the image histogram. The background produced by this method has the large-scale variation present in the original image, and subtracting it produces a leveled image (**Figure 52f**) that clearly defines the features and allows them to be separated from the background by thresholding.

This method is particularly suitable for the quite irregular background brightness variations that occur when looking at details on fracture surfaces. **Figure 53** shows two SEM images in which local ridges and variations produce bright lines on a dark but irregular background. The background in each case was estimated by applying of the ranking operation keeping the darkest pixel in a 7-pixel-wide octagonal neighborhood, followed by smoothing with a Gaussian kernel with a standard deviation of 1.0 pixels. Subtracting this background from the original makes the markings, fatigue striations in one image and brittle quasi-cleavage marks in the other, more visible by removing the overall variation due to surface orientation.

This method is also useful for examination of particles and other surface decorations on freeze-fractured cell walls in biological specimens, examination of surface roughness on irregular particles or pollen, and other similar problems. In some cases it can be used to enhance the visibility of dislocations in transmission electron microscope (TEM) images of materials, which appear as dark lines in different grains whose overall brightness varies due to lattice orientation.

Figure 54 shows an example in which both leveling techniques are used to complement each other. First a ranked background is created by replacing the dark axons with the locally lighter

Figure 52. *Constructing a background image with a rank operation:*
 (a) an image of rice grains with nonuniform illumination;
 (b) each pixel replaced with the darkest neighboring pixel in an octagonal 5×5 neighborhood;
 (c) another repetition of the "darkest neighbor" or grey-scale erosion operation;
 (d) after four repetitions, only the background remains;
 *(e) result of subtracting **d** from **a**;*
 (f) the leveled result with contrast expanded.

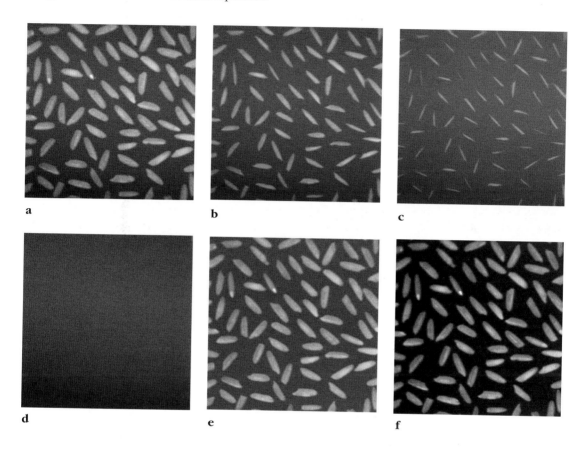

a   b   c

d   e   f

background which is divided into the original image. Then a polynomial fit to the brightest and darkest pixel values is used to locally expand the contrast, which helps to reveal even the small dark axon lines.

The ability to level brightness variations by subtracting a background image, whether obtained by measurement, mathematical fitting, or image processing, is not a cost-free process. Subtraction uses up part of the dynamic range, or grey scale, of the image. **Figure 55** shows an example. The original image has a shading variation that can be fit rather well by a quadratic function, but this has a range of about half of the total 256 grey levels. After the function has been subtracted, the leveled image does not have enough remaining brightness range to show detail in the dark areas of some features. This clipping may interfere with further analysis of the image.

Color shading

Color images present significant problems for shading correction. A typical example of a situation in which this arises is aerial or satellite imagery, in which the irregularity of the ground or the

Figure 53. Application of rank leveling to SEM images:
(a, b) original images of metal fractures showing local brightness variations due to surface orientation;
(c, d) background image produced as described in the text;
(e, f) leveled result after subtraction of the background from the original.

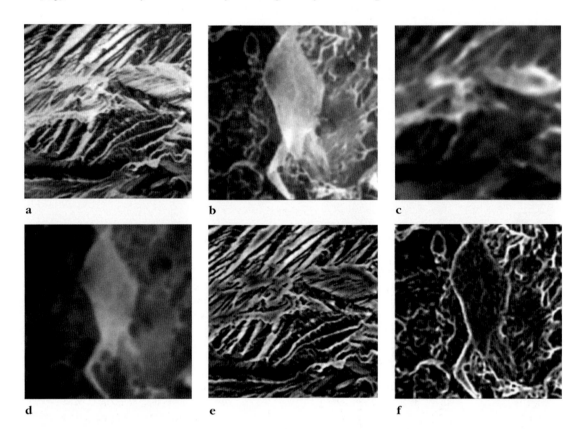

a   b   c

d   e   f

curvature of the planet surface produces an overall shading. In some cases, this affects only the intensity in the image and leaves the color information unaffected; but, depending on the camera response, possible texturing or specular reflection from the surface, atmospheric absorption, and other details of the imaging, it is more common to find that there are also color shifts between the areas in the image that have different illumination.

The same methods used above for grey scale images can be applied to the intensity plane from a color image. In some instances, the same leveling strategies can be applied to the hue plane as shown in **Figure 56**. This is slightly more complicated than leveling brightness since the hue values "warp around" modulo 360°; the simplest solution is to fit the polynomial twice, once with the origin at red and once at cyan, and use whichever gives the better fit. Leveling is practically never useful for application directly to the red, green and blue planes. When (mis)used in this way the operations produce color shifts in pixels that alter the image so that it can not be successfully thresholded, and in most cases does not even "look" right.

Chapter 1 showed an example of another approach. Although the various color planes have each been altered by the effects of geometry and other factors, to a first approximation, the effect is the same across the spectrum of colors. In that case, it is appropriate to use ratios of one color plane to another to level the effects of nonuniform surface orientation or illumination. Filtering the color image in different wavelengths and then dividing one by another cancels out some of the nonuniformity and produces a leveled image in which similar features located in different areas have the same final appearance.

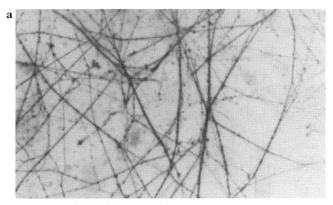

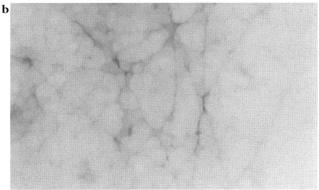

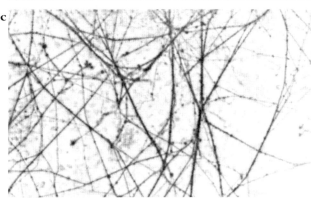

Figure 54. Combined rank and
polynomial methods:
  (a) original TEM image of axons;
  (b) background produced by
replacing dark pixels with their
brightest neighbors within a 5-pixel
radius;
  (c) result of dividing *a* by *b*;
  (d) contrast expanded between
automatically fit polynomial limits.

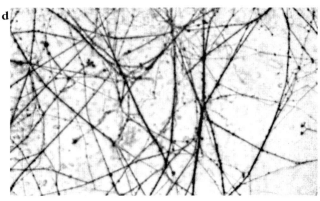

Figure 55. Effect of leveling on an image with limited grey-scale range:
(a) original image;
(b) fitted polynomial background;
*(c) subtracting image **b** from **a** — the background is uniform, but the dark features are not because the original pixels were fully black in the original image.*

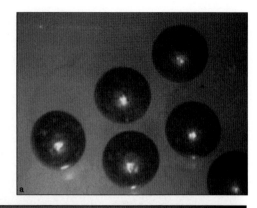

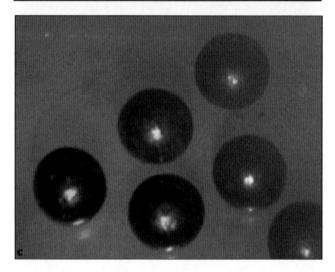

Figure 57 shows an example using a satellite image of the entire earth. The limb darkening around the edges of the globe is due primarily to viewing angle, and secondarily to the effects of atmospheric absorption. Histogram equalization (discussed in Chapter 4) of the individual color planes increases the contrast between features and improves the visibility of structures, but the resulting colors are not "real" and do not have any intrinsic meaning or use. Notice in particular the pink colors that appear in clouds, and the green in the oceans and along cloud edges. Separating the image into

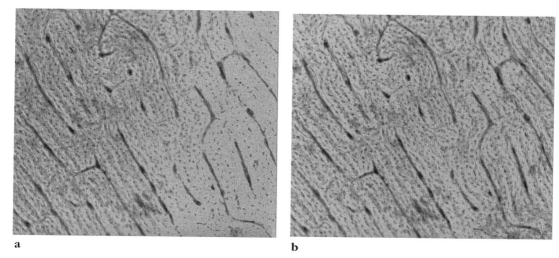

a   b

Figure 56. Leveling hue: (a) light micrograph of bone, showing nonuniform color due to misalignment of the bulb in the illuminator; *(b)* after polynomial leveling of the hue values.

separate color planes and ratioing them reveals fine details and levels the overall contrast range. It does not produce an image of the globe in which pixels near the limb have their colors "corrected" to be similar to those in the center of the field of view.

The rank-based leveling method can also be applied to color images. In the example of **Figure 58**, a red dye has been injected to reveal blood vessels but the background varies, making the smaller vessels and those at the periphery difficult to detect. Removing the blood vessels by replacing each pixel with the color values from its neighbor with the least red (color erosion) followed by the complementary operation in which each pixel is replaced by its neighbor with the greatest red value (color dilation) produces a background. Subtracting this background image from the original produces optimal contrast for the blood vessels.

Color correction of images is a very rich and complicated field. Generally, it requires detailed knowledge of the light source and the camera response, which must be obtained with calibration standards. Accurate colorimetry also requires extreme stability of all components. Colorimetry goes well beyond the capabilities of general-purpose image processing and analysis systems, and is not considered in detail here; however, there is a more routine interest in making some adjustments to color images to permit comparisons between regions or images, or to provide some control over consistency in the printing of color images.

These adjustments are generally accomplished with standardization, at least of a relative kind. For instance, most printers (as discussed in Chapter 2) cannot reproduce the full gamut of colors displayed on the screen or captured by a camera. In order to calibrate the relationship between the display and the input/output devices, some systems create a test pattern that is printed on the system printer, redigitized from the printed output, and compared to the original. This comparison allows the system to construct an internal correction matrix to adjust the colors so that the display and reproduction of colors will be more consistent. It also allows flagging those colors that cannot be printed accurately with a given printer.

Correction for a shift in colors, due for instance to a known change in lighting conditions, is also possible. Acquiring an image from a test card under each of several conditions allows the computer to build a matrix of corrections that may be expressed internally as either RGB or HSI components. These are multiplied by the incoming signal to approximately correct for the change in lighting.

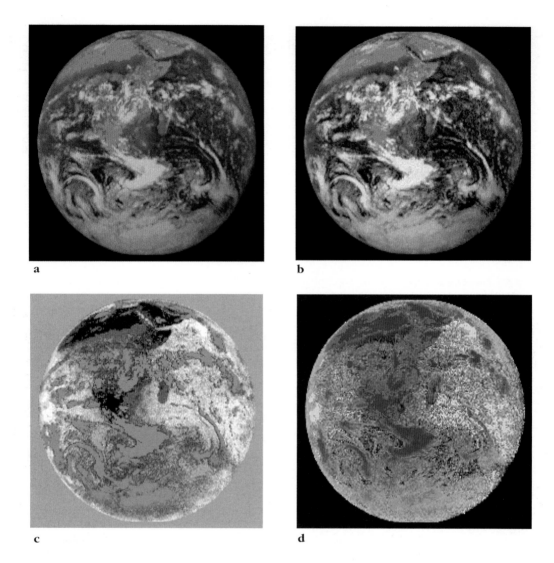

Figure 57. Satellite image of the earth:
   (a) original;
   (b) with contrast increased by histogram equalization of each color plane;
   (c) ratio of the image filtered at 450 nm (blue) to that at 650 nm (orange);
   (d) ratio of the image filtered at 700 nm (red) to that at 550 (green).

One example of the use of this type of correction is to compensate for the yellowing of varnish and other coatings applied to artworks. **Figure 59** shows an example. The painting is "Portrait of a Lady," painted in 1470 by Petrus Christus, a Flemish Renaissance painter (Gemäldegalerie der Staatlichen Museen, Berlin-Dahlem). The painting shows several defects. The two most obvious are the network of fine cracks that have formed in the paint, and the yellowing and fading of the pigments. Measurements on similar pigments freshly made and applied provide color samples that allow compensation for the color change. The application of a median filter allows filling in the cracks without blurring edges, much as the pixel noise was removed from the grey scale images shown previously. The result is a restoration of the appearance of the original painting.

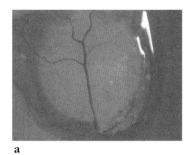
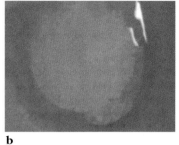
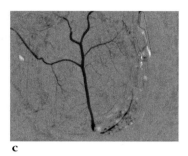

a　　　　　　　　　　　　b　　　　　　　　　　　　c

Figure 58. Example of rank leveling in a color image as described in the text (image courtesy Kathy
　Spencer, The Scripps Research Institute, La Jolla, CA)*:*
　(a) original image;
　(b) background produced by color ranking;
　(c) a minus *b.*

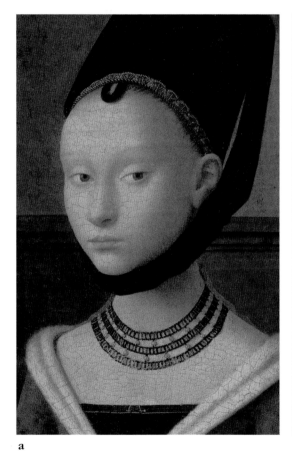
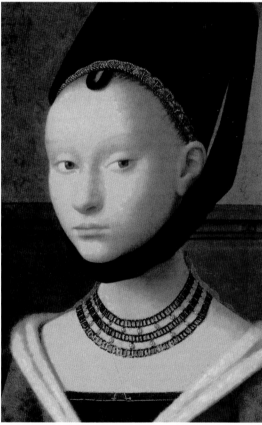

a　　　　　　　　　　　　　　　　　　　　b

Figure 59. Portrait of a Lady, painted in 1470 by Petrus Christus:
　(a) present appearance, showing cracks and fading of the colors;
　(b) application of a median filter to fill in the dark cracks, and color compensation to adjust the colors.

Non-planar views

Computer graphics is much concerned with methods for displaying the surfaces of three-dimensional objects. Some of these methods will be used in Chapter 12 to display representations of three-dimensional structures obtained from a series of 2D image slices, or from direct 3D imaging methods such as tomography.

One particular use of computer graphics which most of us take for granted can be seen each evening on the local news program. Most TV stations in the U.S. have a weather forecast that uses satellite images from the GOES satellite. These pictures show the U.S. as it appears from latitude 0, longitude 108 W (the satellite is shifted to 98 W in summertime to get a better view of hurricanes developing in the south Atlantic), at a geosynchronous elevation of about 22,000 miles.

This image shows cloud patterns, and a series of images taken during the day shows movement of storms and other weather systems. In these images, the coastlines, Great Lakes, and a few other topographic features are evident, but may be partially obscured by clouds. Given the average citizen's geographical knowledge, that picture would not help most viewers to recognize their location. So computer graphics are used to superimpose political outlines, such as the state borders and perhaps other information such as cities, to assist the viewer. Most U.S. TV stations have heavy investments in computer graphics for advertising, news, etc., but they rarely generate these lines themselves, instead obtaining the images with the lines already present from a company which specializes in that niche market.

How are these lines generated? This is not simply a matter of overlaying a conventional map, say a Mercator's projection as used in the school classroom, over the satellite image. The curvature of the earth and the foreshortening of the image need to be taken into account. **Figure 60** shows a weather satellite image of North America that is clearly foreshortened at the top, and also shows noticeable curvature from west to east across the width of the country.

The coordinates, in latitude and longitude, of points on the earth's surface are used to calculate a perspective view of the roughly spherical globe as it is seen from the satellite. Because the viewpoint is constant, this is a one-time calculation, which nevertheless needs to be done for a great many points to construct good outline maps for superposition. The calculation can be visualized as shown in the diagram of **Figure 61**.

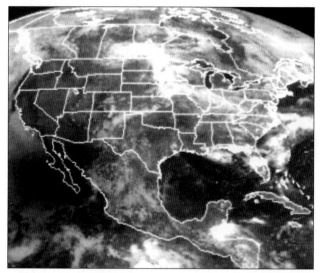

Figure 60. GOES-7 image of North America with political boundary lines superimposed. The dark area just west of Baja California is the shadow of the moon, during the eclipse of June 11, 1991 (image courtesy National Environmental Satellite Data and Information Service).

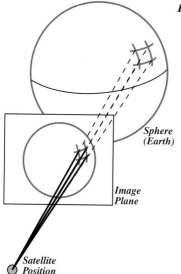

Figure 61. *Diagram of satellite imaging. As in any perspective geometry, the "flat" image is formed by projecting view lines from the three-dimensional object to the viewpoint and constructing the image from the points at which they intersect the image plane.*

Sphere (Earth)

Image Plane

Satellite Position

Figure 62. *Simple trigonometry can be used to calculate the location of points in the image plane from the longitude of the point on the earth, and the location of the satellite. This is the view from the North Pole; a similar view from the equator gives the y-coordinate.*

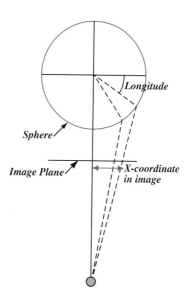

Longitude

Sphere

Image Plane

X-coordinate in image

The location of a point on the spherical earth (specified by its latitude and longitude) is used to determine the intersection of a view line to the satellite with a flat image plane, inserted in front of the sphere. This calculation requires only simple trigonometry as indicated in **Figure 62**. The coordinates of the points in that plane are the location of the point in the viewed image. As shown, a square on the ground is viewed as a skewed trapezoid, and if the square is large enough its sides are noticeably curved.

Computer graphics

Computer graphics is similarly used to construct perspective drawings of three-dimensional objects so that they can be viewed on the computer screen, for instance in CAD (computer aided design) programs. The subject goes far beyond our needs here; the interested reader should refer to standard texts such as Foley and Van Dam (1984) or Hearn and Baker (1986). The display process is the same as that just described, with the addition of perspective control that allows the user to adjust the apparent distance of the camera or viewpoint so as to control the degree of foreshortening that occurs (equivalent to choosing a long or short focal length lens for a camera; the short focal length lens produces more distortion in the image).

Ignoring perspective distortion for the moment (i.e., using a telephoto lens), we can represent the translation of a point in three dimensions by matrix multiplication of its x, y, z coordinates by a set of values that describe rotation and translation. This is simpler to examine in more detail in two dimensions, since our main interest here is with two-dimensional images. Consider a point with Cartesian X, Y coordinates and how it moves when we shift it or rotate it and the other points in the object with respect to the coordinate system.

From simple geometry, we know that a translation of an object simply adds offsets to X and Y, to produce

$$X' = X + \Delta X \qquad (3)$$
$$Y' = Y + \Delta Y$$

while stretching the object requires multiplicative coefficients which may not be the same

$$X' = \alpha\, X \qquad (4)$$
$$Y' = \beta\, Y$$

and rotation of an object by the angle ϑ introduces an interdependence between the original X and Y coordinates of the form

$$X' = X + Y \sin \vartheta \qquad (5)$$
$$Y' = Y - X \cos \vartheta$$

In general, the notation for two-dimensional translations is most commonly written using so-called homogeneous coordinates and matrix notation. The coordinates X, Y are combined in a vector along with an arbitrary constant 1 to allow the translation values to be incorporated into the matrix math, producing the result

$$[X'\ Y'\ 1] = [X\ Y\ 1] \cdot \begin{vmatrix} a & b & 0 \\ c & d & 0 \\ e & f & 1 \end{vmatrix} \qquad (6)$$

which multiplies out to

$$X' = aX + cY + e \qquad (7)$$
$$Y' = bX + dY + f$$

By comparing this matrix form to the examples above, we see that the e and f terms are the translational shift values. The diagonal values a and d are the stretching coefficients, while b and c are the sine and cosine terms involved in rotation. When a series of transformations is combined, including rotation, translation and stretching, a series of matrices is produced that can be multiplied together. When this happens, for instance to produce rotation about some point other than the origin, or to combine nonuniform stretching with rotation, the individual terms are combined in ways that complicate their simple interpretation; however, only the same six coefficients are needed.

If only these terms are used, we cannot produce curvature or twisting of the objects. By introducing higher-order terms, more complex stretching and twisting of figures is possible. This would produce a more complex equation of the form

$$X' = a_1 + a_2X + a_3Y + a_4XY + a_5X^2 + a_6Y^2 + \ldots \tag{8}$$

and a similar relationship for Y'. There is no fundamental reason to limit this polynomial expansion to any particular maximum power, except that as the complexity grows the number of coefficients needed rises (and the difficulty of obtaining them), and the mathematical precision needed to apply the transformation increases. It is unusual to have terms beyond second power, which can handle most commonly encountered cases of distortion and even approximate the curvature produced by looking at a spherical surface, at least over small ranges of angles.

Of course, some surface mappings are better handled by other functions. The standard Mercator's projection of the spherical earth onto a cylinder (**Figure 63**) sends the poles to infinity and greatly magnifies areas at high latitudes. It would require many polynomial terms to approximate it, but since the actual geometry of the mapping is known, it is easy to use the cosecant function that efficiently performs the transformation.

Geometrical distortion

Now we must examine what to do with these mathematical operations. Images are frequently obtained that are not of flat surfaces viewed normally. The example of the satellite image used above is one obvious case. So is viewing surfaces in the SEM, in which the specimen surface is often tilted to increase the contrast in the detected image. If the surface is not flat, different regions may be tilted at arbitrary angles, or continuous curvature may be present. This distortion becomes important if we want to perform any measurements or comparisons within or between images. Many airborne cameras and radars introduce a predictable distortion (which is therefore correctable) due

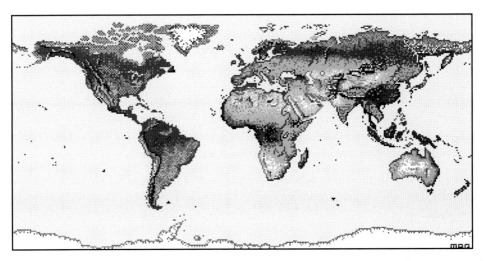

Figure 63. *The standard Mercator's projection of the earth used in maps projects the points on the sphere onto a cylinder, producing distortion at high latitudes.*

to the use of a moving or sideways scan pattern, or by imaging a single line onto continuously moving film. In all of these cases, knowing the distortion is the key to correcting it.

This situation does not commonly arise with light microscopy because the depth of field of the optics is so low that surfaces must be flat and normal to the optical axis to remain in focus. On the other hand, other imaging technologies, frequently encounter non-ideal surfaces or viewing conditions.

Making maps from aerial or satellite images is one application (Thompson, 1966). Of course, there is no perfect projection of a spherical surface onto a flat one, so various approximations and useful conventions are employed. In each case, however, there is a known relationship between the coordinates on the globe and those on the map which can be expressed mathematically. But what about the image? If the viewpoint is exactly known, as for the case of the weather satellite, or can be calculated for the moment of exposure, as for the case of a space probe passing by a planet, then the same kind of mathematical relationship can be determined.

This procedure is usually impractical for aerial photographs, as the plane position is not that precisely controlled. The alternative is to locate a few reference points in the image whose locations on the globe or the map are known, and use them to determine the equations relating position in the image to location on the map. This technique is generally known as image warping or rubber sheeting, and while the equations are the same as those used in computer graphics, the techniques for determining the coefficients are quite different.

We have seen that a pair of equations calculating X', Y' coordinates for a transformed view from original coordinates X, Y may include constants, linear terms in X and Y, plus higher order terms such as XY, X^2, etc. Adding more terms of higher order makes it possible to introduce more complex distortions in the transformation. If the problem is simply one of rotation, only linear terms are needed, and a constraint on the coefficients can be introduced to preserve angles. In terms of the simple matrix shown in **Equation 6**, this would require that the two stretching coefficients a and d must be equal. That means that only a few constants are needed, and they can be determined by locating a few known reference points and setting up simultaneous equations.

More elaborate stretching to align images with each other or with a map requires correspondingly more terms and more points. In electron microscopy, the great depth of field permits acquiring pictures of samples which are locally flat but oriented at an angle to the point of view, producing distortion that is essentially trapezoidal as shown in **Figure 64**. The portion of the surface that is closest to the lens is magnified more than regions farther away, and distances are foreshortened in the direction of tilt. In order to measure and compare features on these surfaces, or even to properly apply image processing methods (which generally assume that the neighbor pixels in various directions are at equal distances from the center), it may be necessary to transform this image to correct the distortion. Since the exact tilt angle and working distance may not be known, a method that uses only reference points within the image itself will be needed.

All that is required here is the ability to identify four points whose real X, Y coordinates on the surface are known, and whose image coordinates X', Y' can be measured. Then the following equations are written

$$X = a_1 + a_2 X' + a_3 Y' + a_4 X'Y' \qquad (9)$$

$$Y = b_1 + b_2 X' + b_3 Y' + b_4 X'Y'$$

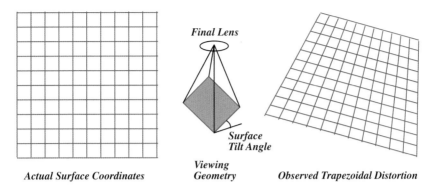

Final Lens

Surface Tilt Angle

Viewing Geometry

Actual Surface Coordinates   **Observed Trapezoidal Distortion**

Figure 64. *Trapezoidal distortion commonly encountered in the electron microscope when observing a tilted surface.*

for each of the four sets of coordinates. This allows solving for the constants a_i and b_i. Of course, if more points are available, then they can be used to obtain a least-squares solution that minimizes the effect of the inevitable small errors in measurement of coordinates in the image.

By limiting the equation to those terms needed to accomplish the rotation and stretching involved in the trapezoidal distortion which we expect to be present, we minimize the number of points needed for the fit. More than the three terms shown above in **Equation 7** are required, because angles are not preserved in this kind of foreshortening. But using the fewest possible is preferred to a general equation involving many higher order terms, both in terms of the efficiency of the calculation (number of reference points) and the precision of the coefficients.

Likewise, if we know that the distortion in the image is that produced by viewing a globe, the appropriate sine and cosine terms can be used in the fitting equations. Of course, if we have no independent knowledge about the shape of the surface or the kind of imaging distortion, then other methods such as stereoscopy represent the only practical approach to determining the geometry.

The chief problem that arises with such perspective correction is for features that do not lie on the tilted planar surface, but extend above or below it. In the example of **Figure 65**, the front of the building is corrected to show the correct angles and dimensions for the structure, but the light pole that extends out over the street in front appears to be at an angle to the building when in fact it is exactly perpendicular.

Alignment

Another very common situation is the alignment of serial section images. In this case, there may be no "ground truth" to align to, but only relative alignment between the successive slices. The alignment is performed either by using features within the image that can be recognized in successive slices, or by introducing fiducial marks such as holes drilled through the specimen block or fibers inserted into it before the sections are cut. The points may be located manually by the user, or automatically by the imaging system, although the latter method works best for artificial markings such as holes, and somewhat poorly when trying to use details within the images which match only imperfectly from one section to the next. Relative alignment is discussed in more detail in Chapter 12.

Serial sections cut with a microtome from a block of embedded biological material commonly are foreshortened in the cutting direction by 5 to 15%, due to compression of the block by the knife.

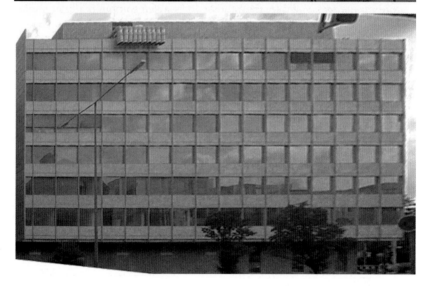

Figure 65. *Correcting trapezoidal distortion due to a non-perpendicular view. Slight distortion remains due to the use of a wide angle lens, and as noted in the text, features out of the plane of the building are incorrectly depicted.*

Then they are rotated arbitrarily before they are viewed. The result is a need for an alignment equation of the form

$$X = a_1 + a_2X' + a_3Y' \qquad (10)$$

with only three constants (and a similar equation for *Y*). Hence, locating three reference points that are common to two sequential images allows one to be rotated and stretched to align with the other. **Figure 66** shows an image in which three points have been marked with vectors to indicate their movement to perform this alignment, and the resulting transformation of the image by stretching.

This kind of warping can be performed to align images with other images, as in serial section reconstruction, or to align images along their edges to permit assembling them as a mosaic (Milgram, 1975). Alignment of side-by-side sections of a mosaic is often attempted with SEM images but fails because of the trapezoidal distortion discussed previously. The result is that features along the

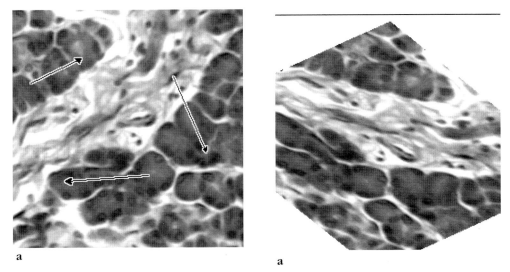

a   a

Figure 66. An image with three displacement vectors (a), and the rotation and stretching transformation which they produce *(b)*. Notice that portions of the original image are lost and some areas of the transformed image have no information.

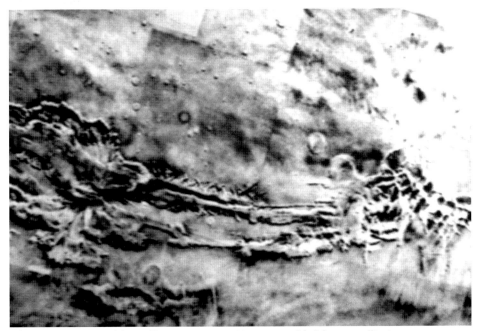

Figure 67. Mosaic image of the Valles Marineris on Mars, assembled from satellite images.

image boundaries do not quite line up, and the mosaic is imperfect. Using rubber sheeting can correct this defect.

Such correction is routinely done for satellite and space probe pictures. **Figure 67** shows an example of a mosaic image constructed from multiple images taken from orbit of the surface of Mars. Boundaries between images are visible because of brightness differences due to variations in illumination or exposure, but the features line up well across the seams. Recently, interest has increased in creating mosaics from separate images to generate panoramic views, and in

Figure 68. Six images that overlap to provide a 3 × 2 array covering a larger scene.

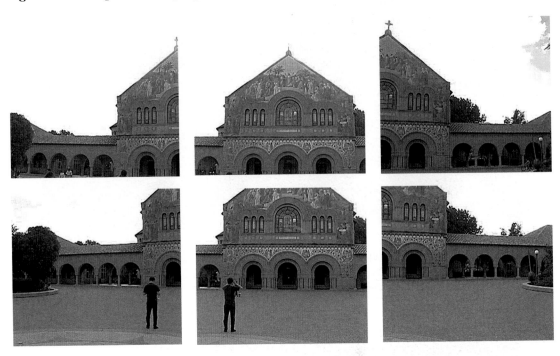

Figure 69. The mosaic produced from the images in Figure 68 (example and software from Enroute Imaging, Palo Alto, CA).

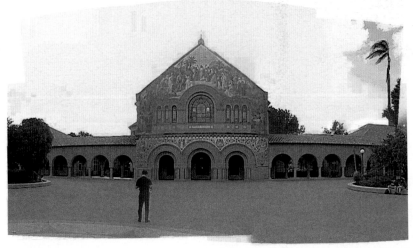

overcoming the limited resolution (as compared with film) of consumer digital cameras. **Figure 68** shows six individual images taken from a single location (by rotating the camera on a tripod) that form a 3 × 2 array with considerable overlap. **Figure 69** shows the resulting mosaic which forms a complete image of the building. Note that the images have been distorted to fit together smoothly, and that their edges do not form straight lines. This image is pleasing visually but not of much use for measurement purposes.

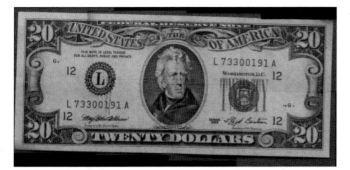

a

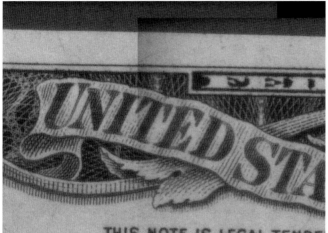

b

Figure 70.
(a) Large mosaic image assembled from eight individual images, each 1600 × 1200 pixels from a digital camera, as discussed in the text; (b) detail of fit between two image tiles.

For scientific imaging purposes, the use of a microscope stage or other specimen positioning device that can shift the sample being imaged with reasonable precision while the camera remains fixed would seem to offer the possibility of acquiring images of unlimited size. More constraints are here to assist in the fitting together of the image. It is known, for example, that the images may be slightly rotated (the mechanism may have slight wobble or misalignment and the shifting cannot be counted on to provide exact edge-to-edge alignment), but they cannot be distorted (i.e., straight lines remain straight and angles are unchanged). Thus, the fitting together process can only shift and rotate the individual image tiles in their entirety.

If the overlap between tiles is between 10 and 20%, and the angular mismatch is no more than a few degrees, matching each of the tiles together can indeed produce large high-resolution mosaics as shown in **Figure 70**. The matching technique is based on cross-correlation (discussed in Chapter 5), and an iterative procedure was used to match all of the tiles together for a best fit. This is particularly effective for images acquired in the atomic force microscope, because the area covered by these devices tends to be rather small, and with the very high spatial resolution it is not feasible to design specimen shifting hardware that is absolutely precise (Condeco et al., 2000).

Interpolation

When images are being aligned, it is possible to write the equations either in terms of the coordinates in the original image as a function of the geometrically corrected one, or vice versa. In practice it is usually preferable to use the grid of x, y coordinates in the corrected image to calculate for

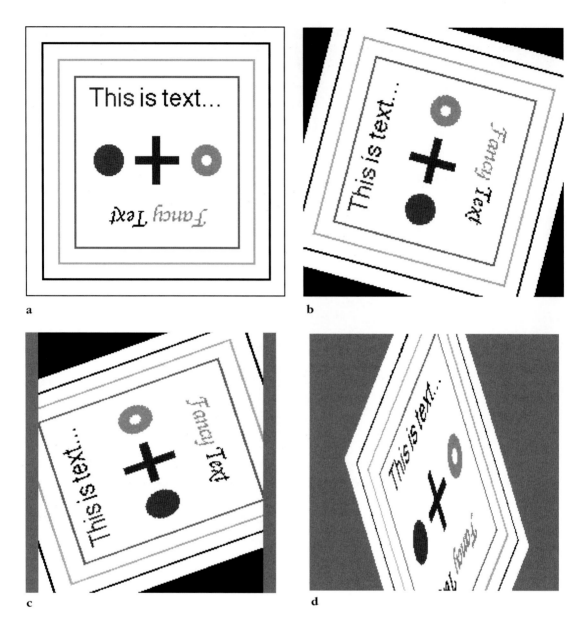

Figure 71. Rotation and stretching of a test image:
    (a) *original;*
    (b) *rotation only, no change in scale;*
    (c) *rotation and uniform stretching while maintaining angles;*
    (d) *general rotation and stretching in which angles may vary (lines remain straight).*

each the coordinates in the original image, and to perform the calculation in terms of actual pixel addresses.

Unfortunately, these calculated coordinates for the original location will only rarely be integers. This means that the location lies "between" the pixels in the original image. Several methods are used to deal with this problem. The simplest is to truncate the calculated values so that the fractional part of the address is discarded and the pixel lying toward the origin of the coordinate system is used. Slightly better results are obtained by rounding the address values to select the nearest pixel, whose brightness is then copied to the transformed image array.

Either method introduces some error in location that can cause distortion of the transformed image. **Figure 71** shows examples using a test pattern in which the biasing of the lines and apparent variations in their width is evident.

When this distortion is unacceptable, another method may be used which requires more calculation. The brightness value for the transformed pixel may be calculated by interpolating between the four pixels surrounding the calculated address. This is called bilinear interpolation, and is calculated simply from the fractional part of the X and Y coordinates. First the interpolation is done in one direction, and then in the other, as indicated in **Figure 72.** For a location with coordinates $j + x$, $k + y$ where x and y are the fractional part of the address, the equations for the first interpolation are

$$B_{j+x,k} = (1-x) \cdot B_{j,k} + x \cdot B_{j+1,k}$$

$$B_{j+x,k+1} = (1-x) \cdot B_{j,k+1} + x \cdot B_{j+1,k+1} \tag{11}$$

and then the second interpolation, in the y direction, gives the final value

$$B_{j+x,k+y} = (1-y) \cdot B_{j+x,k} + y \cdot B_{j+x,k+1} \tag{12}$$

Weighted interpolations over larger regions are also used in some cases. One of the most popular is bicubic fitting. Whereas bilinear interpolation uses a 2×2 array of neighboring pixel values to calculate the interpolated value, the cubic method uses a 4×4 array. Using the same notation as the bilinear interpolation in **Equations 11** and **12**, the summations now go from $k-1$ to $k+2$ and from $j-1$ to $k+2$. The intermediate values from the horizontal interpolation are:

$$B_j +_{x,k} = (1/6)\,(B_{j-1,k} \cdot R_1 + B_{j,k} \cdot R_2 + B_j+1,k \cdot R_3 + Bj+2,k \cdot R_4) \tag{13}$$

and the interpolation in the vertical direction is

$$B_{j+x,k+y} = (1/6)\,(B_j+_{x,k-1} \cdot R_1 + B_{j+x,k} \cdot R_2 + B_{j+x,k+1} \cdot R_3 + B_{j+x,k+2} \cdot R_4) \tag{14}$$

Figure 72. Diagram of pixel interpolation. The brightness values of the neighbors are first interpolated horizontally to determine the brightness values at the locations outlined in red, and then these two values are interpolated vertically to determine the brightness at the target pixel outlined in blue, using the fractional part of the pixel addresses.

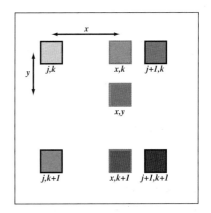

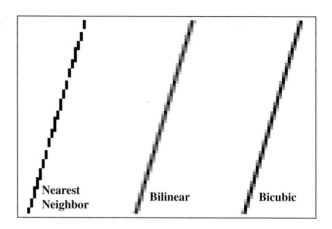

Figure 73. *Effect of rotating a 1-pixel wide black line using nearest neighbor, bilinear, and bicubic interpolation.*

Nearest Neighbor   Bilinear   Bicubic

where the weighting factors R_i are calculated from the real part (x or y respectively) of the address as

$$R_1 = (3+x)^3 - 4 \cdot (2+x)^3 + 6 \cdot (1+x)^3 - 4 \cdot x^3$$
$$R_2 = (2+x)^3 - 4 \cdot (1+x)^3 + 6 \cdot x^3 \tag{15}$$
$$R_3 = (1+x)^3 - 4 \cdot x^3$$
$$R_4 = x^3$$

The bicubic fit is more isotropic than the bilinear method. Interpolation always has the effect of smoothing the image and removing some high frequency information, but minimizes aliasing or "stair-stepping" along lines and edges. **Figure 73** shows the results of rotating a line (originally a black vertical line one pixel wide) by 17° with no interpolation (selecting the nearest neighbor pixel value), bilinear, and bicubic interpolation. The aliasing with the nearest neighbor method is evident. Bilinear interpolation reduces the line contrast more than bicubic, and both assign grey values to adjacent pixels to smooth the appearance of the line.

The advantage of interpolation is that dimensions are altered as little as possible in the transformation, and in particular boundaries and other lines are not biased or distorted. **Figure 74** shows the same examples as **Figure 71**, with bilinear interpolation used. Careful examination of the figure shows that the lines appear straight and not "aliased" or stair-stepped, because some of the pixels along the sides of the lines have intermediate grey values resulting from the interpolation. In fact, computer graphics sometimes uses this same method to draw lines on CRT displays so that the stair-stepping inherent in drawing lines on a discrete pixel array is avoided. The technique is called anti-aliasing and produces lines whose pixels have grey values according to how close they lie to the mathematical location of the line. This fools the viewer into perceiving a smooth line.

Fitting of higher-order polynomials, or adaptive spline fits to the pixel intensity values, can also be used. This can be particularly useful when enlarging images in order to reduce the perceived fuzziness that results when sharp edges are spread out by conventional interpolation. **Figure 75** shows an example (a fragment of the "flowers" image) in which a 4× enlargement has been performed using no interpolation, bilinear interpolation, adaptive spline fitting and fractal interpolation. The latter inserts false "detail" into the image, while spline fitting maintains the sharpness of edges best.

For image warping or rubber-sheeting, interpolation has the advantage that dimensions are preserved, although brightness values are not. With the nearest-pixel method achieved by rounding

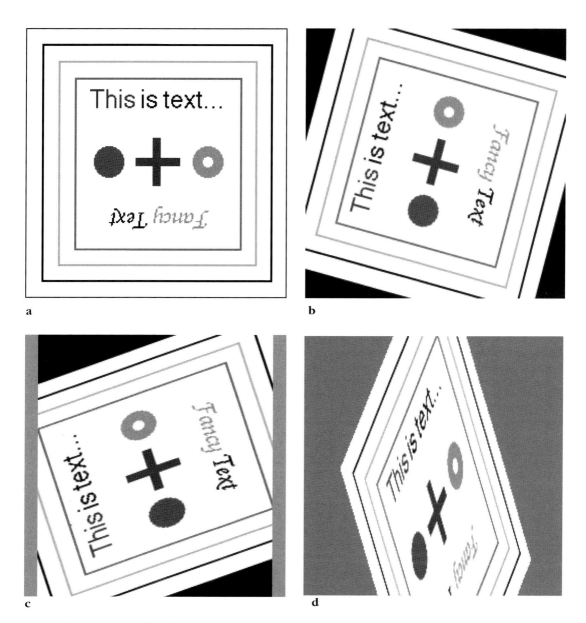

a

b

c

d

Figure 74. *Same generalized rotation and stretching as in* **Figure 71**, *but with bilinear interpolation. Note the smoothing of the lines and boundaries.*

the pixel addresses, the dimensions are distorted but the brightness values are preserved. Choosing which method is appropriate to a particular imaging task depends primarily on which kind of information is more important, and secondarily on the additional computational effort required for the interpolation.

Figure 76 illustrates the effect of adding higher order terms to the warping equations. With quadratic terms, the trapezoidal distortion of a short focal length lens or SEM can be corrected. It is also possible to model the distortion of a spherical surface closely over modest distances. With higher order terms arbitrary distortion is possible, but this is rarely useful in an image processing situation since the reference points to determine such a distortion are not likely to be available.

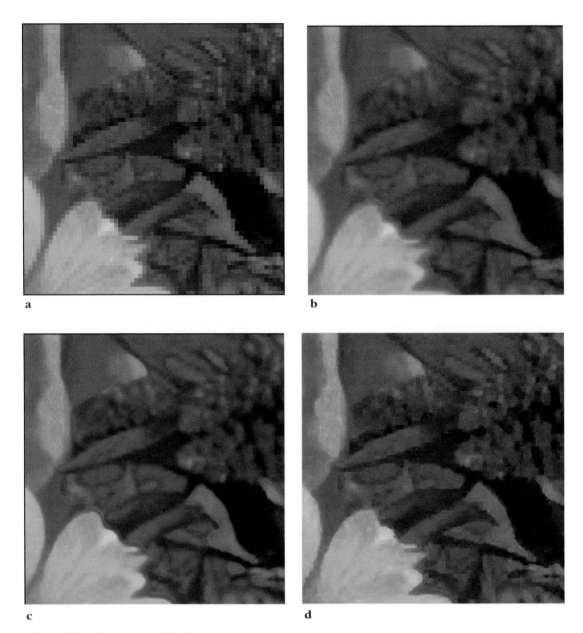

Figure 75. Enlargement of an image:
   (a) *no interpolation;*
   (b) *bilinear interpolation;*
   (c) *spline fitting;*
   (d) *fractal interpolation.*

Morphing

Programs that can perform controlled warping according to mathematically defined relationships, or calculate those matrices of values from a set of identified fiducial or reference marks that apply to the entire image are generally rather specialized. But an entire class of consumer-level programs has become available for performing image morphing based on a net of user-defined control points. The points are generally placed at corresponding locations that are distinctive in the two

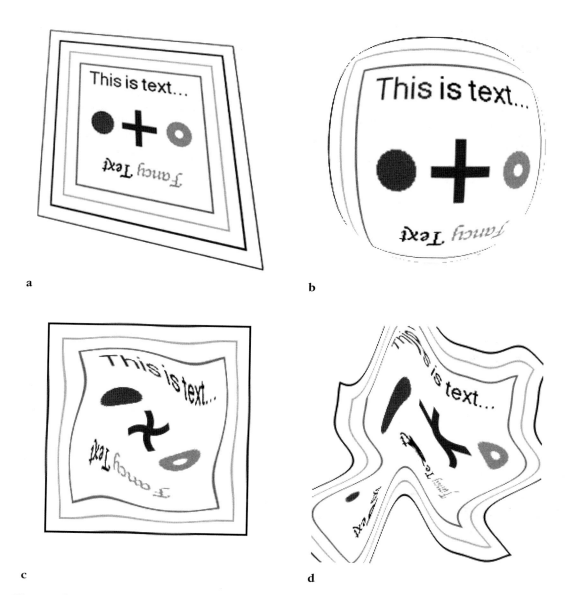

Figure 76. Some additional examples of image warping using the same original image as Figure 71:
   (a) *quadratic warping showing trapezoidal foreshortening;*
   (b) *cubic warping in which lines are curved (approximation here is to a spherical surface);*
   (c) *twisting the center of the field while holding the edges fixed (also cubic warping);*
   (d) *arbitrary warping in which higher order and trigonometric terms are required.*

images. For aligning two faces, for example, points at the tips of the eyes, corners of the mouth, along the hairline and chinline, and so forth are used as shown in the illustration in **Figure 77**.

The program uses the points to form a tesselation of the first image into triangles (technically, the choice of which points to use as corners for the triangles is defined by a procedure called a Voronoi tesselation). Each triangle is uniformly stretched to fit the location of the corner points in the second image. The sides of the triangles are uniformly stretched, so the points along the edges of adjacent triangles are not displaced, although lines may be bent where they cross the boundaries of

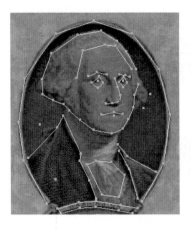
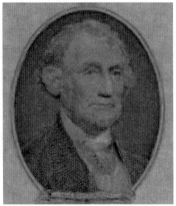
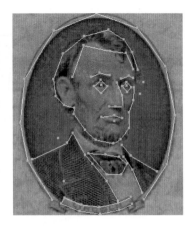

Figure 77. Transformation of George into Abe (pictures from U.S. currency). The corresponding points marked on each original image control the gradual distortion from one to the other. The midpoint frame is plausible as a person and shares feature characteristics with both endpoints.

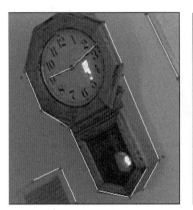
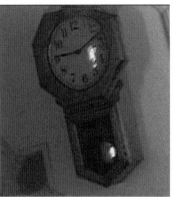
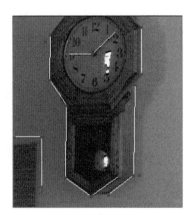

Figure 78. Alignment of two images of a clock. The points shown on the two images control the distortion of one image to fit the second. Within the network of triangles, no abrupt distortions are apparent. Around the edges of the image and where pixels on one do not correspond to locations on the other, however, straight lines show sharp bends.

the triangles. **Figure 78** shows an example of this effect when this procedure is used to rotate one image to match another.

With a triangular mesh and linear stretching of each triangle, lines crossing the boundaries of the triangles would be continuous, but sharply bent. Using spline or cubic equations to control the stretch gives a better appearance by making the curves smooth, but often at the expense of preserving dimensions so that measurements can be made on such images.

The art of using these morphing programs lies primarily in using enough control points, and their careful placement. The results look quite realistic, as shown in the examples. This is especially true when a sequence of images is created with progressive motion of the control points from the original to final locations. These morphing "movies" show one image transforming gradually into the second. These effects are used routinely in creating television advertisements. It is not clear whether there are any technical applications requiring image measurement that can be satisfactorily accomplished with these programs, considering the somewhat arbitrary placement of points and distortion of dimensions and directions.

The ability to use morphing to align images of different objects and produce visually convincing images can be a powerful tool for communicating results to others. This procedure can be useful to show the similarity between two objects, but it is extraordinarily susceptible to misuse, producing apparent matching between different images that are really not the same.

4

Image Enhancement (Processing in the Spatial Domain)

The preceding chapter discussed methods for correcting or alleviating the principal defects in as-acquired images. A fuzzy area exists between simply correcting these defects and going beyond to enhance the images. Enhancement is the subject of this chapter. Methods are available that increase the visibility of one portion, aspect or component of an image, though generally at the expense of others whose visibility is diminished. In this regard, image processing is a bit like word processing or food processing. It is possible to rearrange things to make a product that is more pleasing or interpretable, but the total amount of data does not change. In the case of images, this generally means that the number of bytes (or pixels) is not reduced.

In contrast to image processing, most image analysis procedures attempt to extract only the "important" information from the image. An example would be to identify and count features in an image, reducing the amount of data from perhaps a million bytes to a few dozen, or even a single "Yes" or "No" answer in some quality control, medical, or forensic applications.

Image processing for purposes of enhancement can be performed in either the spatial domain (the array of pixels comprising our conventional representation of the image) or other domains, such as the Fourier domain discussed in Chapter 5. In the spatial domain, pixel values may be modified according to rules that depend on the original pixel value (local or point processes). In addition, pixel values may be combined with or compared with others in their immediate neighborhood in a variety of ways. Examples of each of these approaches were used in Chapter 3, to replace brightness values in order to expand image contrast, or to smooth noise by kernel averaging or median filtering. Related techniques used in this chapter perform further enhancements.

It is worth noting here that two-dimensional (2D) images typically consist of a very large number of pixels, from about 1/4 million to several million. Even a point process that simply modifies the value of each pixel according to its previous contents requires that the computer address each pixel location. For a neighborhood process, each pixel must be addressed many times, and the processing speed slows down accordingly. Fast processors and high speed memory access (and a lot of memory) are essential requirements for this type of work. Some machines use dedicated hardware such as shift registers and array processors, or boards with dedicated memory and custom addressing circuits, or multiple processors with special programming, to permit near-real-time processing of images, when that is economically justified. As CPU speeds have increased, the need for special hardware has diminished. With more memory, entire images can be accessed rapidly without the need to bring in pieces, one at a time, from disk storage.

As desktop computer power has increased, the implementation of increasingly complex algorithms for image enhancement has become practical. Many of these algorithms are not new, dating from decades ago and often developed in conjunction with the need to process images from satellites and space probes, but until recently have only been performed using large computers or special purpose systems. Most can now be satisfactorily applied to images routinely, using personal computers.

Contrast manipulation

Chapter 3 showed examples of expanding the contrast of a dim image by reassigning pixel brightness levels. In most systems, this can be done almost instantaneously by writing a table of values into the display hardware. This lookup table (LUT) substitutes a display brightness value for each stored value and thus does not require actually modifying any of the values stored in memory for the image. Linearly expanding the contrast range by assigning the darkest pixel value to black, the brightest value to white, and each of the others to linearly interpolated shades of grey makes good use of the display and enhances the visibility of features in the image.

It was also shown, in Chapter 1, that the same LUT approach can be used with colors by assigning a triplet of red, green, and blue values to each stored grey scale value. This pseudo-color also increases the visible difference between similar pixels; sometimes it is an aid to the user who wishes to see small or gradual changes in image brightness.

A typical computer display can show 2^8 or 256 different shades of grey, and can produce colors with the same 2^8 brightness values for each of the red, green, and blue components to produce a total of 2^{24} or 16 million different colors. This is often described as "true color," since the gamut of colors that can be displayed is adequate to reproduce most natural scenes. It does not imply, of course, that the colors displayed are photometrically accurate or identical to the original color in the displayed scene. Indeed, that kind of accuracy is very difficult and requires special hardware and calibration. If the original image has more than 256 brightness values (is more than 8 bits deep) in each color channel, some type of lookup table is required even to display it on the screen.

More important, the 16 million different colors that such a system is capable of displaying, and even the 256 shades of grey, are far more than the human eye can distinguish. Under good viewing conditions, we can typically see only a few tens of different grey levels and hundreds of distinguishable colors. That means the display hardware of the image processing system is not being used very well to communicate the image information to the user. If many of the pixels in the image are quite bright, for example, they cannot be distinguished. If there are also some dark pixels present, we cannot simply expand the contrast. Instead, a more complicated relationship between stored and displayed values is needed.

In general, we can describe the manipulation of pixel brightness in terms of a transfer function relating the stored brightness value for each pixel to a displayed value. If this relationship is one-to-one, then for each stored value there will be a unique (although not necessarily visually discernible) displayed value. In some cases, it is advantageous to use transfer functions that are not one-to-one: several stored values are displayed with the same brightness value, so that other stored values can be spread further apart to increase their visual difference.

Figure 1 shows an image in which the 256 distinct pixel brightness values cannot all be discerned even on the display cathode ray tube (CRT); the printed version of the image is necessarily much worse. As discussed in Chapter 2, the number of distinct printed grey levels in a halftone image is determined by the variation in dot size of the printer. For a simple 300-dots-per-inch (dpi) laser writer, this requires a trade-off between grey scale resolution (number of shades) and lateral resolution (number of halftone cells per inch). A typical compromise is 50 cells per inch and more

Figure 1. *An original image with a full range of brightness values, and several examples of arbitrary hand-drawn display transfer functions that expand or alter the contrast in various parts of the range. The plot with each image shows the stored pixel brightness values on the horizontal axis, and the displayed brightness on the vertical axis. Image* **(a)** *has a transfer function that is the identity function, so that actual stored brightnesses are displayed. Images* **(b)** *through* **(f)** *illustrate various possibilities, including reversal and increased or decreased slope over parts of the brightness range.*

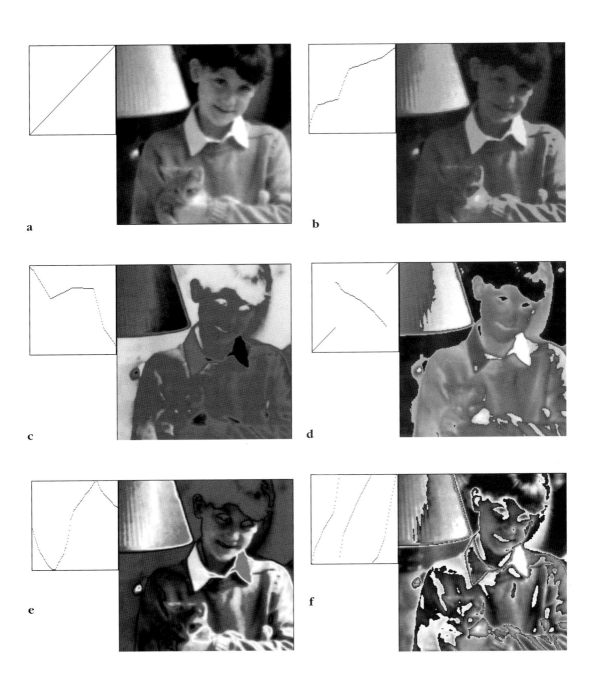

a

b

c

d

e

f

than 30 grey levels, or 75 cells per inch and 17 grey levels. The imagesetter used for this book is capable of much higher resolution and more grey levels, but not as many as a CRT or even a photograph.

For comparison purposes, a good-quality photographic print can reproduce 20 to 40 grey levels (the negative can do much better). An instant print such as the Polaroid film commonly used with laboratory microscopes can show 10 to 15 although both have much higher spatial resolution, making the images appear sharper to the eye.

Even so, looking at the original image in **Figure 1**, the viewer cannot see the detail in the bright and dark regions of the image, even on the video screen (and certainly not on the print). Modifying the LUT can increase the visibility in one region or the other, or in both dark and bright regions, provided something else is given up in exchange. **Figure 1** shows several modifications to the original image produced simply by manipulating the transfer function and the LUT by drawing a new relationship between stored and displayed brightness. In this case, a freehand drawing was made that became the transfer function; it was adjusted purely for visual effect.

Note some of the imaging possibilities. A nonlinear relationship can expand one portion of the grey scale range while compressing another. In photographic processing and also in analog display electronics, this is called varying the gamma (the slope of the exposure-density curve). Using a computer, however, we can draw in transfer functions that are far more complicated, nonlinear, and arbitrary than can be achieved in the darkroom.

Reversing all of the contrast range produces the equivalent of a photographic negative, which sometimes improves the visibility of details. **Figure 2** illustrates this with an example of an X-ray image, which are commonly examined using negatives. Reversing only a portion of the brightness range produces a visually strange effect, called solarization by photographers, that can also be used to show detail in both shadowed and saturated areas.

Increasing the slope of the transfer function so that it "wraps around" produces an image in which several quite different stored brightness values may have the same display brightness. If the overall organization of the image is familiar to the viewer, though, this contouring may not be too

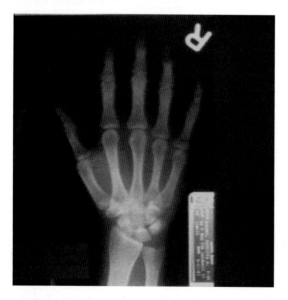
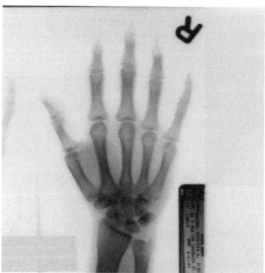

Figure 2. *X-ray image of a human hand, viewed as a positive and a negative.*

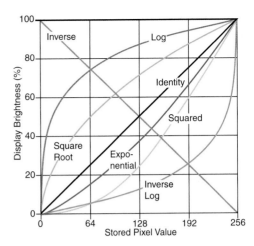

Figure 3. *Examples of display transfer functions.*

disruptive, and it can increase the visibility for small differences; however, as with the use of pseudo-color, this kind of treatment is easily overdone and may confuse rather than enhance most images.

Certainly, experimentally modifying the transfer function until the image "looks good" and best shows those features of most interest to the viewer provides an ultimately flexible (if dangerous) tool. The technique increases the visibility of some image details but hides others, according to the judgment of the operator. Of course, the same can be said of manipulating image contrast in darkroom printing. In most cases, it is desirable to have more reproducible and meaningful transfer functions available which can be applied equally to a series of images, so that proper comparison is possible.

The most common kinds of transfer functions are shown in **Figure 3**. These are curves of displayed vs. stored brightness following simple mathematical relationships such as logarithmic or power law curves. A logarithmic or square root curve will compress the displayed brightnesses at the bright end of the scale, while expanding those at the dark end. This kind of relationship can also convert an image from a camera with a linear response to the more common logarithmic response. An inverse log or squared curve will do the opposite. The error-function curve compresses middle grey values and spreads the scale at both the bright and dark extremes. An inverse curve simply produces a negative image.

Any of these functions may be used in addition to contrast expansion, which stretches the original scale to the full range of the display. Curves or tables of values for these transfer functions are typically precalculated and stored, so that they can be loaded quickly to modify the display LUT. Many systems allow quite a few different tables to be kept on hand for use when an image requires it, just as a series of color LUTs may be available on disk for pseudo-color displays**. Figure 4** illustrates the use of several transfer functions to enhance the visibility of structures in an image.

Histogram equalization

In addition to pre-calculated and stored tables, it is sometimes advantageous to construct a transfer function for a specific image. Unlike the arbitrary hand-drawn functions shown earlier, however, we desire a specific algorithm that gives reproducible and (hopefully) optimal results. The most popular of these methods is called histogram equalization (Stark and Fitzgerald, 1996). To understand it, we must begin with the image brightness histogram.

Figure 5 shows an example of an image with its histogram. The plot shows the number of pixels in the image having each of the 256 possible values of stored brightness. Peaks in the histogram

Figure 4. Manipulation of the grey-scale transfer function:
(a) an original, moderately low contrast transmission light microscope image (prepared slide of a head louse);

(b) expanded linear transfer function adjusted to the minimum and maximum brightness values in the image;

(c) positive gamma (log) function;

(d) negative gamma (log) function;

(e) negative linear transfer function;

(f) nonlinear transfer function (high slope linear contrast over central portion of brightness range, with negative slope or solarization for dark and bright portions).

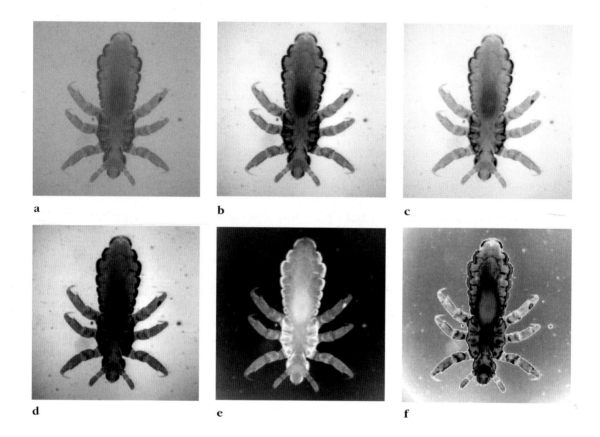

a   b   c

d   e   f

correspond to the more common brightness values, which often identify particular structures that are present. Valleys between the peaks indicate brightness values that are less common in the image. Empty regions at either end of the histogram would show that no pixels have those values, indicating that the image brightness range does not cover the full 0–255 range available.

For a color image, it is possible to show three histograms corresponding to the three color axes or channels. As shown in **Figure 6**, this can be done equally well for RGB, HSI, or YUV color coordinates. Any of these sets of histograms are incomplete, however, in that they do not show the combinations of values that are associated in the same pixels. A three-dimensional histogram in which points in the histogram have coordinates that correspond to the color values and show the number of pixels with each possible combination of values, is illustrated in **Figure 7**. Dark values indicate a large number of pixels with a particular combination of components. The projections of the three-dimensional histogram onto each of the 2D faces of the cube are shown. This tool will

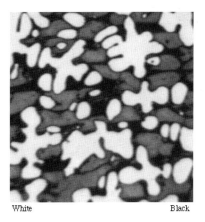

White   Black

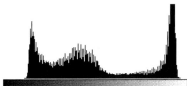

Figure 5. *Metallographic light microscope image of a three-phase metal alloy with its brightness histogram. The plot shows the number of pixels with each of the 256 possible brightness values.*

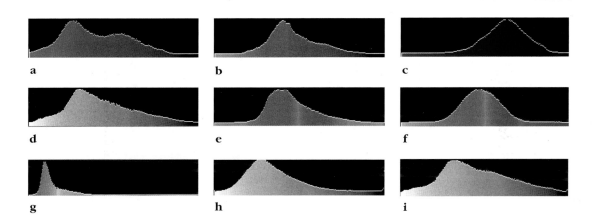

Figure 6. Histograms of individual planes in a color image (the image is a microscopic, thin section of pancreas, which is shown as Figure 52 in Chapter 1):

  (a) *red;*
  (b) *green;*
  (c) *blue;*
  (d) *luminance (Y);*
  (e) *U;*
  (f) *V;*
  (g) *hue;*
  (h) *saturation;*
  (i) *intensity.*

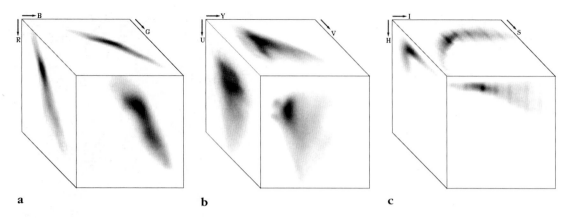

a   b   c

Figure 7. Three-way histograms of the same data shown in Figure 5: (a) RGB; (b) YUV; (c) HSI.

be used again in Chapter 6 in the context of selecting color combinations for thresholding, and in Chapter 7 for measuring the co-localization of intensity in different color channels (e.g., different fluorescent dyes).

Generally, images have unique brightness histograms. Even images of different areas of the same sample or scene, in which the various structures present have consistent brightness levels wherever they occur, will have different histograms, depending on the area fraction of each structure. Changing the overall illumination or camera settings will shift the peaks in the histogram. In addition, most real images exhibit some variation in brightness within features (e.g., from the edge to the center) or in different regions.

From the standpoint of efficiently using the available grey levels on the display, some grey scale values are under-utilized. It might be better to spread out the displayed grey levels in the peak areas selectively, compressing them in the valleys so that the same number of pixels in the display show each of the possible brightness levels. This is called histogram equalization. The transfer function is simply the original brightness histogram of the image, replotted as a cumulative plot as shown in **Figure 8**.

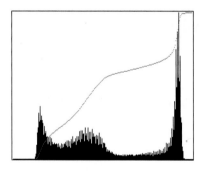

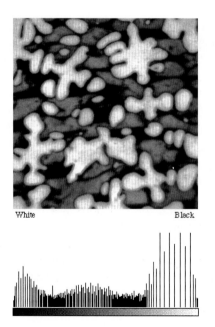

White   Black

Figure 8. The original and cumulative histogram from Figure 5 (a). The cumulative plot (red line) gives the transfer function for histogram equalization. The processed image and its histogram show the result of applying this function.

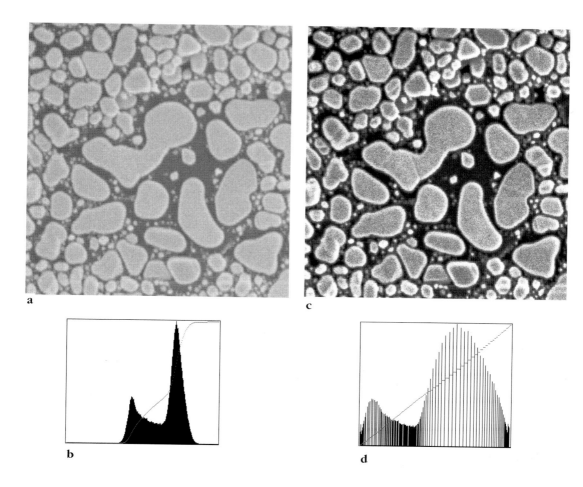

Figure 9. *An SEM image of deposited gold particles* **(a)** *with its histogram shown in conventional and cumulative form* **(b)**. *After histogram equalization* **(c)** *the cumulative histogram is a straight line* **(d)**.

A cumulative histogram helps to understand what histogram equalization does. **Figure 9** shows an SEM image with its original histogram shown in conventional presentation and also as a plot of the total number of pixels less than or equal to each brightness value. After equalization the latter plot is a straight line.

Histogram equalization reassigns the brightness values of pixels based on the image histogram. Individual pixels retain their brightness order (that is, they remain brighter or darker than other pixels) but the values are shifted, so that an equal number of pixels have each possible brightness value. In many cases, this spreads out the values in regions where different regions meet, showing detail in areas with a high brightness gradient.

An image having a few regions in which the pixels have very similar brightness values presents a histogram with peaks. The sizes of these peaks give the relative area of the different phase regions and are useful for image analysis. Performing a histogram equalization on the image spreads the peaks out, while compressing other parts of the histogram by assigning the same or very close brightness values to those pixels that are few in number and have intermediate brightnesses. This equalization makes it possible to see minor variations within regions that appeared nearly uniform in the original image.

The process is quite simple. For each brightness level j in the original image (and its histogram), the new assigned value k is calculated as

$$k = \sum_{i=0}^{j} N_i / T \qquad (1)$$

where the sum counts the number of pixels in the image (by integrating the histogram) with brightness equal to or less than j, and T is the total number of pixels (or the total area of the histogram).

Figure 8 showed an example. The original metallographic specimen has three phase regions with dark, intermediate, and light grey values. These peaks are separated in the histogram by regions having fewer pixels with intermediate brightness values, often because they happen to fall on the boundary between lighter and darker phase regions. Histogram equalization shows the shading within the phase regions, indiscernible in the original image. It also spreads out the brightness values in the histogram, as shown.

Some pixels that originally had different values are now assigned the same value, which represents a loss of information, while other values that were once very close together have been spread out, leaving gaps in the histogram. This image of a polished metal shows well-defined peaks corresponding to different phases present. The histogram-equalized image is less satisfying in terms of showing the distinction between the phases, but much better at showing the gradation in the white phase, which was not visible in the original.

This equalization process need not be performed on an entire image. Enhancing a portion of the original image, rather than the entire area, is also useful in many situations. This is particularly true when large regions of the image correspond to different types of structures or scenes and are generally brighter or darker than the rest of the image. When portions of an image can be selected, either manually or by some algorithm based on the variation in the brightness histogram, a selective equalization can be used to bring out local detail.

Figure 10 shows regions of the same test image used previously, with three regions separately selected and equalized. Two of these regions are arbitrary rectangular and elliptical shapes, drawn by hand. In many cases, this kind of manual selection is the most straightforward way to specify a region. The third area is the lampshade, which can be isolated from the rest of the image because locally the boundary is a sharp transition from white to black. Methods for locating boundary edges are discussed later in the chapter.

Each of the three regions shown was used to construct a brightness histogram, which was then equalized. The resulting reassigned brightness values were then substituted only for the pixels within the region. In the two dark regions (the girl's face and the region near her shoulder), equalization produces an overall brightening as well as spreading out the brightness values so that the small variations are more evident. In the bright area (the lampshade), the overall brightness is reduced; again, more variation is evident.

In all cases, the brightness values in the equalized regions show some contouring, the visible steps in brightness produced by the small number of different values present in these regions in the original image. Contouring is usually considered to be an image defect, since it distorts the actual smooth variation in values present in the image. When it is introduced specifically for effect, it may be called posterization (not to be confused with the use of the same term for the result of repeatedly applying a median filter, discussed in Chapter 3).

It should be noted, of course, that once a region has been selected, either manually or automatically, the contrast can be modified in any way desired: by loading a pre-stored LUT, calculating a

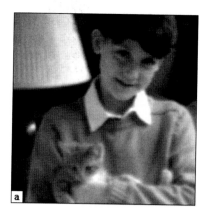 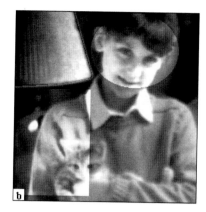

Figure 10. *Selective equalization can be performed in any designated region of an image. In this example, three regions have been selected and histogram equalization performed within each one separately. In the dark regions (the girl's face and the area behind her shoulder), this lightens the image and shows some of the detail that is otherwise not visible. In the light region (the lampshade), this results in an overall average darkening and expansion of the contrast to show shading. In both cases, the process is ultimately limited by the number of discrete grey levels which were actually present in those regions in the original image.*

histogram equalization function, or simply stretching the grey scale linearly to maximize contrast; however, when these operations are applied to only a portion of the entire image, it is not possible to manipulate only the display LUT. Since the stored grey values in other regions of the image are to be shown with their original corresponding display values, it is necessary to actually modify the contents of the stored image to alter the display. This is a very fast operation, since it is performed using a transfer function that is loaded or precalculated from the histogram and each pixel is accessed one time.

Histogram equalization of regions within an image can dramatically improve the local visibility of details, but it usually alters the relationship between brightness and structure. In most cases, it is desirable for the brightness level of pixels associated with a particular type of feature in the image to be the same, wherever in the field of view it may occur. This allows rapid classification of the features for counting or measurement. Local modification of the grey scale relationship voids this assumption, making the display brightness of features dependent on other features that happen to be nearby or in the selected region.

Histogram equalization assigns the same new grey value to each pixel having a given original grey value, everywhere in the region. The result is that regions often have very noticeable and abrupt boundaries, which may or may not follow feature boundaries in the original image. Another approach performs the equalization in a region around each pixel in the image, with the result applied separately to each individual pixel. This is normally done by specifying a neighborhood size (typically round or square). All of the pixels in that region are counted into a histogram, but the equalization procedure is applied only to the central pixel. This process is then repeated for each pixel in the image, always using the original brightness values to construct the histogram.

Figure 11 shows an example in which the neighborhood size used is an approximately circular area 11 pixels wide containing 89 pixels (**Figure 12**). The process is not applied within a distance of five pixels of the edges of the image, where the region cannot be centered on a pixel. Special rules can be made for these points, if required. Some programs implement local equalization using a square neighborhood, which is slightly easier computationally but is less isotropic. The actual calculation is quite simple, because for each pixel the equalized brightness value is just the number of darker pixels in the neighborhood. The neighborhood contains 89

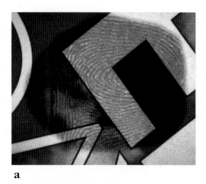
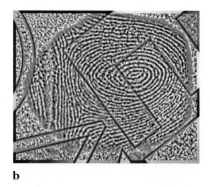

a   b

Figure 11. Local equalization applied to every pixel in an image. This is an image of a fingerprint on a magazine cover, which is difficult to visually distinguish on the dark and light printed regions. For each pixel in the original image (**a**), a 9 × 9 neighborhood has been used to construct a histogram. Equalization of that histogram produces a new brightness value for each pixel, but this is only saved for the central pixel. The process is repeated to apply to each pixel in the original image except those too near the edge, producing the result (**b**). Enlargements to shown individual pixels are shown in (**c**) and (**d**). The effect of this local equalization is to enhance edges, and reveal detail in light and dark regions; however, in the center of uniform regions, it can produce artefacts and noise.

Figure 12. Approximation to a circle 11 pixels wide contains a total of 89 pixels. Using a round neighborhood minimizes directional distortion and artefacts in the image due to local equalization.

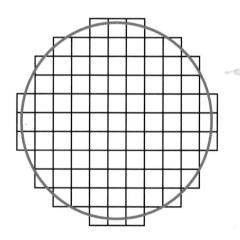

pixels, so the procedure produces an image in which the maximum number of distinct brightness values is 89, instead of the original 256, but this is still more than can be visually distinguished in the display. The process is applied to each pixel in the image, while constructing a new image containing the result, so that only the original values of the neighboring pixels are used to perform the equalization.

The process of local equalization enhances contrast near edges, revealing details in both light and dark regions, although it can be seen in the example that, in nominally uniform regions, this can produce artificial contrast variations that magnify the visibility of noise artefacts in the image. In general, it is important to remove or reduce noise as discussed in Chapter 3 before performing enhancement operations.

Local equalization works by making pixels that are slightly darker than their surroundings much darker, and ones that are slightly lighter, much lighter. Changing the size of the neighborhood used in local equalization offers only a small degree of control over the process. Other modifications that are more effective (and generally combined under the term "adaptive" equalization) are to weight the pixels according to how close they are to the center of the neighborhood, or according to how similar they are in brightness to the central pixel, or to include in the neighborhood only pixels "similar" to the central one. Since equalization is performed by constructing a histogram of the pixels and finding the midpoint of that histogram, the weighting is accomplished by assigning values greater or less than one to the pixels for use in summing up the histogram.

Figure 13 shows an example of adaptive equalization in which center weighting has been used to increase the visibility of fine detail, and value weighting has been used to reduce the effects of noise in the image. In this scanning electron microscope (SEM) image of dried paint, the large contrast range resulting from local variations in surface slope and the difficulty of collecting signal from within deep holes makes it difficult to see local detail. Local equalization (**Figure 13b**) enhances the visibility of the detail, but also the noise. Adaptive equalization (**Figure 13c**) produces a much better result. In both cases, the equalized result was added back to the original image to preserve some of the overall contrast range.

When it is used with color images, local or adaptive equalization is properly applied only to the intensity data. The image is converted from its original RGB format in which it is stored internally, the intensity values are modified and then combined with the original hue and saturation values so that new RGB values can be calculated to permit display of the result. This preserves the color information, which would be seriously altered if the red, green, and blue channels were equalized directly, as shown in **Figure 14** (Buzuloiu et al., 2001).

Laplacian

Local, or neighborhood, equalization of image contrast produces an increase in local contrast at boundaries, as shown in **Figure 15**. This has the effect of making edges easier for the viewer to see, consequently making the image appear sharper (although in the example the increased noise visibility within the uniform grains defeats this improvement). This section will discuss some other approaches to edge enhancement that are less sensitive to overall brightness levels and feature sizes than the equalization discussed above.

The first set of operations uses neighborhoods with multiplicative kernels, usually with integer weights, identical in principle to those used in Chapter 3 for noise smoothing. In the section on smoothing, kernels were written as an array of integers. For example,

$$
\begin{array}{ccc}
1 & 2 & 1 \\
2 & 4 & 2 \\
1 & 2 & 1
\end{array}
$$

This 3×3 kernel is understood to mean that the central pixel brightness value is multiplied by 4, the values of the 4 touching neighbors to the sides and above and below are multiplied by 2, and the 4 diagonally touching neighbors by 1. The total value is added up and then divided by 16 (the sum of the nine weights) to produce a new brightness value for the pixel. Other arrays of weights were also shown, some involving much larger arrays than this simple 3×3. For smoothing, all of the kernels were symmetrical about the center, and the examples shown in Chapter 3 had only positive weight values.

Figure 13. SEM image of dried paint: (a) *original;* **(b)** *conventional local equalization;* **(c)** *adaptive local equalization with center weighting and noise reduction. In both **b** and **c**, the equalized result has been added back to the original image.*

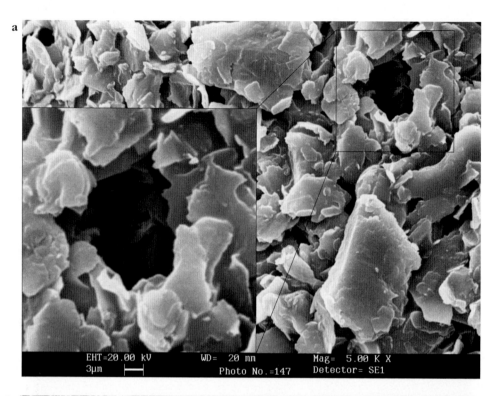

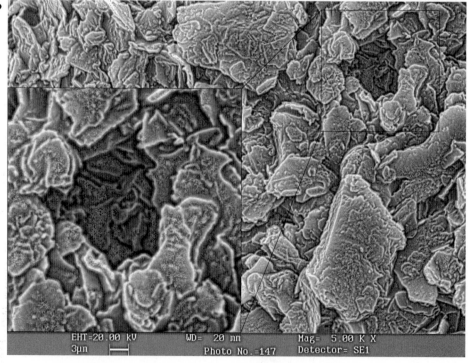

c

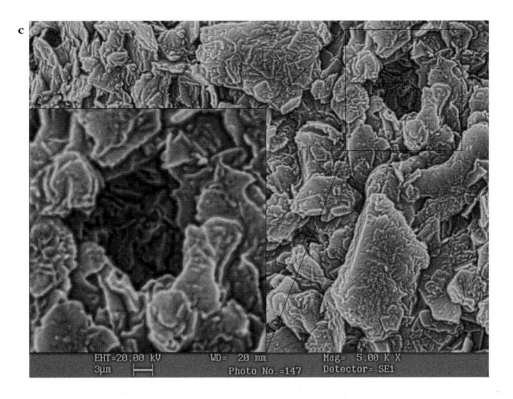

EHT=20.00 kV WD= 20 mm Mag= 5.00 K X
3µm Photo No.=147 Detector= SE1

A very simple kernel that is still symmetrical, but does not have exclusively positive values, is the 3×3 Laplacian operator

$$
\begin{array}{ccc}
-1 & -1 & -1 \\
-1 & +8 & -1 \\
-1 & -1 & -1
\end{array}
$$

This subtracts the brightness values of each of the neighboring pixels from the central pixel. Consequently, in a region of the image that is uniform in brightness or has a uniform gradient of brightness, the result of applying this kernel is to reduce the grey level to zero. When a discontinuity is present within the neighborhood in the form of a point, line, or edge, the result of the Laplacian is a non-zero value. It may be either positive or negative, depending on where the central point lies with respect to edge, etc.

In order to display the result when both positive and negative pixel values arise, it is common to add a medium grey value (128 for the case of a single-byte-per-pixel image with grey values in the range from 0 to 255) so that the zero points are middle grey and the brighter and darker values produced by the Laplacian can be seen. Some systems instead plot the absolute value of the result, but this tends to produce double lines along edges that are confusing both to the viewer and to subsequent processing and measurement operations.

As the name of the Laplacian operator implies, it is an approximation to the linear second derivative of brightness B in directions x and y

$$
\nabla^2 B \equiv \frac{\partial^2 B}{\partial x^2} + \frac{\partial^2 B}{\partial y^2} \tag{2}
$$

Figure 14. Color
photograph (courtesy
Eastman Kodak Co.):
(a) original;
(b) adaptive equalization
of the individual red,
green, and blue channels;
(c) adaptive equalization
of intensity, leaving hue
and saturation
unchanged. Note the
increased visibility of
figures and detail in
shadow areas, and the
false color variations
present in **b**.

a

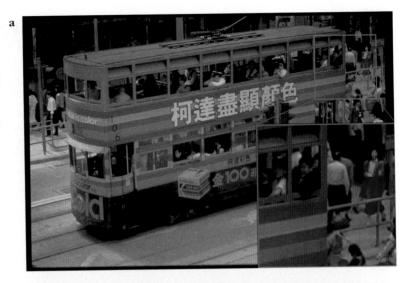

b

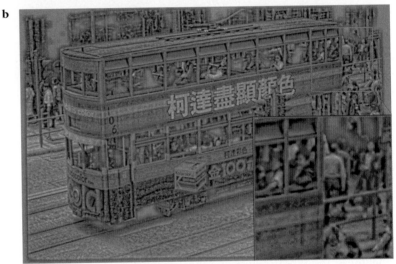

c

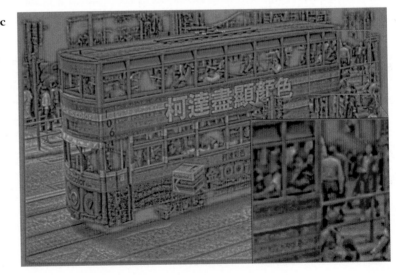

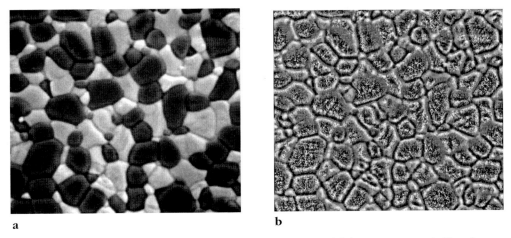

Figure 15. Local (not adaptive) equalization of a two-phase material (alumina-zirconia). Note the increased contrast at boundaries, and the noise artefacts within the grains.

which is invariant to rotation, and hence insensitive to the direction in which the discontinuity runs. This highlights the points, lines, and edges in the image and suppresses uniform and smoothly varying regions, with the result shown in **Figure 16**. By itself, this Laplacian image is not very easy to interpret. Adding the Laplacian enhancement of the edges from the original image restores the overall grey scale variation, which the human viewer can comfortably interpret. It also sharpens the image by locally increasing the contrast at discontinuities as shown in the figure. This can be done simply by changing the weights in the kernel, so that it becomes

$$\begin{array}{ccc} -1 & -1 & -1 \\ -1 & +9 & -1 \\ -1 & -1 & -1 \end{array}$$

This kernel is often described as a sharpening operator, because of the improved image contrast that it produces at edges. Justification for the procedure can be found in two different explanations. First, consider blur in an image to be modeled by a diffusion process in which brightness spreads out across the image, which would obey the partial differential equation

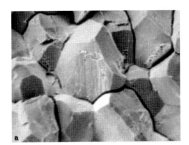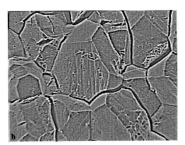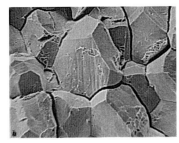

Figure 16. **Enhancement of contrast at edges, lines, and points using a Laplacian:** (a) original SEM image of ceramic fracture; (b) application of Laplacian operator; (c) addition of the Laplacian to the original image.

$$\frac{\partial f}{\partial t} = k\nabla^2 f \qquad (3)$$

where the blur function is $f(x,y,t)$ and t is time. If this is expanded into a Taylor series around time τ, we can express the unblurred image as

$$B(x,y) = f(x,y,\tau) - \tau\frac{\partial f}{\partial t} + \frac{\tau^2}{2}\frac{\partial^2 f}{\partial t^2} - \ldots \qquad (4)$$

If the higher-order terms are ignored, this is just

$$B = f - k\tau\nabla^2 f \qquad (5)$$

In other words, the unblurred image B can be restored by subtracting the Laplacian (times a constant) from the blurred image. While the modeling of image blur as a diffusion process is at best approximate and the scaling constant is unknown or arbitrary, this at least gives some plausibility to the approach.

At least equally important is the simple fact that the processed image "looks good." **Figure 17** illustrates this with an astronomical photograph of Saturn. The visibility of the fine detail in the rings and atmosphere is enhanced by processing. The human visual system itself concentrates on

Figure 17. Application of a Laplacian operator to enhance the visibility of band structures in the rings and atmosphere of Saturn:
(a) original image;
(b) application of Laplacian operator (notice the haloes around the tiny moons);
(c) addition of the Laplacian to the original image.

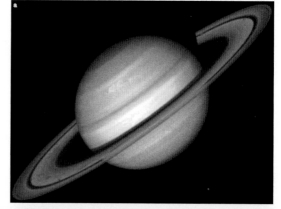

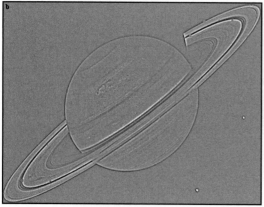

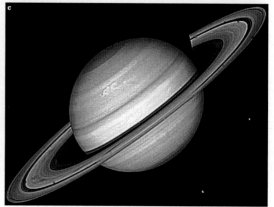

edges and ignores uniform regions (Marr and Hildreth, 1980; Marr, 1982; Hildreth, 1983). This capability is hard-wired into our retinas. Connected directly to the rods and cones of the retina are two layers of processing neurons that perform an operation very similar to the Laplacian. The horizontal cells in the second layer average together the signals from several neighboring sensors in the first layer, and the bipolar cells in the third layer combine that signal with the original sensor output. This is called local inhibition and helps us to extract boundaries and edges. It also accounts for some of the visual illusions shown in Chapter 1.

At a more practical level, consider the ability of the eye to respond to cartoons and line drawings. These are highly abstracted bits of information about the original scene, yet they are entirely recognizable and interpretable. The cartoon provides the eye with exactly the minimum information it would otherwise have to extract from the scene itself to transmit up to higher levels of processing in the brain. (Similar inhibition in the time domain, using the next two layers of retinal neurons, helps us detect motion.)

One characteristic of human vision that confirms this behavior is the presence of Mach bands, a common illusion resulting from local brightness inhibition (Mach, 1906; Cornsweet, 1970). **Figure 18** shows a series of vertical bands of uniform intensity. The human viewer does not perceive them as uniform, but sees an undershoot and overshoot on each side of the steps as shown in the plot. This increases the contrast at the step, and hence its visibility.

To see how this works using the Laplacian, we will use a one-dimensional kernel of the form

$$-1 \qquad +2 \qquad -1$$

and apply it to a series of brightness values along a line profile, across a step of moderate steepness

$$2 \qquad 2 \qquad 2 \qquad 2 \qquad 2 \qquad 4 \qquad 6 \qquad 6 \qquad 6 \qquad 6 \qquad 6$$

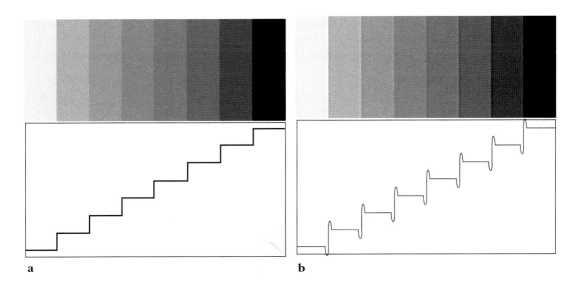

a   b

Figure 18. Illustration of Mach bands: (a) uniform grey bands with the brightness profile of the bands; *(b)* application of a Laplacian to the bands in image a with the brightness profile, showing increased contrast at the boundaries (this is the way the human eye perceives the uniform bands in image *a*.

Shifting the kernel to each position, multiplying the kernel values times the brightness values, then adding, gives the result

| 0 | 0 | 0 | 0 | −2 | 0 | +2 | 0 | 0 | 0 | 0 |

which can be added to the original to give

| 2 | 2 | 2 | 2 | 0 | 4 | 8 | 6 | 6 | 6 | 6 |

The undershoot and overshoot in brightness on either side of the step correspond to the Mach band effect.

Local inhibition also influences our perception of brightness and color. **Figure 19** shows the effect of the surrounding grey scale value on the apparent brightness and size of the central square (the two central grey squares are identical). This also happens in color. **Figure 20** illustrates several effects of local inhibition. In **Figure 20a** the reddish lines appear to change in color, brightness and thickness according to the varying colors of the intervening cyan/blue lines. In **Figure 20b**, the three identical central squares appear to vary in size, color and brightness according to the color of the surrounding square. In **Figure 20c**, the size of the two central squares appears different, and the color of the central square appears brighter and more saturated than when the same color occupies the surrounding outer patch. Similar visual illusions based on inhibition are commonly shown in many books and articles on vision and perception.

Inhibition is a process that takes place within the eye itself. Connections between the neurons within the retina suppress the output from one region according to its neighbors. Inhibition is useful for edge detection, but also affects our visual comparisons of size and orientation. **Figure 21** shows a typical result from an experiment in which the output from a single retinal ganglion in the optic nerve (shown as a time sequence across the top) is plotted as a small white target is slowly moved across the visual field. The cluster of white dots shows the location of the corresponding receptor on the retina. Notice the zone around the receptor that is very poor in white dots. Light shining on neighboring receptors inhibits the output from the central receptor. Presenting a dark spot in the visual field produces additional output from the receptor when it lies within the zone of inhibition, and suppresses output when it lies on the receptor. Selecting different ganglia will map other receptor cells, including those that surround the one shown. Each cell inhibits output from its neighbors. Other ganglia show temporal inhibition, in which output from a cell ignores the steady presence of either light or dark, and responds only to changes in illumination. You can demonstrate this effect by staring at a bright red pattern and then looking away; the afterimage will appear in your eye as green.

Another way to describe the operation of the Laplacian is as a high-pass filter. In Chapter 5, image processing in the Fourier domain is discussed in terms of the high- and low-frequency components of the image brightness. A low-pass filter, such as the smoothing kernels discussed in Chapter 3, removes the high-frequency variability associated with random noise, which can cause nearby pix-

Figure 19. Visual inhibition causes the brightness of the central grey square to appear different depending on the brightness of the surroundings.

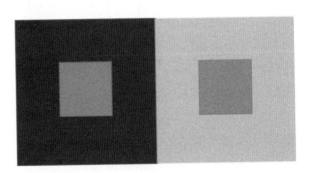

Figure 20. Inhibition in color images:
(a) *the red lines are constant in color and width, but appear to vary because of changes in the blue/cyan lines;*
(b) *the central square appears to change in size and color with variations in the surroundings;*
(c) *the color of the central square looks brighter and more saturated than the same color when it appears in the surroundings.*

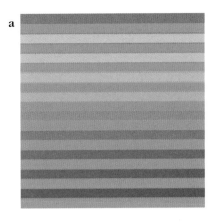

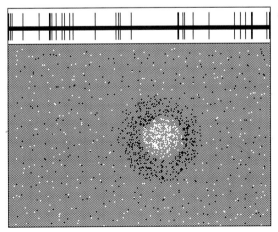

Figure 21. *Experimental results plotting the output from a single retinal ganglion in the optic nerve as targets consisting of small white or black circles are moved slowly across the visual field. The central cluster of white dots shows a positive response to the white circle, and the reduction in pulses when the white target lies in the field of a neighboring receptor. The dark target gives a complementary result.*

els to vary in brightness. Conversely, a high-pass filter allows these high frequencies to remain (pass through the filter), while removing the low frequencies corresponding to the gradual over-all variation in brightness.

As with smoothing kernels, there are many different sets of integers and different-size kernels that can be used to apply a Laplacian to an image. The simplest just uses the four immediately touching pixels that share a side with the central pixel

$$
\begin{array}{ccc}
 & -1 & \\
-1 & +4 & -1 \\
 & -1 &
\end{array}
$$

Larger kernels may combine a certain amount of smoothing by having positive weights for pixels in a small region near the central pixel, surrounded by negative weights for pixels farther away. Several examples are shown below. Because of the shape of these kernels when they are plotted as isometric views (**Figure 22**), they are sometimes described as a Mexican hat or sombrero filter; this name is usually reserved for kernels with more than one positive-weighted pixel at the center.

As in the discussion of Gaussian filters in Chapter 3, the restriction of these kernels to integer values is arbitrary based on the historic cost of computing with real (floating point) values. By using real numbers it is possible to construct smoother kernels that better fit the ideal functional shapes, which are closely approximate the difference of two Gaussians of different standard deviation, as discussed in the next section.

Figure 22. *Isometric and contour plot views of the 17 × 17 Mexican hat kernel.*

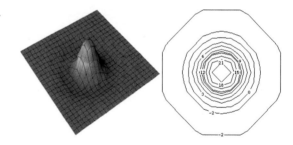

5 × 5 Laplacian kernel
```
 0  0 -1  0  0
 0 -1 -2 -1  0
-1 -2 16 -2 -1
 0 -1 -2 -1  0
 0  0 -1  0  0
```

7 × 7 Mexican hat kernel
```
 0  0 -1 -1 -1  0  0
 0 -1 -3 -3 -3 -1  0
-1 -3  0  7  0 -3 -1
-1 -3  7 24  7 -3 -1
-1 -3  0  7  0 -3 -1
 0 -1 -3 -3 -3 -1  0
 0  0 -1 -1 -1  0  0
```

13 × 13 Mexican hat kernel

```
0  0  0  0  0 -1 -1 -1  0  0  0  0  0
0  0  0 -1 -1 -2 -2 -2 -1 -1  0  0  0
0  0 -2 -2 -3 -3 -4 -3 -3 -2 -2  0  0
0 -1 -2 -3 -3 -3 -2 -3 -3 -3 -2 -1  0
0 -1 -3 -3 -1  4  6  4 -1 -3 -3 -1  0
-1 -2 -3 -3  4 14 19 14  4 -3 -3 -2 -1
-1 -2 -4 -2  6 19 24 19  6 -2 -4 -2 -1
-1 -2 -3 -3  4 14 19 14  4 -3 -3 -2 -1
0 -1 -3 -3 -1  4  6  4 -1 -3 -3 -1  0
0 -1 -2 -3 -3 -3 -2 -3 -3 -3 -2 -1  0
0  0 -2 -2 -3 -3 -4 -3 -3 -2 -2  0  0
0  0  0 -1 -1 -2 -2 -2 -1 -1  0  0  0
0  0  0  0  0 -1 -1 -1  0  0  0  0  0
```

17 × 17 Mexican hat kernel

```
0  0  0  0  0  0 -1 -1 -1 -1 -1  0  0  0  0  0  0
0  0  0  0 -1 -1 -1 -1 -1 -1 -1 -1 -1  0  0  0  0
0  0 -1 -1 -1 -2 -3 -3 -3 -3 -3 -2 -1 -1 -1  0  0
0  0 -1 -1 -2 -3 -3 -3 -3 -3 -3 -2 -1 -1  0  0
0 -1 -1 -2 -3 -3 -3 -2 -3 -2 -3 -3 -3 -2 -1 -1  0
0 -1 -2 -3 -3 -3  0  2  4  2  0 -3 -3 -3 -2 -1  0
-1 -1 -3 -3 -3  0  4 10 12 10  4  0 -3 -3 -3 -1 -1
-1 -1 -3 -3 -2  2 10 18 21 18 10  2 -2 -3 -3 -1 -1
-1 -1 -3 -3 -3  4 12 21 24 21 12  4 -3 -3 -3 -1 -1
-1 -1 -3 -3 -2  2 10 18 21 18 10  2 -2 -3 -3 -1 -1
-1 -1 -3 -3 -3  0  4 10 12 10  4  0 -3 -3 -3 -1 -1
0 -1 -2 -3 -3 -3  0  2  4  2  0 -3 -3 -3 -2 -1  0
0 -1 -1 -2 -3 -3 -3 -2 -3 -2 -3 -3 -3 -2 -1 -1  0
0  0 -1 -1 -2 -3 -3 -3 -3 -3 -3 -2 -1 -1  0  0
0  0 -1 -1 -1 -2 -3 -3 -3 -3 -3 -2 -1 -1 -1  0  0
0  0  0  0 -1 -1 -1 -1 -1 -1 -1 -1 -1  0  0  0  0
0  0  0  0  0  0 -1 -1 -1 -1 -1  0  0  0  0  0  0
```

Derivatives

The Laplacian is a high-pass filter, but not a particularly good tool for demarcating edges (Berzins, 1984; Heath et al., 1997). In most cases, boundaries or edges of features or regions appear at least locally as a step in brightness, sometimes spread over several pixels. The Laplacian gives a larger response to a line than to a step, and to a point than to a line. In an image that contains noise, which is typically present as points varying in brightness due to counting statistics, detector characteristics, etc., the Laplacian will show such points more strongly than the edges or boundaries that are of interest.

Another approach to locating edges uses first derivatives in two or more directions. It will be helpful to first examine simple, one-dimensional first derivatives. Some images are essentially one-dimensional, such as chromatography preparations in which proteins are spread along lanes in an electrical field (**Figure 23**) or tree ring patterns from drill cores (**Figure 24**). Applying a first derivative to such an image, in the direction of important variation, demarcates the boundaries and enhances the visibility of small steps and other details, as shown in the figures. Of course, for an

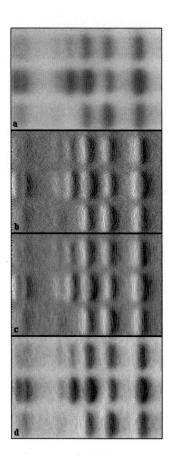

Figure 23. Image of a protein separation gel:
(a) original;
(b) difference between each pixel and its neighbor to the left;
(c) vertical averaging of image **b** to reduce noise;
(d) horizontal derivative using a 3 × 3 kernel as discussed in the text.

Figure 24. Image of tree rings in a drill core:
(a) original;
(b) difference between each pixel and its neighbor to the left;
(c) vertical averaging of image **b** to reduce noise;
(d) horizontal derivative using a 3 × 3 kernel as discussed in the text.

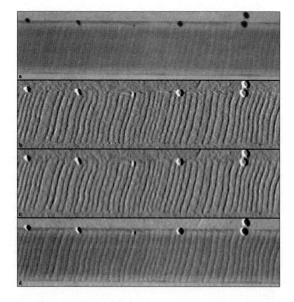

image with digitized finite pixels, a continuous derivative cannot be performed. Instead, the difference value between adjacent pixels can be calculated as a finite derivative. This difference is somewhat noisy, but averaging in the direction perpendicular to the derivative can smooth the result, as shown in the figures.

A derivative image with smoother appearance can be produced with fewer steps by applying an asymmetric kernel. Consider a set of kernels of the form shown below. Eight rotational orientations of this kernel about the center are possible.

1	0	−1		2	1	0		1	2	1
2	0	−2		1	0	−1		0	0	0 …
1	0	−1		0	−1	−2		−1	−2	−1

Applying the first pattern of values shown to the tree ring and protein separation images is shown in **Figures 23** and **24**.

One improvement comes from averaging together the adjacent pixels in each vertical column before taking the difference; this reduces noise in the image. A second, more subtle effect is that these kernels are 3 pixels wide and thus replace the central pixel with the difference value. The simple subtraction described previously causes a half-pixel shift in the image, which is absent with this kernel. Finally, the method shown here is fast, requiring only a single pass through the image.

Obviously, other kernel values can be devised that will also produce derivatives. As the kernel size increases, more different directions are possible. Because this is fundamentally a one-dimensional derivative, it is possible to directly use the coefficients of Savitsky and Golay (1964), which were originally published for use with such one-dimensional data as spectrograms or other strip-chart recorder output. These coefficients, like the smoothing weights shown in Chapter 3, are equivalent to least-squares fitting a high-order polynomial to the data. In this case, however, the first derivative of the polynomial is evaluated at the central point. Both second degree (quadratic) and fourth degree (quartic) polynomials are shown in **Tables 1** and **2**.

Figure 25 shows a fragment of the brightness profile along the center of the tree ring image in **Figure 24**. The first derivative plots shown were obtained by using the pixel difference approximation, and by using these weights to fit quadratic and quartic polynomials over widths of 5, 9, and 13 pixels around each point. The fits produce much smoother results and suppress noise; however, by increasing the fitting width, the small-scale real variations in the data are suppressed. It is generally necessary, as in any fitting or smoothing operation, to keep the kernel size smaller than the features of interest.

Using one-dimensional derivatives to extract one-dimensional data from two-dimensional images is a relatively specialized operation, although extending the same principles to locating boundaries with arbitrary orientations in two-dimensional images is one of the most common of all image enhancement operations. The problem, of course, is finding a method that is insensitive to the (local) orientation of the edge.

One of the earliest approaches to this task was the Roberts' Cross operator (Roberts, 1965). It uses the same difference technique shown above for the one-dimensional case, but with two pixel differences at right angles to each other, as diagrammed in **Figure 26**. These two differences represent a finite approximation to the derivative of brightness. Two-directional derivatives can be combined to obtain a magnitude value that is insensitive to the orientation of the edge by squaring, adding, and taking the square root of the total.

Table 1. Coefficients for First Derivative Quadratic Fit

No.	5	7	9	11	13	15	17	19	21	23	25
−12											−.0092
−11										−.0109	−.0085
−10									−.0130	−.0099	−.0077
−9								−.0158	−.0117	−.0089	−.0069
−8							−.0196	−.0140	−.0104	−.0079	−.0062
−7						−.0250	−.0172	−.0123	−.0091	−.0069	−.0054
−6					−.0330	−.0214	−.0147	−.0105	−.0078	−.0059	−.0046
−5				−.0455	−.0275	−.0179	−.0123	−.0088	−.0065	−.0049	−.0038
−4			−.0667	−.0364	−.0220	−.0143	−.0098	−.0070	−.0052	−.0040	−.0031
−3		−.1071	−.0500	−.0273	−.0165	−.0107	−.0074	−.0053	−.0039	−.0030	−.0023
−2	−.2000	−.0714	−.0333	−.0182	−.0110	−.0071	−.0049	−.0035	−.0026	−.0020	−.0015
−1	−.1000	−.0357	−.0250	−.0091	−.0055	−.0036	−.0025	−.0018	−.0013	−.0010	−.0008
0	0	0	0	0	0	0	0	0	0	0	0
+1	+.1000	+.0357	+.0250	+.0091	+.0055	+.0036	+.0025	+.0018	+.0013	+.0010	+.0008
+2	+.2000	+.0714	+.0333	+.0182	+.0110	+.0071	+.0049	+.0035	+.0026	+.0020	+.0015
+3		+.1071	+.0500	+.0273	+.0165	+.0107	+.0074	+.0053	+.0039	+.0030	+.0023
+4			+.0667	+.0364	+.0220	+.0143	+.0098	+.0070	+.0052	+.0040	+.0031
+5				+.0455	+.0275	+.0179	+.0123	+.0088	+.0065	+.0049	+.0038
+6					+.0330	+.0214	+.0147	+.0105	+.0078	+.0059	+.0046
+7						+.0250	+.0172	+.0123	+.0091	+.0069	+.0054
+8							+.0196	+.0140	+.0104	+.0079	+.0062
+9								+.0158	+.0117	+.0089	+.0069
+10									+.0130	+.0099	+.0077
+11										+.0109	+.0085
+12											+.0092

This method has the same problems as the difference method used in one dimension. Noise in the image is magnified by the single-pixel differences, and the result is shifted by half a pixel in both the x and y directions. In addition, the result is not invariant with respect to edge orientation. As a practical matter, the computers in common use when this model was first proposed were not very fast, nor were they equipped with separate floating-point math coprocessors. This made the square root of the sum of the squares impractical to calculate. Two alternatives were used: adding the absolute values of the two directional differences, or comparing the two absolute values of the differences and keeping the larger one. Both of these methods make the result quite sensitive to direction. In addition, even if the square root method is used, the magnitude of the result will vary because the pixel spacing is not the same in all directions, and edges in the vertical and horizontal directions spread the change in brightness over more pixels than edges in the diagonal directions.

In several of the comparison sequences that follow, the Roberts' Cross image will be shown (**Figures 29b** and **44c**). In all cases, the square root of the sum of squares of the differences was used. Even so, the images are characterized by varying sensitivity with respect to edge orientation, as well as a high noise sensitivity.

The Sobel and Kirsch operators

Just as for the example of the horizontal derivative described earlier, the use of a larger kernel offers reduced sensitivity to noise by averaging several pixels and eliminating image shift. In fact, the

Table 2. Coefficients for First Derivative Quartic Fit

No.	5	7	9	11	13	15	17	19	21	23	25
−12											+.0174
−11										+.0200	+.0048
−10									+.0231	+.0041	−.0048
−9								+.0271	+.0028	−.0077	−.0118
−8							+.0322	−.0003	−.0119	−.0159	−.0165
−7						+.0387	−.0042	−.0182	−.0215	−.0209	−.0190
−6					+.0472	−.0123	−.0276	−.0292	−.0267	−.0231	−.0197
−5				+.0583	−.0275	−.0423	−.0400	−.0340	−.0280	−.0230	−.0189
−4			+.0724	−.0571	−.0657	−.0549	−.0431	−.0335	−.0262	−.0208	−.0166
−3		+.0873	−.1195	−.1033	−.0748	−.0534	−.0388	−.0320	−.0219	−.0170	−.0134
−2	+.0833	−.2659	−.1625	−.0977	−.0620	−.0414	−.0289	−.0210	−.0157	−.0120	−.0094
−1	−.6667	−.2302	−.1061	−.0575	−.0346	−.0225	−.0154	−.0110	−.0081	−.0062	−.0048
0	0	0	0	0	0	0	0	0	0	0	0
+1	+.6667	+.2302	+.1061	+.0575	+.0346	+.0225	+.0154	+.0110	+.0081	+.0062	+.0048
+2	−.0833	+.2659	+.1625	+.0977	+.0620	+.0414	+.0289	+.0210	+.0157	+.0120	+.0094
+3		−.0873	+.1195	+.1033	+.0748	+.0534	+.0388	+.0320	+.0219	+.0170	+.0134
+4			−.0724	+.0571	+.0657	+.0549	+.0431	+.0335	+.0262	+.0208	+.0166
+5				−.0583	+.0275	+.0423	+.0400	+.0340	+.0280	+.0230	+.0189
+6					−.0472	+.0123	+.0276	+.0292	+.0267	+.0231	+.0197
+7						−.0387	+.0042	+.0182	+.0215	+.0209	+.0190
+8							−.0322	+.0003	+.0119	+.0159	+.0165
+9								−.0271	−.0028	+.0077	+.0118
+10									−.0231	−.0041	+.0048
+11										−.0200	−.0048
+12											−.0174

derivative kernels shown above, or other similar patterns using different sets of integers, are widely used. Some common examples of these coefficients are shown in **Table 3** below.

Table 3. Examples of derivative filter weights

+1	0	−1		+1	0	−1		+1	−1	−1		+5	−3	−3
+1	0	−1		+2	0	−2		+2	+1	−1		+5	0	−3
+1	0	−1		+1	0	−1		+1	−1	−1		+5	−3	−3
+1	+1	0		+2	+1	0		+2	+1	−1		+5	+5	−3
+1	0	−1		+1	0	−1		+1	+1	−1		+5	0	−3
0	−1	−1		0	−1	−2		−1	−1	−1		−3	−3	−3
+1	+1	+1		+1	+2	+1		+1	+2	+1		+5	+5	+5
0	0	0		0	0	0		−1	+1	−1		−3	0	−3
−1	−1	−1		−1	−2	−1		−1	−1	−1		−3	−3	−3

and so forth for eight rotations.

It actually makes little difference which of these patterns of values is used, as long as the magnitude of the result does not exceed the storage capacity of the computer being used. This is often

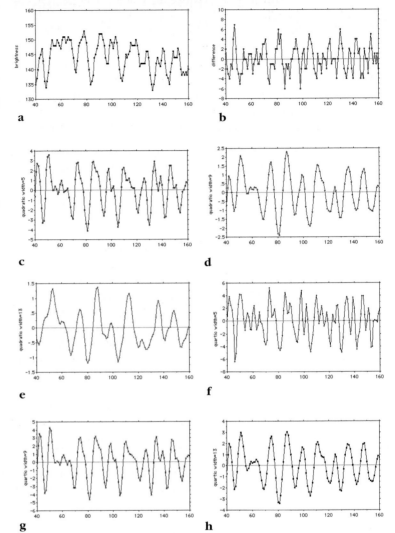

Figure 25. Horizontal brightness profile for a line in the center of the tree ring image (Figure 25), and its derivatives:
(a) original brightness plotted for each pixel along a fragment of the line;
(b) finite difference plot showing the difference between adjacent pixels;
(c) derivative calculated using the weights for a quadratic polynomial fit to 5 points;
(d) a quadratic fit to 9 points;
(e) a quadratic fit to 13 points;
(f) derivative calculated using the weights for a quartic polynomial fit to 5 points;
(g) a quartic fit to 9 points;
(h) a quartic fit to 13 points.

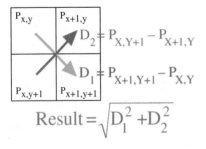

Figure 26. Diagram of Roberts' Cross operator. Two differences in directions at right angles to each other are combined to determine the gradient.

a single byte per pixel, which, because the result of the previous operation may be either negative or positive, can handle only values between –127 and +128. If large steps in brightness are present, this may result in the clipping of the calculated values, so that major boundaries are broadened or distorted in order to see smaller ones. The alternative is to employ automatic scaling, using the maximum and minimum values in the derivative image to set the white and dark values. To avoid loss of precision, this requires two passes through the image: one to perform the calculations and find the extreme values and the second to actually compute the values and scale the results for storage, or one to perform the calculations and temporarily store intermediate results with full precision, and a second to rescale the values to fit the range for pixel values.

As for the Roberts' Cross method, if the derivatives in two orthogonal directions are computed, they can be combined as the square root of the sums of their squares to obtain a result independent of orientation.

$$\text{Magnitude} = \sqrt{\left(\frac{\partial B}{\partial x}\right)^2 + \left(\frac{\partial B}{\partial y}\right)^2} \tag{6}$$

This is the Sobel (1970) method. It is one of the most commonly used techniques, even though it requires a modest amount of computation to perform correctly. (As for the Roberts' Cross, some computer programs attempt to compensate for hardware limitations by adding or comparing the two values, instead of squaring, adding, and taking the square root.)

With appropriate hardware, such as a shift register or array processor, the Sobel operation can be performed in essentially real time. This usually means 1/30th of a second per image, so that conventional video images can be processed and viewed. It often means viewing one frame while the following one is digitized, but in the case of the Sobel, it is even possible to view the image live, delayed only by two video scan lines. Two lines of data can be buffered and used to calculate the derivative values using the 3 × 3 kernels shown previously. Specialized hardware to perform this real-time edge enhancement is used in some military applications, making it possible to locate edges in images for tracking, alignment of hardware in midair refueling, and other purposes.

At the other extreme, some general-purpose image analysis systems that do not have hardware for fast math operations perform the Sobel operation using a series of operations. First, two derivative images are formed, one using a horizontal and one a vertical orientation of the kernel. Then each of these is modified using a LUT to replace the value of each pixel with its square. The two resulting images are added together, and another LUT is used to convert each pixel value to its square root. No multiplication or square roots are needed. However, if this method is applied in a typical system with 8 bits per pixel, the loss of precision is severe, reducing the final image to no more than 4 bits (16 grey levels) of useful information.

A more practical way to avoid the mathematical operations needed to calculate the square root of the sum of squares needed by the Sobel is the Kirsch operator (1971). This method applies each of the eight orientations of the derivative kernel and keeps the maximum value. It requires only integer multiplication and comparisons. For many images, the results for the magnitude of edges are very similar to the Sobel. **Figure 27** shows an example. Vertical and horizontal derivatives of the image, and the maximum derivative values in each of eight directions, are shown.

Figures 28 and **29** illustrate the formation of the Sobel edge-finding image and compare it to the Laplacian, Roberts' Cross, and Kirsch operators. The example image contains many continuous edges running in all directions around the holes in the carbon film, as well as some straight edges at various orientations along the asbestos fibers. The Laplacian image is quite noisy, and the Roberts' Cross does not show all of the edges equally well. The individual vertical and horizontal

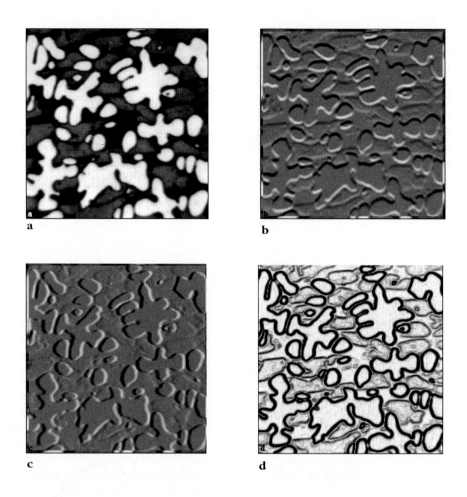

a

b

c

d

Figure 27. *A metallographic image* **(a)** *with two directional derivatives* **(b** *and* **c),** *and the Kirsch image* **(d)** *produced by keeping the maximum value from each direction.*

Figure 28. *Original image (asbestos fibers on a holey carbon film, imaged in a TEM). This image is the basis for the processing shown in* **Figure 29**.

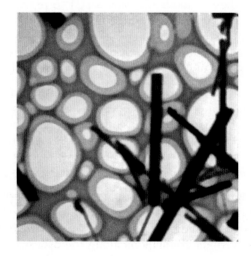

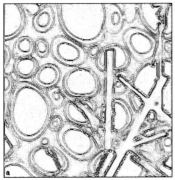

Figure 29. Edge enhancement of the image in Figure 28:
(**a**) *Laplacian operator;*
(**b**) *Roberts' Cross operator;*
(**c**) *horizontal derivative, scaled to full grey-scale range;*
(**d**) *absolute value of image **c**;*
(**e**) *vertical derivative, scaled to full grey-scale range;*
(**f**) *absolute value of image **e**;*
(**g**) *sum of absolute values from images **d** and **f**;*
(**h**) *maximum of values in images **d** and **f**, pixel by pixel;*
(**i**) *Sobel operator (square root of sum of squares of values);*
(**j**) *Kirsch operator.*

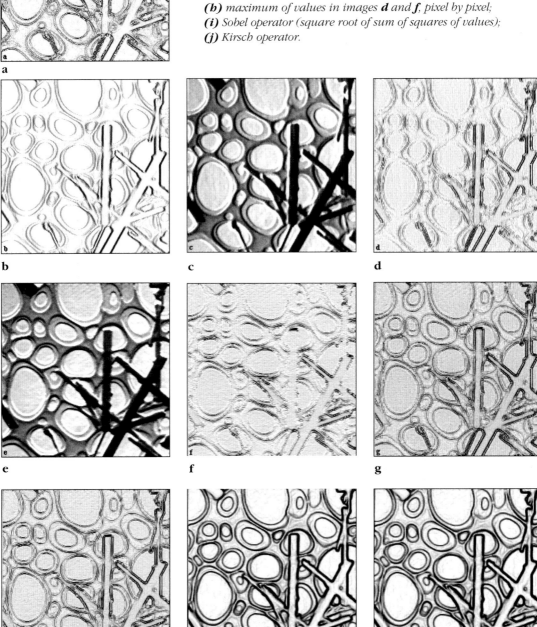

derivatives are shown with the zero value shifted to an intermediate grey, so that both the negative and positive values can be seen. The absolute values are also shown.

Combining the two directional derivatives by a sum, or maximum operator, produces quite noisy and incomplete boundary enhancement. The square root of the sum of squares produces a good image, with little noise and continuous edge markings. The result from the Kirsch operator is very similar to the Sobel for this image.

In addition to the magnitude of the Sobel operator, it is also possible to calculate a direction value (Lineberry, 1982) for each pixel as:

$$\text{Direction} = \text{Arc Tan}\left(\frac{\partial B / \partial y}{\partial B / \partial x}\right) \tag{7}$$

This assigns a value to each pixel for the gradient direction, which can be scaled to the grey scale of the image. **Figure 30** shows the vector results from applying the Sobel operator to the image of **Figure 29**. The magnitude and direction are encoded, but the vector field is too sparse to show any image details.

Figure 31 shows only the direction information for the image in **Figure 27**, using grey values to represent the angles. The progression of values around each more-or-less circular hole is evident. The use of a pseudo-color scale for this display is particularly suitable, since a rainbow of hues can show the progression without the arbitrary discontinuity required by the grey scale (in this example, at an angle of zero degrees). Unfortunately, the pixels within relatively homogeneous areas of the features also have colors assigned, because at every point there is some direction to the gradient, and these colors tend to overwhelm the visual impression of the image. A solution is to combine the magnitude of the gradient with the direction, as shown in **Figure 32**. This is the dendrite image from **Figure 28**, processed to show the magnitude and the direction of the Sobel edge gradient, the latter in color. These two images are then multiplied together so that the intensity of the color is proportional to the magnitude of the gradient. The result clearly shows the orientation of boundaries.

The magnitude and direction information can also be combined in an HSI representation of the image. In **Figure 33,** the original grey-scale image (the SEM image from **Figure 9**) has been processed to obtain the Sobel magnitude and direction. The direction information is then assigned to the hue plane and the magnitude to saturation and intensity.

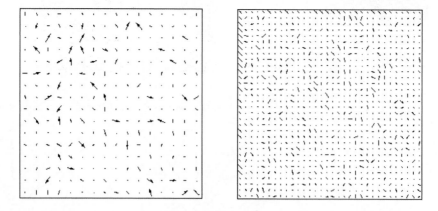

Figure 30. *Applying a Sobel operator to the image in* **Figure 27**. *Each vector has the direction and magnitude given by the operator, but even the fine vector field is too sparse to show any details of the image.*

Figure 31. Direction of the Sobel operator for the image in *Figure 28.*

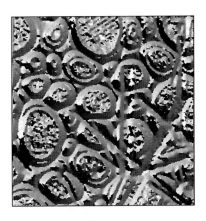

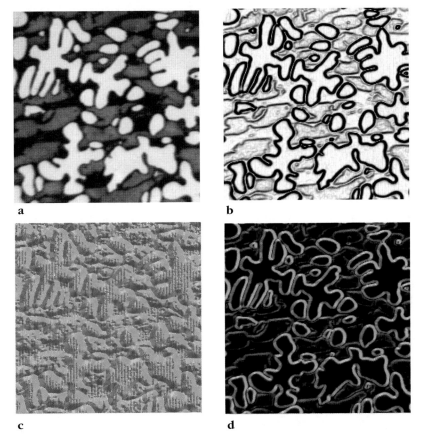

a

b

c

d

Figure 32. Combining the magnitude and direction information from the Sobel gradient operator:
- **(a)** *original grey scale image (from* **Figure 28***);*
- **(b)** *Sobel gradient magnitude;*
- **(c)** *Sobel direction (color coded);*
- **(d)** *product of* **b** *times* **c***.*

Another way to improve the resulting image is to show the direction information only for those pixels which also have a strong magnitude for the brightness gradient. In **Figure 34,** this is done by using the magnitude image as a mask, selecting (by thresholding as discussed in Chapter 6) the 40% of the pixels with the largest gradient magnitude, and showing the direction only for those

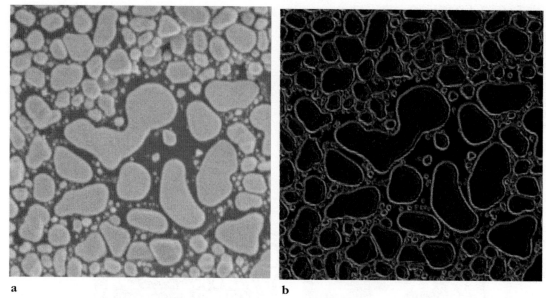

a   b

Figure 33. HSI representation of the gradient vector, with hue representing direction and the magnitude shown by saturation and intensity: (a) original image; (b) result.

pixels. This is particularly suitable for selecting pixels to be counted as a function of color (direction) for analysis purposes.

Figure 34 also shows a histogram plot of the preferred orientation in the image. This kind of plot is particularly common for interpreting the orientation of lines, such as dislocations in metals and the traces of faults in geographic maps. In **Figure 35**, the orientation of the collagen fibers is measured using this same technique. The plot shows that they are not isotropically oriented, with about twice as many pixels showing an orientation of about 70 degrees. Further examples of

a
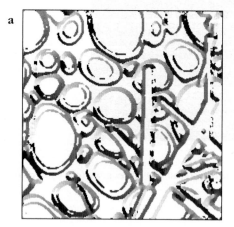

Figure 34. Uses of the edge-orientation image in Figure 31:
(a) masking only those pixels whose edge magnitude is large (the 40% of the pixels with the largest magnitude);
(b) generating a histogram of orientation values, in which the horizontal axis of the histogram (255 brightness values) represents the angular range 0–360°.

b
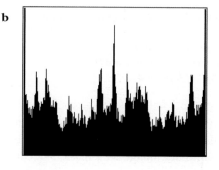

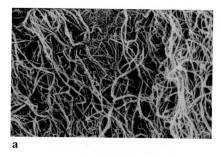

a

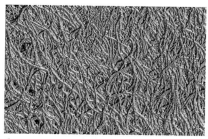

b

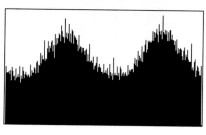

c

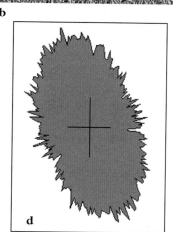

d

Figure 35. Image of collagen fibers (a), with the *Sobel orientation values (b) plotted as a conventional histogram (c) and as a rose plot (d).*

measurement using this tool will be discussed below, as will the use of the direction image to reveal image texture, or to select regions of the image based on the texture or its orientation.

When the oriented features do not fill the image, but are either isolated fibers or edges of features, they can be selected for measurement by using the Sobel magnitude image. Thresholding this image to select only the points whose gradient vector is large, and applying the resulting binary image as a selection mask to eliminate pixels that are not of interest for orientation measurement, produces a result as shown in **Figure 36**.

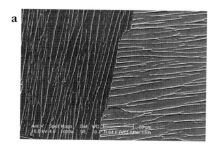

a

b

Figure 36. Lamellar structure in a titanium alloy:
(a) SEM image (courtesy H. Fraser, Ohio State University);
(b) edges color coded with orientation and selected by magnitude of the Sobel gradient;
(c) histogram of orientations from 0–180°.

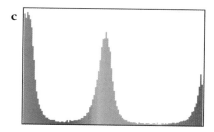

c

Figure 37. *Sobel magnitude images on a noisy test image (**a**) using 3 × 3 (**b**) and 5 × 5 (**c**) kernels.*

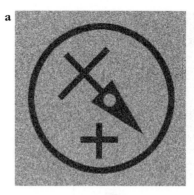

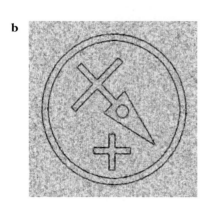

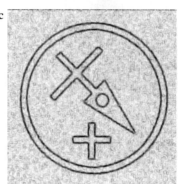

Orientation determination using the angle calculated from the Sobel derivatives is not a perfectly isotropic or unbiased measure of boundary orientations because of the effects of the square pixel grid and limited number of points sampled. With a larger kernel of values, weights can be assigned to better correspond to how far away the pixels are from the center. With a 5 × 5 array a more smoothly varying and isotropically uniform result can be obtained. **Figure 37** shows an example with a circle and some lines with superimposed image noise as a test object; the definition of the edge using the Sobel magnitude is improved by the larger neighborhood, and the effect of random noise in the image is minimized, although the line breadth becomes greater.

The use of an edge-enhancing operator to modify images is useful in many situations. We have already seen examples of sharpening using the Laplacian, to increase the contrast at edges and make images appear sharper to the viewer. Gradient or edge-finding methods also do this, but they also modify the image so that its interpretation becomes somewhat different. This contrast increase is selective; therefore, it responds to local information in the image in a way that manipulating the brightness histogram cannot.

For example, **Figure 38** shows several views of galaxy M51. In the original image, it is quite impossible to see the full range of brightness, even on a high-quality photographic negative. It is even less possible to print it. The extremely light and dark areas simply cover too great a range. Compressing the range nonlinearly, using a logarithmic transfer function, can make it possible to see both ends of the scale at the same time. However, this is accomplished by reducing small variations, especially at the bright end of the scale, so that they are not visible.

The gradient enhancement shown in **Figure 38c** uses a Sobel operator to mark edges. This shows the structure within the galaxy in a different way, by emphasizing local spatial variations regardless of the absolute value of the brightness. This produces a distinctly different result than the unsharp masking shown in **Figure 38b**.

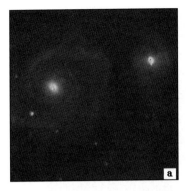

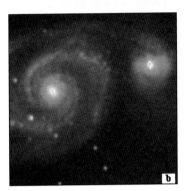

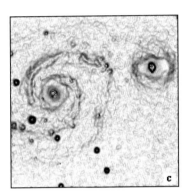

Figure 38. Enhancing an astronomical image (Messier 51):
(a) original telescope image, with brightness range too great for printing;
(b) application of "unsharp masking" by subtracting a smoothed image to reduce contrast selectively and show detail;
(c) gradient of original image using a Sobel operator, which also shows the fine structure of the galaxy.

Unsharp masking has traditionally been applied using photographic darkroom techniques. First, a contact print is made from the original negative onto film, leaving a small gap between the emulsion on the original and that on the film so that the image is blurred. After the film is developed, a new print is made with the two negatives clamped together. The light areas on the original negative are covered by dark areas on the printed negative, allowing little light to come through. Only regions where the slightly out-of-focus negative does not match the original are printed. This is functionally similar to the Laplacian, which subtracts a smoothed (out of focus) image from the original to suppress gradual changes and pass high frequencies or edges.

Applying the unsharp mask operator increases the visibility of fine detail, while suppressing overall variations in brightness. **Figure 39** shows an example using the same x-ray image from **Figure 2**. In the original image the bones in the fingers are thinner and hence not as dense as those in the wrist, and the written label is hardly visible. The processed image makes these more readily visible.

Closely related to unsharp masking, in fact the most general form of this technique, is the subtraction of one smoothed version of the image from another having a different degree of smoothing. This is called the Difference of Gaussians (DOG) method and is believed (Marr, 1982) to be similar to the way the human visual system locates boundaries and other features (the effect of inhibition increasing contrast at boundaries was shown above). Smoothing an image using a Gaussian kernel with an appropriate standard deviation suppresses high-frequency information, which corresponds to small details and spacings that are present. Large structures are not affected. The difference between the two images smoothed with two different Gaussians keeps only those structures (lines, points, etc.) that are in the intermediate size range between the two operators. A plot of two Gaussian curves with different standard deviations, and their difference, is shown in **Figure 40**; the difference is very similar to a cross section of the Laplacian when both

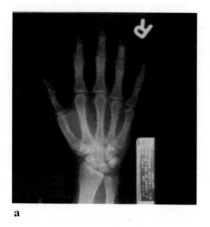
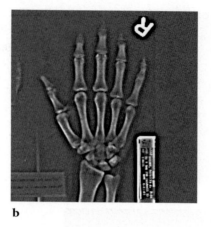

a

b

Figure 39. Application of an unsharp mask to an x-ray image of a human hand: (a) *original;* ***(b)*** *processed.*

Figure 40. *The Difference-of-Gaussian (DOG) operator in one dimension. Two Gaussian curves with different standard deviations are shown, with their difference. The result is a sharpening operation much like the Laplacian.*

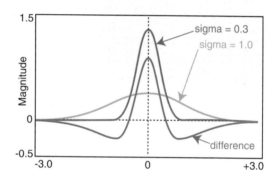

standard deviations are small, and to the unsharp mask when the smaller one is negligible. This edge extractor is also sometimes called a Marr–Hildreth operator. In terms of the frequencies involved, and for comparison to the Fourier-space filtering discussed in Chapter 5, this is a band pass method. Examples are shown in **Figure 41** for comparison with other methods (some of which are discussed later).

Performing derivative operations using kernels can be considered a template matching or convolution process. The pattern of weights in the kernel is a template that gives the maximum response when it matches the pattern of brightness values in the pixels of the image. The number of different kernels used for derivative calculations indicates that there is no single best definition of what constitutes a boundary. Also, it might be helpful at the same time to look for other patterns that are not representative of an edge.

These ideas are combined in the Frei and Chen algorithm (1977), which applies a set of kernels to each point in the image. Each kernel extracts one kind of behavior in the image, only a few of which are indicative of the presence of an edge. For a 3 × 3 neighborhood region, the kernels, which are described as orthogonal or independent basis functions, are shown in the following table:

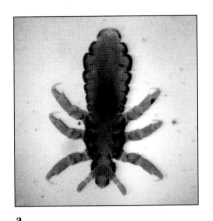

a

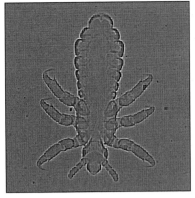

b

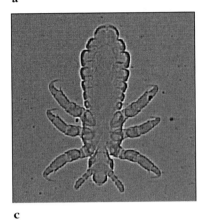

c

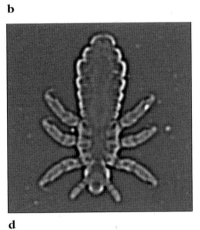

d

Figure 41. Difference of Gaussians applied to a test image:
(a) original image;
(b) original minus 3×3 Gaussian smooth;
(c) difference between smoothing with $\sigma = 0.625$ and $\sigma = 1.0$ pixels;
(d) difference between smoothing with $\sigma = 1.6$ and $\sigma = 1.0$ pixels.

Number	Kernel			Number	Kernel		
0	1	1	1	4	$\sqrt{2}$	−1	0
	1	1	1		−1	0	1
	1	1	1		0	1	$-\sqrt{2}$
1	−1	$-\sqrt{2}$	−1	5	0	1	0
	0	0	0		−1	0	1
	1	$\sqrt{2}$	1		0	−1	0
2	−1	0	1	6	−1	0	1
	$-\sqrt{2}$	0	$\sqrt{2}$		0	0	0
	−1	0	1		1	0	−1
3	0	−1	$\sqrt{2}$	7	1	−2	1
	1	0	−1		−2	4	−2
	$-\sqrt{2}$	1	0		1	−2	1
				8	−2	1	−2
					1	4	1
					−2	1	−2

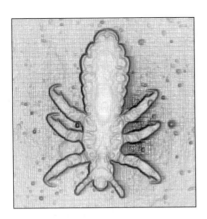

Figure 42. Application of the Frei and Chen edge detector to the test image from Figure 41a.

Only kernels 1 and 2 are considered to indicate the presence of an edge. The results of applying each kernel to each pixel are therefore summed to produce a ratio of the results using kernels 1 and 2 to those for the other kernels. The cosine of the square root of this value is the vector projection of the information from the neighborhood in the direction of "edgeness," and is assigned to the pixel location in the derived image.

The advantage compared to more conventional edge detectors such as the Sobel is sensitivity to a configuration of relative pixel values independent of the magnitude of the brightness, which may vary from place to place in the image. **Figure 42** shows an example of the use of the Frei and Chen operator. This may be compared to other edge-finding processing, shown in **Figures 41** through **44**, which apply some of the other operations discussed in this chapter to the same image.

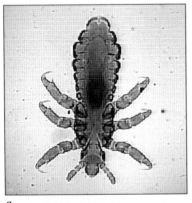

a

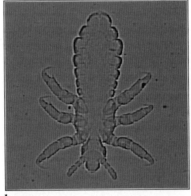

b

Figure 43.
Application of Laplacian difference operations to the test image from Figure 41a:
(a) Sharpening (addition of the 3 × 3 Laplacian to the original grey-scale image);
(b) 5 × 5 Laplacian;
(c) 7 × 7 Laplacian;
(d) 9 × 9 Laplacian.

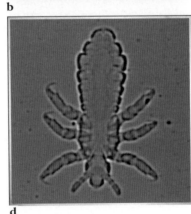

c

d

Figure 44: Derivative edge finding applied to the test image from Figure 41a:
(a) single derivative *(from the upper left);* *(b)* brightest value at each point after applying two crossed derivatives; *(c)* Roberts' Cross operator; *(d)* Sobel operator.

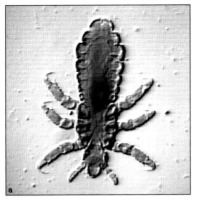
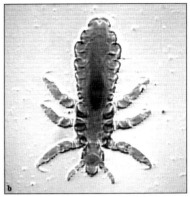
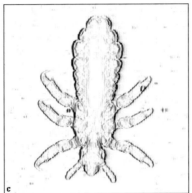
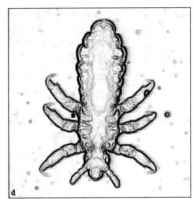

The noise or blurring introduced by some of the operations is evident, as is the ability of the Frei and Chen procedure to reveal even the rather subtle edge information present in the original. **Figure 43** shows the application of a Laplacian operator, or high-pass filter, using different-sized kernels; note the similarity to the difference of Gaussians results in **Figure 41**. The use of derivatives, including the Roberts' Cross and Sobel methods, is shown in **Figure 44**.

Most of the edge-finding processing operations involve square or circular neighborhoods, with a large number of multiplications and other operations. The Canny filter produces results similar to Kirsch or Sobel operators, but is separable (Canny, 1986; Olsson, 1993). This means that it can be performed in two passes, one of which requires only values from pixels in a horizontal line adjacent to the central pixel, and the other requires only values from pixels in a vertical line. From both a computational point of view, and in terms of the complexity of addressing a large number of neighbor pixels, this offers a significant speed advantage.

The Canny filter is based on finding the zero crossing of the Laplacian of Gaussian (LoG, also called a Marr–Hildreth operator), a bandpass filter that calculates the second derivative of a smoothed image. Because of its shape, this is sometimes called a Mexican hat or sombrero operator. It is very similar in shape and performance to the difference of Gaussians (DOG filter). In the example of a 17×17 set of weights shown above, it is presented as a full 2D array of weights, but it can be applied as a separable operation (one-dimensional filters applied to the rows and then to the columns of pixels in an image). **Figure 45** shows the zero crossings of the L.o.G. Typically this operation is performed with several different size filters to isolate edges at different dimensional scales.

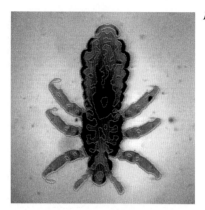

Figure 45. Zero crossings obtained after application of the LoG filter to the image from *Figure 41a.*

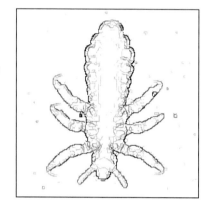

Figure 46. Canny edge detector applied to the test image from *Figure 41a.*

The Canny then adds the additional step of thinning the edge results to single pixel width us a thinning method described below. As shown in **Figure 46**, this is attractive from the standpoint of locating the edge, but tends in many cases to break the line up into discontinuous pieces.

Figure 47 shows an example using a different method. The specimen is a polished aluminum metal examined in the light microscope. The individual grains exhibit different brightnesses because their crystallographic lattices are randomly oriented in space so that the etching procedure used darkens some grains more than others. It is the grain boundaries that are usually important in studying metal structures, since the configuration of grain boundaries results from prior heat treatment and processing and controls many mechanical properties.

The human visual process detects the grain boundaries using its sensitivity to boundaries and edges. Most image analysis systems use a gradient operation, such as a Sobel, to enhance the boundaries prior to measuring them. In the example in **Figure 47**, a statistical method has been employed instead. This is still a local neighborhood operation, but does not use a kernel of weights. The variance operator calculates the sum of squares of the brightness differences for the neighborhood of pixels surrounding each pixel in the original image (in the example, a circular neighborhood with a radius of 2.5 pixels). The variance value, like the other edge-enhancement operators, is very small in uniform regions of the image and becomes large whenever a step is present. In this example, the dark lines (large magnitudes of the variance) are further processed by thinning to obtain the single pixel lines that are superimposed on the original image. This thinning or ridge-finding method is discussed in the next section.

Rank operations

The neighborhood operations discussed in the preceding section use linear arithmetic operations to combine the values of various pixels. Another class of operators that also use neighborhoods

Figure 47. Delineating boundaries between grains:
(a) *Aluminum metal, polished and etched to show different grains (contrast arises from different crystallographic orientation of each grain, so that some boundaries have less contrast than others);*
(b) *Variance edge-finding algorithm applied to image **a***;
(c) *grey-scale skeletonization (ridge finding) applied to **b** (points not on a ridge are suppressed);*
(d) *thresholding and skeletonization of the boundaries to a single line of pixels produces the grain boundaries, shown superimposed on the original image.*

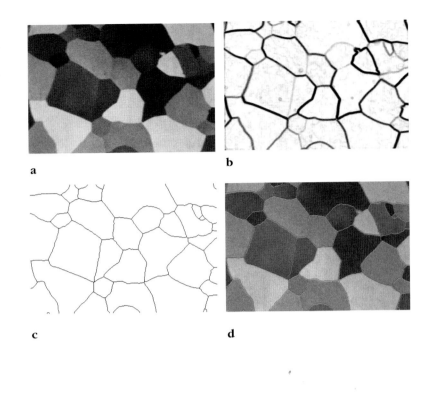

instead performs comparisons and ranking. In Chapter 3, the median filter was introduced. This sorts the pixels in a region into brightness order, finds the median value, and replaces the central pixel with that value. Used to remove noise from images, this operation completely eliminates extreme values from the image.

Rank operations also include the maximum and minimum operators, which find the brightest or darkest pixels in each neighborhood and place that value into the central pixel. By loose analogy to the erosion and dilation operations on binary images, which are discussed in Chapter 7, these are sometimes called grey scale erosion and dilation (Heijmans, 1991). The erosion effect of this ranking operation was demonstrated in Chapter 3, in the context of removing features from an image to produce a background for leveling.

Rank operators can be used to produce an edge-enhancement filter conceptually similar in some ways to a Sobel filter. The horizontal "derivative" is calculated as the difference between the median value of the right hand column of pixels and that of the left hand column, in the neighborhood. A vertical derivative is obtained in the same way, and the edge strength is then computed as the square root of the sum of squares. This does not perform well on diagonal lines, so two more differences are calculated in the diagonal directions to determine another square root value, and the greater of the two is used. The method requires more computation than a traditional Sobel and does not generally produce superior results.

One of the important variables in the use of a rank operator is the size of the neighborhood. Generally, shapes that are squares (for convenience of computation) or approximations to a circle (to minimize directional effects) are used. As the size of the neighborhood is increased, however, the computational effort in performing the ranking increases rapidly. Also, these ranking operations

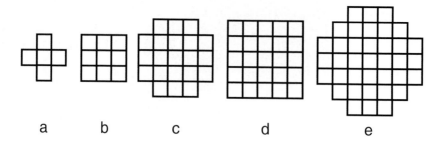

Figure 48. Neighborhood patterns used for ranking operations: (a) 4 nearest-neighbor cross; *(b)* 3 × 3 square containing nine pixels; *(c)* 5 × 5 octagonal region with 21 pixels; *(d)* 5 × 5 square containing 25 pixels; *(e)* 7 × 7 octagonal region containing 37 pixels.

cannot be easily programmed into specialized hardware, such as array processors. In typical cases, regions such as those shown in **Figure 48** are used.

Several uses of rank operators are appropriate for image enhancement and the selection of one portion of the information present in an image. For example, the top hat operator (Bright and Steel, 1987) has been implemented in various ways, but can be described using two different-size regions, as shown in **Figure 49**. If we assume that the goal of the operator is to find bright points, then the algorithm compares the maximum brightness value in a small central region to the maximum brightness value in a larger surrounding one. If the difference between these two values exceeds some arbitrary threshold, then the value of the central pixel is retained. Otherwise it is removed. This principle was also illustrated in Chapter 3.

Figure 50 shows the application of a top hat filter, in which the bright points in the diffraction pattern (calculated using a fast Fourier transform as discussed in Chapter 5) are retained and the overall variation in background brightness is suppressed. A top hat with inner radius of 2 pixels and outer radius of 4 pixels was used. Performing the inverse transform on only the major points provides an averaged image, combining the repetitive information from many individually noisy atom images.

The top hat filter is basically a point or feature finder. The size of the feature is defined by the smaller of the two neighborhood regions and may be as small as a single pixel in some cases. The larger region defines the local background, which the points of interest must exceed in brightness. Unlike the Laplacian, which subtracts the average value of the surrounding background from the central point, the top hat method finds the maximum brightness in the larger surrounding region (the "brim" of the hat) and subtracts that from the brightest point in the interior region. If the difference exceeds some arbitrary threshold (the "height" of the hat's crown), then the central pixel is kept.

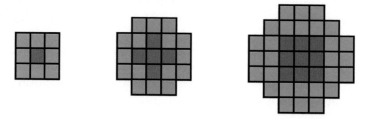

Figure 49. Neighborhood patterns used for a top hat filter. The brightest (or darkest) value in the outer (green) region is subtracted from the brightest (or darkest) value in the inner (red) region. If the difference exceeds a threshold, then the central pixel is kept. Otherwise it is erased.

Figure 50. Application of a top hat filter to select points in a diffraction pattern: *(a)* *high resolution TEM image of silicon nitride, showing atomic positions;* *(b)* *FFT magnitude image calculated from image **a**;* *(c)* *application of a top hat filter to image **b**, selecting the locally bright points on a nonuniform background;* *(d)* *inverse transform using only the points selected in image **c**, enlarged to show detail.*

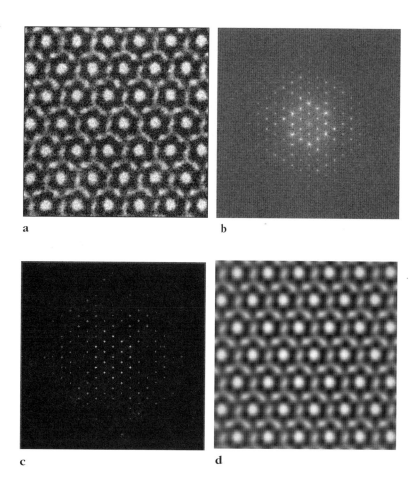

a

b

c

d

In the usual description of the operation of the algorithm, the brim rests on the data and any point that pokes through the crown of the hat is kept. If the central region is larger than a single pixel, though, this depiction is not quite accurate. When any of the points in the central region exceeds the brim value, the central pixel value (which may not be the bright one) is kept. This may produce small haloes around single bright points that are smaller than the central neighborhood region, although any bright point that is part of a feature larger than the central region will not be found by the top hat filter.

Of course, it should be noted that some images have features of interest that are darker rather than lighter than their surroundings. The logic of the top hat filter works just as well when it is inverted, and darkness rather than lightness is the test criterion. **Figure 51** shows such a case, in which the small (and quite uniformly sized) dark features are gold particles in Golgi stained muscle tissue. In this example, simply thresholding the dark particles does not work, because other parts of the image are just as dark. A linear filter method (convolution) such as unsharp masking, accomplished in the example by subtracting the average value (using a Gaussian smoothing filter with a standard deviation of 0.6 pixels) from the original, produces an image in which the particles are quite visible to a human viewer, but are still not distinguishable to a computer program.

It is possible to apply a top hat filter to one-dimensional data. The method is sometimes used, for instance, to select peaks in spectra. **Figure 52** shows an example. The brim of the hat rests on the profile and in only a few places does the plot poke through the crown. Peaks that are too low, too broad, or adjacent to others are not detected.

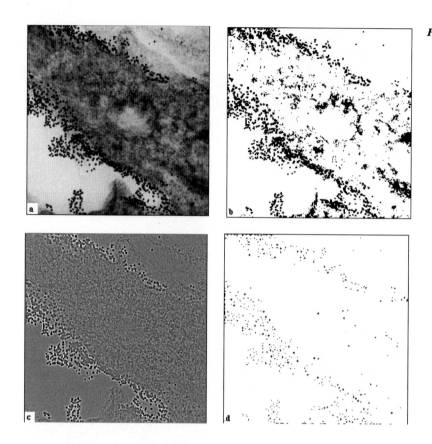

Figure 51. Application of a top-hat filter: (a) *TEM image of golgi-stained rat skeletal muscles, with gold particles (dark) on variable background;* (b) *thresholding of image a selects dark pixels, but cannot isolate the particles;* (c) *unsharp masking, produced by subtracting a smoothed version of the image from the original;* (d) *the top hat filter finds (most of) the particles in spite of the variation in the background.*

Figure 52. Diagram of application of the top-hat filter to one-dimensional data (a brightness profile). Several placements of the filter are shown, but only for those marked with a green dot does the central value exceed the threshold.

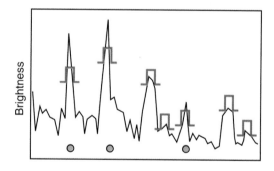

It is also possible, in principle, to design a top hat filter that is not circularly symmetrical, but has regions shaped to select particular features of interest, even lines. Of course, the orientation of the feature must match that of the filter, so this is not a very general operation, although it is sometimes used to locate and remove scratches in movie film as mentioned in Chapter 3. When features with a well-defined shape and orientation are sought, cross-correlation in either the spatial or frequency domain is generally more appropriate.

A close relative of the top hat filter is the rolling ball filter described in Chapter 3 as a noise removal tool. Instead of selecting points that exceed the local background, this filter eliminates them, replacing those pixel values with the neighborhood value. In **Figure 53** this filter has been used to remove the dark gold particles from the image to produce a background image with just the cell organelles. The ratio of the original image to the background isolates just the gold particles.

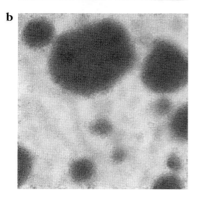

a

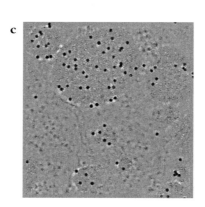

b

c

Figure 53. Application of a rolling-ball filter:
  (a) image of immuno-gold particles attached to cell organelles;
  (b) removal of the dark gold particles (inner radius is 4 pixels; outer radius is 5 pixels);
  *(c) dividing image **a** by image **b**.*

The top hat filter is an example of a suppression operator. It removes pixels from the image if they do not meet some criteria of being "interesting" and leaves alone those pixels that do. Another operator of this type, which locates lines rather than points, is variously known as ridge-finding or grey-scale skeletonization (by analogy to skeletonization of binary images, discussed in Chapter 7). We have already seen a number of edge-finding and gradient operators that produce bright or dark lines along boundaries. These lines are often wider than a single pixel and it may be desirable to reduce them to a minimum width (Bertrand et al., 1997).

The ridge-finding algorithm suppresses pixels (by reducing their value to zero) if they are not part of the center ridge of the line. **Figure 46** showed an example of the application as part of the Canny edge finding filter. When the method is applied to any of the edge-finding gradient operations, it tends to reduce the image to a sketch. **Figure 54** shows an example using a color image, in which the Sobel gradient filter was first applied to the individual red, green, and blue channels, followed by ridge-finding.

Many structures are best characterized by a continuous network, or tesselation, of boundaries. **Figure 55** shows an example, a ceramic containing grains of two different compositions (the dark grains are alumina and the light ones are zirconia). The grains are easily distinguishable by the viewer, but it is the grain boundaries that are important for measurement to characterize the structure, not just the boundaries between light and dark grains, but also those between light and light or dark and dark grains.

Figure 56 shows the application of various edge-finding operators to this image. In this case, the variance produces the best boundary demarcation without including too many extraneous lines due to the texture within the grains. Thresholding this image (as discussed in Chapter 6) and processing the binary image (as discussed in Chapter 7) to thin the lines to single pixel width produces an image of only the boundaries, as shown in **Figure 57**. It is then possible to use the brightness

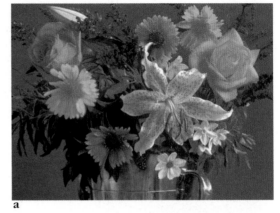

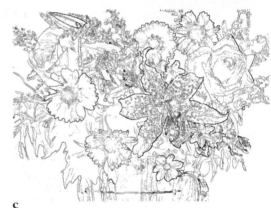

a

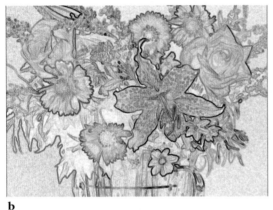

b

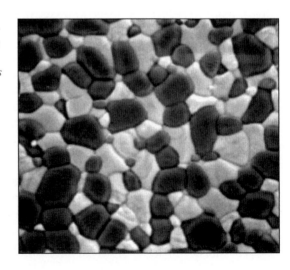

c

Figure 54. Thinning or ridge-finding applied to a color image:
(a) *original;*
(b) *Sobel gradient filter applied to the R, G, B channels;*
(c) *each color channel thinned.*

of the pixels in the original image to classify each grain as either α or β. Images of only those boundaries lying between α and α, β and β, or α and β can then be obtained (as shown in the figure and discussed in Chapter 7). It is also possible to count the number of neighbors around each grain and use a color or grey scale to code them, as shown in **Figure 58**. This goes beyond the usual scope of image processing, however, and into the realm of image measurement and analysis, which is taken up in Chapter 9.

Figure 55. *SEM image of thermally etched alumina-zirconia multiphase ceramic. The two phases are easily distinguished by brightness, but the boundaries between two light or two dark regions are not. (Image courtesy of Dr. K. B. Alexander, Oak Ridge National Labs, Oak Ridge, TN)*

Figure 56. Processing of Figure 55 to enhance edges (all operations performed on 3 × 3 neighborhood regions):
(a) absolute value of the Laplacian;
(b) absolute value of the difference between original and Gaussian smooth;
(c) Sobel gradient operator;
(d) Frei and Chen edge operator;
(e) variance operator;
(f) range operator.

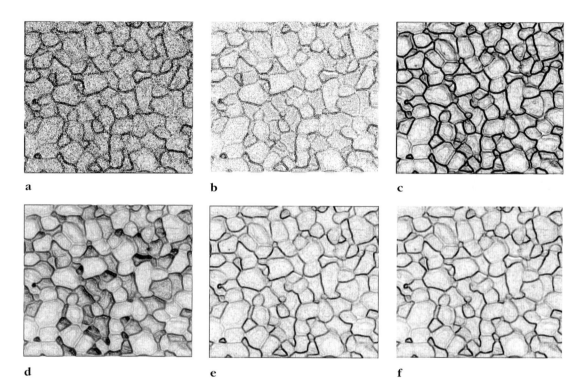

a   b   c

d   e   f

A range image, such as those from the atomic force microscope (AFM) or interference microscope, or from radar imaging, assigns each pixel a brightness value representing elevations, so it is not necessary to arbitrarily interpret the grey-scale brightness as such a structure. Rank operations are particularly well suited to such images, and can often be used to locate boundaries. **Figure 59** shows an example, an AFM image of the topography of a deposited coating. There is some variation in elevation from noise in the image, producing a local variation in grey levels that "roughens" the surface. This can be reduced with a rolling ball filter as shown.

Performing a grey-scale dilation (replacing each pixel with the brightest pixel in a 5-pixel wide neighborhood) and subtracting the original produces a set of bright lines along the boundaries. Thresholding and skeletonizing this image (using techniques discussed in Chapters 6 and 7) produce a network of lines as shown in the figure. Overlaying these lines on the original shows that the correspondence to the visual boundaries between regions is not perfect. This is due primarily to the fact that the surface slope on each side of the boundaries is different, and the subtraction process therefore produces an asymmetric border that has a midline that is offset from the boundary. Nevertheless, the tesselation of lines is useful for counting and measuring the individual structures in the coating.

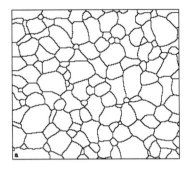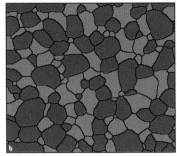

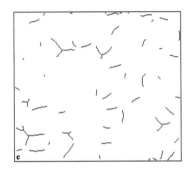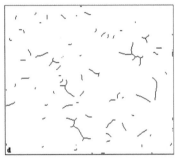

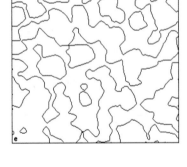

Figure 57. Grain boundary images derived from the variance image in Figure 56e by thresholding and skeletonization:
(a) boundaries between the grains;
(b) grains grey-scale coded to show phase identification;
(c) only those boundaries between two dark (alumina) grains, making up 16.2% of the total;
(d) only those boundaries between two light (zirconia) grains, making up 15.2% of the total;
(e) only those boundaries between a light and dark grain, making up 68.6% of the total boundary.

Figure 58. *These grains from* **Figure 57** *are color-coded to show the number of neighbors touching each and a plot of the frequency of each number of neighbors. Further analysis shows that both the size and the number of neighbor plots are different for the two different phases.*

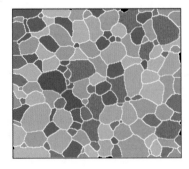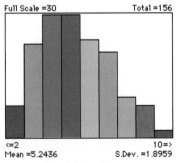

***Figure 59. An atomic force microscope (AFM) image of a deposited coating, showing a series of
gently rounded bumps:***
(a) the original range image (grey scale proportional to elevation);
(b) noise smoothed by the application of a rolling ball filter;
(c) use of a rank filter to replace each pixel with its brightest neighbor;
*(d) difference between **b** and **c**, showing boundary delineation;*
*(e) thresholding and skeletonizing image **d** to get lines;*
(f) boundary lines overlaid on the original image.

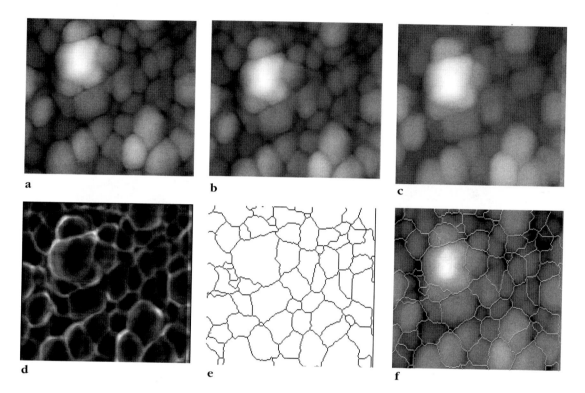

For range images (particularly radar images used in surveillance), searching for a target pattern can
be accomplished using a special class of adaptive operators. A top hat filter of the right size and
shape can be used for the task, but better performance can be achieved by adjusting the parameters of size and especially height according to the local pixel values (Verly and Delanoy, 1993). For
example, the threshold difference in brightness between the inner and outer regions could be
made a percentage of the brightness rather than a fixed value. In principle, the more knowledge
available about the characteristics of the target and of the imaging equipment, the better an adaptive filter can be made to find the features and separate them from background. In practice, these
approaches seem to be little used, and are perhaps too specific for general applications.

Texture

Many images contain regions characterized not so much by a unique value of brightness, but by
a variation in brightness that is often called texture. This is a somewhat loosely defined term that
refers to the local variation in brightness from one pixel to the next or within a small region. If the
brightness is interpreted as elevation in a representation of the image as a surface, then the texture
is a measure of the surface roughness, another term without a single accepted or universal quantitative meaning.

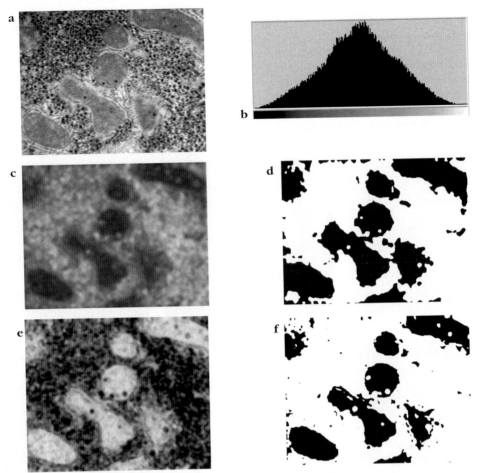

Figure 60. Enhancement of texture:

   (a) transmission electron microscope image of liver thin section;

   (b) histogram of a;

   (c) range image (difference between maximum and minimum brightness values in a neighborhood with 3.5-pixel radius);

   (d) binary image produced by automatic thresholding of c;

   (e) variance of pixel values in a neighborhood with 3.5-pixel radius;

   (f) binary image produced by automatic thresholding of e.

Rank operations are also used to detect this texture in images. One of the simplest of the texture operators is simply the range or difference between maximum and minimum brightness values in the neighborhood. For a flat or uniform region, the range is small. Larger values of the range correspond to surfaces with a larger roughness. The size of the neighborhood region must be large enough to include dark and light pixels, which generally means being larger than any small uniform details that may be present. **Figure 60** shows an example in which the original image has a histogram with a single broad peak and no ability to distinguish the visually smooth and textured regions based on brightness. The range image produces different brightness values which allow thresholding. A second texture extraction method, also shown in the figure, is the calculation of the statistical variance of the pixel values in a moving neighborhood, which also is able to distinguish the regions in this image. Note that both the range and variance operators are also sometimes used with a smaller neighborhood size to locate edges, as shown in **Figure 61**.

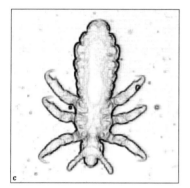

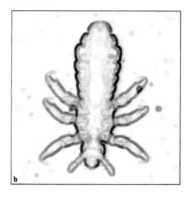

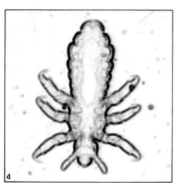

Figure 61. Application of range and variance operators to the test image from Figure 41a:
(a) range (3 × 3 neighborhood);
(b) range (5-pixel-wide circular neighborhood);
(c) variance (3 × 3 neighborhood);
(d) variance (5-pixel-wide circular neighborhood).

When visual examination of an image suggests that the basis for discriminating various structural regions is a texture rather than color or brightness, it is often possible to use a simple texture operator such as the range to extract it. This is often the case in biological specimens, and particularly in foods. **Figure 62** shows another example, a microscope image of the curds and whey protein in cheese. The smooth regions (curds) produce a low range value, while the highly textured whey produces a larger range value. The overall shading of the image has also been removed.

Satellite images are especially appropriate for characterization by texture operators. Categorization of crops, construction, and other land uses produces distinctive textures that humans can recognize. Therefore, methods have been sought that duplicate this capability in software algorithms. In a classic paper on the subject, Haralick listed 14 such texture operators that utilize the pixels within a region and their brightness differences (Haralick et al., 1973; Haralick, 1979; Weszka et al., 1976). This region is not a neighborhood around each pixel, but comprises all of the pixels within a contiguous block delineated by some boundary or other identifying criterion such as brightness, etc. A table is constructed with the number of adjacent pixel pairs within the region as a function of their brightnesses. This pixel table is then used to calculate the texture parameters.

In the expressions below, the array $P(i,j)$ contains the number of nearest-neighbor pixel pairs (in 90-degree directions only) whose brightnesses are i and j, respectively. R is a renormalizing constant equal to the total number of pixel pairs in the image or any rectangular portion used for the calculation. In principle, this can be extended to pixel pairs that are separated by a distance d and to pairs aligned in the 45-degree direction (whose separation distance is greater than ones in the 90-degree directions). The summations are carried out for all pixel pairs in the region. Haralick applied this to rectangular regions, but it is equally applicable to pixels within irregular outlines.

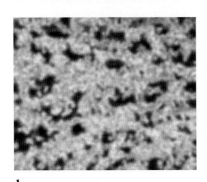

a

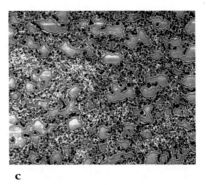

Figure 62. Application of a range operator to an image of curds and whey protein: (a) original; (b) range operator applied (5-pixel-wide circular neighborhood); (c) region outlines from thresholding superimposed on original.

b

c

The first parameter shown is a measure of homogeneity using a second moment. Since the terms are squared, a few large differences will contribute more than many small ones. The second one shown is a difference moment, which is a measure of the contrast in the image. The third is a measure of the linear dependency of brightness in the image, obtained by correlation.

$$f_1 = \sum_{i=1}^{N} \sum_{j=1}^{N} \left(\frac{P(i,j)}{R} \right)^2$$

$$f_2 = \sum_{n=0}^{N-1} n^2 \left\{ \sum_{|i-j|=n} \left(\frac{P(i,j)}{R} \right) \right\}$$

$$f_3 = \frac{\sum_{i=1}^{N} \sum_{j=1}^{N} [i \cdot j \cdot P(i,j)/R] - \mu_x \cdot \mu_y}{\sigma_x \cdot \sigma_y}$$

(8)

In these expressions, N is the number of grey levels, and μ and σ are the mean and standard deviation, respectively, of the distributions of brightness values accumulated in the x and y directions. Additional parameters describe the variance, entropy, and information measure of the brightness value correlations. Haralick has shown that when applied to large rectangular areas in satellite photos, these parameters can distinguish water from grassland, different sandstones from each other, and woodland from marsh or urban regions.

Some of these operations are easier to calculate than others for all of the pixels in an image. The resulting values can be scaled to create a derived image that can be discriminated with brightness

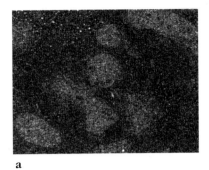 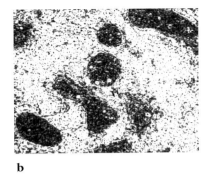

a   b

Figure 63. Application of Haralick texture operators to the image from Figure 60:
  (a) homogeneity;
  (b) difference moment.

thresholding. In any given instance, it sometimes requires experimentation with several texture operators to find the one that gives the best separation between the features of interest and their surroundings.

Some of these same operations can be applied to individual pixels to produce a new image, in which the brightness is proportional to the local texture. **Figure 63** illustrates the use of the Haralick homogeneity and angular second moment operators (f_1 and f_2 above) applied in a moving neighborhood centered on each pixel to calculate a texture value, which is then assigned to the pixel. This result can be compared to **Figure 60**.

Fractal analysis

The characterization of surface roughness by a fractal dimension has been applied to fracture surfaces, wear and erosion, corrosion, etc. (Mandelbrot et al., 1984; Underwood and Banerji, 1986; Mecholsky and Passoja, 1985; Mecholsky et al., 1986, 1989; Srinivasan et al., 1991; Fahmy et al., 1991). It has also been shown (Pentland, 1983; Peleg et al., 1984) that the brightness pattern in images of fractal surfaces is also mathematically a fractal and that this also holds for SEM images (Russ, 1990a). A particularly efficient method for computing the fractal dimension of surfaces from elevation images is the Hurst coefficient, or rescaled range analysis (Hurst et al., 1965; Feder, 1988; Russ, 1990c). This procedure plots the greatest difference in brightness (or elevation, etc.) between points along a linear traverse of the image or surface as a function of the search distance, on log-log axes. When the range is scaled by dividing by the standard deviation of the data, the slope of the resulting line is directly related to the fractal dimension of the profile.

Performing such an operation at the pixel level is interesting, because it may permit local classification that can be of use for image segmentation. Processing an image so that each pixel value is converted to a new brightness scale indicating local roughness (in the sense of a Hurst coefficient) permits segmentation by simple brightness thresholding. It uses two-dimensional information on the brightness variation, compared to the one-dimensional comparison used in measuring brightness profiles.

Figure 64 shows a neighborhood region consisting of 37 pixels in a 7-pixel-wide octagonal shape. The size is a compromise between the desire to include many pixel values (for accurate results) and the need for a local operator. Qualitatively similar results are obtained with 5-, 9-, and 11-pixel-wide regions. Unlike some neighborhood operators, such as smoothing kernels, the use of progressively larger neighborhood regions for the Hurst operator does not select information with different dimensions or scales in the image. Instead, it increases the precision of the fit and reduces

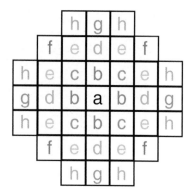

Figure 64. *Octagonal 7-pixel-wide neighborhood (37 pixels total) used for local rescaled-range (Hurst coefficient) calculation. Pixel labels identify groups with the same distance from the central pixel.*

the noise introduced by individual light or dark pixels, at least up to a region size as large as the defined structures in the image. Each of the pixels in the diagram is labeled to indicate its distance from the center of the octagon. The distances (in pixel units) range from 1 pixel (the 4 touching neighbors sharing a side with the central pixel) to 3.162 pixels ($\sqrt{10}$).

Application of the operator proceeds by examining the pixels in the neighborhood around each pixel in the original image. The brightest and darkest pixel values in each of the distance classes are found and their difference used to construct a Hurst plot. Performing a least-squares fit of the slope of the log (brightness difference) vs. log (distance) relationship is simplified because the distance values (and their logarithms) are unvarying and can be stored beforehand in a short table. It is also unnecessary to divide by the standard deviation of pixel brightnesses in the image, since this is a constant for each pixel in the image and the slope of the Hurst plot will be scaled to fit the brightness range of the display anyway. Building the sums for the least-squares fit and performing the necessary calculations is moderately complex. Thus, it is time consuming compared to simple neighborhood operations such as smoothing, etc., but still well within the capability of typical desktop computer systems.

Figure 65 shows a portion of the TEM image of a thin section of liver tissue, used in **Figures 60** and **63**. The conversion of the original image based on the texture information permits thresholding of the

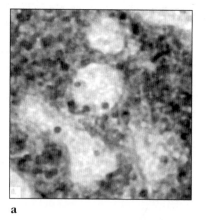

a

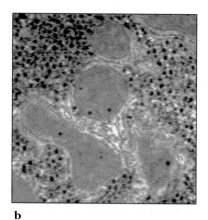

b

Figure 65. Application of the Hurst texture operator to the image from Figure 60 (a), *and the region outlines from thresholding superimposed on the original* **(b)**.

regions is shown in the figure. **Figure 66** shows highly magnified images of two representative locations in each of these regions, with outlines showing specific locations of the octagonal neighborhood. Sorting through the pixels in each distance class, finding the brightest and darkest and their difference, and constructing a plot of log (brightness range) vs. log (distance) is shown for these two specific pixel locations in **Figure 67**. Notice that the slopes of the Hurst plots are quite different and that the lines fit the points rather well. Scaling the Hurst values to the brightness range of an image and applying the operation to each pixel in the image produces the result shown in **Figure 65**.

Figure 68 shows an image of the broken end of a steel test specimen. Part of the surface was produced by fatigue and part by the terminal tearing failure. Visual examination easily distinguishes the two regions based on texture. Measuring the area of the fatigue crack is important for determining the mechanical properties of the steel, although the boundary is quite difficult to locate by computer processing. The brightness histograms of two regions of the image overlap extensively, so that simple thresholding is not possible. Applying the local Hurst operator to this image produces the result shown, in which the two regions are clearly delineated.

Implementation notes

Many of the techniques discussed in this chapter and in Chapter 3 are neighborhood operators that access pixels in a small area around each central pixel, perform some calculation or comparison with those values, and then derive a new value for the central pixel. In all cases, this new value is used to produce a new image, and it is the original values of pixels which are used in the neighborhood around the next pixel as the operation is repeated throughout the image.

Figure 66. Expanded detail of two locations in the image from Figure 65a, with positions of the measurement neighborhood inidcated.

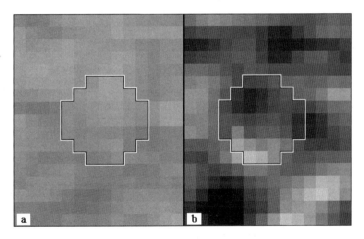

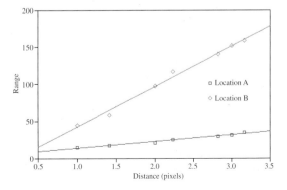

Figure 67. Hurst plots of the logarithm of the maximum brightness range vs. log of distance for the two locations shown in Figure 66.

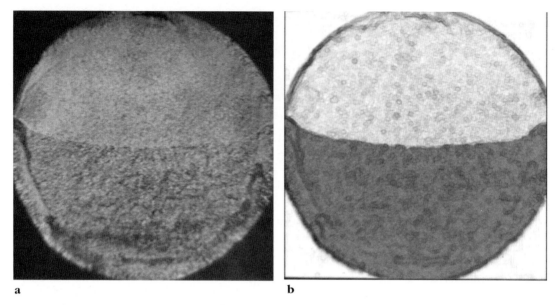

a   b

Figure 68. Fracture surface of a steel test specimen. The smooth portion of the fracture occurred by fatigue, and the rougher portion by tearing:
(**a**) *original;*
(**b**) *after application of the Hurst texture operator.*

Most image analysis systems, particularly those operating in desktop computers, have limited memory (particularly when the large size of images is considered). Creating a new image for every image processing operation is an inefficient use of this limited resource. Consequently, the strategy generally used is to perform the operation "in place," to process one image and replace it with the result.

This requires only enough temporary memory to hold a few lines of the image. The operations are generally performed left to right along each scan line and top to bottom through the image. Duplicating the line that is being modified, and keeping copies of the preceding lines whose pixels are used, allows the new (modified) values to be written back to the original image memory. The number of lines is simply $(n + 1)/2$ where n is the neighborhood dimension (e.g., 3×3, 5×5, etc.). Usually, the time required to duplicate a line from the image is small and by shuffling through a series of pointers, it is only necessary to copy each line once when the moving process reaches it, then re-use the array for subsequent vertical positions.

Some of the image processing methods described above create two or more intermediate results. For example, the Roberts' Cross or Sobel filters apply two directional derivatives whose magnitudes are subsequently combined. It is possible to do this pixel by pixel, so that no additional storage is required; however, in some implementations, particularly those that can be efficiently programmed into an array processor (which acts on an entire line through the image at one time), it is faster to obtain the intermediate results for each operator applied to each line and then combine them for the whole line. This requires only a small amount of additional storage for the intermediate results.

Another consideration in implementing neighborhood operations is how to best treat pixels near the edges of the image. Many of the example images shown here are taken from the center of larger original images, so edge effects are avoided. In others, a band around the edge of the image is skipped, which is one of the most common ways to respond to the problem. With this approach, the programs skip pixels within a distance of $(n - 1)/2$ pixels from any edge, where n is the total width of the neighborhood.

Other possibilities include having special neighborhood rules near edges to sort through a smaller set of pixels, duplicating rows of pixels at edges (i.e., assuming each edge is a mirror), or using wrap-around addressing (i.e., assuming that the left and right edges and the top and bottom edges of the image are contiguous). None of these methods is particularly attractive, in general. Since the largest and smallest brightness values are used to find the maximum range, the duplication of rows of pixels would not provide any extra information for range operations. In all cases, the use of fewer pixels for calculations would degrade the precision of the results. There is no reason whatsoever to assume that the image edges should be matched, and indeed, quite different structures and regions will normally occur there. The most conservative approach is to accept a small shrinkage in useful image size after processing, by ignoring near-edge pixels.

Image math

The image processing operations discussed so far in this chapter operate on one image and produce a modified result, which may be stored in the same image memory. Another class of operations uses two images to produce a new image (which may replace one of the originals). These operations are usually described as image arithmetic, since operators such as addition, subtraction, division, and multiplication are included. They are performed pixel by pixel, so that the sum of two images simply contains pixels whose brightness values are the sums of the corresponding pixels in the original images. There are some additional operators used, as well, such as comparing two images to keep the brighter (or darker) pixel, obtaining the absolute difference, or basing the comparison on neighborhood values (for instance, keeping the pixel with the greater local variance, illustrated in Chapter 3 as a means of combining images with different focus settings). Other two-image operations, such as Boolean OR or AND logic, are generally applied to binary images; they will be discussed in that context in Chapter 7.

Actually, image addition has already been used in a method described previously. In Chapter 3, the averaging of images to reduce noise was discussed. The addition operation is straightforward, but a decision is required about how to deal with the result. If two 8-bit images (with brightness values from 0 to 255 at each pixel) are added together, the resulting value can range from 0 to 510. This exceeds the capacity of the image memory. One possibility is simply to divide the result by two, obtaining a resulting image that is correctly scaled to the 0 to 255 range. This is what is usually applied in image averaging, in which the N images added together produce a total, which is then divided by N to rescale the data.

Another possibility is to find the largest and smallest actual values in the sum image, and then dynamically rescale the result to this maximum and minimum, so that each pixel is assigned a new value B = range × (sum − minimum)/(maximum − minimum), where range is the capacity of the image memory, typically 255. This is superior to performing the division by two and then subsequently performing a linear expansion of contrast, as discussed in Chapter 3, because the precision of the resulting values is higher. When the integer division by two is performed, fractional values are truncated and some information may be lost.

On the other hand, when dynamic ranging or automatic scaling is performed, it becomes more difficult to perform direct comparison of images after processing, since the brightness scales may not be the same. In addition, autoscaling takes longer, since two complete passes through the image are required: one to determine the maximum and minimum and one to apply the autoscaling calculation. Many of the images printed in this book have been autoscaled in order to maximize printed contrast. In most cases this operation has been performed as part of the processing operation to maintain precision.

Adding together images superimposes information and can in some cases be useful to create composites, which help to communicate complex spatial relationships. We have already seen that adding the Laplacian or a derivative image to the original can help provide some spatial guidelines to interpret the information from the filter. Usually, this kind of addition is handled directly in the processing by changing the central value of the kernel. For the Laplacian, this modification is called a sharpening filter, as noted previously.

Subtracting images

Subtraction is widely used and more interesting than the addition operation. In Chapter 3, subtraction was used to level images by removing background. This chapter has already mentioned uses of subtraction, such as that employed in unsharp masking, where the smoothed image is subtracted, pixel by pixel, from the original. In such an operation, the possible range of values for images whose initial range is 0 to 255 becomes –255 to +255. The data can be rescaled to fit into a single byte, replacing the original image, by dividing by two and adding 128, or the same autoscaling method described above for addition may be employed. The same advantages and penalties for fixed and flexible scaling are encountered.

In some cases, the absolute difference may be preferred to simple subtraction of a background. **Figure 69** shows a phase-contrast image of cells on a slide. Images such as this in which features have pronounced bright and dark shadows on opposite sides are very difficult to measure, because on two sides there are different criteria to define an edge, and on the top and bottom the edges are not revealed at all but are inferred by the viewer. Using a large median filter to remove the shadows produces a "background" image without the features. The absolute difference between this and the original shows both shadows as bright. Thresholding this image produces two disconnected arcs, but dilation of the binary image (discussed in Chapter 7) merges the two sides. After filling and eroding this back to the original size, the outlines of the cells are adequately delineated for useful measurement.

Subtraction is primarily a way to discover differences between images. **Figure 70** shows two images of coins and their difference. The parts of the picture that are essentially unchanged in the two images cancel out and appear as a uniform medium grey except for minor variations due to the precision of digitization, changes in illumination, etc. The coin that has been moved between the two image acquisitions is clearly shown. The dark image shows where the feature was; the bright one shows where it has gone.

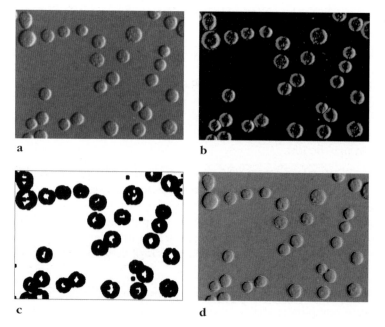

a   b

c   d

Figure 69. Isolating cells in a phase contrast image:
(a) original image;
(b) absolute difference between original and a median-filtered copy;
(c) image *b* thresholded and dilated (as discussed in Chapter 6) to join left and right shadows;
(d) resulting cell boundaries superimposed on the original image.

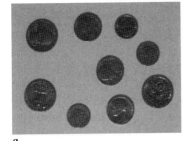

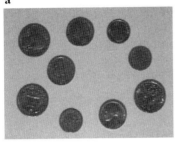

a

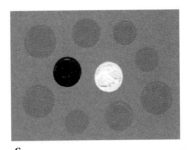

Figure 70. Showing image differences by subtraction:
(a) original image;
(b) image after moving one coin;
(c) difference image after pixel by pixel subtraction.

b   c

Subtracting one image from another effectively removes from the difference image all features that do not change, while highlighting those that do. If the lighting and geometry of view is consistent, the only differences in pixel values where no changes occur are statistical variations in the brightness, due to camera or electronic noise. The bright and dark images show features that have been removed from or added to the field of view, respectively.

Even in the presence of some noise, subtraction of two images can be an effective way to identify small differences that might otherwise escape notice. **Figure 71** shows an example. The image shows two films from a Debye–Scherer x-ray camera. The vertical lines show the exposure of the film by x-rays that were diffracted from a tiny sample, each line corresponding to reflection from one plane of atoms in the structure of the material. Comparing the films from these similar samples shows that most of the lines are similar in position and intensity, because the two samples are in fact quite similar in composition. The presence of trace quantities of impurities is revealed by additional faint lines in the image. Subtraction of one set of lines from the second increases the relative amount of noise, but reveals the presence of lines from the trace compounds. These can then be measured and used for identification.

Figure 71. Image subtraction to enhance the visibility of details: (a, b) scanned images of films from a Debye–Scherer x-ray camera, taken with similar compounds; *(c)* the difference between *b* and *a* showing the low intensity lines present in one film due to the presence of trace compounds in the sample.

a

b

c

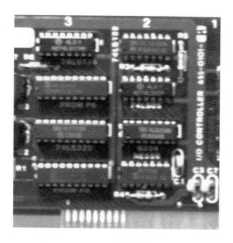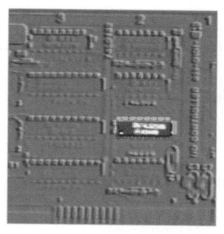

Figure 72. Difference images for quality control. A master image is subtracted from images of each subsequent part. In this example, the missing chip in a printed circuit board is evident in the difference image.

A major use of image subtraction is quality control. A master image is acquired and stored that shows the correct placement of parts on circuit boards (**Figure 72**), the alignment of labels on packaging, etc. When the image is subtracted from a series of images acquired from subsequent objects, the differences are strongly highlighted, revealing errors in production. This subtraction is often carried out at video frame rates using dedicated hardware. Since it is unrealistic to expect parts to be exactly aligned, a tolerance can be specified by the area of bright and dark (mismatched) pixels present after the subtraction.

The same technique is used in reconnaissance photos to watch for the appearance or disappearance of targets in a complex scene. Image warping, as discussed in Chapter 3, may be required to align images taken from different points of view before the subtraction can be performed. A similar method is used in astronomy. "Blinking" images taken of the same area of the sky at different times is the traditional way to search for moving planets or asteroids. This technique alternately presents each image to a human viewer, who notices the apparent motion of the point of light that is different in the two images while ignoring the stationary stars. Some use of computer searching using subtraction has been used, but, for dim objects in the presence of background noise, has not proved as sensitive as a human observer.

In the example of **Figure 73**, two images were acquired about 1 minute apart. The difference between the two clearly shows the motion of the minute hand and the change in position of the pendulum. The very small motion of the hour hand is also shown, which would be much too small to be noticed by viewing the images side by side.

Object motion can be measured using subtraction, if the features are large enough and the sequential images are acquired fast enough that they overlap in successive frames. In this case, the subtraction shows a bright area of mismatch that can be measured. The length of the unmatched region divided by the elapsed time gives the velocity; direction can be determined by the orientation of the region. This technique is used at microscopic scales to track the motion of cells on slides (**Figure 74**) in response to chemical cues.

At the other extreme, subtraction is used to track ice floes in the north Atlantic from satellite photos. For motion between two successive images that is too large for this method, it may be possible to identify the same objects in successive images based on size, shape, etc. and thus track motion. Or, one can assume that where paths cross, the points causing the least deviation of the path give the correct match (**Figure 75**); however, the direct subtraction technique is much simpler and more direct.

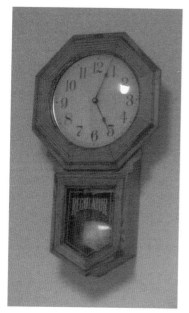
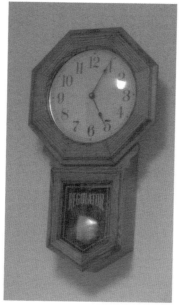
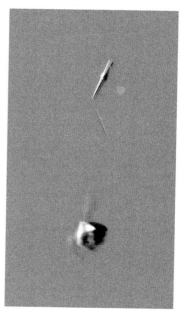

Figure 73. *Difference between two images of a clock taken 1 minute apart. The motion of the hands is evident.*

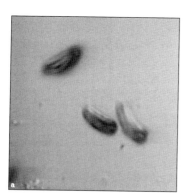
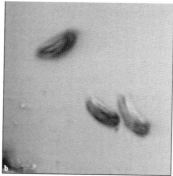
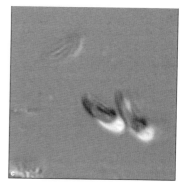

Figure 74. *Two frames from a videotape sequence of free swimming single-celled animals in a drop of pond water and the difference image. The length of the white region divided by the time interval gives the velocity.*

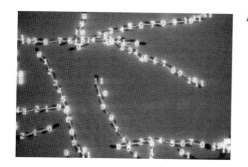

Figure 75. *Analysis of motion in a more complex situation than shown in* **Figure 74.** *Where the paths of the swimming microorganisms cross, they are sorted out by assuming that the path continues in a nearly straight direction (from Gualtieri and Coltelli, 1991).*

Multiplication and division

Image multiplication is perhaps the least used of the mathematics modes, but it is generally included for the sake of completeness in systems offering the other arithmetic operations. Multiplication was used above in **Figure 32** to combine the edge magnitude and direction data from the Sobel operator. Another possible use is superimposing one image on another in the particular case when the superimposed data is proportional to the absolute brightness of the original image. An example is texture; **Figure 76** shows an illustration of what is often called "bump-mapping." A brightness pattern (generated using fractal iteration) is superimposed on the smooth polygonal approximation of a shaded sphere in order to provide an impression of roughness. Similar multiplicative superimposition may be used to add fluorescence or other emission images to a reflection or transmission image.

One of the difficulties with multiplication is the extreme range of values that may be generated. With 8-bit images whose pixels can have a range between 0 and 255, the possible products can range from 0 to more than 65,000. This is a 2-byte product, only the high byte of which can be stored back into the same image memory unless automatic scaling is used. A significant loss of precision may result for values in the resulting image.

The magnitude of the numbers also creates problems with division. First, division by 0 must be avoided. This is usually done by adding 1 to all brightness values, so that the values are interpreted as 1 to 256 instead of 0 to 255. Then it is necessary to first multiply each pixel in the numerator by some factor that will produce quotients covering the 0 to 255 range, while maintaining some useful precision for the ends of the range. Automatic scaling is particularly useful for these situations, but it cannot be used in applications requiring comparison of results to each other or to a calibration curve.

An example of division in which automatic scaling is useful is the removal of background (as discussed in Chapter 3) when linear detectors or cameras are used. An example of division when absolute values are required is calculating ratios of brightness from two or more Landsat bands (an example is shown in Chapter 1) or two or more filter images when examining fluorescent probes in the light microscope. In fluorescence microscopy, the time variation of emitted light intensity is normalized by alternately collecting images through two or more filters at different wavelengths above and below the line of interest, and calibrating the ratio against the activity of the element(s)

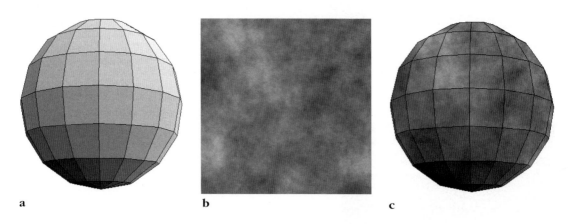

a   b   c

Figure 76. Multiplication of images can be used to superimpose texture on an image:
    (a) smooth faceted globe;
    (b) iterated midpoint displacement (fractal) pattern;
    (c) product of a times b.

of interest. In satellite imagery, ratios of intensities (particularly Band 4 = 0.5 to 0.6 μm, Band 5 = 0.6 to 0.7 μm, Band 6 = 0.7 to 0.8 μm, and Band 7 = 0.8 to 1.1 μm) are used for terrain classification and the identification of some rock types. The thermal inertia of different rock formations may also be determined by ratioing images obtained at different local times of day, as the formations heat or cool.

As an example of mineral identification, silicates exhibit a wavelength shift in the absorption band with composition. Granites, diorites, gabbros, and olivene peridotes have progressively decreasing silicon content. The absorption band shifts to progressively longer wavelengths in the 8 to 12 µm thermal infrared band as the bond-stretching vibrations between Si and O atoms in the silicate lattice change. The Thermal Infrared Multispectral Mapper satellite records six bands of image data in this range, which are combined and normalized to locate the absorption band and identify rock formations. Carbonate rocks (dolomite and limestone) have a similar absorption response in the 6 to 8 µm range, but this is difficult to measure in satellite imagery because of atmospheric absorption. At radar wavelengths, different surface roughnesses produce variations in reflected intensity in the Ka, X, and L bands and can be combined in the same ways to perform measurements and distinguish the coarseness of sands, gravels, cobbles, and boulders (Sabins, 1987).

In the same way, Bands 1 (0.55 to 0.68 µm, or visible red) and 2 (0.72 to 1.10 µm, or reflected infrared) from multispectral satellite imagery are used to recognize vegetation. Band 1 records the chlorophyll absorption and Band 2 gives the reflection from the cell structure of the leaves. The ratio (B2 − B1)/(B2 + B1) eliminates variations due to differences in solar elevation (illumination angle) and is used to measure the distribution of vegetation in images. Typically, this approach also combines data from successive scans to obtain the spectral vegetation index as a function of time. Other ratios have been used to image and to measure chlorophyll concentrations due to phytoplankton in the ocean (Sabins, 1987). **Figure 77** shows a simplified approximation of this method using the ratio of near infrared to blue to isolate vegetation from satellite imagery.

Ratios are also used in astronomical images. **Figure 78** shows infrared images of the star-forming region in NGC-2024. Infrared light penetrates the dust that blocks much of the visible light. Ratios or differences of the different wavelength images show details in the dust and enhance the visibility of the young stars.

Image math also includes the logical comparison of pixel values. For instance, two images may be combined by keeping the brighter (or darker) of the corresponding pixels at each location. This is used, for instance, to build up a confocal scanning light microscope (CSLM) image with great depth of field. Normal light microscope images have limited depth of field because of the high numerical aperture of the lenses. In the CSLM, the scanning light beam and aperture on the detector reduce this depth of field even more by eliminating light scattered from any point except the single point illuminated in the plane of focus.

A single, two-dimensional image is formed by scanning the light over the sample (or, equivalently, by moving the sample itself with the light beam stationary). For a specimen with an irregular surface, this image is very dark, except at locations where the surface lies in the plane of focus. By moving the specimen vertically, many such planar images can be acquired. The display of a complete three-dimensional set of such images is discussed in Chapter 10, although at each pixel location, the brightest value of light reflectance occurs at the in-focus point. Consequently, the images from many focal depths can be combined by keeping only the brightest value at each pixel location to form an image with an unlimited depth of field. **Figure 79** shows an example.

An additional effect can be produced by shifting each image slightly before performing the comparison and superposition. **Figure 80** shows an example. The 26 individual images, four of which

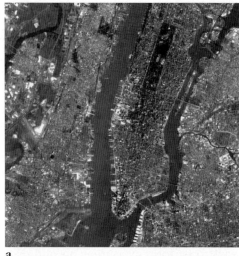

a

*Figure 77. Landsat thematic mapper images of
New York City:*
(a) Band 1 (visible blue);
(b) Band 4 (near infrared);
(c) ratio of Band 4 to Band 1 (showing
vegetation areas).

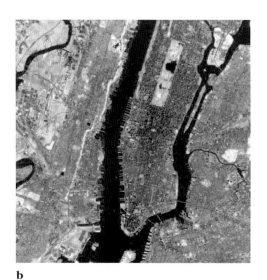

b

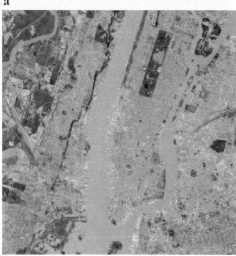

c

are shown, are combined in this way to produce a perspective view of the surface (this image was also shown in Chapter 1 as an example of one mode of collecting and displaying three-dimensional imaging information).

Another use of combining several images arises in polarized light microscopy. As shown in **Figure 81**, the use of polarizer and analyzer with specimens such as mineral thin sections produces images in which some grains are colored and others dark, as a function of analyzer rotation. Combining images from many rotations and keeping just the brightest pixel value produces an image that shows all of the grains. The same technique can be used with transmission electron microscope images of thin metal foils, to combine images in which some grains are darkened due to electron diffraction effects, or to remove dark contours that result from bending of the foil.

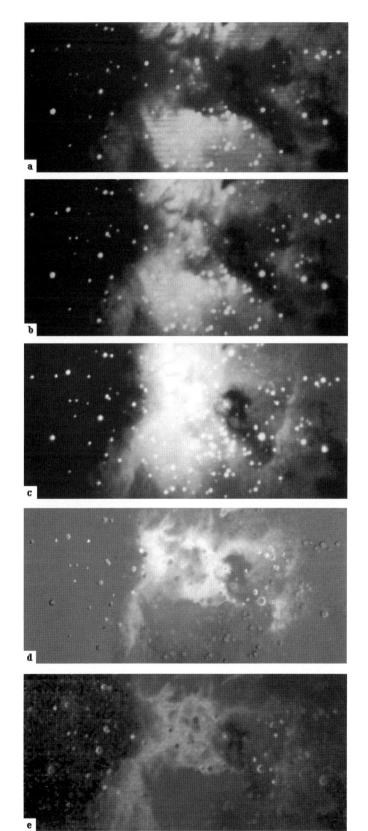

Figure 78. Combining views of NGC-2024 to show star-forming regions and dust:
(a) 1.2 µm infrared image;
(b) 1.6 µm infrared image;
(c) 2.2 µm infrared image;
(d) 2.2 µm image minus 1.6 µm image;
(e) 1.6 µm image divided by 1.2 µm image.

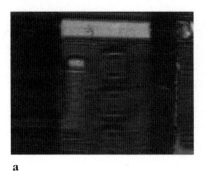 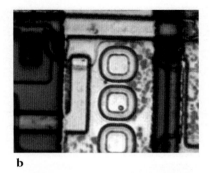

a   b

*Figure 79. Combining CSLM images by keeping the brightest value at each pixel location. Image **a** shows one individual focal plane image from a series of 25 on an integrated circuit. Only the portion of the surface which is in focus is bright. Because the in-focus point is brightest, combining all of the individual planes produces image **b**, which shows the entire surface in focus.*

Figure 80. *Four individual focal sections from a confocal light microscope series on a ceramic fracture surface. The images are 40 μm wide, and the stack of 26 images are spaced 1 μm apart in depth. Generating a surface reconstruction from the images (shown in e) shifts each image two pixels to the right and up, keeping the brightest value at each pixel location. The result is a perspective view of the entire surface.*

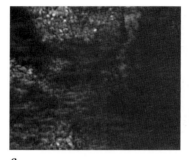

a

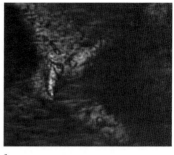

b

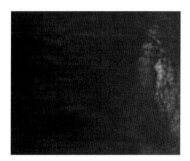

c

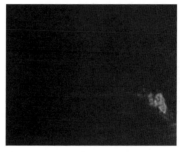

d

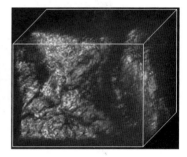

e

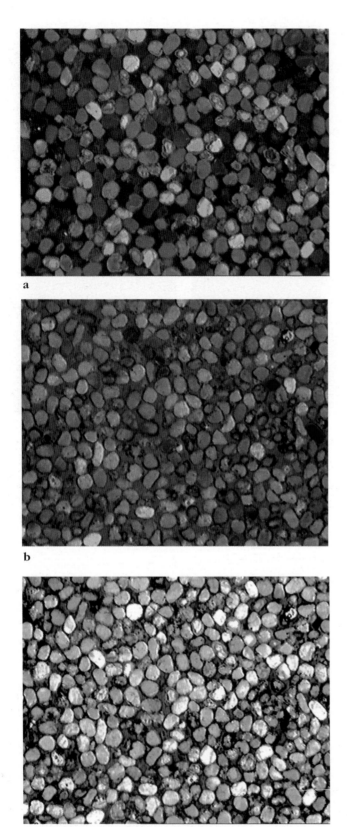

a

b

c

Figure 81. Thin section of sandstone viewed by polarized light. (a, b) different orientations of the analyzer; *(c)* maximum brightness image from six rotations.

5

Processing Images in Frequency Space

Some necessary mathematical preliminaries
What frequency space is all about

I t is unusual to pick up a book on image analysis without finding at least a portion of it devoted to a discussion of Fourier transforms (see especially Pratt, 1991; Gonzalez and Wintz, 1987; Jain, 1989). In part, this is due to the utility of working in frequency space to perform certain image measurement and processing operations. Many of these same operations can be performed in the original (spatial or pixel domain) image only with significantly greater computational effort. Another reason for the lengthy sections on these methods is that the authors frequently come from a background in electrical engineering and signal processing and so are familiar with the mathematics and the use of these methods for other types of signals, particularly the one-dimensional (time varying) electrical signals that make up much of our modern electronics.

The typical image analyst interested in applying computer methods to images for purposes of enhancement or measurement, however, may not be comfortable with the pages of mathematics (and intimidating notation) used in these discussions. Furthermore, he or she may not have the fortitude to relate these concepts to the operation of a dedicated image analysis computer. Unable to see the connection between the topics discussed and the typical image problems encountered in real life, the potential user might therefore find it easier to skip the subject. This is a loss, because the use of frequency space methods can offer benefits in many real-life applications, and it is not essential to deal deeply with the mathematics to arrive at a practical working knowledge of these techniques.

The Fourier transform and other frequency space transforms are applied to two-dimensional images for many different reasons. Some of these have little to do with the purposes of enhancing visibility and selection of features or structures of interest for measurement. For instance, some of these transform methods are used as a means of image compression, in which less data than the original image may be transmitted or stored. In this type of application, it is necessary to reconstruct the image (bring it back from the frequency to the spatial domain) for viewing. It is desirable to be able to accomplish both the forward and reverse transform rapidly and with a minimum loss of image quality. Image quality is a somewhat elusive concept that certainly includes the alteration of grey levels and color values, definition and location of feature boundaries, and introduction or removal of fine-scale texture in the image. Usually, the greater the degree of compression, the greater the loss of image fidelity, as shown in Chapter 2.

Speed is usually a less important concern to image measurement applications, since the acquisition and subsequent analysis of the images are likely to require some time anyway, but the computational advances (both in hardware and software or algorithms) made to accommodate the requirements of the data compression application help to shorten the time for some other processing operations, as well. On the other hand, the amount of image degradation that can be tolerated by most visual uses of the compressed and restored images is far greater than is usually acceptable for image analysis purposes. Consequently, the amount of image compression that can be achieved with minimal loss of fidelity is rather small, as discussed in Chapter 2.

In most cases, the transmission of an image from the point of acquisition to the computer used for analysis is not a major concern; therefore, we will ignore this entire subject here and assume that the transform retains all of the data, even if this means that there is no compression at all. Indeed, most of these methods are free from any data loss. The transform encodes the image information completely and it can be exactly reconstructed, at least to within the arithmetic precision of the computer being used (which is generally better than the precision of the original image sensor or analog-to-digital converter).

Although many different types of image transforms can be used, the best known (at least, the one with the most recognizable name) is the Fourier transform. This is due in part to the availability of a powerful and very efficient algorithm for computing it, known as the fast Fourier transform (FFT) (Cooley and Tukey, 1965; Bracewell, 1989), which we will encounter in due course. Although some programs actually perform the computation using the Fast Hartley Transform or FHT (Hartley, 1942; Bracewell, 1984, 1986; Reeves, 1990), the frequency space images are usually presented in the same form that the Fourier method would yield. For the sake of explanation, it is easiest to describe the better-known method.

The usual approach to developing the mathematical background of the Fourier transform begins with a one-dimensional waveform and then expands to two dimensions (an image). In principle, this can also be extended to three dimensions, although it becomes much more difficult to visualize or display. Three-dimensional transforms between the spatial domain (now a volume image constructed of voxels instead of pixels) and the three-dimensional frequency space are used, for example, in some tomographic reconstructions.

The mathematical development that follows has been kept as brief as possible, but if you suffer from "integral-o-phobia" then it is permitted to skip this section and go on to the examples and discussion, returning here only when (and if) a deeper understanding is desired.

The Fourier transform

Using a fairly standard nomenclature and symbology, begin with a function $f(x)$, where x is a real variable representing either time or distance in one direction across an image. It is very common to refer to this function as the spatial or time domain function and the transform F introduced below as the frequency space function. The function f is a continuous and well-behaved function. Do not be disturbed by the fact that in a digitized image, the values of x are not continuous but discrete (based on pixel spacing), and the possible brightness values are quantized as well. These values are considered to sample the real or analog image that exists outside the computer.

Fourier's theorem states that it is possible to form any one-dimensional function $f(x)$ as a summation of a series of sine and cosine terms of increasing frequency. The Fourier transform of the function $f(x)$ is written $F(u)$ and describes the amount of each frequency term that must be added together to make $f(x)$. It can be written as

$$F(u) = \int\limits_{-\infty}^{+\infty} f(x)e^{-2\pi iux}\,dx \qquad (1)$$

where i is (as usual) $\sqrt{-1}$. The use of the exponential notation relies on the mathematical identity (Euler's formula)

$$e^{-2\pi iux} = \cos(2\pi ux) - i\sin(2\pi ux) \qquad (2)$$

One of the very important characteristics of this transform is that given $F(u)$, it is possible to recover the spatial domain function $f(x)$ in the same way.

$$f(x) = \int\limits_{-\infty}^{+\infty} F(u)e^{2\pi iux}\,du \qquad (3)$$

These two equations together comprise the forward and reverse Fourier transform. The function $f(x)$ is generally a real function, such as a time-varying voltage or a spatially-varying image brightness; however, the transform function $F(u)$ is generally complex, the sum of a real part R and an imaginary part I.

$$F(u) = R(u) + iI(u) \qquad (4)$$

It is usually more convenient to express this in polar rather than Cartesian form

$$F(u) = |F(u)| \cdot e^{i\Phi(u)} \qquad (5)$$

where $|F|$ is called the magnitude and ϕ is called the phase. The square of the magnitude $|F(u)|^2$ is commonly referred to as the power spectrum, or spectral density of $f(x)$.

The integrals from minus to plus infinity will in practice be reduced to a summation of terms of increasing frequency, limited by the finite spacing of the sampled points in the image. The discrete Fourier transform is written as

$$F(u) = \frac{1}{N}\sum_{x=0}^{N-1} f(x) \cdot e^{-i2\pi ux/N} \qquad (6)$$

where N depends on the number of sampled points along the function $f(x)$, which are assumed to be uniformly spaced. Again, the reverse transform is similar (but not identical; note the absence of the $1/N$ term and the change in sign for the exponent).

$$f(x) = \sum_{u=0}^{N-1} F(u) \cdot e^{i2\pi ux/N} \qquad (7)$$

The values of u from 0 to $N-1$ represent the discrete frequency components added together to construct the function $f(x)$. As in the continuous case, $F(u)$ is complex and may be written as real and imaginary or as magnitude and phase components.

The summation is normally performed over terms up to one-half the dimension of the image (in pixels), since it requires a minimum of two pixel brightness values to define the highest frequency present. This limitation is described as the Nyquist frequency. Because the summation has half as many terms as the width of the original image, but each term has a real and imaginary part, the total number of values produced by the Fourier transform is the same as the number of pixels in the original image width, or the number of samples of a time-varying function. Since the original pixel values are usually small integers (0..255 for an 8-bit image), while the values produced by the Fourier transform are floating point numbers (and double precision ones in the best implementations), this actually represents an expansion in the storage requirements for the data.

In both the continuous and the discrete cases, a direct extension from one-dimensional functions to two- (or three-) dimensional ones can be made by substituting $f(x,y)$ for $f(x)$ and $F(u,v)$ for $F(u)$, and performing the summation or integration over two (or three) variables instead of one. Because the dimensions x,y,z are orthogonal, so are the u,v,w dimensions. This means that the transformation can be performed separately in each direction. For a two-dimensional image, for example, it would be possible to perform a one-dimensional transform on each horizontal line of the image, producing an intermediate result with complex values for each point. Then a second series of one-dimensional transforms can be performed on each vertical column, finally producing the desired two-dimensional transform.

The program fragment listed below shows how to compute the FFT of a function. It is written in Fortran, but can be translated into any other language (you may have to define a type to hold the complex numbers). On input to the subroutine, F is the array of values to be transformed (usually the imaginary part of these complex numbers will be 0) and LN is the power of 2 (up to 10 for the maximum 1024 in this implementation). The transform is returned in the same array F. The first loop reorders the input data, the second performs the successive doubling that is the heart of the FFT method, and the final loop normalizes the results.

```
      SUBROUTINE FFT(F,LN)
      COMPLEX F(1024),U,W,T,CMPLX
      PI=3.14159265
      N=2**LN
      NV2=N/2
      NM1=N-1
      J=1
      DO 3 I=1,NM1
            IF (I.GE.J) GOTO 1
            T=F(J)
            F(J)=F(I)
            F(I)=T
1           K=NV2
2           IF (K.GE.J) GOTO 3
            J=J-K
            K=K/2
            GOTO 2
3           J=J+K
      DO 5 L=1,LN
            LE=2**L
            LE1=LE/2
            U=(1.0,0.0)
            W=CMPLX(COS(PI/LE1),-SIN(PI/LE1))
            DO 5 J=1,LE1
                  DO 4 I=J,N,LE
                        IP=I+LE1
                        T=F(IP)*U
                        F(IP)=F(I)-T
```

```
4                                      F(I)=F(I)+T
5                      U=U*W
          DO 6 I=1MN
6              F(I)=F(I)/FLOAT(N)
          RETURN
          END
```

Applying this one-dimensional transform to each row and then each column of a two-dimensional image is not the fastest way to perform the calculation, but it is by far the simplest and is actually used in many programs. A somewhat faster approach, known as a butterfly because it uses various sets of pairs of pixel values throughout the two-dimensional image, produces identical results. Storing the array of W values can also provide a slight increase in speed. Many software math packages include highly optimized FFT routines. Some of these allow for array sizes that are not an exact power of two.

The resulting transform of the original image into frequency space has complex values at each pixel. This is difficult to display in any readily interpretable way. In most cases, the display is based on only the magnitude of the value, ignoring the phase. If the square of the magnitude is used, this may be referred to as the image's power spectrum, because different frequencies are represented at different distances from the origin, different directions represent different orientations in the original image, and the power at each location shows how much of that frequency and orientation is present in the image. This display is particularly useful for isolating periodic structures or noise, which is discussed below; however, the power spectrum by itself cannot be used to restore the original image. The phase information is also needed, although it is rarely displayed and is usually difficult or impossible to interpret visually.

Fourier transforms of real functions

A common illustration in introductory-level math textbooks on the Fourier transform (which usually deal only with the one-dimensional case) is the quality of the fit to an arbitrary, but simple, function by the sum of a finite series of terms in the Fourier expansion. **Figure 1** shows the familiar case of a step function, illustrating the ability to add up a series of sine waves to produce the desired step. The coefficients in the Fourier series are the magnitudes of each increasing frequency needed to produce the fit. **Figure 2a** shows the result of adding together the first 4, 10, and 25 terms. Obviously, the greater the number of terms included, the better the fit (especially at the sharp edge). **Figure 2b** shows the same comparison for a ramp function. One of the important characteristics of the Fourier transform is that the first few terms include much of the information and adding more terms progressively improves the quality of the fit.

Notice in both of these cases that the function is actually assumed to be repetitive or cyclical. The fit goes on past the right and left ends of the interval as though the function were endlessly repeated in both directions. This is also the case in two dimensions; the image in the spatial domain is effectively one tile in an endlessly repeating pattern. If the right and left edges or the top and bottom edges of the image are different, this can produce very noticeable effects in the resulting transform. One solution is to embed the image in a larger one consisting of either zeroes or the average brightness value of the pixels. This kind of padding makes the image twice as large in each direction, requiring four times as much storage and calculation. It is needed particularly when correlation is performed, as discussed below. Padding out to a larger size is also the simplest way to deal with an image that does not have dimensions that are an exact power of two.

The magnitude of the Fourier coefficients from the transforms shown in **Figure 2** is plotted as amplitude vs. frequency (**Figure 3**). Notice that the step function consists only of odd terms, while the magnitudes for the ramp function transform decrease smoothly. Rather than the magnitudes, it

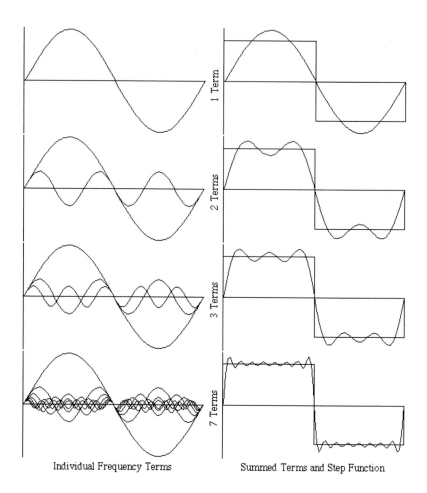

Figure 1. *Summation of Fourier frequency terms to fit a simple step function.*

Individual Frequency Terms

Summed Terms and Step Function

1 Term

2 Terms

3 Terms

7 Terms

is somewhat more common to plot the power spectrum of the transform, and to plot it as a symmetric function extending to both sides of the origin (zero frequency, or the DC level). As noted above, the power is simply the square of the magnitude. Because the range of values can be very large, the power spectrum is often plotted with a logarithmic or other compressed vertical scale to show the smaller terms usually present at high frequencies, along with the lower frequency terms.

Figure 4 reiterates the duality of the Fourier transform process. The spatial and frequency domains show the information in very different ways, but the information is the same. Of course, the plot of amplitude or power in the frequency transform does not show the important phase information, but we understand that the values are actually complex. Shifting the spatial domain image does not alter the amplitude values, but does change the phase values for each sinusoidal component.

It is important to recall, in examining these transforms, that the axes represent frequency. The low-frequency terms provide the overall shape of the function, while the high-frequency terms are needed to sharpen edges and provide fine detail. The second point to be kept in mind is that these terms are independent of each other (this is equivalent to the statement that the basis functions — the sinusoidal waves — are orthogonal). Performing the transform to determine coefficients to higher and higher frequencies does not change the previous ones, and selecting any particular range of terms to reconstruct the function will do so to the greatest accuracy possible with those frequencies.

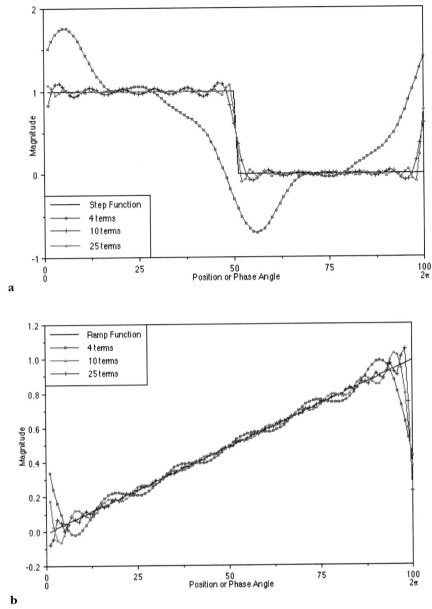

Figure 2. *Match between a step function (**a**) and a ramp function (**b**) and the first 4, 10, and 25 Fourier terms.*

Proceeding to two dimensions, **Figure 5** shows four images of perfectly sinusoidal variations in brightness. The first three vary in spacing (frequency) and orientation; the fourth is the superposition of all three. For each, the two-dimensional frequency transform is particularly simple. Each of the pure tones has a transform consisting of a single point (identifying the frequency and orientation). Because of the redundancy of the plotting coordinates, the point is shown in two symmetrical locations around the origin, which by convention lies at the center of the power spectrum plot.

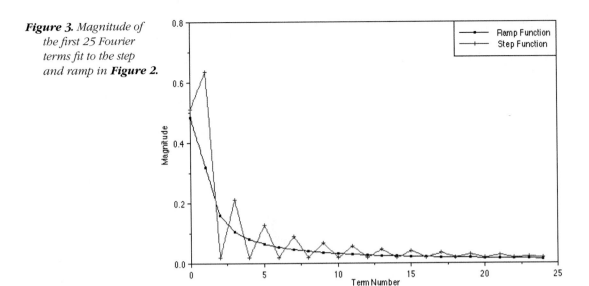

Figure 3. Magnitude of the first 25 Fourier terms fit to the step and ramp in Figure 2.

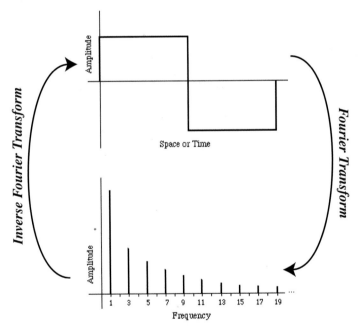

Figure 4. Role of the forward and inverse transform and the spatial and frequency domain representations of a step function.

Two-dimensional power spectra are easiest to describe using polar coordinates. The frequency increases with radius ρ, and the orientation depends on the angle θ. It is common to display the two-dimensional transform with the frequencies plotted from the center of the image, which is consequently redundant (the top and bottom or left and right halves are simply duplicates, with symmetry about the origin). In some cases, this image is shifted so that the origin is at the corners of the image and the highest frequencies are in the center. One format can be converted to the other by swapping quadrants of the display. For the purposes of image processing (removing or selecting specific frequencies, etc.) the display with the origin centered is simplest to use and has been adopted here.

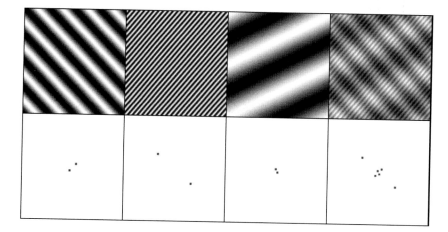

Figure 5. Three sinusoidal patterns, their frequency transforms, and their sum.

The power spectrum of the low frequency (greatest spacing) sinusoid has a point close to the origin, and the higher frequency sinusoids have points farther away, and in directions that identify the orientation of the lines. The superposition of the three sinusoids produces an image whose frequency transform is simply the sum of the three individual transforms. This principle of additivity will be important for much of the discussion in the following paragraphs. Subtracting the information from a location in the frequency transform is equivalent to removing the corresponding information from every part of the spatial-domain image. **Figure 6** shows two images with the same shape in different orientations. The frequency transforms rotate with the feature.

Figure 7 shows a two-dimensional step consisting of a rectangle. The two-dimensional frequency transform of this image produces the same series of diminishing peaks in the x and y axis directions as the one-dimensional step function. The darkness of each point in the power spectrum display represents the log of the square of the amplitude of the corresponding frequency. Limiting the reconstruction to only the central (low-frequency) terms produces the reconstructions shown. Just as for the one-dimensional case, this limits the sharpness of the edge of the step and produces some ringing (oscillations near the edge) in the overall shape. The line profiles through the image show the same shape as previously discussed for the one-dimensional case.

Figure 6. Rotation of a spatial domain image (left), and the corresponding rotation of the frequency transform (right).

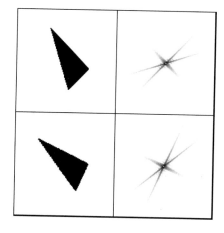

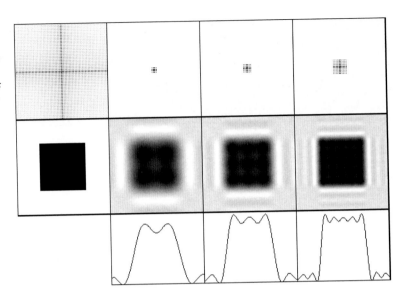

Figure 7. *A two-dimensional step function and its frequency transform (left), and reconstructions with different numbers of terms (shown as a portion of the frequency transform). Bottom row shows horizontal line profiles through the center of the reconstructed spatial image.*

Frequencies and orientations

It is helpful to develop a little familiarity with the power spectrum display of the frequency-space transform of the image using simple images. In **Figure 8a**, the lines can be represented by a single peak because their brightness profile is perfectly sinusoidal; thus only a single frequency is present. If the line profile is different, more terms are needed to represent the shape and consequently more peaks appear in the power spectrum. **Figure 8b** shows an example in which the frequency transform consists of a series of peaks at multiples of the lowest frequency, in the same orientation (perpendicular to the line angle).

In **Figure 8c,** the lines have the aliasing common in computer displays (and in halftone printing technology), in which the lines at a shallow angle on the display are constructed from a series of steps corresponding to the rows of display pixels. This further complicates the frequency transform, which now has additional peaks representing the horizontal and vertical steps in the image that correspond to the aliasing, in addition to the main line of peaks seen in the figure.

It is possible to select only the peaks along the main row and eliminate the others with a mask or filter, as will be discussed in the next section. After all, the frequency-domain image can be modified just like any other image. If this is done and only the peaks in the main row are used for the inverse transformation (back to the spatial domain), the aliasing of the lines is removed. In fact, that is how the images in **Figures 8a** and **8b** were produced. This will lead naturally to the subject of filtering (discussed in a later section): removing unwanted information from spatial-domain images by operating on the frequency transform. For example, it offers one practical technique to remove aliasing from lines and make them visually smooth.

Measuring images in the frequency domain
Orientation and spacing

The idealized examples shown in the preceding tutorial show that any periodic structure in the original spatial-domain image will be represented by a peak in the power spectrum image at a radius corresponding to the spacing and a direction corresponding to the orientation. In a real image, which typically consists of mostly non-periodic information, any such peaks will be superimposed on a broad and sometimes noisy background, although, finding the peaks is generally much

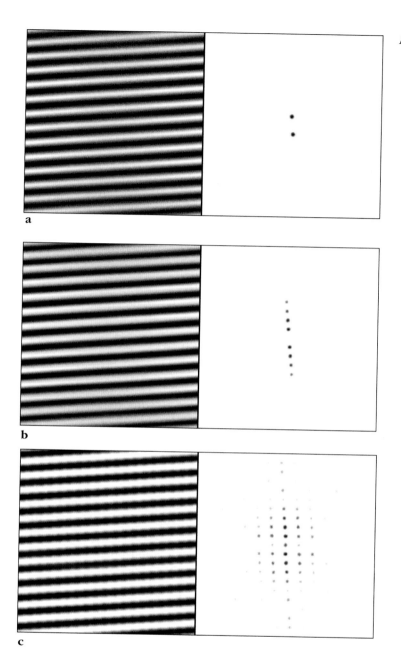

Figure 8. A set of lines (left) and their frequency transform (right):
(a) *sinusoidal lines;*
(b) *with a non-sinusoidal brightness profile;*
(c) *the lines from b with aliasing.*

a

b

c

easier than finding the original periodic structure. Also, measuring the peak locations accurately is much easier and more accurate than trying to extract the same information from the original image, because all of the occurrences are effectively averaged together in the frequency domain.

Figure 9 shows an example of this kind of peak location measurement. The spatial-domain image is a high-resolution transmission electron microscope (TEM) image of the lattice structure in pure silicon. The regular spacing of the bright spots represents the atomic structure of the lattice. Measuring all of the individual spacings of the spots would be very time-consuming and not particularly accurate. The frequency-domain representation of this image shows the periodicity clearly. The series of peaks indicates that the variation of brightness is not a simple sine wave, but contains many higher harmonics. The first-order peak gives the basic atomic spacing (and orientation),

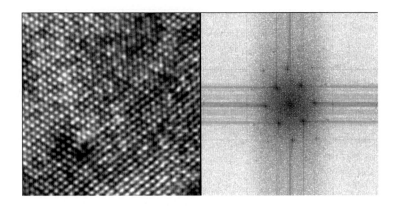

Figure 9. *High resolution TEM image of atomic lattice in silicon (left), with the frequency transform (right) (image courtesy Sopa Chevacharoenkul, Microelectronics Center of North Carolina).*

which can be measured by interpolating the peak position to a fraction of a pixel width, corresponding to an accuracy for the atom spacing of a few parts in 10,000. The spacing of the features that produce the point in the power spectrum is simply the width of the image (e.g., 256 pixels in the example, times whatever calibration applies) divided by the distance from the origin to the center of the peak in the power spectrum.

To the electron microscopist, the power spectrum image of the frequency-domain transform looks just like an electron diffraction pattern, which in fact it is. The use of microscope optics to form the diffraction pattern is an analog method of computing the frequency-domain representation. This can be done with any image by setting up suitable optics. While it is a fast way to obtain the frequency-domain representation, this method has two serious drawbacks for use in image processing.

First, the phase information is lost when the diffraction pattern is recorded, so it is not possible to reconstruct the spatial-domain image from a photograph of the diffraction pattern. (Recording the entire diffraction pattern including the phase information results in a hologram, from which the original image *can* be reconstructed.) It is possible to perform the reconstruction from the diffraction pattern in the microscope by using suitable lenses (indeed, that is how the microscope functions), so in principle it is possible to insert the various masks and filters discussed below. Making these masks and filters is difficult and exacting work, however, which must usually be performed individually for each image to be enhanced. Consequently, it is much easier (and more controllable) to use a computer to perform the transform and to apply any desired masks.

It is also easier to perform measurements on the frequency-domain representation using the computer. Locating the centers of peaks by curve fitting would require recording the diffraction pattern (typically with film, which may introduce nonlinearities or saturation over the extremely wide dynamic range of many patterns), followed by digitization to obtain numerical values. Considering the speed with which a spatial-domain image can be recorded, the frequency transform calculated, and interactive or automatic measurement performed, the computer is generally the tool of choice. This analysis is made easier by the ability to manipulate the display contrast so that both brighter and dimmer spots can be seen, and to use image processing tools such as background leveling and a top hat filter to isolate the peaks of interest.

When spots from a periodic structure are superimposed on a general background, the total power in the spots expressed as a fraction of the total power in the entire frequency transform gives a useful quantitative measure of the degree of periodicity in the structure. This may also be used to compare different periodicities (different spacings or orientations) by comparing summations of values in the power spectrum. For electron diffraction patterns, this is a function of the atomic density of various planes and the atomic scattering cross sections.

Although the display of the power spectrum corresponds to a diffraction pattern and is the most familiar presentation of frequency-space information, it must not be forgotten that the phase information is also needed to reconstruct the original image. **Figure 10** shows a test image, consisting of a regular pattern of spots, and its corresponding power spectrum and phase values. If the phase information is erased (all phases set to zero), the reconstruction (**Figure 11**) shows some of the same periodicity, but the objects are no longer recognizable. The various sine waves have been shifted in phase, so that the feature boundaries are not reconstructed.

The assumption that the image is one repetition of an endless sequence is also important. Most real images do not have perfectly matching left and right or top and bottom edges. This produces a large step function at the edge, which is more apparent if the image is shifted by an arbitrary offset (**Figure 12**). As noted previously, this does not alter the power spectrum image, although the phase image is shifted. The discontinuity requires high-frequency terms to fit, and since the edges are precisely horizontal and vertical, the power spectrum display shows a central cross superimposed on the rest of the data, which is visible in **Figure 10**. For the test pattern, the result of eliminating these lines from the original frequency transform and then retransforming is shown in **Figure 13**. The central portion of the image is unaffected, but at the edges the discontinuity is no longer sharp because the many frequencies needed to create the step functions at the edges are missing. The pattern from each side has been reproduced on the other side of the boundary, superimposed on the correct data.

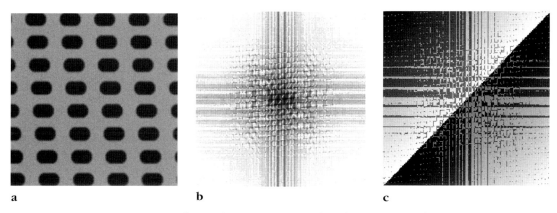

a   b   c

Figure 10. *Test image consisting of a regular pattern (**a**), with its frequency transform power spectrum (**b**) and phase values (**c**).*

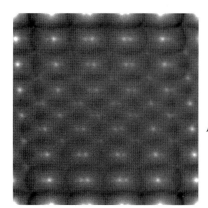

Figure 11. *Retransformation of **Figure 10** with all phase information set to zero.*

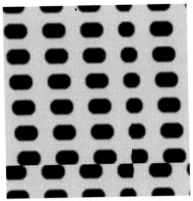

*Figure 12. The test image of **Figure 10** with an arbitrary spatial shift, showing the discontinuities at the image boundaries*

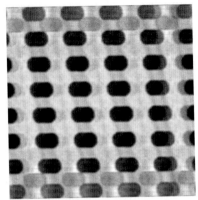

*Figure 13. Retransformation of **Figure 10** with the central cross (horizontal and vertical lines) reduced to zero magnitude, so that the left and right edges of the image, and the top and bottom edges, are forced to match.*

Preferred orientation

Figure 14 shows another example of a periodic structure, only much less perfect and larger in scale than the lattice images above. The specimen is a thin film of magnetic material viewed in polarized light. The stripes are oppositely oriented magnetic domains in the material that are used to store information in the film. The frequency transform of this image clearly shows the width and spacing of the domains. Instead of a single peak, some arcs show the variation in orientation of the stripes, which is evident in the original image but difficult to quantify.

The length of the arcs and the variation of brightness (power) with angle along them can be easily measured to characterize the preferred orientation in the structure. Even for structures that are not perfectly periodic, the integrated power as a function of angle can be used to measure the preferred orientation. This is identical to the results of autocorrelation operations carried out in the spatial domain, in which a binary image is shifted and combined with itself in all possible displacements to obtain a matrix of fractional values, but it is much faster to perform with the frequency-domain representation. Also, this makes it easier to deal with grey scale values.

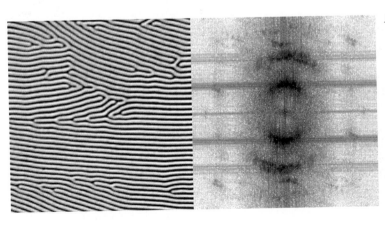

Figure 14. Polarized light image of magnetic domains in thin film material (left), with the frequency transform (right).

Reconstructing periodic structures that are not perfectly aligned can be performed by selecting the entire arc in the frequency transform. **Figure 15** illustrates this with a virus particle. The TEM image hints at the internal helical structure, but does not show it clearly. In the frequency transform, the periodic spacing and the variation in direction is evident. The spacing can be measured (2.41 nm) and the helix angle determined from the length of the arc. Retransforming only these arcs shows the periodicity, but this is not limited spatially to the virus particle. Using the spatial-domain image as a mask (as discussed in Chapter 7) makes the internal helical pattern evident.

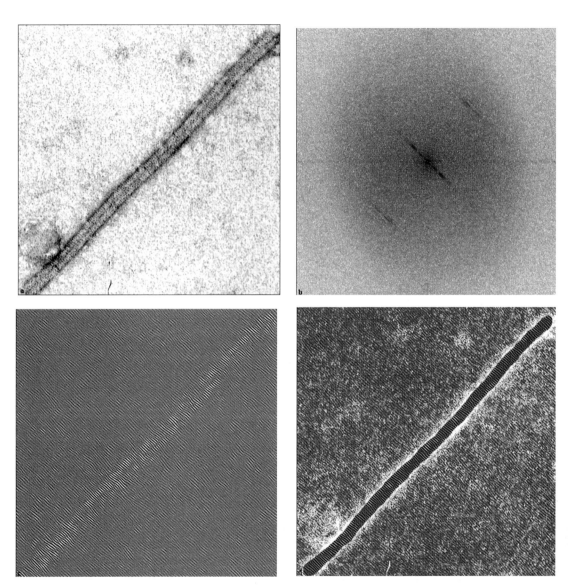

Figure 15. TEM image of a virus *(courtesy Dr. R. L. Grayson, Virginia Polytechnic Institute, Blacksburg, VA):*
   (a) original image, in which the internal helical structure is difficult to discern;
   (b) frequency transform of image a, in which the regular repeating structure of the virus and its angular variation in orientation is evident;
   (c) retransformation of just the peaks in the frequency transform, in which the periodic lines are not limited to the virus;
   (d) using the virus particle as a mask, the helical pattern becomes evident.

One particular type of preferred orientation in images, which arises not from the specimen but rather from the imaging system itself, is astigmatism. This is a particular problem with electron microscopes because of the operating principles of electromagnetic lenses. Even skilled operators devote considerable time to making adjustments to minimize astigmatism, and it is often very difficult to recognize it in images in order to correct it. Astigmatism results in the defocusing of the image and a consequent loss of sharpness in one direction, sometimes with an improvement in the perpendicular direction. This becomes immediately evident in the frequency transform, since the decrease in brightness or power falls off radially (at higher frequencies) and the asymmetry can be noted.

Figure 16 shows an example. The specimen is a cross section with three layers. The bottom is crystalline silicon, above which is a layer of amorphous (non-crystalline) silicon, followed by a layer of glue used to mount the sample for thinning and microscopy. The glue is difficult to distinguish by eye from the amorphous silicon. Frequency transforms for the three regions are shown. The regular structure in the pattern from the crystalline silicon gives the expected diffraction pattern. While the two regions above do not show individual peaks from periodic structures, they are not the same. The amorphous silicon has short-range order in the atomic spacings based on strong covalent bonding that is not visible to the human observer because of its chaotic overall pattern. This shows up in the frequency transform as a white cross in the dark ring, indicating that in the 45-degree directions there is a characteristic distance and direction to the next atom. This pattern is absent in the glue region, where there is no such structure.

In both regions, the dark circular pattern from the amorphous structure is not a perfect circle, but an ellipse. This indicates astigmatism. Adjusting the microscope optics to produce a uniform circle will correct the astigmatism and provide uniform resolution in all directions in the original image. It is much easier to observe the effects of small changes in the frequency-space display than in the spatial-domain image.

The frequency transform of an image can be used to optimize focus and astigmatism. When an image is in focus, the high-frequency information is maximized in order to sharply define the edges.

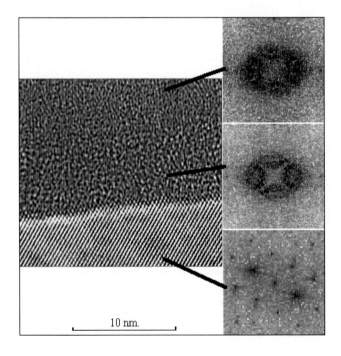

Figure 16. TEM image of cross section of crystalline and amorphous silicon, and glue, with frequency transforms of each region shown at right (image courtesy Sopa Chevacharoenkul, Microelectronics Center of North Carolina).

10 nm.

This provides a convenient test for sharpest focus. **Figure 17** shows a light microscope image that is in focus. The line profiles of the power spectrum in both the vertical and horizontal directions show a more gradual drop-off at high frequencies than **Figure 18**, which is the same image out of focus. When astigmatism is present (**Figure 19**), the power spectrum is asymmetric, as shown by the profiles.

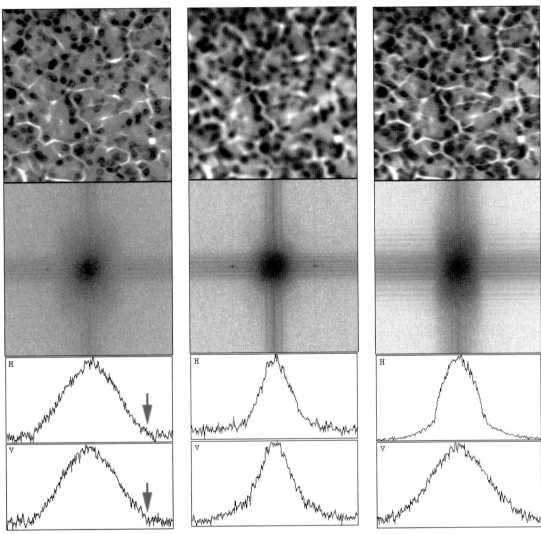

Figure 17. Out-of-focus image with its power spectrum and horizontal and vertical line profiles, showing presence of high-frequency information as compared with **Figure 18**. Red arrows indicate actual resolution limit as discussed in text.

Figure 18. Out-of-focus image with its power spectrum and horizontal and vertical line profiles, showing loss of high frequency information as compared to **Figure 17**.

Figure 19. Astigmatic image produced by misaligning lens, with its power spectrum and horizontal and vertical line profiles showing different high-frequency components.

Profiles of the power spectrum also provide a convenient tool for measuring the actual resolution of images, to characterize various types of cameras and acquisition devices as discussed in Chapter 1. Most image acquisition procedures store an image that has somewhat more pixels than the actual resolution. As shown by the red arrows in **Figure 17**, the power spectrum shows a definite break in slope. This indicates the frequency at which the real information in the image ends; only noise is present at higher frequencies (smaller spacings).

Figure 20 shows a test pattern of radial lines. Due to the finite spacing of detectors in the video camera used, as well as limitations in electronics bandwidth that eliminate the very high frequencies required to resolve small details, these lines are incompletely resolved where they are close together. **Figure 21** shows the two-dimensional Fourier transform power spectrum of this image. The power spectrum is plotted isometrically in **Figure 22** to emphasize the drop-off in magnitude, which is different in the horizontal and vertical directions. As is common in video, the resolution along each scan line is poorer than the vertical resolution. **Figure 23** shows the complete set of data using color. One image shows the real and imaginary components of the transform

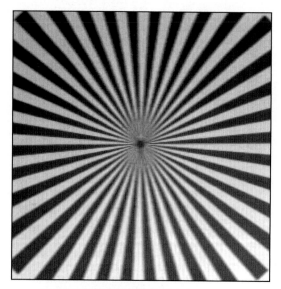

Figure 20. *Test pattern image.*

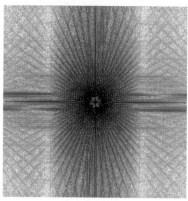

a

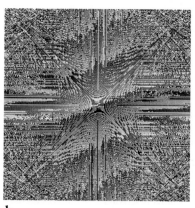

b

Figure 21. Fourier transform of the test image in Figure 20:
    (a) *power spectrum magnitude;*
    (b) *phase (angles from 0 to 180° displayed as grey-scale values from black to white).*

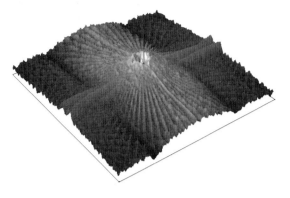

Figure 22. *The power spectrum from* **Figure 21** *presented as an isometric view.*

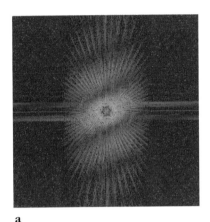

a

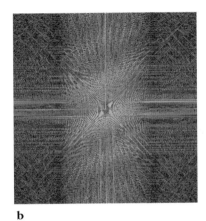

b

Figure 23. Color representations of the Fourier transform from Figure 21:
   (a) *YUV image in which U = Real,V = Imaginary;*
   (b) *RGB image in which Intensity = Magnitude, Hue = Phase.*

and the other the magnitude and phase, encoded in different color channels. Although technically complete, these displays are rarely used because the phase information is confusing to the viewer.

In the power spectrum, it is evident that there is a well-defined boundary, different in the x and y directions, beyond which the magnitude drops abruptly. This corresponds to the image resolution, which is different in the horizontal and vertical directions. In many cases, it is not so obvious where the physical source of resolution limitation lies. It can arise from the finite spacing of detectors in the camera, or various electronic effects in the amplification and digitization process; however, the Fourier transform power spectrum will still show the limit, permitting the resolution of any imaging system to be ascertained.

Texture and fractals

Besides the peaks in the power spectrum resulting from periodic structures that may be present and the ultimate limitation at high frequencies due to finite image resolution, it may seem as though there is only a noisy background containing little useful information. This is far from true. Many images represent the brightness of light scattered from surfaces, or other data such as surface elevation. In these images, the roughness or texture of the surface is revealed and may be measured from the power spectrum.

The concept of a fractal surface dimension will not be explained here in detail, but is discussed in Chapter 13. Surfaces that are fractal have an area that is mathematically undefined. It is greater than the projected area covered by the irregular surface and increases as the measurement scale becomes finer. The fractal dimension may be determined the slope of a line on a log-log plot of measured area vs. the size of the measuring tool. Many naturally occurring surfaces resulting from wear, erosion, agglomeration of particles, or fracture are observed to have this character. It has also been shown that images of these surfaces, whether produced by the scattering of diffuse light or the production of secondary electrons in an scanning electron microscope (SEM), are also fractal. That is, the variation of brightness with position obeys the same mathematical relationship. The fractal dimension is an extremely powerful and compact representation of the surface roughness, which can often be related to the history of the surface and the properties that result.

Measuring surface fractals directly is rarely practical, although it can be done physically by determining the number of molecules of various gases that can adhere to the surface as a function of their size. One common imaging approach is to reduce the dimensionality and measure the fractal dimension of a boundary line produced by intersecting the surface with a sampling plane. This may either be produced by cross sectioning or by polishing down into the surface to produce islands. In either case, the rougher the surface, the more irregular the line. In the case of polishing parallel to the surface to produce islands, the perimeter line also has a fractal dimension (the slope of a log-log plot relating the measured line length and the length of the measurement tool), which is just 1.0 less than that of the surface.

For a fractal surface, the power spectrum shows the superposition of sinusoids of all frequencies and orientations to have a specific shape: the magnitudes of the coefficients in a Fourier transform of a fractal curve decrease exponentially with the log of frequency, while the phases of the terms are randomized. This can be understood qualitatively, since by definition a fractal curve is self-similar and has detail extending to ever-finer scales (or higher frequencies). This also implies that the proportion of amplitudes of higher frequency terms must be self-similar. An exponential curve satisfies this criterion.

Plotting the log of the amplitude (or the power spectrum, which is the square of the amplitude) versus the logarithm of frequency produces a straight line plot, which is easily analyzed. There is a simple relationship between the fractal dimension of a profile and the exponential decrease in magnitude of the terms in a Fourier expansion, as had been predicted by Feder (1989). This correlation makes it practical to use the radial decrease of magnitude in a two-dimensional Fourier-transform image as a measure of roughness and the directional variation of that decrease as a measure of orientation (Mitchell and Bonnell, 1990; Russ, 1990; Russ, 1994).

Figure 24 shows a range image (brightness represents elevation) for a fractal surface, with its Fourier transform power spectrum. Plotting log (amplitude) vs. log (frequency) as shown in **Figure 25** produces a straight line, and a plot of the histogram of the phase values shows a uniform random distribution, which confirms the fractal geometry of the surface. The slope of the plot gives the dimension of the surface (which must lie between 2.0 for a Euclidean surface and 2.999, for one so irregular that it effectively fills three-dimensional space) as Fractal Dimension = (6 + Slope)/2, or about 2.2 for the example shown. This is an isotropic surface produced by shotblasting a metal, so the slope is the same in all directions.

Figure 26 shows another surface, this produced by machining, with tool marks oriented in a specific direction. Similar analysis of this surface shows (**Figure 27**) that while it is still fractal (with average dimension about 2.25), it is not isotropic. Actually, two methods are used to depart from isotropy: one is changing the slope of the Log (amplitude) vs. Log (frequency) plot, and the other its intercept, as a function of direction. Chapter 13 discusses fractal surface geometry in more detail (see also Russ, 1994 and Russ, 2001b).

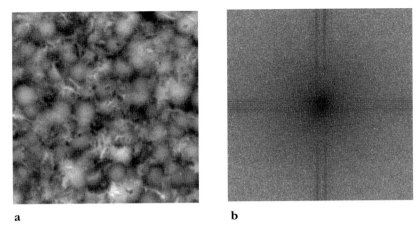

a   b

Figure 24. Range image of a shotblasted metal surface, with its Fourier transform power spectrum.

Figure 25. Analysis of the Fourier transform data showing the isotropic fractal nature of the surface in Figure 24.

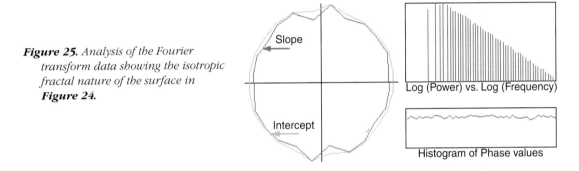

Measuring the two-dimensional Fourier transform is more efficient than measuring many individual brightness profiles in the original image. It also allows any periodic structures that may be present to be ignored, since these show up as discrete points in the frequency-transform image and can be skipped in determining the overall exponential decrease in the magnitude values. In other words, it is possible to look beyond the periodic structures or noise (e.g., arising from electronic components) in the images and still characterize the underlying chaotic but self-similar nature of the surface.

Filtering images
Isolating periodic noise

It was noted earlier (and shown in **Figure 5** for a simple case) that the frequency transform has a property of separability and additivity. Adding together the transforms of two original images or functions produces the same result as the transform of the sum of the originals. This idea opens the way to using subtraction to remove unwanted parts of images. It is most commonly used to remove periodic noise, which can be introduced by the devices used to record or transmit images. We will see some examples below. If the frequencies associated with the noise can be determined (often possible directly from the Fourier transform), then setting the amplitude of those terms to zero will leave only the desired part of the information. This can then be inverse transformed back to the spatial domain to produce a noise-free image.

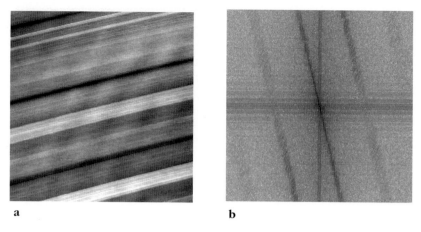

a   b

Figure 26. *Range image of a machined metal surface, with its Fourier transform power spectrum.*

Figure 27. *Analysis of the Fourier transform data showing the anisotropic fractal nature of the surface in* **Figure 26.**

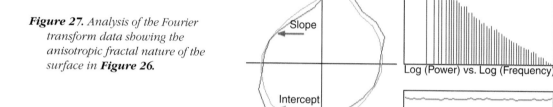

The same method of removing selected frequencies can be used for a more basic type of filtering as well. **Figure 28** shows an image with its Fourier transform power spectrum. There are no evident "spikes" or noise peaks, just the usual gradual reduction in the amplitude of higher frequencies. Keeping the low frequencies and removing the high frequencies can be accomplished by zeroing the amplitude of all sinusoids above a selected frequency. The red circle in **Figure 28b** was used to perform this "low-pass" filtering operation (i.e., passing or keeping the low frequencies), to produce the result in **Figure 28c**. Conversely, keeping the high frequencies and removing the low frequencies (a "high-pass" filter) produces the result in **Figure 28d**.

Except for the ringing around boundaries (discussed below), the results are exactly the same as those for Gaussian smoothing and Laplacian sharpening, shown in the two preceding chapters. In fact, it can be shown mathematically that the operations are exactly the same whether performed in the frequency domain or in the pixel domain.

In this illustration of filtering, portions of the Fourier-transform image were selected based on frequency, which is why these filters are generally called low-pass and high-pass filters. Usually, selecting arbitrary regions of the frequency domain for reconstruction produces artefacts, unless some care is taken to shape the edges of the filter region to attenuate the data smoothly. This can be seen in the one-dimensional example of the step function in **Figure 1** and the corresponding two-dimensional example of **Figure 7**. If only the first few terms are used then, in addition to not

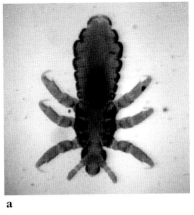

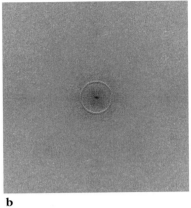

a

b

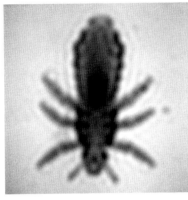

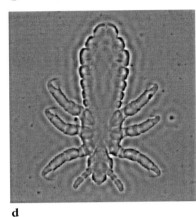

c

d

Figure 28. Frequency filtering using the Fourier transform: (**a**) *original image;* (**b**) *power spectrum with a circular frequency cutoff;* (**c**) *retransforming just the low frequencies inside the circle (a low-pass filter);* (**d**) *retransforming just the high frequencies outside the circle (a high-pass filter).*

modeling the steepness of the step, the reconstruction has oscillations near the edge, which are generally described as ringing.

It is necessary to shape the edge of the filter to prevent ringing at sharp discontinuities. This behavior is well-known in one-dimensional filtering (used in digital signal processing, for example). Several different shapes are commonly used. Over a specified width (usually given in pixels, but of course ultimately specified in terms of frequency or direction), the filter magnitude can be reduced from maximum to minimum using a weighting function. The simplest function is linear interpolation (also called a Parzen window function). Better results can be obtained using a parabolic or cosine function (also called Welch and Hanning window functions, respectively, in this context). The most elaborate filter shapes do not drop to the zero or minimum value, but extend a very long tail beyond the cutoff point. One such shape is a Gaussian. **Figure 29** shows several of these shapes.

Another filter shape often used in these applications is a Butterworth filter, with a magnitude that can be written as

$$H = 1 / \left[1 + C \left(\frac{R}{R_0} \right)^{2n} \right] \tag{8}$$

where R is the distance from the center of the filter (usually the center of the power spectrum image, or zero-frequency point), and R_0 is the nominal filter cutoff value. The constant C is often set equal to 1.0 or to 0.414; the value defines the magnitude of the filter at the point where $R = R_0$ as either 50% or $1/\sqrt{2}$. The integer n is the order of the filter; its most common values are 1 or 2.

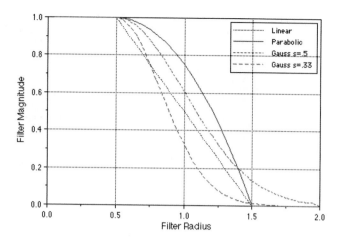

Figure 29. Some common filter edge profiles.

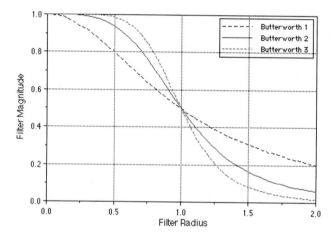

Figure 30. Shapes for Butterworth filter profiles of order 1, 2, and 3.

Figure 30 shows comparison profiles of several Butterworth low-pass filters (ones that attenuate high frequencies). The converse shape having negative values of *n* passes high frequencies and attenuates low ones. **Figure 31** shows the effect that shaping the frequency cutoff has on the quality of the retransformed images from **Figure 28**.

To illustrate the effects of these filters on ringing at edges, **Figure 32** shows a simple test shape and its two-dimensional FFT power spectrum image. The orientation of principal terms perpendicular to the major edges in the spatial-domain image is evident. Performing a reconstruction using a simple aperture with a radius equal to 25 pixels (called an ideal filter) produces the result shown in **Figure 33a**. The oscillations in brightness near the edges are quite visible.

Ringing can be reduced by shaping the edge of the filter, as discussed above. The magnitudes of frequency terms near the cutoff value are multiplied by factors less than one, whose values are based on a simple function. If a cosine function is used, which varies from 1 to 0 over a total width of 6 pixels, the result is improved (**Figure 33b**). In this example, the original 25-pixel radius used for the ideal filter (the sharp cutoff) is the point at which the magnitude of the weighting factor drops to 50%. The weights drop smoothly from 1.0 at a radius of 22 pixels to 0.0 at a radius of 28 pixels.

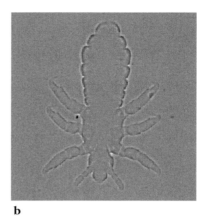
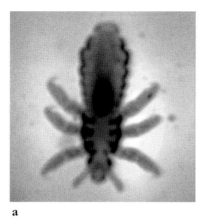

a   b

Figure 31. Shaping the frequency cutoff with a Butterworth filter:
  (a) low-pass filter (compare with **Figure 28c**);
  (b) high-pass filter (compare with **Figure 28d**).

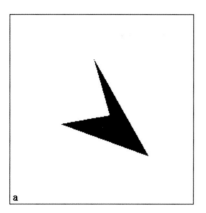
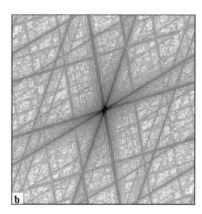

a   b

Figure 32. *Test shape with its frequency transform power spectrum.*

Increasing the distance over which the transition takes place further reduces the ringing, as shown in **Figure 33c**. Here, the 50% point is still at 25 pixels but the range is from 15 to 35 pixels. Note that the improvement is not achieved simply by increasing the high-frequency limit, which would improve the sharpness of the feature edges but would not by itself reduce the ringing. **Figure 33d** shows the same reconstruction using a second-degree Butterworth filter shape whose 50% point is set at 25 pixels.

Figure 34 shows an image with both fine detail and some noise along with its frequency transform. Applying Butterworth low-pass filters with radii of 10 and 25 pixels in the frequency-domain image smooths the noise with some blurring of the high-frequency detail (**Figure 35**), while the application of Butterworth high-pass filters with the same radii emphasizes the edges and reduces the contrast in the large (low-frequency) regions (**Figure 36**). All of these filters were applied to the amplitude values as multiplicative masks. Adjusting the radius of the filter cutoff controls the range of frequencies in the inverse transformed image, just as changing the size of the convolution kernel alters the degree of smoothing or sharpening when the equivalent procedure is carried out in the spatial or pixel domain.

Of course, it is not necessary for the variation in magnitude to be from 1 to 0. Sometimes the lower limit is set to a fraction, so that the high (or low) frequencies are not completely attenuated.

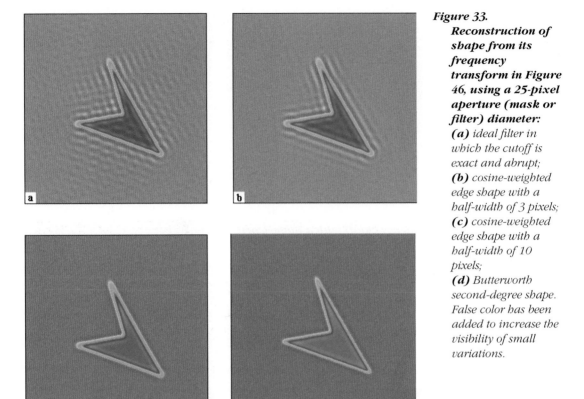

Figure 33.
Reconstruction of shape from its frequency transform in Figure 46, using a 25-pixel aperture (mask or filter) diameter: *(a) ideal filter in which the cutoff is exact and abrupt; (b) cosine-weighted edge shape with a half-width of 3 pixels; (c) cosine-weighted edge shape with a half-width of 10 pixels; (d) Butterworth second-degree shape. False color has been added to increase the visibility of small variations.*

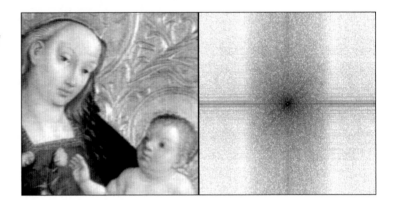

Figure 34. *Image and its transform used for filtering in **Figures 35** and **36**.*

It is also possible to use values greater than 1. A high-frequency emphasis filter with the low-frequency value set to a reduced value, such as 0.5, and a high-frequency value greater than 1, such as 2, is called a homomorphic filter. It is usually applied to an image whose brightness values have previously been converted to their logarithms (using a LUT). This filtering operation will simultaneously increase the high-frequency information (sharpening edges) while reducing the overall brightness range to allow edge brightness values to show. The physical reasoning behind the homomorphic filter is a separation of illumination and reflectance components in the image. As with most of these filters, though, the real justification is that it improves the appearance of many images of practical interest.

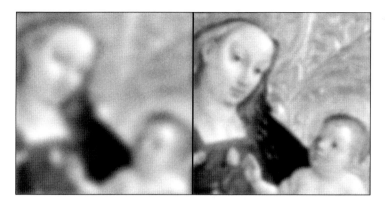

*Figure 35. Filtering of **Figure 34** with low-pass Butterworth Filters having 50% cutoff diameters of 10 (left) and 25 pixels (right).*

*Figure 36. Filtering of **Figure 34** with high-pass Butterworth Filters having 50% cutoff diameters of 10 (left) and 25 pixels (right).*

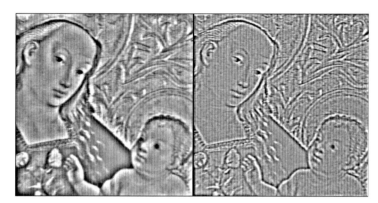

It is also possible to select a region of the Fourier transform image that is not centered on the origin. **Figure 37** shows a selection of intermediate frequency values lying in a particular direction on the transform in **Figure 20**, along with the resulting reconstruction. This kind of filtering may be useful to select directional information from images. It also demonstrates the basic characteristic of Fourier transform images: locations in the Fourier transform image identify periodicity and orientation information from any or all parts of the spatial-domain image. Note that the correct shape for off-centered regions is a combination of annuli and wedges that have cutoffs corresponding to frequencies and angles, rather than the more easily constructed circles or rectangles, and that the edges require the same type of smoothing shown previously.

Masks and filters

Once the location of periodic noise in an original image is isolated into a single point or a few points in the Fourier-transform image, it becomes possible to remove the noise by removing those sinusoidal terms. A filter removes selected frequencies and orientations by reducing the magnitude values for those terms, either partially or to zero, while leaving the phase information alone (which is important in determining where in the image that information appears).

Many different ways are used to specify and to apply this reduction. Sometimes it is practical to specify a range of frequencies and orientations numerically, but most often it will be convenient to do so using the magnitude or power spectrum display of the Fourier transform image. Manually or automatically selecting regions on this display allows specific peaks in the power spectrum, corresponding to the periodic information, to be selected for elimination.

Rather than the use of combinations of arcs and radial lines, for isolated noise peaks (often referred to as noise "spikes") it is convenient and usually acceptable to use small circles to define the

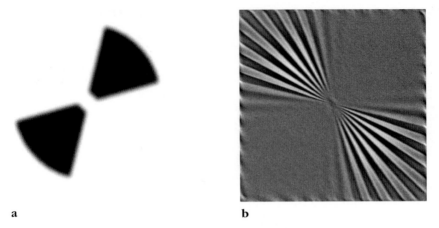

a   b

Figure 37. Inverse transform of the Fourier transform of Figure 20 (b) through a filter selecting a range of frequencies and angles (a).

regions. It is important to use a smoothing function to modify the edges of the regions. When the transition takes place over a distance of only a few pixels, the differences between the various transition curves described previously are of little importance, and a simple Gaussian smooth is most commonly applied.

Usually, it is only by first examining the transform-image power spectrum that the presence and exact location of these points can be determined. **Figure 38** shows an image of a halftone print from a magazine. The pattern results from the halftone screen used in the printing process. In the frequency transform of the image, this regular pattern shows up as well-defined narrow peaks or spikes. Filtering removes the peaks by setting the magnitude at those locations to zero (but not altering any of the phase information). This allows the image to be retransformed without the noise. The filtered Fourier transform image power spectrum shown in **Figure 39** shows the circular white spots where filtering was performed.

It is interesting to note that image compression does not necessarily remove these noise spikes in the Fourier transform. Compression is generally based on discarding the terms in the transform (Fourier, Cosine, etc.) whose magnitudes are small. The halftone pattern or other periodic noise is interpreted as an important feature of the image by these compression methods. The need to preserve the periodic noise spikes actually reduces the amount of other useful detail that can be retained.

The effects of compression are best examined in the frequency transform. **Figure 40** shows a portion of the image of Saturn used in Chapter 4, before and after compression by the JPEG algorithm. Some differences, particularly in the rings, can be seen. The frequency transforms of the two images show that this is due to the loss of lines of high frequency information that are needed to define the profiles of the rings and the detail within them.

The example in **Figure 39** relied on human observation of the peaks in the Fourier transform image, recognition that the peaks were responsible for the periodic noise, and selecting them to produce the filter. In some cases, it is possible to construct an appropriate image filter automatically from the Fourier transform power spectrum. The guiding principle is that peaks in the power spectrum that are narrow and rise significantly above the local background should be removed. If the Fourier transform magnitude image is treated like an ordinary spatial-domain grey scale image, this peak removal can often be accomplished automatically using a rank-based filter like the top hat.

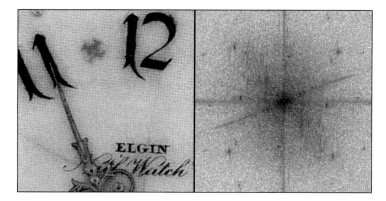

Figure 38. A halftoned printed image (left) and its frequency transform (right).

Figure 39. Removal of periodic information from Figure 38 by reducing the magnitude (left) and retransforming (right).

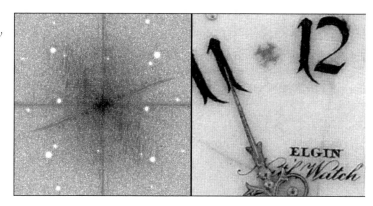

Figure 41 shows the power spectrum from the image in **Figure 38** and the result of applying a top hat filter with an inner radius of 3 pixels, an outer radius of 5 pixels, and a height of 8 grey-scale values. The brim of the hat rests on the background that drops off gradually and smoothly as frequency (radius) increases. The located features correspond to the noise spikes. Enlarging the spots by a few pixels and applying a smoothing to the edges, and inverting this result creates a mask that will remove the spikes. The figure shows the resulting modified power spectrum and the retransformed result.

Sometimes, the process of determining where the noise peaks are located can be simplified by selecting a region of the image that exhibits the noise pattern in an otherwise uniform area. This sequence is demonstrated in **Figure 42** for the same image as in **Figures 38** and **41**. A region of halftone periodic noise is selected and the rest of the image cleared. The transform of this image is then processed by smoothing and leveling, and then thresholded to locate the peaks. The inverse of this mask is then smoothed and multiplied by the frequency transform of the original image to produce the filtered result.

Removal of noise spikes is not always enough to restore an image completely. The example in **Figure 43** shows an example of an image scanned in from a newspaper; the halftone dots are very evident. The dark spots ("spikes") in the power spectrum (**Figure 43b**) correspond to the periodic structure in the image. They align with the repetitive pattern of dots, and their darkness indicates how much of various frequencies are present. Removing them is equivalent to removing the periodic component. In this case a top hat filter was used to locate the spikes and create a mask (**Figure 43c**). The result of applying this mask as a filter to remove the spikes shows that the periodic noise has been removed without affecting any of the other information present (**Figure 43d**). There is still some pixel-to-pixel noise because the image has been scanned at a higher magnification than it was printed, and the halftone cells in the original image are separated.

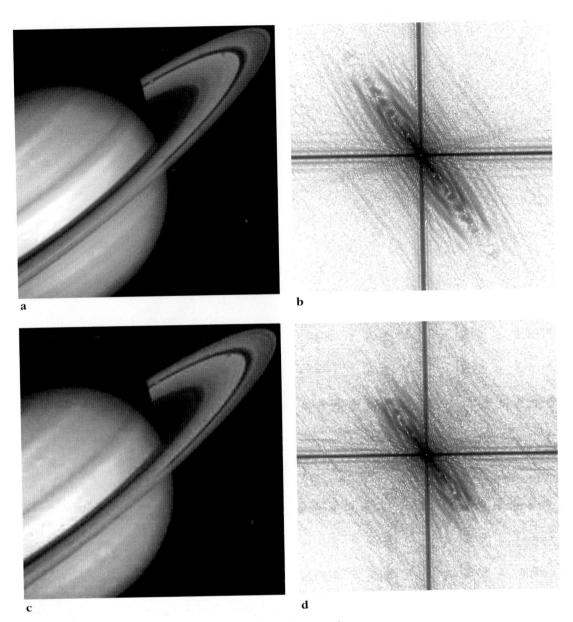

Figure 40. Portion of the image of Saturn from Chapter 4:
(a) original;
(b) FT power spectrum showing high frequencies needed for detail in rings;
(c) image after JPEG compression (factor of 12);
*(d) FT power spectrum of **c** showing loss of high-frequency information.*

An additional filter can be employed to fill in the space between cells. A Butterworth second-order, high-frequency cutoff filter keeps low frequencies (gradual variations in grey scale) while progressively cutting off higher ones. In this case the midpoint of the cutoff was set to the spacing of the halftone dots in the original image. The final version of the power spectrum (**Figure 43e**) shows the periodic spots removed and the high frequencies attenuated. An inverse transform produces the final image (**Figure 43f**). Note that even the cat's whiskers which are barely discernible in the original image can be clearly seen.

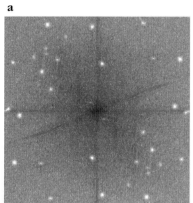

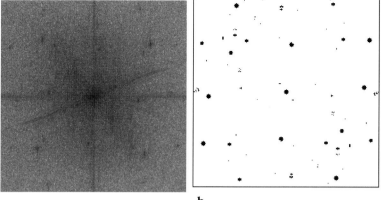

a

b

Figure 41. Automatic location and removal of noise spikes: (a) original power spectrum from *Figure 38; (b)* top hat filter applied to *a; (c)* modified power spectrum after removal of spikes found in *b; (d)* retransformed image.

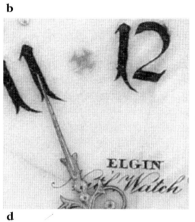

c

d

Figure 42. Identification of noise spikes by selecting image regions that exhibit the noise pattern (a): (b) Fourier transform power spectrum from the selected areas; *(c)* mask created by processing *b; (d)* result of applying the filter from *c* to the Fourier transform of the entire original image.

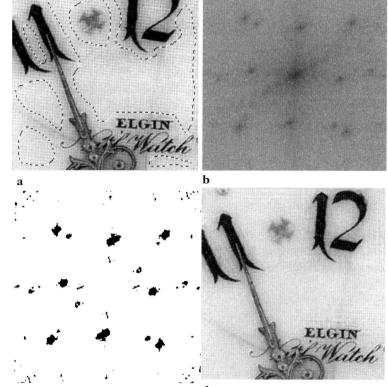

a

b

c

d

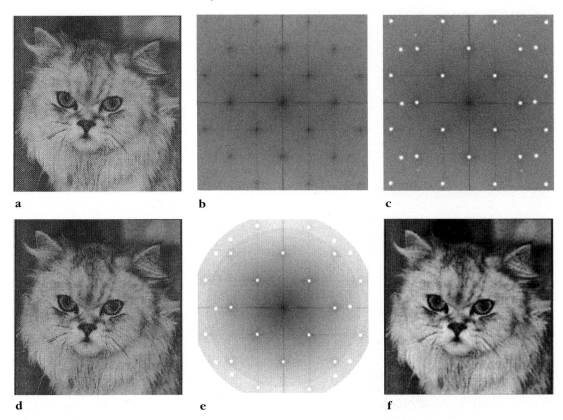

Figure 43. Removal of halftone pattern:
(a) original scanned image;
(b) power spectrum;
(c) mask applied to remove spikes;
(d) inverse transform with spikes removed;
(e) Butterworth low-pass filter applied to power spectrum;
(f) final result.

A common recommendation (found in internet newsgroups, for instance) for dealing with scanned halftone images or ones with moiré patterns from the scanner is to use smoothing to eliminate the pattern (sometimes by scanning the image at an angle and rotating it in software, using the interpolation as a low-pass filter, sometimes by scanning at a larger size and again depending on the filtering effects of interpolation as the image size is reduced, and sometimes by the overt application of a smoothing algorithm). This is a flawed strategy. The use of a smoothing or blur function in this image would have erased these fine lines long before the halftone dots were smoothed out.

When the original image has been scanned in from a color print, the situation is slightly more complicated. As mentioned in Chapter 2 and shown in **Figure 44**, colored halftone prints are typically made using cyan, magenta, yellow, and black inks, with each color having a halftone screen oriented at a different angle. The procedure required is to separate the color channels, process each one, and then recombine them for the final result. In the figure, the power spectra for each of the channels is shown superimposed, in the corresponding color, to show the different screen orientations. A top hat filter was applied to the Fourier transform power spectrum from each channel to select the noise peaks, which were then removed. Recombining the resultant color channel images produces the result shown.

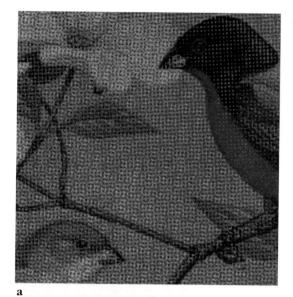

a

Figure 44. Halftone removal in a color image:
(**a**) *original image (a portion of a postage stamp, printed in CMYK);*
(**b**) *Fourier transform power spectra for each color channel, superimposed in color;*
(**c**) *removal of noise from each channel and recombining the color channels.*

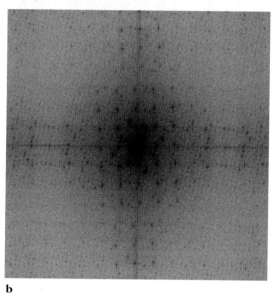

b

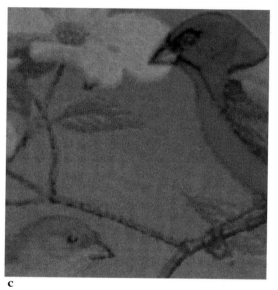

c

Selection of periodic information

In some types of images, it is the periodic information that is useful and the non-periodic noise that must be suppressed. The methods for locating the periodic peaks, constructing filters, smoothing the filter edges, and so forth are unchanged. The only difference is that the filter sense is changed and in the case of a multiplicative mask, the values are inverted.

Figure 45 shows a one-dimensional example. The image is a light micrograph of stained skeletal muscle, in which there is a just-visible band spacing that is difficult to measure because of the spotty staining contrast (even with contrast expansion). The FT image shows the spots that identify the band structure. Reconstruction with only the first harmonic shows the basic band structure, and adding the second and third harmonics defines the band shape fairly well.

Figure 46 shows a high-resolution TEM lattice image from a crystalline ceramic (mullite). The two-dimensional periodicity of the lattice can be seen, but it is superimposed on a variable and

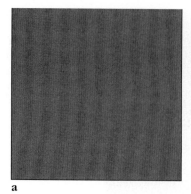

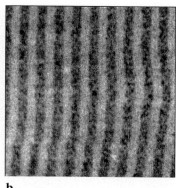

Figure 45. Light micrograph of stained (toluidine blue) 1μm section of skeletal muscle:
(a) original image;
(b) expanded contrast (the band spacing is still difficult to measure due to spotty stain contrast);
(c) the FT power spectrum shows spots that identify the band spacing;
(d) reconstruction with just the first harmonic shows the basic band spacing;
(e) adding the second and third harmonics defines the band shape well.

a

b

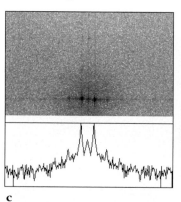

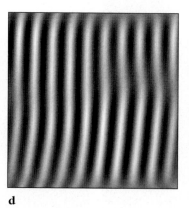

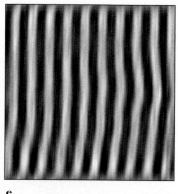

c

d

e

noisy background, which alters the local contrast making it more difficult to observe the details in the rather complex unit cell of this material. The Fourier transform image has peaks that correspond to the periodic structure. As noted before, this image is essentially the same as would be recorded photographically using the TEM to project the diffraction pattern of the specimen to the camera plane. Of course, retransforming the spatial-domain image from the photographed diffraction pattern is not possible because the phase information has been lost. In addition, more control over the Fourier transform display is possible because a log scale or other rule for converting magnitude to screen brightness can be selected.

A filter mask is constructed to select a small circular region around each of the periodic spots. This was done, as before, by using a top hat filter with size just large enough to cover the peaks. In this case the filter is used to keep the amplitude of terms in the peaks but reduce all of the other terms to zero, which removes the random or non-periodic noise, both the short-range (high-frequency) graininess and the gradual (low-frequency) variation in overall brightness. Retransforming this image produces a spatial-domain image which shows the lattice structure clearly.

Figure 47 shows an even more dramatic example. In the original image (a cross section of muscle myofibrils) it is practically impossible to discern the periodic structure due to the presence of noise. In isolated locations, a few of the fibrils can be seen to have a regular spacing and arrangement, but human observers do not easily see through the noise and variability to find this regularity. The Fourier transform image shows the peaks from the underlying regularity,

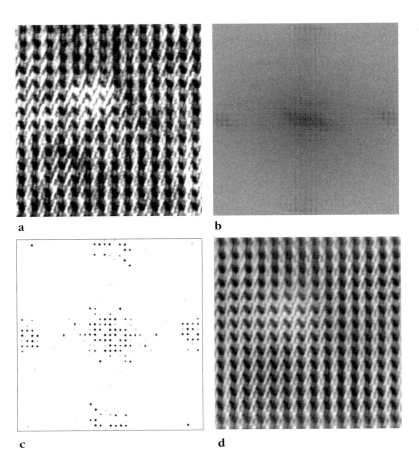

a

b

Figure 46. Transmission electron microscope lattice image of the mullite (ceramic):
(a) original;
(b) Fourier transform power spectrum;
(c) result of applying top hat filter to **b** to construct a filter;
(d) retransformation of just the selected periodic information.

c

d

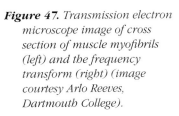

Figure 47. Transmission electron microscope image of cross section of muscle myofibrils (left) and the frequency transform (right) (image courtesy Arlo Reeves, Dartmouth College).

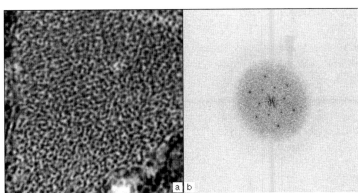

however. Selecting only these peak points in the magnitude image (with their original phase information) and reducing all other magnitude values to zero produces the result shown in **Figure 48**. The retransformed image clearly shows the sixfold symmetry expected for the myofibril structure. The inset shows an enlargement of this structure in even finer detail, with both the thick and thin filaments shown. The thin filaments, especially, cannot be seen clearly in the original image.

A caution is needed in using this type of filtering to extract periodic structures. It is possible to construct a mask that will eliminate real information from the image while keeping artefacts and noise.

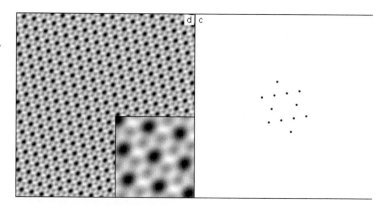

Figure 48. Retransformation of *Figure 46* (left) with only the principal periodic peaks in the frequency transform (right). The points in the filter mask have been enlarged for visibility.

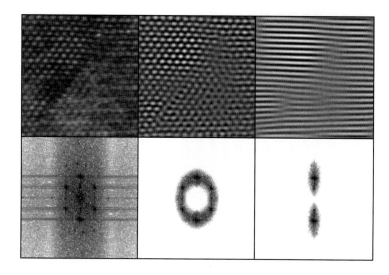

Figure 49. Noisy high-resolution TEM image (left), and the results of applying an annular filter to select atomic spacings (center), and a slit filter to select vertical spacings only (right). Top images show the spatial domain, and bottom row shows frequency domain.

Selecting points in the power spectrum with sixfold symmetry ensured that the filtered and retransformed spatial image would show that type of structure. This means that the critical step is the recognition and selection of the peaks in the Fourier transform image. Fortunately, many suitable tools are available for finding and isolating such points, because they are narrow peaks that rise above a gradually varying local background. The top hat filter illustrated previously is an example of this approach.

It is also possible to construct a filter to select a narrow range of spacings, such as the interatomic spacing in a high-resolution image. This annular filter makes it possible to enhance a selected periodic structure. **Figure 49** shows a high-resolution TEM image of an atomic lattice. Applying an annular filter that blocks both the low and high frequencies produces the result shown, in which the atom positions are more clearly defined. If the filter also selects a particular orientation (a slit or wedge filter), however, then the dislocation that is difficult to discern in the original image becomes clearly evident.

As for the case of removing periodic noise, a filter that selects periodic information and reveals periodic structure can often be designed by examining the Fourier transform power spectrum image itself to locate peaks. The mask or filter can be constructed either manually or automatically. In some cases, there is *a priori* information available (such as lattice spacings of crystalline specimens).

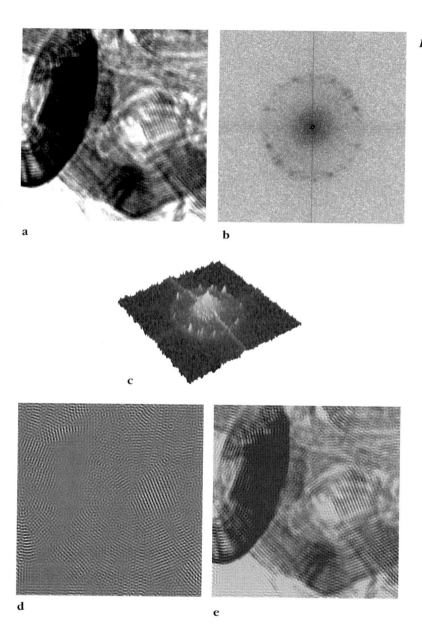

Figure 50. Transmission electron microscope (TEM) image of graphitized carbon (a): (b) the FT power spectrum from image a showing the broken ring of spots corresponding to the 3.5 Angstrom plane spacing in the graphite; (c) the power spectrum plotted as a perspective drawing to emphasize the ring of peaks; (d) inverse transform of just the ring of spots; (e) image d added to the original image a to enhance the visibility of the lattice.

a

b

c

d

e

In **Figure 50**, the structure (of graphitized carbon in particles used for tire manufacture) shows many atomic lattices in different orientations. In this case, the diffraction pattern shows the predominant atom plane spacing of 3.5 Ångstroms, in the form of a ring of spots. Applying an annular filter to select just that spacing, retransforming and adding the atom positions to the original image, enhances the visibility of the lattice structure.

The use of filtering in FT space is also useful for isolating structural information when the original image is not perfectly regular. **Figure 51** shows the same skeletal muscle tissue shown in **Figure 45**, but cross-sectioned and stained with uranyl acetate/lead citrate. The black dots are immuno-gold labeling for fast myosin, involved in muscle contraction. The spots are more or less regularly spaced because of the uniform diameters of the muscle fibers, but have no regular order to their arrangement. Sharpening the image using a top hat filter, as discussed above and in Chapter 4,

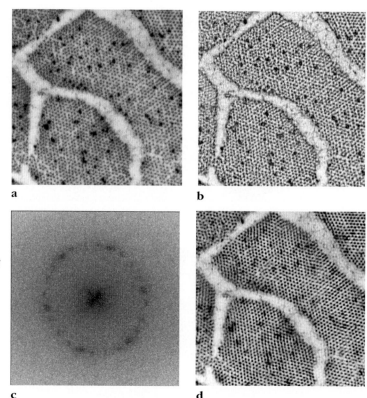

Figure 51. Light micrograph of cross section of the same skeletal muscle as in Figure 62, cross-sectioned and uranyl acetate/lead citrate stained. Black dots are immunogold labeling for fast myosin:
(a) original;
(b) top hat filter applied to the image, as shown in Chapter 4;
(c) the power spectrum from the Fourier transform, showing a broken ring of spots corresponding to the average diameter of the fibers;
(d) retransforming the ring of spots with an annular filter that selects just the spacings of the gold particles and adding this back to the original image increases the contrast of the fibers.

improves the visibility of the spots as compared to the original image. So does the use of an annular Fourier filter that selects just the ring of spots corresponding to the fiber diameter.

Similarly, measurement of "quasi-periodic" structures can also be performed in Fourier space. In **Figure 52**, the packed arrays of latex spheres are not perfectly regular, but the Fourier transform power spectrum shows the rings of nearest neighbors, second-nearest, third-nearest, and so forth. Measuring the spacing is simplified by using a plot of the circularly averaged power spectrum values, as shown.

Convolution and correlation

Fundamentals of convolution

One of the very common operations on images performed in the spatial domain is convolution, in which a kernel of numbers is multiplied by each pixel and its neighbors in a small region, the results summed, and the result placed in the original pixel location. This is applied to all of the pixels in the image. In all cases, the original pixel values are used in the multiplication and addition, and the new derived values are used to produce a new image, although as a practical matter of implementation the operation may be performed a few lines at a time, so that the new image ultimately replaces the old one.

This type of convolution is particularly common for the smoothing and derivative operations illustrated in Chapter 3 and 4. For instance, a simple smoothing kernel might contain the following values:

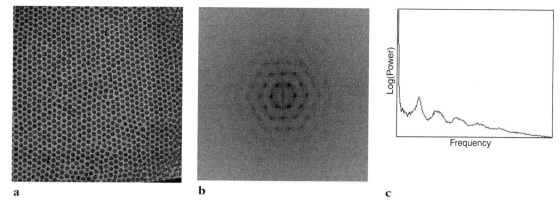

Figure 52. Quasi-periodic arrays of latex spheres:
  (a) original image;
  (b) Fourier transform power spectrum;
  (c) circularly averaged plot of the power spectrum, in which peak locations identify the distances of first, second-, etc., neighbors.

$$
\begin{array}{ccc}
1/16 & 2/16 & 1/16 \\
2/16 & 4/16 & 2/16 \\
1/16 & 2/16 & 1/16
\end{array}
$$

In practice, the fastest implementation would be to multiply the pixel and its 8 immediate neighbors by the integers 1, 2, or 4, sum the products, then divide the total by 16. In this case, using integers that are powers of 2 allows the math to be extremely fast (involving only bit shifting), and the small size of the kernel (3 × 3) makes the application of the smoothing algorithm on the spatial-domain image very fast, as well.

Many spatial-domain kernels are used, including kernels that apply Gaussian smoothing (to reduce noise), take first derivatives (for instance, to locate edges), and take second derivatives (for instance, the Laplacian, which is a non-directional operator that acts as a high-pass filter to sharpen points and lines). They are usually presented as a set of integers, although greater accuracy is attainable with floating point numbers, with it understood that there is a divisor (usually equal to the sum of all the positive values) that normalizes the result. Some of these operators may be significantly larger than the 3 × 3 example shown previously, involving the adding together of the weighted sum of neighbors in a much larger region that is usually, but not necessarily, square.

Applying a large kernel takes time. **Figure 53** illustrates the process graphically for a single placement of the kernel. Even with very fast computers and with careful coding of the process to carry out additions and multiplications in the most efficient order, performing the operation with a 25 × 25 kernel on a 1024 × 1024 image would require a significant amount of time (and even larger kernels and images are often encountered). Though it can be speeded up somewhat by the use of special hardware, such as a pipelined array processor, a special-purpose investment is required. A similar hardware investment can be used to speed up the Fourier transform. Our interest here is in the algorithms, instead of their implementation.

For any computer-based system, increasing the kernel size eventually reaches a point at which it is more efficient to perform the operation in the Fourier domain. The time needed to perform the FFT transformation from the spatial domain to the frequency domain and back is more than balanced by the speed with which the convolution can be carried out. If any other reasons are needed to perform

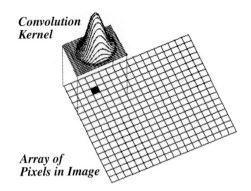

Figure 53. *Illustration of applying a convolution kernel to an image in the spatial domain (illustration courtesy Arlo Reeves, Dartmouth College).*

Convolution Kernel

Array of Pixels in Image

the transformation to the frequency-domain representation of the image, then even small kernels can be most efficiently applied there.

This is because the equivalent operation to spatial-domain convolution is a single multiplication of each pixel in the magnitude image by the corresponding pixel in a transform of the kernel. The transform of the kernel can be obtained and stored beforehand just as the kernel is stored. If the kernel is smaller than the image, it is padded with zeroes to the full image size. Convolution in the spatial domain is exactly equivalent to multiplication in the frequency domain. Using the notation presented before, in which the image is a function $f(x,y)$ and the kernel is $g(x,y)$, we describe the convolution operation in which the kernel is positioned everywhere on the image and multiplied by it as

$$g(x,y) * f(x,y) = \iint (f(\alpha,\beta) \cdot g(x-\alpha, y-\beta) d\alpha\, d\beta \qquad (9)$$

where α and β are dummy variables for the integration, the range of which is across the entire image, and the symbol * indicates convolution. If the Fourier transforms of $f(x,y)$ and $g(x,y)$ are $F(u,v)$ and $G(u,v)$, respectively, then the convolution operation in the Fourier domain is simple point-by-point multiplication, or

$$g(x,y) * f(x,y) \Leftrightarrow G(u,v)F(u,v) \qquad (10)$$

A few practical differences exist between the two operations. The usual application of a kernel in the spatial domain avoids the edge pixels (those nearer to the edge than the half-width of the kernel), since their neighbors do not exist. As a practical alternative, a different kernel that is one-sided and has different weights can be applied near edges, or the edge can be considered to be a mirror. In transforming the image to the frequency domain, however, the assumption is made that the image wraps around at edges, so that the left edge is contiguous with the right and the top edge is contiguous with the bottom. Applying a convolution by multiplying in the frequency domain is equivalent to addressing pixels in this same wraparound manner when applying the kernel to the spatial image. It will usually produce some artefacts at the edges. The most common solution for this problem is to embed the image of interest in a larger one in which the borders are either filled with the mean brightness value of the image, or smoothly interpolated from the edge values.

Figure 54 shows the equivalence of convolution in the spatial domain and multiplication in the frequency domain, for the case of a smoothing kernel. The kernel, a Gaussian filter with standard deviation of 2.0 pixels, is shown as an array of grey-scale values, along with its transform. Applying the kernel to the image in the spatial domain produces the result shown in the example.

Figure 54. Smoothing by applying a large kernel in the spatial domain and convolution in the frequency domain:
  (a) *original image;*
  (b) *smoothing kernel (Gaussian, standard deviation = 2.0 pixels), with enlargement to show pixel detail;*
  (c) *smoothed image produced by spatial convolution with kernel or inverse Fourier transform of* ***e****;*
  (d) *Fourier transform of* ***a****;*
  (e) *Fourier transform of* ***b****;*
  (f) *product of* ***d*** *and* ***e****.*

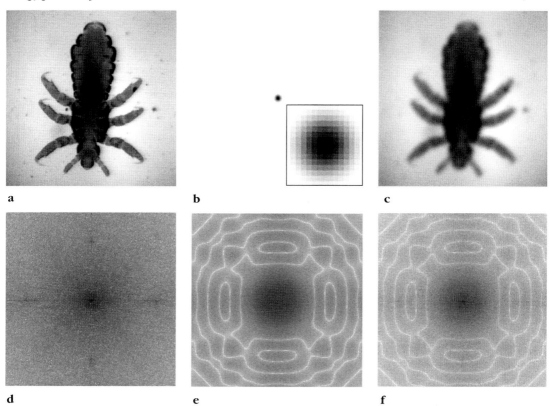

a   b   c

d   e   f

Multiplying the kernel transform by the image transform produces the frequency-domain image with the power spectrum shown. Retransforming this image produces the identical result to the spatial-domain operation.

Notice that the equivalence of frequency-domain multiplication to spatial-domain convolution is restricted to multiplicative filters, which are also known as "linear" filters. Other neighborhood operations, such as rank filtering (saving the brightest, darkest, or median brightness value in a neighborhood) and histogram modification (e.g., local adaptive equalization), are nonlinear and have no frequency-domain equivalent.

Imaging system characteristics

Convolution can also be used as a tool to understand how imaging systems alter or degrade images. For example, the blurring introduced by imperfect lenses can be described by a function $H(u,v)$ which is multiplied by the frequency transform of the image (**Figure 55**). The operation of physical optics is readily modeled in the frequency domain. Sometimes it is possible to determine the separate characteristics of each component of the system; often it is not. In some cases,

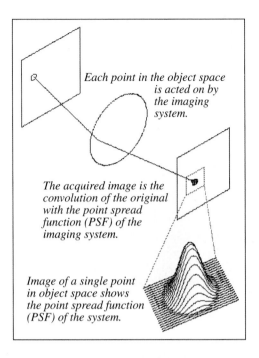

Figure 55. *System characteristics introduce a point spread function into the acquired image (illustration courtesy Arlo Reeves, Dartmouth College).*

Each point in the object space is acted on by the imaging system.

The acquired image is the convolution of the original with the point spread function (PSF) of the imaging system.

Image of a single point in object space shows the point spread function (PSF) of the system.

determining the point-spread function of the system (the degree to which a perfect point in the object plane is blurred in the image plane) may make it possible to sharpen the image by removing some of the blur. This is done by dividing the transform of the point-spread image by $H(u,v)$.

To illustrate this sharpening we can use the one of the best-known examples of correction of an out-of-focus condition due to an imperfect imaging system. As originally deployed, the Hubble telescope had an incorrectly figured main mirror that produced poorly focused images. Eventually a compensating optical device was installed in the imaging system to correct most of the defect, but even with the original telescope it was possible to obtain high resolution results by using deconvolution with the known point spread function (PSF). The corrected optical package, however, restored much of the telescope's light-gathering power, which was severely reduced due to the incorrect mirror curvature.

In this particular instance, it was possible to calculate the PSF from available measurement data on the mirror, but in many astronomical situations, the problem is simplified because the point spread function can be measured by examining the image of a single star, which is effectively a point as seen from earth. This requires a considerable grey-scale depth to the image, but in astronomy, cooled cameras often deliver 12 or 14 bits of information, which is also important for obtaining enough precision to perform the deconvolution.

Figure 56 shows the result of this method. The original, blurred image is sharpened by dividing its Fourier transform by that of the measured PSF, and the resulting inverse transform shows a considerably sharpened image.

For deconvolution, we divide the complex frequency-domain image from the out-of-focus test pattern by the image for the point spread function. This is complex division, performed by dividing the magnitude values and subtracting the phase values. One of the problems with division is that division by very small values can cause numeric overflow problems, and the Fourier transform of a symmetrical and well behaved point spread function often contains zero values. The usual

Figure 56. Hubble telescope image sharpening:
- ***(a)*** *original;*
- ***(b)*** *measured point spread function, with enlargement to show pixel detail;*
- ***(c)*** *deconvolution result obtained as inverse transform of* ***f***;
- ***(d)*** *Fourier transform of* ***a***;
- ***(e)*** *Fourier transform of* ***b***;
- ***(f)*** ***d*** *divided by* ***e***.

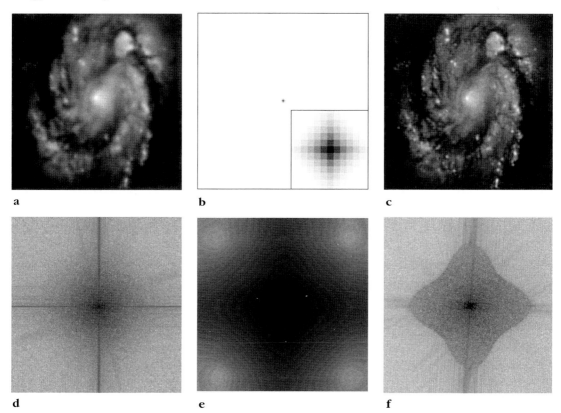

a   b   c

d   e   f

solution to this problem is apodization to restrict the division operation to those pixels in the complex transform images that will not cause overflow.

Deconvolution of image blur, which may arise from out-of-focus optics, motion, the size and arrangement of transistors in the camera chip, insufficient bandwidth in the electronics, or other causes, is an imperfect science. A mathematically optimum procedure neither exists, nor is there a proof that one exists in all cases. The practical techniques that are used have been developed under a variety of assumptions and apply to many real situations, producing impressive improvements in image quality. The results, although good, represent trade-offs between different limitations, one of which is the time required for the computations.

Deconvolution is discussed here in terms of grey scale images. In most cases, color images need to be separated into discrete color channels that correspond to the physics of the acquisition device, usually red, green and blue, and each one deconvolved separately. It is usual to find that the point spread function is different for each channel, especially if a single-chip camera with a Bayer pattern color filter has been used for acquisition (see Chapter 2).

It is important to always start with the best image possible. This means obtaining the best focus, least motion blur, etc., that you can achieve. Deconvolution is never as good a solution as correcting the source of the problem beforehand. Next, capture the image with the best possible range of contrast, from nearly full white to nearly full black without clipping. The tonal or gray scale range should have good precision and a wide dynamic range. Eight-bit images from uncooled digital cameras are marginal, and poorer images from video cameras usually unacceptable unless special procedures such as averaging multiple frames are used. It is particularly important to have high precision and bit depth for the point spread function, whether it is obtained by measurement or by calculation.

Finally, random pixel noise (speckle) must be minimized. Noise in either the acquired image or (especially) in the point spread function is significantly amplified in the deconvolution process and will dominate the result if it is too great. Long exposures and image averaging may be useful in some cases. The usual description of the magnitude of image noise is a signal-to-noise ratio expressed in decibels. This is defined in terms of the standard deviation of values in the blurred image and in the noise (which of course may not be known).

$$SNR[\text{dB}] = 10 \cdot \log_{10}\left(\frac{\sigma_{image}}{\sigma_{noise}}\right) \qquad (11)$$

When the signal-to-noise ratio is in the range of 40–50 dB, the noise is, practically speaking, invisible in the image and has a minimal effect on deconvolution. On the other hand, a low signal-to-noise ratio of 10–20 dB makes the noise so prominent that deconvolution becomes quite impractical.

The ideal and simplest form of deconvolution is to measure (or in a few cases calculate from known optical parameters) the point spread function of the system. Computing the Fourier transform of the blurred image and that of the PSF, dividing the second into the first, and performing an inverse transform, produces the deconvolved result as shown previously. The key requirement is that the blur due to the imaging system is assumed to be the same everywhere in the image, which is a good assumption for telescope images (**Figure 56**). When some portion of the blur is due to the passage of light through the sample itself, as occurs in thick sections examined in the light microscope, the blur can vary from point to point and this method becomes less useful.

An indirect measurement of the PSF can be accomplished by capturing an image of a precisely known object using the same optical setup as that used for the real image. Dividing the Fourier transform of the image of the object by that of the ideal shape, and inverse transforming the result, produces the system PSF, which can then be used to deconvolve images obtained with the optical system.

In some microscope situations, the insertion of fluorescing microbeads, or even an image of a small dust particle on the slide, may be useful as an estimate of the PSF. In the atomic force microscope, a direct measurement of the PSF may be accomplished by scanning an image of a known shape, usually a circular test pattern produced expressly for this purpose by the same methods used to etch integrated circuits. As shown in **Figure 57**, if the resulting image is deconvolved by dividing its Fourier transform by that for the ideal shape, the result is an image of the point spread function, which in this case corresponds to the shape of the scanning tip. This shape can then be used to deconvolve other images, at least until the tip is further damaged or replaced.

If an image contains many edges oriented in different directions, and the actual edge shape is known (ideally a perfectly sharp knife-edge transition in grey level), then the PSF can be determined at least in principle by measuring the actual transition across each edge, and combining the various profiles to form a PSF image. In practice this usually requires assuming that the function is symmetrical and of known shape (usually a Gaussian as a convenient approximation to the central portion of the Airy disk produced by real optics), so that measurements on a few edges can be generalized to an entire two-dimensional PSF image.

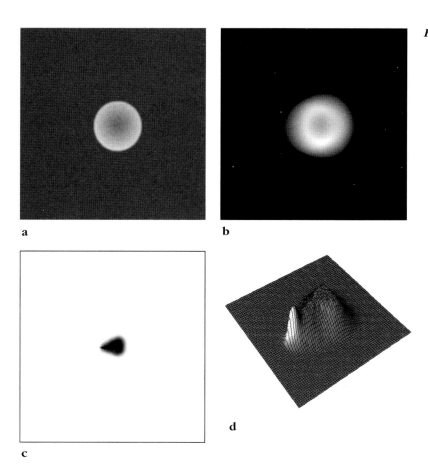

a

b

Figure 57. Measuring the PSF of an atomic force microscope: (a) ideal image of a circular test pattern; (b) measured image using an imperfect tip; (c) deconvolution of b by a, producing an image of the tip; (d) perspective view of the shape in c.

c

d

If it is not possible to obtain a PSF by measurement, it may be possible to calculate a useful approximate one based on assumptions such as a Gaussian blur function or straight line motion. Real optical defocusing does not produce an ideal Gaussian blur, but it is not necessary in many cases to have the exact PSF, just a sufficiently useful approximation to remove most of the blur by deconvolution. Sometimes important insight into the nature of the PSF can be obtained by examining the Fourier transform of the blurred image. The presence of zeroes (or near-zero values) in lines, arcs, etc., is a powerful clue to the nature of the blur. Straight lines indicate motion blur, in a direction orthogonal to the lines. Arcs indicate non-Gaussian blurring (e.g., by a uniform disk). These can be used to estimate a PSF which can be used to perform a deconvolution, perhaps iterating the estimated PSF either automatically using one of the convergence methods discussed below, or by interactive selection, to reach a satisfactory result.

The blur produced by purely optical effects is frequently uniform in all directions, although astigmatism can modify this; however, the tip shape in scanned probe microscopes can produce arbitrarily shaped point spread functions. In many cameras the shape and spacing of the transistors produces different blur magnitudes in the horizontal and vertical directions, and the effects of the color filter pattern used can also alter the shape of the PSF. In any scanned image acquisition, the electronic parameters of the amplifiers used can produce different amounts of blur in the fast scan direction (generally horizontal) as compared to the slow scan direction (vertical). Time constants in phosphors, amplifiers or other components can also produce asymmetrical blurs ("comet tails") in the output signal.

Noise and Wiener deconvolution

If there is significant noise content in the image to be sharpened or, worse yet, in the measured PSF, it can exacerbate the numerical precision and overflow problems and greatly degrades the resulting inverse transform. Removal of more than a portion of the blurring in a real image is almost never possible, but of course, some situations exist in which even a small improvement may be of considerable practical importance.

Division by the frequency transform of the blur is referred to as an inverse filter. Using the notation introduced previously, it can be written as

$$F(u,v) \approx \left[\frac{1}{H(u,v)}\right] G(u,v)$$

(12)

If the presence of noise in the blurred image prevents satisfactory deconvolution by simply dividing the Fourier transforms, then it may be practical to perform a Wiener deconvolution. Instead of calculating the deblurred image by dividing the Fourier transform of the original image by that of the blur function, a scalar value is used to increase the denominator. Theoretically, the additive factor K is dependent on the statistical properties of the images and their relative noise contents, but in practice these are not usually known and so the additive constant is typically treated as an adjustable parameter that controls the tradeoff between sharpening and noise.

$$F(u,v) \approx \left[\frac{1}{H(u,v)}\right] \cdot \left[\frac{|H(u,v)|^2}{|H(u,v)|^2 + K}\right] \cdot G(u,v)$$

(13)

Figure 58 shows an example of the effect of additive random noise on a image with out-of-focus blur. In the absence of any noise, a direct deconvolution using a Gaussian model for the PSF produces useful results. The addition of random Gaussian noise (SNR = 15 dB) to the image results in a deconvolution using the same PSF that is dominated by noise and ringing that obscures the features. Wiener filtering (**Figure 59**) reduces this problem and allows adjustment which trades off the sharpness of the restoration (higher K values leave more blurring) against the amount of noise (higher K values reduce the noise). Because of the low signal-to-noise ratio, it is not possible in this case to recover all the internal details of the original image.

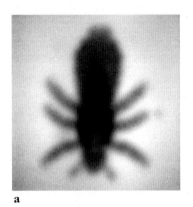 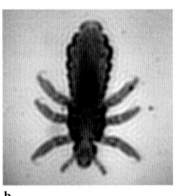 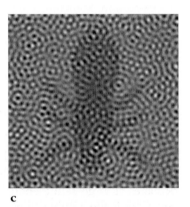

a   b   c

Figure 58. Effect of noise on deconvolution: (a) severely blurred image of the bug in Figure 54 with added random noise; (b) deconvolution that can be achieved in the absence of noise; (c) deconvolution with noise present.

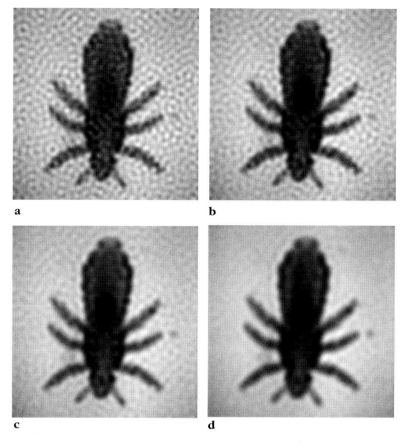

Figure 59. Wiener filtering of the image in Figure 58a: (a–d) *increasing the empirical K value reduces noise at the expense of sharpness.*

a   b

c   d

The Wiener deconvolution has a long history as a practical method for achieving useful, if not perfect blur removal. Another approach of long standing is the Van Cittert iterative technique. This method has apparently been discovered many times and is also known as a Bially or Landweber iteration. Instead of trying to remove the entire blur in one step, a series of iterative removal steps are performed. In the limit, this iteration would reach the same result as an ideal deconvolution, but instead it is terminated before convergence, resulting in a (partially) deblurred image that does not exhibit an unacceptable noise level. The quality of the results is generally similar to that of the Wiener method.

Many other methods are used, and most of them are much more complicated mathematically (and require much more computation and time). Many of them are iterative, trying to find the best form of the blur function and the deblurred image. Typically this involves trying to solve a very large number of simultaneous equations, which may be over- or under-determined. The techniques for such solutions occupy a significant mathematical literature, and are discussed further in Chapter 11. One of the issues is how to efficiently guide the iteration and how to determine when to terminate it. Another related question is the best measure of image quality, which in different implementations may be based on Bayesian statistics, maximization of entropy, etc. The calculations may be performed in either the frequency or the spatial domain. Even a small PSF in the spatial domain becomes as large as the entire image in the frequency domain, and the number of simultaneous equations is the number of pixels in the image.

Most of these methods are highly specific to particular types of applications, and depend on the *a priori* information that can be supplied, usually in the form of constraints on the solution of the equations. For example, a commonly used constraint is that negative values for pixels have no physical meaning and so values are not permitted to become negative. If more information on the image, such as the presence of substantial background (as in astronomical or fluorescence images), or known specific pixel values that are permitted, can be incorporated it improves the quality of the result and the efficiency of reaching it. The details of these methods are far beyond the scope of this text, but a very clear and comprehensive revue and comparison can be found in Lagendijk and Biemond (1991).

Another area of current interest is the deconvolution of multiple images that are related to each other. This includes multiple channel images (e.g., different wavelengths or colors) of the same scene, or a series of images from parallel closely spaced planes in semi-transparent specimens (e.g., a series of focal planes in the light microscope). Information from one channel or plane can be used to guide the deconvolution of another.

If the blur is not known *a priori*, it can often be estimated from the power spectrum or by trial and error to find an optimum (or at least useful) result. A recent development in deconvolution that has great efficiency because it is not an iterative method has been published by Carasso (2001). Analysis of the shape of radial profile of the values in the Fourier transform of the blurred image (avoiding the regions dominated by noise) allows constructing an approximate PSF that can be used for deconvolution. This method cannot be used for all types of blur functions (particularly motion blur) but produces very good results for those situations where it is applicable.

An important area for these image restoration techniques is deblurring the images formed by optical sectioning. This is the technique in which a series of images are recorded from different depths of focus in a semitransparent specimen using a light microscope. The passage of light through the overlying layers of the specimen cause a blurring that adversely affects the sharpness and contrast of the images, preventing their being assembled into a three-dimensional stack for visualization and measurement of the three-dimensional structures present.

The confocal light microscope overcomes some of these problems by rejecting light from points away from the point of focus, which improves the contrast of the images (it also reduces the depth of field of the optics, producing higher resolution in the depth axis, but this is important only at the highest magnifications); but the scattering and diffraction of light by the upper layers of the specimen still degrade the image resolution.

In principle, the images of the upper layers contain information that can be used to deconvolute those from below. This would allow sharpening of those images. The entire process is iterative and highly computer-intensive, more so because the blurring of each point on each images may be different from other points. In practice, it is usual to make some assumptions about the blurring and noise content of the images which are used as global averages for a given specimen or for a given optical setup.

Even with these assumptions, the computations are still intensive and iterative. A considerable theoretical and limited practical literature has been published in this field (Carrington, 1990; Holmes et al., 1991; Monck et al., 1992; Joshi and Miller, 1993; Richardson, 1972; Snyder et al., 1992) A review of several of the leading methods can be found in (Van Kempen et al., 1997). The examples shown deal only with idealized structures and averaging assumptions about the noise characteristics of the images and the point spread function of the microscope, which suggests that restoration of real images will not be as good as the examples shown. Similar concerns and methods can in principle be applied to other *in situ*, three-dimensional imaging techniques such as tomography and seismic imagery.

Motion blur

Additional defects besides out-of-focus optics can be corrected by deconvolution as well. These operations are not always performed in the frequency domain, but the basic understanding of the process of removing the blur convolution imposed by the system is most clearly illustrated there. One of the most common defects is blur caused by motion. This is rarely a problem in microscopy applications, but can be very important in remote sensing, in which light levels are low and the exposure time must be long enough for significant camera motion to occur with respect to the scene. Fortunately, in most of these circumstances the amount and direction of motion is known. That makes it possible to draw a line in the spatial domain that defines the blur. The frequency transform of this line is then divided into the transform of the blurred image. Retransforming the resulting image restores the sharp result. **Figure 60** illustrates the method.

It is important to note the similarity and the difference between this example and the removal of out-of-focus blur. Both involve dividing the transform of the blurred image by that of the defect. This follows directly from the equation presented for convolution, in which the transform of the convolved image is the product of those from the original image and the defect. The major difference is that in the motion blur case we can sometimes calculate the exact blurring vector to be removed, while in the out-of-focus blur case we must estimate the blur from an actual image. This estimation introduces unavoidable noise in the image, which is greatly magnified by the division.

As in the example shown previously for out-of-focus blur, the use of a Wiener deconvolution can partially alleviate the effects of noise. In the example of **Figure 61**, the motion blur can be estimated from the orientation and spacing of the lines of zero (or near zero) values in the power spectrum of the Fourier transform of the blurred image. Using this to determine the motion vector as the point spread function allows performing a deconvolution. Increasing the Wiener K factor controls the tradeoff between image sharpness and noise as shown in **Figure 62**. This factor is usually treated as an empirical adjustment. Human observers generally prefer an image that is noisier but less blurred than a theoretical K value based on the noise content delivers.

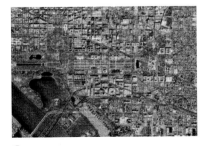

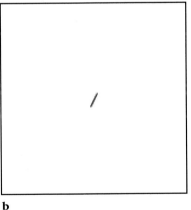

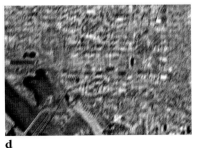

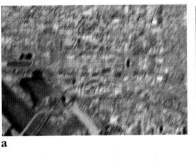

Figure 60. Removal of motion blur:
(a) original image (the Mall and tidal basin in Washington, D.C.);
(b) motion vector based on airplane speed, direction, and exposure time;
(c) deconvolution result;
(d) deconvolution result using 8-bit images and single-precision arithmetic.

Figure 61. Motion blur:
(a) unblurred image;
(b) uniform motion blur;
(c) power spectrum of the Fourier transform of b;
(d) motion vector shown as a point spread function (enlarged to show pixels).

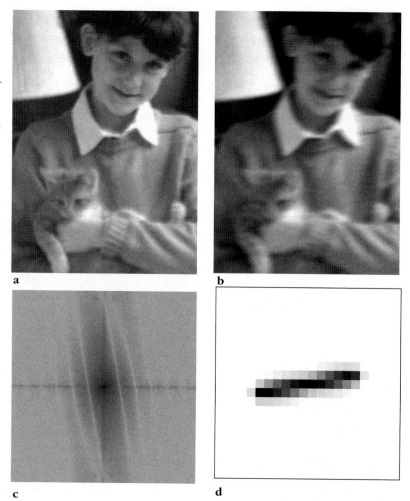

a

b

c

d

Increasing the value of the constant K in the denominator of equation 13 reduces the magnitude of all terms in the complex Fourier transform that is inverted to obtain the restored image, but it reduces terms that were originally small more than it does large ones. These terms are the ones most likely to be dominated by random noise. One effect of this reduction is the elimination of more of the small terms by apodization. **Figure 63** shows the terms eliminated in the Wiener filtered restoration of the image (compare it to the FT power spectrum of the original image in **Figure 61c**).

Additional limitations arise from the finite internal precision in computer implementation of the Fourier transform and the storage of the complex frequency-transform image. Programs may use either floating-point or fixed-point notation, the latter requiring less storage space and offering somewhat greater speed; double precision internal values give the best results because the minimum magnitude values that can be accurately recorded generally occur at higher frequencies, controlling the appearance of sharp edges in the spatial-domain image. Too small a precision in either the image or the calculation limits the ability to sharpen images by removing degrading blur due to the imaging system. To illustrate the problems introduced by images with insufficient precision, in **Figure 60d**, the original image was reduced from a bit depth of 12 (more than 4000 grey scale values obtained by scanning a 35-mm film negative) to 6 bits (the performance of a typical video camera). Note the vastly inferior (even useless) quality of the results.

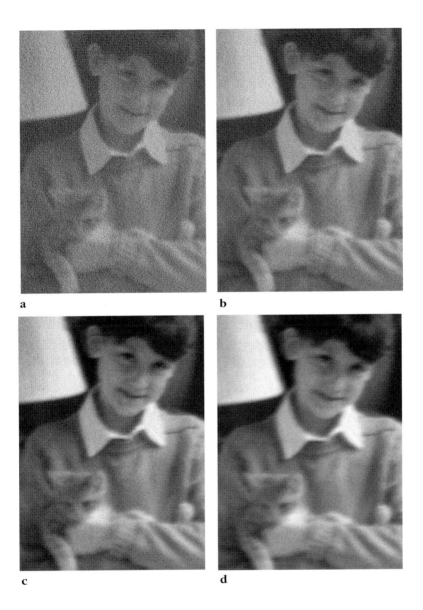

a

b

c

d

Figure 62.
Deconvolution of the image in Figure 61b: *(a)* Wiener constant K set to zero; *(b–d)* increasing K values covering the range from too noisy to too blurred.

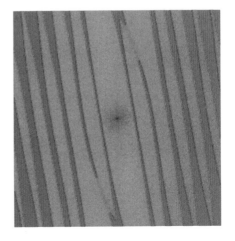

Figure 63. Power spectrum of the image in *Figure 62* showing in red the values eliminated from the restored image by apodization (compare with *Figure 61c*).

Template matching and correlation

Closely related to the spatial-domain application of a kernel for smoothing, derivatives, etc. is the idea of template matching or cross-correlation. In this case, a target pattern is shifted to every location in the image, the values are multiplied by the pixels that are overlaid, and the total is stored at that position to form an image showing where regions identical or similar to the target are located. **Figure 64** illustrates this process. The multiplication and summation process is identical to convolution, except that the target is rotated 180° first, so that the upper left corner value in the target pattern is multiplied by the lower right value in the neighborhood on the image and so forth. When the process is performed in frequency space, this amounts to a phase shift of the Fourier transform values.

This method is used in many contexts to locate features within images. One is searching reconnaissance images for particular objects such as vehicles. Tracking the motion of hurricanes in a series of weather satellite images or cells moving on a microscope slide can also use this approach. Modified to deal optimally with binary images, it can be used to find letters in text. When the target is a pattern of pixel brightness values from one image in a stereo pair and the searched image is the second image from the pair, the method can be used to perform fusion (locating matching points in the two images) to measure parallax and calculate range, as shown in Chapter 13.

For continuous two-dimensional functions, the cross-correlation image is calculated as

$$c(i, j) = \iint f(x, y) g(x - i, y - j) dx\, dy \tag{14}$$

Replacing the integrals by finite sums over the dimensions of the image gives **Equation 15**. In order to normalize the result of this template matching or correlation without the absolute brightness value of the region of the image biasing the results, the operation in the spatial domain is usually calculated as the sum of the products of the pixel brightnesses divided by their geometric mean.

$$\frac{\displaystyle\sum_{i,j} f_{x+i,y+j} \cdot g_{i,j}}{\sqrt{\displaystyle\sum_{i,j} f^2_{x+i,y+j} \cdot \sum_{i,j} g^2_{i,j}}} \tag{15}$$

When the dimensions of the summation are large, this is a slow and inefficient process compared to the equivalent operation in frequency space. The frequency-space operation is simply

Figure 64. *Cross-correlation matches a pattern of grey scale values to many points in the target image to find the location with the best match. In the tiny example shown here, the 3 × 3 target is applied to every possible position in the image to produce the line of values shown. The marked location is most similar (but not identical) to the target.*

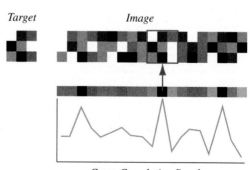

Target *Image*

Cross-Correlation Result

$$C(u,v) = F(u,v)G*(u,v) \qquad (16)$$

where * indicates the complex conjugate of the function values. The complex conjugate of the pixel values affects only the phase of the complex values. The operation is thus seen to be very similar to convolution, and indeed it is often performed using many of the same program subroutines. Operations that involve two images (division for deconvolution, multiplication for convolution, and multiplication by the conjugate for correlation) are sometimes called dyadic operations, to distinguish them from filtering and masking operations (monadic operations) in which a single frequency transform image is operated on (the filter or mask image is not a frequency-domain image nor does it contain complex values).

Usually, when correlation is performed, the wraparound assumption joining the left and right edges and the top and bottom of the image is not acceptable. In these cases, the image should be padded by surrounding it with zeroes to bring it to the next larger size for transformation (the next exact power of two, required by many FFT routines). Because the correlation operation also requires that the actual magnitude values of the transforms be used, slightly better mathematical precision can be achieved by padding with the average values of the original image brightnesses rather than with zeroes. It may also be useful to subtract the average brightness value from each pixel, which removes the zeroth (DC) term from the transformation. This value is usually the largest in the transform (it is the value at the central pixel), so its elimination allows the transform data more dynamic range.

Figure 65. Cross-correlation example:
(a) *image containing many letters with superimposed random noise;*
(b) *target letter;*
(c) *cross-correlation result (grey-scale representation of goodness of match);*
(d) *isometric view of* **c** *showing peaks on the A's in the original;*
(e) *thresholded peaks in* **c** *superimposed on* **a** *— note that only the letters in the same size and font have been located.*

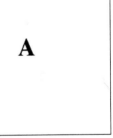

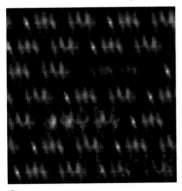

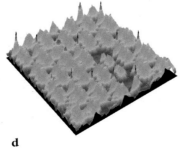

Correlation is primarily used for locating features in one image that appear in another. **Figure 65** shows an example. The image contains text, while the target contains the letter "A" by itself. The result of the cross-correlation after retransforming the image to the spatial domain shows peaks where the target letter is found, which may be more apparent when the same image presented as an isometric display. The brightest points in the correlation image correspond to the occurrences of the letter "A" in the same size and font as the target. Lower but still significant peaks exist, corresponding to two of the other letter As, in different fonts. In general, however, cross-correlation is quite size- and shape-specific as discussed in Chapter 10.

When combined with other image processing tools to analyze the cross-correlation image, this is an extremely fast and efficient tool for locating known features in images. In the example of **Figure 66**, a very large number of SEM images of Nuclepore filters with latex spheres presented a problem for automatic counting because of the variation in contrast and noise, the presence of dirt, and the texture presented by the filters. Also, the contrast of an isolated sphere is consistently different than that of one surrounded by other spheres.

A target image (**Figure 66a**) was created by averaging together ten representative latex spheres. This was then cross-correlated with each image, a top-hat filter (inner radius = 3 pixels; outer radius = 5 pixels; height = 8 grey scale values) applied to isolate each peak in the image, and the resulting spots counted automatically. The figure shows a few example images from the set, with marks showing the particles that were found and counted. After the top hat has been applied to select the peaks in the cross-correlation image, the resulting spots can be convolved with the stored target image to produce the result shown in **Figure 67**, which is just the latex spheres without the other features present in the original image.

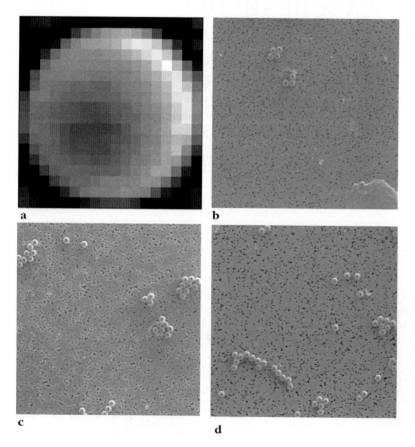

a

b

c

d

Figure 66. Cross-correlation to detect and count latex spheres on Nuclepore filters: (a) average of ten representative latex spheres, used as a target; *(b–d)* representative example images, with red spots marking the result of the procedure described in the text.

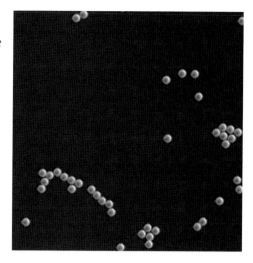

Figure 67. Convolution of the target image from Figure 66a with the binary image of peaks found by the top hat filter applied to the cross-correlation image (the red marks superimposed on Figure 66d), showing just the latex spheres.

Cross-correlation is also used as a tool for aligning serial section images. Even if the images are not identical (as in general they are not), enough common features exist so that a sharp cross-correlation peak occurs when two successive images are in best x,y alignment. The location of the peak can be determined to sub-pixel accuracy and used to shift the images into optimum alignment. The method does not deal with rotation, but it is possible to iteratively rotate the images and use the peak cross-correlation value as a measure of quality to determine the best value. Serial section alignment is discussed further in Chapter 12.

Autocorrelation

In the special case when the image functions f and g (and their transforms F and G) are the same, the correlation operation is called autocorrelation. This is used to combine together all parts of the image, in order to find repetitive structures. In Chapter 13, this method is used to measure the texture of surface roughness in terms of the characteristic distance over which amplitude of the peak drops. **Figure 68** shows another use of the autocorrelation function, to measure preferred orientation. The image is a felted textile material. Due to the fabrication process the fibers have neither a randomized nor uniform orientation; neither are they regularly arranged. The frequency transform shown indicates a slightly asymmetric shape. Performing the cross-correlation and re-transforming to the spatial domain gives the image shown in **Figure 69**. The brightness profiles of the central spot along its major and minor axes show the preferred orientation quantitatively. This is the same result achieved by cross-correlation in the spatial domain (rotating the image by 180° and sliding the image across itself while recording the area of feature overlap as a function of relative offset) to determine preferred orientation.

Figure 68. Image of felted textile fibers (left) and the frequency transform (right).

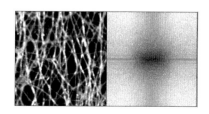

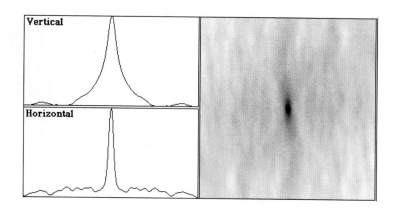

Figure 69. *Autocorrelation image from **Figure 68** (right), and its horizontal and vertical brightness profiles (left) along the major and minor axes of the peak.*

Conclusion

Processing images in the frequency domain is useful for removing certain types of noise and image blur, applying large convolution kernels, enhancing periodic structures, and locating defined structures in images. It can also be used to measure images to determine periodicity or preferred orientation. All these operations can be carried out in the spatial domain, but are often much more efficient in the frequency domain. The FFT operations can be efficiently computed in small (desktop) systems. This makes frequency-domain operations useful and important tools for image analysis.

6

Segmentation and Thresholding

One of the most critical steps in the process of reducing images to information is segmentation: dividing the image into regions that presumably correspond to structural units in the scene or distinguish objects of interest. Segmentation is often described by analogy to visual processes as a foreground/background separation, implying that the selection procedure concentrates on a single kind of feature and discards the rest.

This is not quite true for computer systems, which can generally deal much better than humans with scenes containing more than one type of feature of interest. **Figure 1** shows a common optical illusion that can be seen as a vase or as two facing profiles, depending on whether we concentrate on the white or black areas as the foreground. It appears that humans are unable to see both interpretations at once, although we can flip rapidly back and forth between them once the two have been recognized. This is true in many other illusions as well. **Figure 2** shows two others. The cube can be seen in either of two orientations, with the dark corner close to or far from the viewer; the sketch can be seen as either an old woman or a young girl. In both cases, we can switch between versions very quickly, but we cannot perceive them both at the same time.

These illusions work because human vision interprets the image in terms of the relationships between structures, which have already been unconsciously constructed at lower levels in the visual pathway. In computer-based image analysis systems, we must start at those low levels and work upwards. The initial decisions must be made at the level of individual pixels.

Thresholding

Selecting features within a scene or image is an important prerequisite for most kinds of measurement or understanding of the scene. Traditionally, one simple way this selection has been accomplished is to define a range of brightness values in the original image, select the pixels within this range as belonging to the foreground, and reject all of the other pixels to the background. Such an image is then usually displayed as a binary or two-level image, using black and white or other colors to distinguish the regions. (There is no standard convention on whether the features of interest are white or black; the choice depends on the particular display hardware in use and the designer's preference. In the examples shown here, the features are black and the background is white.)

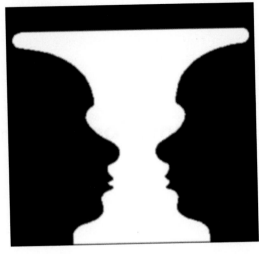

Figure 1. *The "Vase" illusion. Viewers may see either a vase or two human profiles in this image, and can alternate between them, but cannot see both interpretations at the same time.*

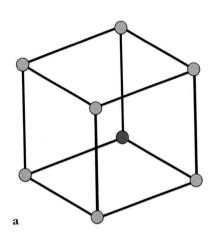

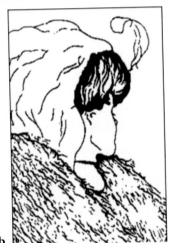

a

b

Figure 2. Examples of either/or interpretation:
  (a) *the Necker cube, in which the dark corner may appear close to or far from the viewer;*
  (b) *the "old woman/young girl" sketch.*

This operation is called thresholding. Thresholds may be set interactively by a user watching the image and using a colored overlay to show the result of turning a knob or otherwise adjusting the settings. As a consequence of the ubiquitous use of a mouse as the human interface to a graphical computer display, the user may adjust virtual sliders or mark a region on a histogram to select the range of brightness values. The brightness histogram of the image (or a region of it) is often useful for making adjustments. As discussed in earlier chapters, this is a plot of the number of pixels in the image having each brightness level. For a typical 8-bit monochrome image, this equals 2^8 or 256 grey scale values. The plot may be presented in a variety of formats, either vertical or horizontal, and some displays use color or grey scale coding to assist the viewer in distinguishing the white and black sides of the plot.

Systems that also handle images with a greater tonal range than 256 grey levels (8 bits per color channel), as are obtained from scanners, some digital cameras, and other instruments, may allow up to 16 bits (65,536 distinct pixel values). As a matter of convenience and consistency, both for thresholding purposes and to preserve the meaning of the various numeric constants introduced in preceding chapters, such images may still be described as having a brightness range of 0–255 to cover the range from black to white. But instead of being limited to integer brightness values the greater precision of the data allows brightnesses to be reported as real numbers (e.g., a pixel value of 31,605 out of 65,536 would be divided by 256 and reported as 123.457). This does not solve the problem of displaying such a range of values in a histogram. A full histogram of more than 65,000 values would be too wide for any computer screen, and for a typical image size would have so few counts in each channel as to be uninterpretable. One solution is to divide the data down into a conventional 256 channel histogram for viewing, but allow selective expansion of any part of it for purposes of setting thresholds, as indicated in **Figure 3**.

Examples of histograms have been shown in earlier chapters. Note that the histogram counts pixels in the entire image (or in a defined region of interest), losing all information about the original location of the pixels or the brightness values of their neighbors. Peaks in the histogram often identify the various homogeneous regions (often referred to as phases, although they correspond to a phase in the metallurgical sense only in a few applications) and thresholds can then be set between the peaks. There are also automatic methods to adjust threshold settings (Prewitt and Mendelsohn, 1966; Weszka, 1978; Otsu, 1979; Kittler et al., 1985; Russ and Russ, 1988a; Rigaut, 1988; Lee et al., 1990; Sahoo et al., 1988; Russ, 1995c), using either the histogram or the image itself as a guide, as we will see in the following paragraphs. Methods that compare to *a priori* knowledge the measurement parameters obtained from features in the image at many threshold levels (Wolf, 1991) are too specialized for discussion here.

Many images have no clear-cut set of histogram peaks that correspond to distinct phases or structures in the image. **Figure 4** shows a real-world image in which this is the case. Under the more controlled lighting conditions of a microscope, and with sample preparation that includes selective staining or other procedures, this condition is more likely to be met. In some of the difficult cases, direct thresholding of the image is still possible but the settings are not obvious from examination of the histogram peaks. In many situations, the brightness levels of individual pixels are not uniquely related to structure. In some of these instances, prior image processing can be used to transform the original brightness values in the image to a new image, in which pixel brightness represents some derived parameter such as the local brightness gradient or direction.

Histogram analysis is sometimes done by fitting Gaussian (or other shape) functions to the histogram. Given the number of Gaussian peaks to combine for a best overall fit, the position, width and height of each can be determined by multiple regression. This permits estimating the area of each phase but of course cannot determine the spatial position of the pixels in each phase if the peaks overlap. And the result is generally poor because few real imaging situations produce ideally

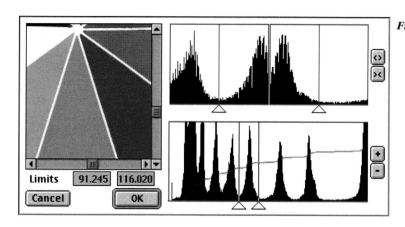

Figure 3. *Example of thresholding a histogram of a 16-bit image, with the bottom graph representing a 256-bin brightness distribution and the top graphs showing expanded details of the values near the threshold settings.*

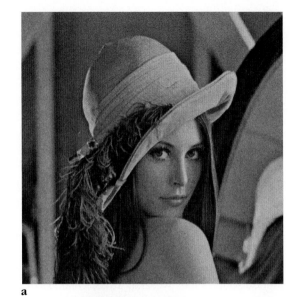

Figure 4. Thresholding a real-world image based on a histogram peak: *(a) the "Lena" image, widely used in the image processing field (original copyright Playboy Magazine); (b) histogram showing a peak with threshold limits; (c) resulting binary image, showing that the locations of pixels with the selected brightness value do not correspond to any obvious structural unit in the original scene.*

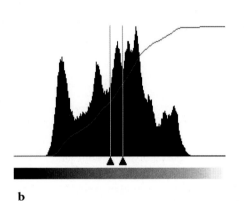

b

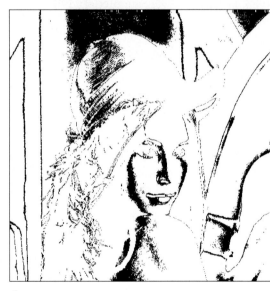

c

Gaussian peaks (or any other consistent shape). One exception is magnetic resonance imaging (MRI), where this method has been applied to produce images in which pixels in the overlap areas are not converted to black or white, but shaded according to the relative contributions of the two overlapping Gaussian peaks at that brightness value (Frank et al., 1995). This does not, of course, produce a segmented image in the conventional sense, but it can produce viewable images that delineate the overlapped structures (e.g., dark matter and white matter in brain scans).

Multiband images

In some cases, segmentation can be performed using multiple original images of the same scene. The most familiar example is that of color imaging, which uses different wavelengths of light. For satellite imaging in particular, this may include several infrared bands containing important information for selecting regions according to vegetation, types of minerals, and so forth (Haralick and

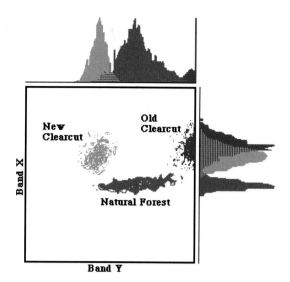

Figure 5. *Example of terrain classification from satellite imagery using multiple spectral bands. Overlaps in each band require that both be used to distinguish the types of terrain.*

Dinstein, 1975). **Figure 5** shows an example. A series of images obtained by performing different processing operations on the same original image can also be used in this way. Examples include combining one image containing brightness data, a second containing local texture information, etc., as will be described in the following paragraphs.

In general, the more independent color bands or other images that are available, the easier and better the job of segmentation that can be performed. Points that are indistinguishable in one image may be fully distinct in another; however, with multispectral or multilayer images, it can be difficult to specify the selection criteria. The logical extension of thresholding is simply to place brightness thresholds on each image, for instance to specify the range of red, green, and blue intensities. These multiple criteria are then usually combined with an AND operation (i.e., the pixel is defined as part of the foreground if its three RGB components all lie within the selected ranges). This is logically equivalent to segmenting each image plane individually, creating separate binary images, and then combining them with a Boolean AND operation afterward. Such operations to combine multiple binary images are discussed in Chapter 7.

The reason for wanting to combine the various selection criteria in a single process is to assist the user in defining the ranges for each. The optimum settings and their interaction are not particularly obvious when the individual color bands or other multiple image brightness values are set individually. Indeed, simply designing a user interface which makes it possible to select a specific range of colors for thresholding a typical visible light image (usually specified by the RGB components) is not easy. A variety of partial solutions are in use.

This problem has several aspects. First, while red, green, and blue intensities represent the way the detector works and the way the data are stored internally, they do not correspond to the way that people recognize or react to color. As discussed in Chapter 1, a system based on hue, saturation, and intensity (HSI) or lightness is more familiar. It is sometimes possible to perform satisfactory thresholding using only one of the hue, saturation or intensity planes as shown in **Figure 6**, but in the general case it may be necessary to use all of the information. A series of histograms for each of the RGB color planes may show peaks, but the user is not often able to judge which of the peaks correspond to individual features of interest.

Even if the RGB pixel values are converted to the equivalent HSI values and histograms are constructed in that space, the use of three separate histograms and sets of threshold levels still does

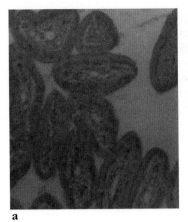 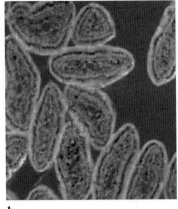 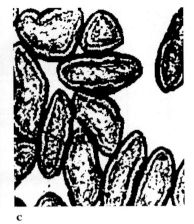

a   b   c

Figure 6. Thresholding a color image using a single channel:
(a) original stained biological thin section;
(b) hue values calculated from stored red, green, and blue values;
(c) thresholding on the hue image delineates the stained structures.

little to help the user see which pixels have various combinations of values. For a single mono-chrome image, various interactive color-coded displays allow the user either to see which pixels are selected as the threshold levels are adjusted or to select a pixel or cluster of pixels and see where they lie in the histogram. **Figure 7** shows an example, though because it consists of still im-ages, it cannot show the live, real-time feedback possible in this situation.

For a three-dimensional color space, either RGB or HSI, interactive thresholding is more difficult. There is no easy or obvious way with present display or control facilities to interactively enclose an arbitrary region in three-dimensional space and see which pixels are selected, or to adjust that region and see the effect on the image. It is also helpful to mark a pixel or region in the image and see the color values (RGB or HSI) labeled directly in the color space. For more than three colors (e.g., the multiple bands sensed by satellite imagery), the situation is even worse.

Using three one-dimensional histograms and sets of threshold levels, for instance in the RGB case, and combining the three criteria with a logical AND selects pixels that lie within a portion of the color space that is a simple prism, as shown in **Figure 8.** If the actual distribution of color values has some other shape in the color space, for instance if it is elongated in a direction not parallel to one axis, then this simple rectangular prism is inadequate to select the desired range of colors.

Two-dimensional thresholds

A somewhat better bound can be set by using a two-dimensional threshold. This can be done in any color coordinates (RGB, HSI, etc.), but in RGB space it is difficult to interpret the meaning of the settings. This is one of the (many) arguments against the use of RGB for color images; how-ever, the method is well-suited for color images encoded by hue and saturation (HS). The HS plane can be represented as a circle, in which direction (angle) is proportional to hue and radius is proportional to saturation (**Figure 9**). The intensity or lightness of the image is perpendicular to this plane and requires another dimension to show or to control.

Instead of a one-dimensional histogram of brightness in a monochrome image, the figure shows a two-dimensional display in the HS plane. The number of pixels with each pair of values of hue and saturation can be plotted as a brightness value on this plane, representing the histogram with its dark peaks. Thresholds can be selected as a region that is not necessarily simple, convex, or even connected, and so can be adapted to the distribution of the actual data. **Figure 9b** illustrates this

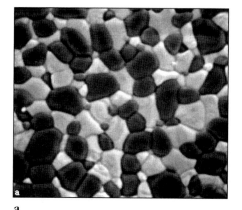

a

Figure 7. Thresholding a grey-scale image:
(a) original SEM image of a two-phase ceramic;
(b) typical thresholding user dialog with upper and lower limits and a preview of the results;
(c) several threshold ranges marked on the image histogram;
(d–g) corresponding binary images produced by changing the settings of the threshold values used to select pixels, as shown on the histogram. The area fraction of the light phase varies with these setting from about 33 to 48% in these results.

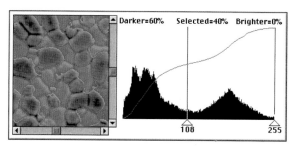

b

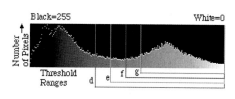

c

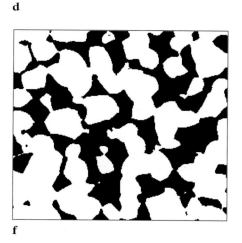

d

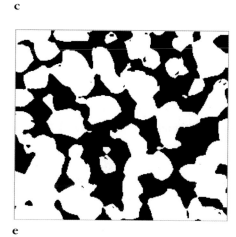

e

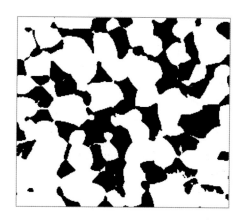

f

g

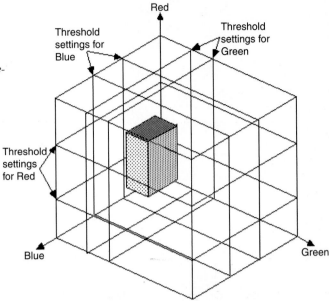

Figure 8. *Illustration of the combination of separate thresholds on individual color planes. The shaded area is the "AND" of the three threshold settings for red, green, and blue. The only shape that can be formed in the three-dimensional space is a rectangular prism.*

method. It is also possible to find locations in this plane as a guide to the user in the process of defining the boundary, by pointing to pixels in the image so that the program can highlight the location of the color values on the HS circle. In the figure, the third axis (intensity) is shown with a conventional histogram and adjustable limits.

Similar histogram displays and threshold settings can be accomplished using other planes and coordinates. For color images, the HS plane is sometimes shown as a hexagon (with red, yellow, green, cyan, blue, and magenta corners). The CIE color diagram shown in Chapter 1 is also a candidate for this purpose. For some satellite images, the near and far infrared intensities form a plane in which combinations of thermal and reflected IR can be displayed and selected.

As a practical matter, the HS plane is sometimes plotted as a square face on a cube that represents the HSI space. This is simpler for the computer graphics display and is used in several of the examples that follow. The HSI cube with square faces is topologically different, however, from the cone or bi-cone used to represent HSI space in Chapter 1, and the square HS plane is topologically different from the circle in **Figure 9**. In the square, the minimum and maximum hue edges (400 nm = red and 700 nm = violet) are far apart, whereas in the circle, hue is a continuous function that wraps around. This makes using the square for thresholding somewhat less intuitive, but it is still superior in most cases to the use of RGB color space.

For the two-dimensional square plot, the axes may have unusual meanings, but the ability to display a histogram of points based on the combination of values and to select threshold boundaries based on the histogram is a significant advantage over multiple one-dimensional histograms and thresholds, even if it does not generalize easily to the n-dimensional case.

The dimensions of the histogram array are usually somewhat reduced from the actual resolution (typically one part in 256) of the various RGB or HSI values for the stored image. This is not only because the array size would become very large (256^2 = 65,536 for the square, 256^3 = 16,777,216 for the cube). Another reason is that for a typical real image, there are simply not that many distinct pairs or triples of values present, and a useful display showing the locations of peaks and clusters can be presented using fewer bins. The examples shown here use 32 × 32 bins for each of the square faces of the RGB or HSI cubes, each of which thus requires 32^2 = 1024 storage locations.

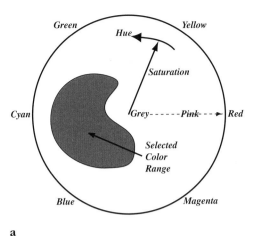

a

Figure 9. Illustration of selecting an arbitrary region in a two-dimensional parameter space (here, the hue/saturation circle) to define a combination of colors to be selected for thresholding:
(a) schematic view;
(b) implementation in which the HSI values for a single crayon are selected from the histogram (which is shown on the hue-saturation circle as grey-scale values representing the number of image pixels — note the clusters for each crayon color);
(c) resulting image in which the selected pixels are outlined in white.

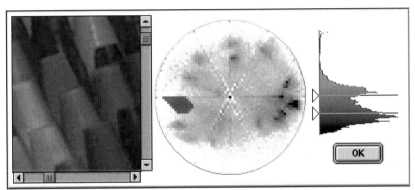

b

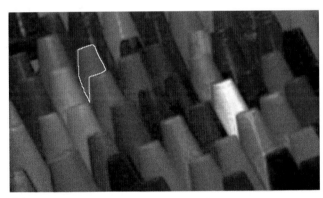

c

It is possible to imagine a system in which each of the two-dimensional planes defined by pairs of signals is used to draw a contour threshold, then project all of these contours back through the multi-dimensional space to define the thresholding, as shown in **Figure 10**. As the dimensionality increases, however, so does the complexity for the user, and the AND region defined by the multiple projections still cannot fit irregular or skewed regions very satisfactorily.

Multiband thresholding

Figure 6 showed a color image from a light microscope. The microtomed thin specimen of intestine has been stained with two different colors, so that there are variations in shade, tint, and tone.

Figure 10. *Illustration of the combination of 2-parameter threshold settings. Outlining of regions in each plane defines a shape in the three-dimensional space which is more adjustable than the Boolean combination of simple one-dimensional thresholds in* **Figure 8***, but still cannot conform to arbitrary three-dimensional cluster shapes.*

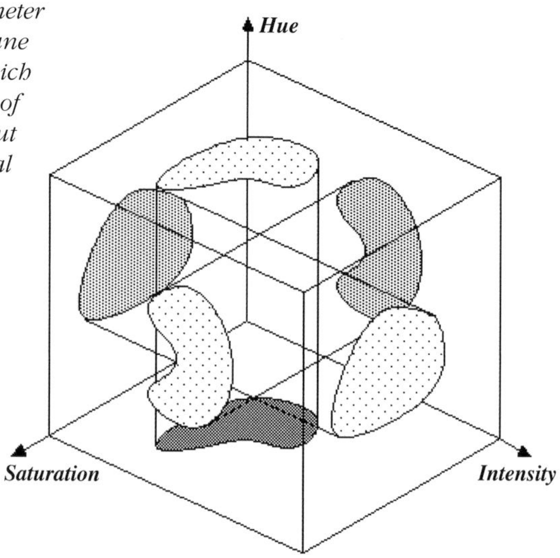

Figure 10 shows the individual red, green, and blue values. The next series of figures illustrates how this image can be segmented by thresholding to isolate a particular structure using this information.

Figure 11 shows the individual brightness histograms of the red, green, and blue color planes in the image, and **Figure 12** shows the histograms of pixel values, projected onto the red/green, green/blue, and blue/red faces of the RGB color cube. Notice that there is a trend on all faces for the majority of pixels in the image to cluster along the central diagonal in the cube. In other words,

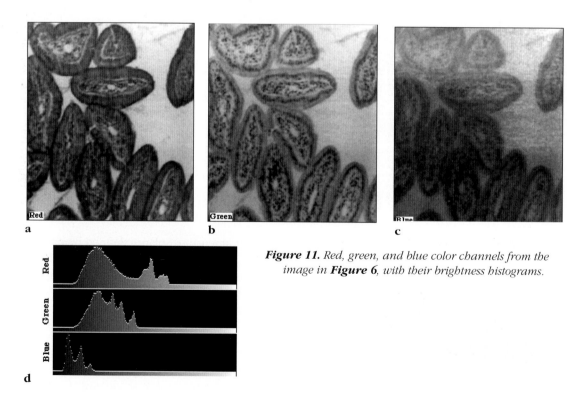

a

b

c

Figure 11. *Red, green, and blue color channels from the image in* **Figure 6***, with their brightness histograms.*

d

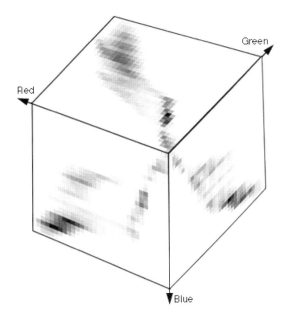

Figure 12. Pairs of values for the pixels in the images of Figure 11, plotted on RG, BG, and RB planes and projected onto the faces of a cube.

for most pixels, the trend toward more of any one color is part of a general increase in brightness by increasing the values of all colors. This means that RGB space poorly disperses the various color values and does not facilitate setting thresholds to discriminate the different regions present.

Figure 13 shows the conversion of the color information from **Figure 11** into hue, saturation, and intensity images, and the individual brightness histograms for these planes. **Figure 14** shows

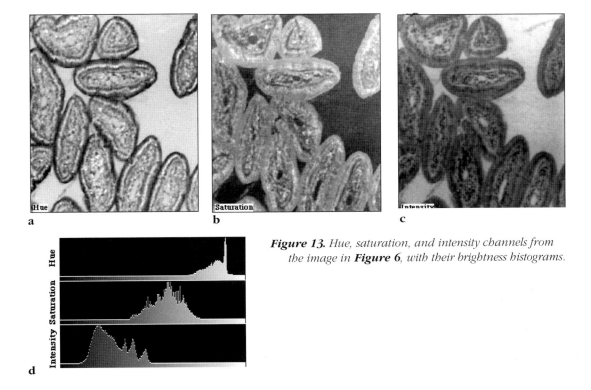

Figure 13. Hue, saturation, and intensity channels from the image in Figure 6, with their brightness histograms.

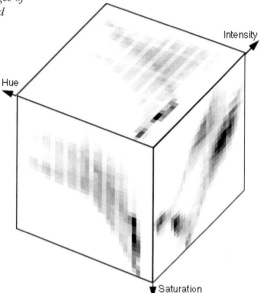

Figure 14. *Pairs of values for the pixels in the images of* **Figure 13,** *plotted on HS, SI, and HI planes and projected onto the faces of a cube.*

the values projected onto individual two-dimensional hue/saturation, saturation/intensity, and intensity/hue square plots. Notice how the much greater dispersion of peaks in the various histograms uses more of the color space and separates several different clusters of values.

In general, for stains used in biological samples, the hue image identifies where a particular stain is located while the saturation image corresponds to the amount of the stain, and the intensity image indicates the overall density of the stained specimen. Combining all three planes as shown in **Figure 15** can often select particular regions that are not well delineated otherwise.

Multiband images are not always simply different colors. A very common example is the use of multiple elemental x-ray maps from the scanning electron microscope (SEM), which can be combined to select phases of interest based on composition. In many cases, this combination can be accomplished simply by separately thresholding each individual image and then applying Boolean logic to combine the images. Of course, the rather noisy original x-ray maps may first require image processing (such as smoothing) to reduce the statistical variations from pixel to pixel (as discussed in Chapters 3 and 4), and binary image processing (as illustrated in Chapter 7).

Using x-rays or other element-specific signals, such as secondary ions or Auger electrons, essentially the entire periodic table can be detected. It becomes possible to specify very complicated combinations of elements that must be present or absent, or the approximate intensity levels needed (because intensities are generally roughly proportional to elemental concentration) to specify the region of interest. Thresholding these combinations of elemental images produces results that are sometimes described as chemical maps. Of course, the fact that several elements may be present in the same area of a specimen, such as a metal, mineral, or block of biological tissue, does not directly imply that they are chemically combined.

In principle, it is possible to store an entire analytical spectrum for each pixel in an image and then use appropriate computation to derive actual compositional information at each point, which is eventually used in a thresholding operation to select regions of interest. At present, this approach is limited in application by the large amount of storage and lengthy calculations required. As faster and larger computers and storage devices become common, however, such methods will become more widely used.

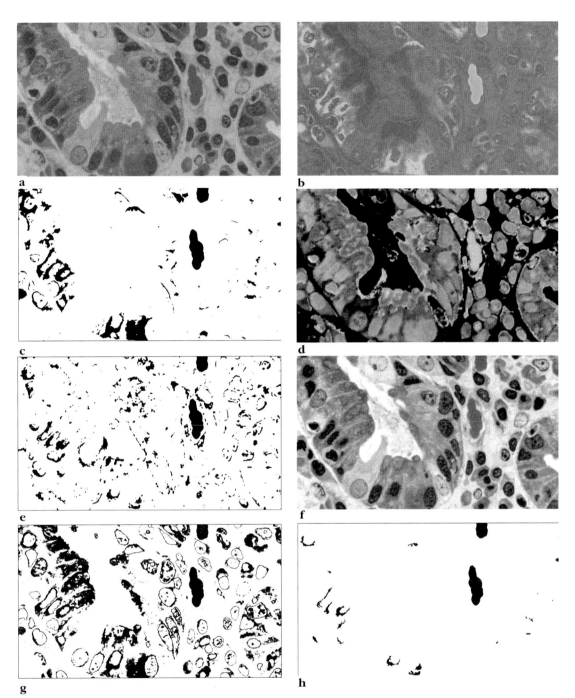

Figure 15. Light micrograph of stomach epithelium with a polychromatic stain, showing thresholding and color separations in HSI space:

    (a) original;

    (b) hue image;

    (c) thresholded hue image;

    (d) saturation image;

    (e) thresholded saturation image;

    (f) intensity image;

    (g) thresholded intensity image;

    (h) Boolean AND applied to combine three binary images produced by thresholding H, S, and I planes.

Visualization programs used to analyze complex data may also employ Boolean logic to combine multiple parameters. A simple example would be a geographical information system, in which such diverse data as population density, mean income level, and other census data were recorded for each city block (which would be treated as a single pixel). Combining these different values to select regions for test marketing commercial products is a standard technique. Another example is the rendering of calculated tensor properties in metal beams subject to loading, as modeled in a computer program. Supercomputer simulations of complex dynamical systems, such as evolving thunderstorms, produce rich data sets that can benefit from such analysis.

Other uses of image processing derive additional information from a single original grey-scale image to aid in performing selective thresholding of a region of interest. The processing produces additional images that can be treated as multiband images useful for segmentation.

Thresholding from texture

Few real images of practical interest can be satisfactorily thresholded using simply the original brightness values in a monochrome image. The texture information present in images is one of the most powerful additional tools available. Several kinds of texture may be encountered, including different ranges of brightness, different spatial frequencies, and different orientations (Haralick et al., 1973). The next few figures show images that illustrate these variables and the tools available to utilize them.

Figure 16 shows a test image containing five irregular regions that can be visually distinguished by texture. The average brightness of each of the regions is identical, as shown by the brightness histograms. Region (**e**) contains pixels with uniformly random brightness values covering the entire 0–255 range. Regions (**a**) through (**d**) have Gaussian brightness variations, which for regions (**a**) and (**d**) are also randomly assigned to pixel locations. For region (**b**) the values have been spatially averaged with a Gaussian smooth, which also reduces the amount of variation. For region (**c**) the pixels have been averaged together in one direction to create a directional texture.

One tool that is often recommended (and sometimes useful) for textural characterization is the two-dimensional frequency transform. **Figure 17** shows these power spectra for each of the

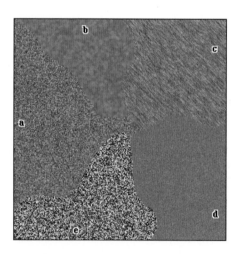
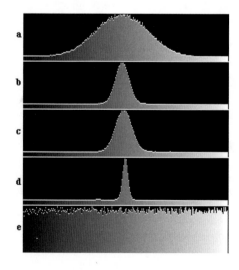

Figure 16. Test image containing five different regions to be distinguished by differences in the textures. The brightness histograms are shown; the average brightness of each region is the same.

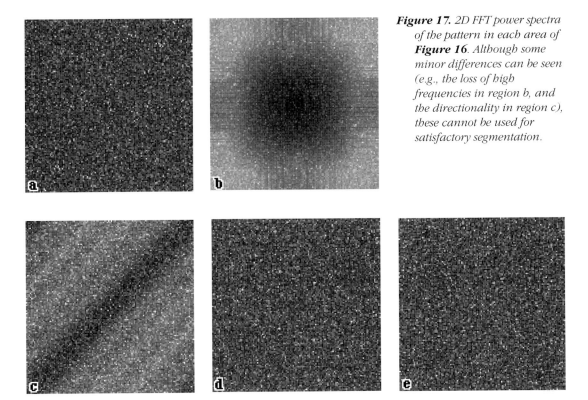

patterns in **Figure 16**. The smoothing in region (**b**) acts as a low-pass filter, so the high frequencies are attenuated. In region (**c**), the directionality is visible in the frequency transform image. For the other regions, the random pixel assignments do not create any distinctive patterns in the frequency transforms. They cannot be used to select the different regions in this case.

Several spatial-domain, texture-sensitive operators are applied to the image in **Figure 18**. The Laplacian shown in (**a**) is a 3×3 neighborhood operator; it responds to very local texture values and does not enhance the distinctions between the textures present here. All the other operators act on a 5×5 pixel octagonal neighborhood and transform the textures to grey-scale values with somewhat different levels of success. Range (**d**) and variance (**f**), both discussed in Chapter 4, give the best distinction between the different regions.

Some variation still occurs in the grey values assigned to the different regions by the texture operators, because they work in relatively small neighborhoods where only a small number of pixel values control the result. Smoothing the variance image (**Figure 19a**) produces an improved image that has unique grey-scale values for each region. **Figure 20** shows the brightness histogram of the original variance image and the result after smoothing. The spatial smoothing narrows the peak for each region by reducing the variation within it. The five peaks are separated and allow direct thresholding. **Figure 21a** shows a composite image with each region selected by thresholding the smoothed variance image.

Figure 19b shows the application of a Sobel edge (gradient) operator to the smoothed gradient image. Thresholding and skeletonizing (as discussed in Chapter 7) produces a set of boundary lines, which are shown superimposed on the original image in **Figure 21b**. Notice that because the spatial scale of the texture is several pixels wide, the location of the boundaries of regions is necessarily uncertain by several pixels. It is also difficult to estimate the proper location visually, for the same reason.

Figure 18. Application of various texture-sensitive operators to the image in Figure 16:
  (a) Laplacian;
  (b) Frei and Chen;
  (c) Haralick;
  (d) range;
  (e) Hurst;
  (f) variance.

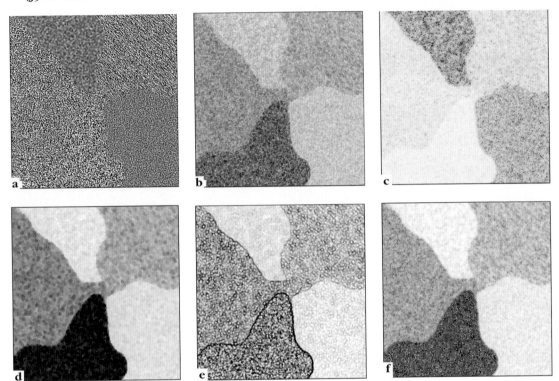

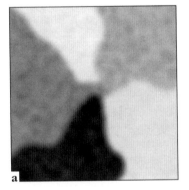

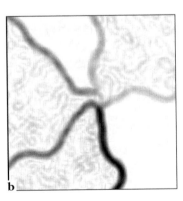

Figure 19. *Result of smoothing the variance image (**Figure 18f**) with a Gaussian kernel with standard deviation equal to 1.6 pixels (**a**), and the Sobel edge detector applied to the smoothed image (**b**).*

Figure 22 shows an image typical of many obtained in microscopy. The preparation technique has used a chemical etch to reveal the microstructure of a metal sample. The lamellae indicate islands of eutectic structure, which are to be separated from the uniform light regions to determine the volume fraction of each. The brightness values in regions of the original image are not distinct, but a

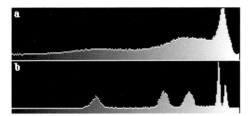

Figure 20. Histograms of the variance image (*Figure 18f*) before (*a*) and after (*b*) smoothing the image with a Gaussian kernel with 1.6-pixel standard deviation. The five regions are now distinct in brightness and can be thresholded successfully.

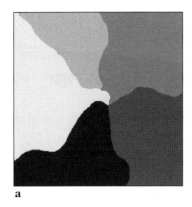

a

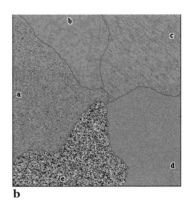

b

Figure 21. Segmentation of the texture image:
   (*a*) *thresholding the smoothed variance image (**Figure 19a**) for each of the peaks in the histogram delineates the different texture regions;*
   (*b*) *skeletonizing the edge from the Sobel operator in **Figure 19b**.*

texture operator is able to convert the image to one that can be thresholded. Chapter 4 showed additional examples of converting texture to brightness differences.

Multiple thresholding criteria

Figure 23a shows a somewhat more complex test image, in which some of the regions are distinguished by a different spatial texture and some by a different mean brightness. No single parameter can be used to discriminate all four regions. The texture values are produced by assigning Gaussian random values to the pixels. As before, a variance operator applied to a 5 × 5 octagonal neighborhood produces a useful grey-scale distinction. **Figures 23b–d** show the result of smoothing the brightness values and the variance image.

It is necessary to use both images to select individual regions. This can be done by thresholding each region separately and then using Boolean logic (discussed in Chapter 7) to combine the two binary images in various ways. Another approach is to use the same kind of two-dimensional histogram as described earlier for color images (Panda and Rosenfeld, 1978). **Figure 24** shows the individual image-brightness histograms and the two-dimensional histogram. In each of the individual histograms, only three peaks are present because the regions are not all distinct in either brightness or variance. In the two-dimensional histogram, individual peaks are visible for each of the four regions.

Figure 25a shows the result of thresholding the intermediate peak in the histogram of the brightness image, which selects two of the regions of medium brightness. **Figure 25b** shows the result of selecting a peak in the two-dimensional histogram to select only a single region. The outlines around each of the regions selected in this way are shown superimposed on the original image in **Figure 25c.**

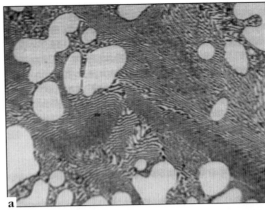

Figure 22. Application of the Hurst texture operator to a microscope image of a metal containing a eutectic:

(a) original image, with light single-phase regions and lamellae corresponding to the eutectic;

(b) application of a Hurst operator (discussed in Chapter 4) to show the local texture in image **a**;

(c) binary image formed by thresholding image b to select the low-texture (single phase) regions.

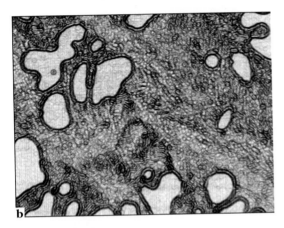

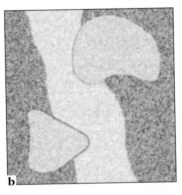

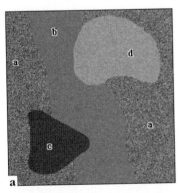

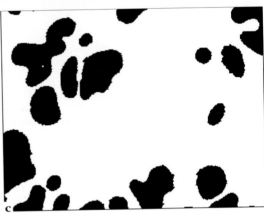

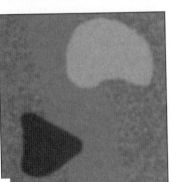

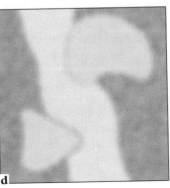

Figure 23. Another segmentation test image, in which some regions have different textures and some different mean brightness:

(a) original;

(b) variance;

(c) smoothing **a** with Gaussian filter, standard deviation = 1.6 pixels;

(d) same smoothing applied to **b**.

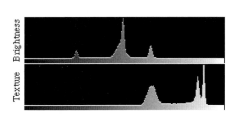

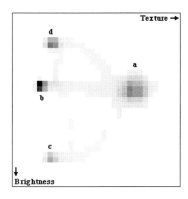

Figure 24. *Histograms of the images in **Figure 23c** and **23d**, and the two way histogram of the pixels showing the separation of the four regions.*

The different derived images used to successfully segment an image such as this one are sometimes displayed using different color planes. This is purely a visual effect, of course, because the data represented have nothing to do with color. However, it does take advantage of the fact that human vision distinguishes colors well (for most people, at least) and uses color information for segmentation, and it also reveals the similarity between this example of thresholding based on multiple textural and brightness criteria with the more commonplace example of thresholding color images based on the individual color channels. **Figure 25d** shows the information from the images in **Figures 25a** and **25b**, with the original image in the Luminance plane, the smoothed brightness values in the a plane, and the texture information from the variance operator in the b plane of an L·a·b color image.

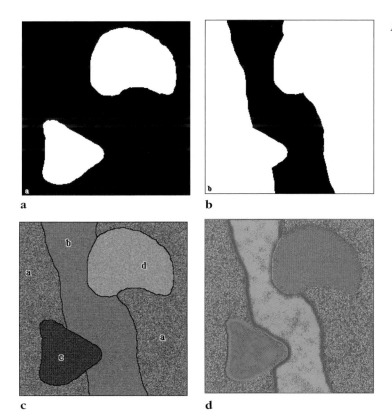

a

b

c

d

Figure 25. Thresholding of images in Figure 23:
(a) *selecting intermediate brightness values (regions **a** and **b**);*
(b) *selecting only region **b** by its brightness and texture;*
(c) *region definition achieved by selection ANDing binary images thresholded individually;*
(d) *color coding of the images from **Figure 23** as described in the text.*

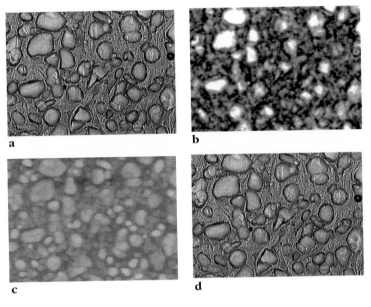

Figure 26. Segmentation of ice crystals in a food product:
(a) *original image;*
(b) *Hurst texture operator applied to the intensity channel;*
(c) *hue channel;*
(d) *final result shown as outlines on the original image.*

a

b

c

d

Figure 26 shows an application of thresholding using two criteria, one of them texture, to a real image. The sample is ice crystals in a food product. The Hurst texture operator partially delineates the ice crystals, as does the use of the hue channel. Thresholding each, and then combining them with Boolean logic and applying a closing (discussed in Chapter 7) produces a useful segmentation of the crystals, as shown by the outlines on the figure.

Textural orientation

Figure 27 shows another test image containing regions having different textural orientations but identical mean brightness, brightness distribution, and spatial scale of the local variation. This rather subtle texture is evident in a two-dimensional frequency transform, as shown in **Figure 28a**. The three ranges of spatial-domain orientation are revealed in the three spokes in the transform.

Using a selective wedge-shaped mask with smoothed edges to select each of the spokes and re-transform the image produces the three spatial-domain images shown in **Figure 28**. Each texture orientation in the original image is isolated, having a uniform grey background in other locations. These images cannot be directly thresholded because the brightness values in the textured regions cover a range that includes the surroundings. Applying a range operator to a 5 × 5-pixel octagonal neighborhood, as shown in **Figure 29**, suppresses the uniform background regions and highlights the individual texture regions.

Thresholding these images and applying a closing operation (discussed in Chapter 7) to fill in internal gaps and smooth boundaries, produces images of each region. **Figure 29d** shows the composite result. Notice that the edges of the image are poorly delineated, a consequence of the inability of the frequency transform to preserve edge details, as discussed in Chapter 5. Also, the boundaries of the regions are rather irregular and only approximately rendered in this result.

In many cases, spatial-domain processing is preferred for texture orientation. **Figure 30** shows the result from applying a Sobel operator to the image, as discussed in Chapter 4. Two directional first derivatives in the x and y directions are obtained using a 3 × 3 neighborhood operator. These are then combined using the arc tangent function to obtain an angle that is the direction of maximum brightness gradient. The resulting angle is scaled to fit the 0 to 255 brightness range of the image, so that each step in brightness corresponds to about 1.4 degrees.

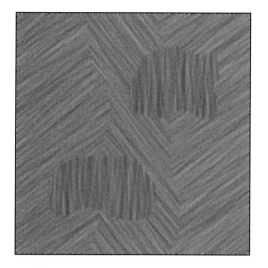

Figure 27. An image containing regions that have different textural orientations, but the same average brightness, standard deviation, and spatial scale.

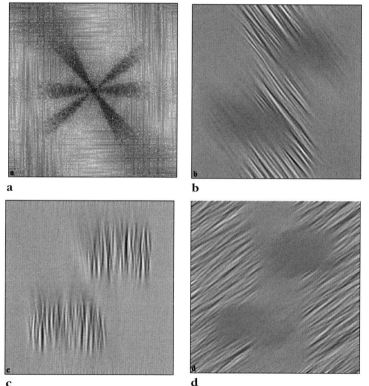

a b c d

Figure 28. Isolating the directional texture in frequency space: *(a)* two-dimensional frequency transform of the image in *Figure 27*, showing the radial spokes corresponding to each textural alignment; *(b–d)* retransformation using masks to select each of the orientations.

The brightness histogram shown in **Figure 30b** shows six peaks. These occur in pairs 180 degrees apart, since in each texture region the direction of maximum gradient may lie in either of two opposite directions. This image can be reduced to three directions in several ways. One is to use a grey-scale LUT, as discussed in Chapter 4, which assigns the same grey-scale values to the highest and lowest halves of the original brightness (or angle) range; this converts the 0–360 degree range to 0–180 degrees and permits thresholding a single peak for each direction. A second method is to set two different threshold ranges on the paired peaks and then combine the two resulting binary images using a Boolean "OR" operation (see Chapter 7). A third approach is to set a multiple-threshold range on the two complementary peaks. All these methods are functionally equivalent.

*Figure 29. Application of a range operator to the images in **Figure 28b, 28c**, and **28d**, and the combination of the regions selected by thresholding these images.*

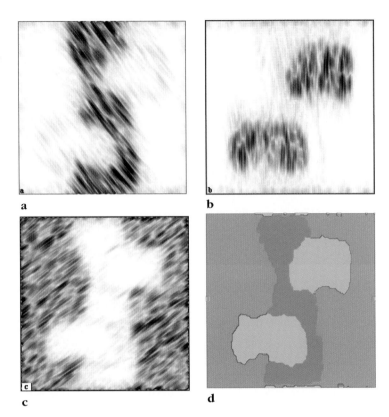

a

b

c

d

Figure 31 shows the results of three thresholding operations to select each of the three textural orientations. Some noise occurs in these images, consisting of white pixels within the dark regions and vice versa, but these are much fewer and smaller than in the case of thresholding the results from the frequency-transform method shown previously. After applying a closing operation (a dilation followed by an erosion, as discussed in Chapter 7), the regions are well delineated, as shown by the superposition of the outlines on the original image (**Figure 31d**). This result is superior to the frequency transform and has smoother boundaries, better agreement with the visual judgment of location, and no problems at the image or region edges.

Figure 32 shows a scanned stylus image of a flycut metal surface. Two predominant directions of machining marks are present, and applying the Sobel direction operator produces an image

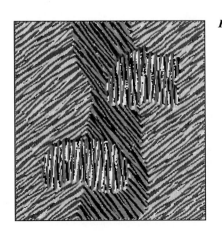

*Figure 30. Application of the Sobel direction operator to the image in **Figure 27**, calculating the orientation of the gradient at each pixel by assigning a grey level to the arc tangent of $(\partial B / \partial y) / (\partial B / \partial x)$. The brightness histogram shows six peaks, in pairs for each principal textural orientation, because the directions are complementary.*

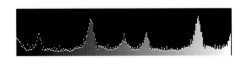

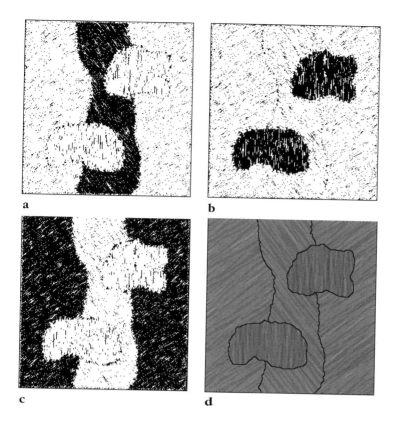

a b

c d

Figure 31. *Thresholded binary images from* ***Figure 30****, selecting the grey values corresponding to each pair of complementary directions, and the outlines showing the regions defined by applying a closing operation to each of the binary images.*

(**Figure 33**) with the expected four peaks, because the grey scale values represent directions covering 360 degrees. This can be reduced to 180 degrees by using a lookup table that replaces the original grey scale with the values shown in **Figure 33b**, which range from black to white over the first 128 values and then again over the second 128 values. Thresholding this produces a binary image (**Figure 34a**) that can be processed with a median filter to remove the speckle noise (**Figure 34b**), resulting in good delineation of the regions in the original image (**Figure 34c**).

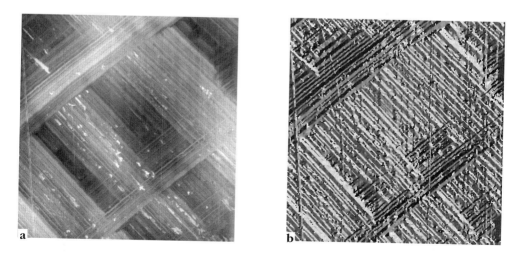

a b

Figure 32. Surface of flycut metal (a), *and the result of applying the Sobel direction operator **(b)** to show the directionality of the machining marks.*

Figure 33. *Histogram of the image in* **Figure 32b,** *showing two pairs of peaks. The application of a look-up table (**b**) converts the image as shown in* **Figure 34.**

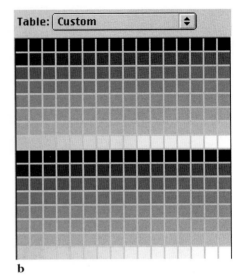

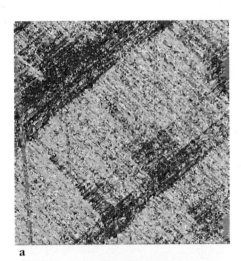

a

b

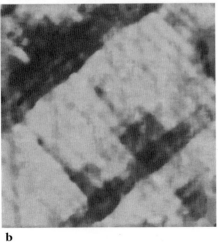

a

Figure 34. Direction information for the surface machining marks:
(**a**) *as produced from* **Figure 31b** *using the lookup table in* **Figure 33b;**
(**b**) *application of a median filter to remove speckle noise;*
(**c**) *segmentation of the original image produced by thresholding* **b.**

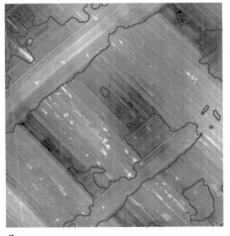

b

c

Note that applying any neighborhood processing operation such as smoothing or median filtering to an image in which grey scale represents direction requires special rules to account for the modulo change in values at 0. For example, the average value in a neighborhood containing pixel values of 15 and 251 is 5, not 133. A simple but effective way to accomplish this is to process each neighborhood twice, once with the stored values and once with the values shifted to become (P + 128) mod 255, and then keep whichever result is smaller.

Figure 35 shows another example, a metallographic sample with a lamellar structure. This requires several steps to segment into the various regions. Brightness thresholding can delineate one region directly. Applying the Sobel orientation operator produces an image that can be thresholded to delineate the other two regions, but as before each region has pairs of grey-scale values that are 180 degrees or 128 grey values apart. Thresholding the various regions produces a complete map of the sample as shown.

Accuracy and reproducibility

In one or more dimensions, the selection of threshold values discussed so far has been manual. An operator interactively sets the cutoff values so that the resulting image is visually satisfying and the correspondence between what the user sees in the image and the pixels the thresholds select is as close as possible. This is not always consistent from one operator to another, or even for the same person over a period of time. The difficulty and variability of thresholding represents a serious source of error for further image analysis.

Two slightly different requirements have been established for setting threshold values. Both have to do with the typical use of binary images for feature measurement. One is to achieve reproducibility, so that variations due to the operator, lighting, etc. do not affect the results. The second

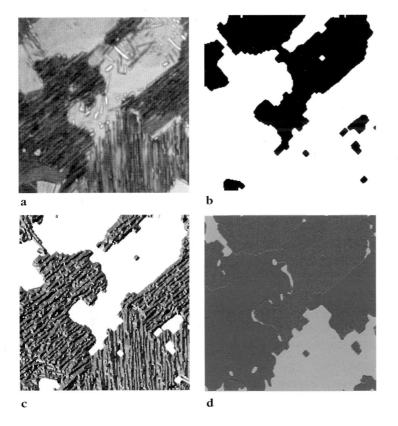

Figure 35. Thresholding on multiple criteria:
(a) original metallographic image;
(b) one region selected by brightness thresholding;
(c) Sobel orientation operator applied to the remaining region;
(d) final segmentation result with regions color coded.

a

b

c

d

goal of setting threshold values is to achieve accurate boundary delineation so that measurements are accurate.

Because pixel-based images represent, at best, an approximation to the continuous real scene being represented, and because thresholding classifies each pixel as either part of the foreground or the background, only a certain level of accuracy can be achieved. An alternate representation of features based on boundary lines can be more accurate. These may be polygons with many sides and corner points defined as x, y coordinates of arbitrary accuracy, or spline curves, etc., as compared with the comparatively coarse pixel spacing.

Such boundary-line representation is superior for accurate measurement because the line itself has no width, although determining the line is far from easy. The location of individual points can be determined by interpolation between pixels, perhaps fitting mathematical functions to pixels on either side of the boundary to improve the results. This type of approach is commonly used geographic applications in which elevation values measured at discrete points are used to construct topographic maps. It is also used in metrology applications, such as measuring dimensions of microelectronic circuit elements on silicon wafers, and is possible because the shape of the features (usually straight lines) is known *a priori*. This type of application goes beyond the typical image processing operations dealt with in this chapter.

One approach to interpolating a smoothed boundary line through the pixels is used by the super-resolution perimeter measurement routine used in Chapter 9 for feature measurement. This uses neighborhood processing (the Laplacian of a Gaussian) to fit an adaptive boundary line through each pixel, achieving improved precision and fractional-pixel accuracy.

Thresholding produces a pixel-based representation of the image that assigns each pixel to either the feature(s) or the surroundings. The finite size of the pixels allows the representation only a finite accuracy, but we would prefer to have no bias in the result. This means that performing the same operation on many repeated images of the same scene should produce an average result that approaches the true value for size or other feature measurements. This is not necessary for quality control applications in which reproducibility is of greater concern than accuracy, and some bias (as long as it is consistent) can be tolerated. Many things can contribute to bias in setting thresholds. Human operators are not very good at setting threshold levels without bias. In most cases, they are more tolerant of settings that include additional pixels from the background region along with the features than they are of settings that exclude some pixels from the features.

As indicated at the beginning of this chapter, the brightness histogram from the image can be an important tool for setting threshold levels. In many cases, it will show distinct and separated peaks from the various phases or structures present in the field of view, or it can be made to do so by prior image processing steps. In this case, it seems that setting the threshold level somewhere between the peaks should produce consistent, and perhaps even accurate, results.

Unfortunately, this idea is easier to state than to accomplish. In many real images, the peaks corresponding to particular structures are not perfectly symmetrical or ideally sharp, particularly when there may be shading either of the entire image or within the features (e.g., a brightness gradient from center to edge). Changing the field of view or even the illumination may cause the peak to shift and/or to change shape. Nonlinear camera response or automatic gain circuits can further distort the brightness histogram. If the area fraction of the image that is the bright (or dark) phase changes from one field of view to another, some method is needed to maintain a threshold setting that adapts to these changes and preserves precision and accuracy.

If the peaks are consistent and well-defined, then choosing an arbitrary location at some fixed fraction of the distance between them is a rapid method often satisfactory for quality control work. In many cases, it is necessary to consider the pixels whose brightness values lie between the peaks

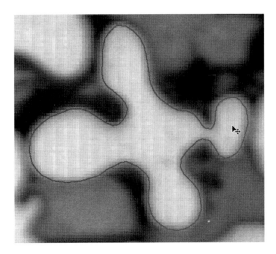

in the brightness histogram. In most instances, these are pixels that straddle the boundary and have averaged together the two principal brightness levels in proportion to the area subtended within the pixel, as indicated in **Figure 36**.

Asymmetric boundaries (for example, a metallographic specimen in which etching has attacked the softer of two phases so that the boundary is skewed) can introduce bias in these brightness values, and so can prior processing steps, such as those responding to texture in the image. Many of these operations work on a finite and perhaps rather large neighborhood, so the boundary position becomes somewhat uncertain. If the processing operation responds nonlinearly to differences, as the variance operator does, the apparent boundary location will shift toward the most different pixel in the neighborhood.

Including position information

The histogram display shows only the frequency of occurrence of different values and does not preserve any information about position, the brightness of neighboring pixels, and other factors. Yet, it is this spatial information that is important for determining boundary location. It is possible, in principle, to build a co-occurrence matrix for the image in which all possible combinations of pixel brightness are counted in terms of the distance between them. This information is used to select the pixels that are part of the feature instead of simply the pixel brightness values, but this is equivalent to a processing operation that uses the same co-occurrence matrix to construct a texture image for which simple thresholding can be used.

One possible algorithm for threshold settings is to pick the minimum point in the histogram (**Figure 37**). This should correspond to the value that affects the fewest pixels and thus gives the lowest expected error in pixel classification when the image is segmented into features and background. The difficulty is that because this region of the histogram is (hopefully) very low, with few pixels having these values, the counting statistics are poor and the shape of the curve in the histogram is poorly defined. Consequently, the minimum value is hard to locate and may move about considerably with only tiny changes in overall illumination, a change in the field of view to include objects with a different shape, or more or fewer pixels along the boundary. Smoothing the histogram with a polynomial fit may provide a somewhat more robust location for a minimum point.

Figure 38 shows an image having two visibly distinguishable regions. Each contains a Gaussian noise pattern with the same standard deviation but a different mean, though the brightness values in the two regions overlap. This means that setting a threshold value at the minimum between the two peaks causes some pixels in each region to be misclassified, as shown.

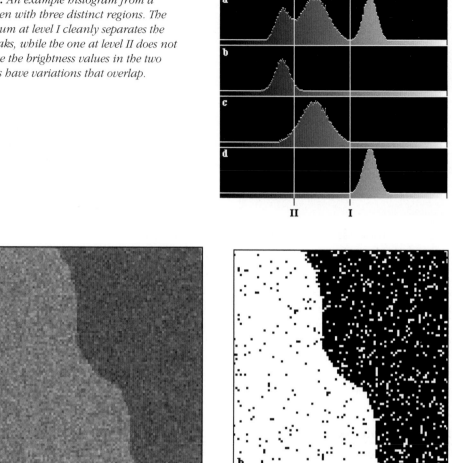

Figure 37. *An example histogram from a specimen with three distinct regions. The minimum at level I cleanly separates the two peaks, while the one at level II does not because the brightness values in the two regions have variations that overlap.*

Figure 38. A test image containing two regions whose mean brightness levels are different, but which have variations in individual pixels that overlap:
 (a) *original image (enlarged to show pixels);*
 (b) *result of setting a simple threshold at the minimum point.*

This type of image often results from situations in which the total number of photons or other signals is low and counting statistics cause a variation in the brightness of pixels in uniform areas. Counting statistics produce a Poisson distribution, but when moderately large numbers are involved, this is very close to the more convenient Gaussian function used in these images. For extremely noisy images, such as x-ray dot maps from the SEM, some additional processing in the spatial domain may be required before attempting thresholding (O'Callaghan, 1974).

Figure 39 shows a typical sparse dot map. Most of the pixels contain 0 counts, and a few contain 1 count. The boundaries in the image are visually evident, but their exact location is at best approximate, requiring the human visual computer to group the dots together. Imaging processing can do this by counting the number of dots in a circular neighborhood around each pixel. Convolution with a kernel consisting of "ones" in a 15-pixel-diameter circle accomplishes this, producing the result shown. This grey-scale image can be thresholded to locate the boundaries shown, but there is inadequate data to decide whether the small regions, voids, and irregularities in the

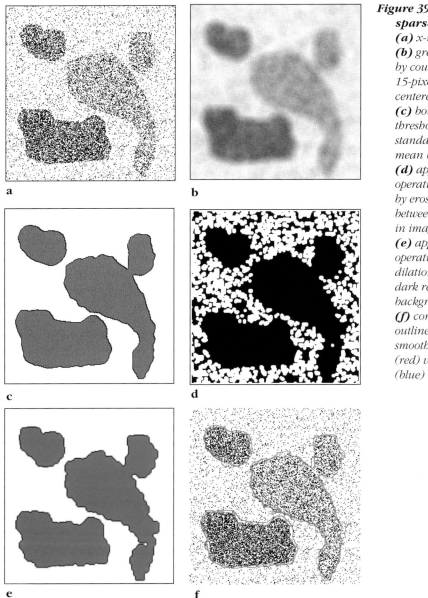

Figure 39. Thresholding a sparse dot image:
(a) x-ray dot map;
(b) grey-scale image formed by counting the dots within a 15-pixel-diameter circle centered on each pixel;
(c) boundary determined by thresholding image **b** at 4 standard deviations above the mean background level;
(d) application of a closing operation (dilation followed by erosion) to fill the gaps between closely spaced pixels in image **a**;
(e) application of an opening operation (erosion followed by dilation) to remove small dark regions in the background in image **d**;
(f) comparison of the feature outlines determined by the smoothing and thresholding (red) vs. closing and opening (blue) methods.

boundaries are real or simply due to the limited counting statistics. Typically, the threshold level will be set by determining the mean brightness level in the background region, and then setting the threshold several standard deviations above this to select just the significant regions.

The figure compares this approach to one based on the binary editing operations discussed in Chapter 7. Both require making some assumptions about the image. In the smoothing and thresholding case (**Figures 39b** and **c**), some knowledge about the statistical meaning of the data is required. For x-rays, the standard deviation in the count rate is known to vary in proportion to the square root of the number of counts, which is the brightness in the smoothed image. Erosion and dilation are based on assumptions about the distances between dots in the image. Closing (dilation followed by erosion) fills in the gaps between dots to create solid areas corresponding to the features, as shown in **Figure 39d**. In the background regions, this does not produce a continuous dark region and so an opening (erosion followed by dilation) can remove it (**Figure 39e**). Adding

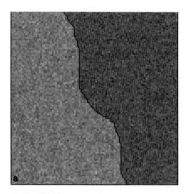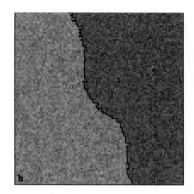

Figure 40. The boundary in the image of Figure 38:
(a) thresholding at the minimum point in the histogram followed by closing (dilation and erosion);
(b) iteratively setting the minimum entropy point.

and then removing pixels produces the final result shown. The boundaries are slightly different from those produced by smoothing and thresholding, but the original image does not contain enough data to distinguish between them.

Several possible approaches may be used to improve the segmentation of noisy regions, using **Figure 38** as a test case. Chapter 7 discusses binary image editing operations, including morphological processing. The sequence of a dilation followed by an erosion, known as a closing, fills holes, erases isolated pixels, and smooths the boundary line to produce the result shown in **Figure 40a**. By contrast, a much more complicated operation reassigns pixels from one region to the other to achieve minimum entropy in both regions. Entropy methods are generally a very computer-intensive approach to image restoration. They function to improve degraded grey-scale images, as discussed in Chapter 3.

In this case, the collection of pixels into two regions can be described as an entropy problem as follows (Kanpur et al., 1985): The total entropy in each region is calculated as $-\Sigma p_i \log_e p_i$, where p_i is the fraction of pixels having brightness i. Solving for the boundary that classifies each pixel into one of two groups to minimize this function for the two regions, subject to the constraint that the pixels in each region must touch each other, produces the boundary line shown in **Figure 40b**. Additional constraints, such as minimizing the number of touching pixels in different classes, would smooth the boundary. The problem is that such constraints are ad hoc, make the solution of the problem very difficult, and can usually be applied more efficiently in other ways (for instance by smoothing the binary image).

Setting a threshold value at the minimum in the histogram is sometimes described as selecting for minimum area sensitivity in the value (Weszka, 1978; Wall et al., 1974). This means that changing the threshold value causes the least change in the feature (or background) area, although, as noted previously, this says nothing about the spatial arrangement of the pixels that are thereby added to or removed from the features. Indeed, the definition of the histogram makes any minimum in the plot a point of minimum area sensitivity.

For the image shown in **Figure 38**, the histogram can be changed to produce a minimum that is deeper, broader, and has a more stable minimum value by processing the image. **Figure 41** shows the results of smoothing the image (using a Gaussian kernel with a standard deviation of 1 pixel) or applying a median filter (both methods are discussed in Chapters 3 and 4). The peaks are narrower and the valley is broader and deeper. The consequences for the image, and the boundary that is selected by setting the threshold level between the peaks, are shown in **Figure 42**.

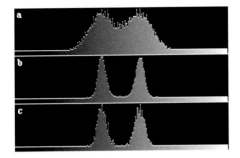

Figure 41. Histogram of the image in Figure 38:
(a) *original, with overlapped peaks;*
(b) *after smoothing;*
(c) *after median filtering.*

Figure 42. Processing the image in Figure 38 to modify the histogram:
(a) *Smoothing with a Gaussian kernel, standard deviation = 1 pixel;*
(b) *the boundary produced by thresholding image **a**, superimposed on the original;*
(c) *median processing (iteratively applied until no further changes occurred);*
(d) *the boundary produced by thresholding image **c**, superimposed on the original.*

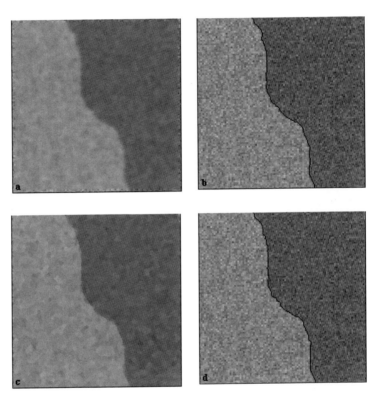

It appears that this is not the criterion used by human operators, especially when they watch an image and interactively adjust a threshold value. Instead of the total area of features changing minutely with adjustment, which is difficult for humans to judge, another approach is to use the total change in perimeter length around the features (Russ and Russ, 1988a). This may, in fact, be the criterion actually used by skilled operators. The variation in total perimeter length with respect to threshold value provides an objective criterion that can be efficiently calculated. The minimum in this response curve provides a way to set the thresholds that is reproducible, adapts to varying illumination, etc., and mimics to some extent the way humans set the values. For the case in which both upper and lower threshold levels are to be adjusted, this produces a response surface in two dimensions (the upper and lower values), which can be solved to find the minimum point as indicated in **Figure 43**.

Figure 44 shows an image whose brightness threshold has been automatically positioned to minimize the variation in total boundary length. The brightness histogram shown in the figure has a very long valley between the two phase peaks, neither of which has a symmetric or

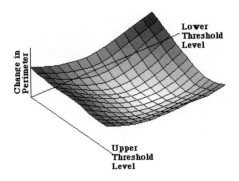

Figure 43. *A two-way plot of the change in perimeter length vs. the settings of upper and lower level brightness thresholds. The minimum indicates the optimal settings.*

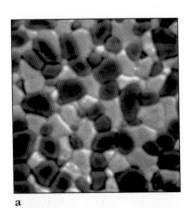

a

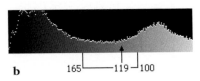

b   165 —119— 100

Figure 44. *A test image for automatic threshold adjustment (**a**), and its brightness histogram (**b**). The optimum threshold point within the search range marked, based on minimizing the change in perimeter length is shown on the histogram, with the thresholded binary result (**c**) and the boundary overlaid on the original (**d**).*

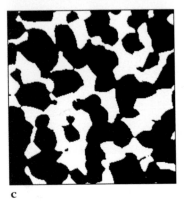

c

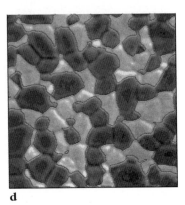

d

Gaussian shape. The selected threshold point is not at the lowest point in the histogram. Repeated measurements using this algorithm on many images of the same objects show that the reproducibility in the presence of finite image noise and changing illumination is rather good. Length variations for irregular objects varied less than 0.5%, or 1 pixel in 200 across the major diameter of the object.

Many of the algorithms developed for automatic setting of thresholds are intended for the discrimination of printed text on paper, as a first step in programs that scan pages and convert them to text files for editing or communication. **Figure 45** shows an example of a page of scanned text with the results of several of these algorithms, as summarized in Parker (Parker, 1997; Yager, 1979; Otsu, 1979; Trussell, 1979). Note that there is no "valley between two peaks" present in this histogram. Each method makes different assumptions about the nature of the histogram and the appropriate statistical or other tests that can be used to divide it into two parts, each representing one

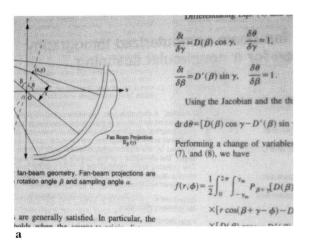

a

Figure 45. Automatic thresholding of printed text on paper using algorithms from Parker (1997):
(a) *original grey-scale scan;*
(b) *histogram;*
(c) *Yager algorithm, threshold = 134;*
(d) *Trussell method, threshold = 172;*
(e) *Shannon entropy algorithm; threshold = 184;*
(f) *Kittler algorithm, threshold = 196.*

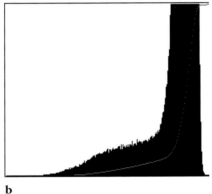

b

Using the Jacobian and the th

$$dt\,d\theta = [D(\beta)\cos\gamma\quad D'(\beta)\sin$$

Performing a change of variables (7), and (8), we have

c

Using the Jacobian and the thi

$$dt\,d\theta = [D(\beta)\cos\gamma - D'(\beta)\sin$$

Performing a change of variables (7), and (8), we have

d

Using the Jacobian and the thi

$$dt\,d\theta = [D(\beta)\cos\gamma - D'(\beta)\sin$$

Performing a change of variables (7), and (8), we have

e

Using the Jacobian and the thi

$$dt\,d\theta = [D(\beta)\cos\gamma - D'(\beta)\sin$$

Performing a change of variables (7), and (8), we have

f

of the two structures present (paper and ink). Many of the algorithms summarized in Parker produce closely similar results on this image, but some of the results do not separate the characters entirely and others cause them to break up. No single method will work for all types of printing, paper, and image acquisition settings. Even if a single method did exist, the problem being addressed is more specialized than the general range of images containing just two types of structures, while many images contain more than two.

The Trussell algorithm (Trussell, 1979) is probably the most widely used automatic method, because it usually produces a fairly good result (**Figure 45d**) and is easy to implement. It finds the threshold setting that produces two populations of pixels (brighter and darker) with the largest value of the student's t statistic, which is calculated from the difference between the means of the two groups and their standard deviations. This is a fairly standard statistical test, but it really should only be applied when the groups are known to have normal or Gaussian distributions, which is rarely the case for the distribution of pixel brightness values in typical images. Another algorithm that often produces good results (slightly different from the Trussell method) minimizes the entropy of the two sets of pixels (above and below the threshold setting), and is illustrated in **Figure 45e**.

Selective histograms

Most of the difficulties with selecting the optimum threshold brightness value between two peaks in a typical histogram arise from the intermediate brightness values of the histogram. These pixels lie along the boundaries of the two regions, so methods that eliminate them from the histogram will contain only peaks from the uniform regions and can be used to select the proper threshold value (Weszka and Rosenfeld, 1979; Milgram and Herman, 1979).

One way to perform this selection is to use another derived image, such as the Sobel gradient or any of the other edge-finding operators discussed in Chapter 4. Pixels having a high gradient value can be eliminated from the histogram of the original image to reduce the background level in the range between the two phase peaks. **Figure 46** shows an example. The original image contains three phases with visually distinct grey-levels. Several methods can be used to eliminate edge pixels. It is most straightforward to threshold a gradient image, selecting pixels with a high values. This produces a binary image that can be used as a mask, as discussed in Chapter 7. This mask restricts which pixels in the original image are to be used for the histogram to be analyzed.

As an example, using the image from **Figure 46**, the 20% of the pixels with the largest magnitude in the Sobel gradient image were selected to produce a mask used to remove those pixels from the original image and the histogram. The result, shown in **Figure 47**, is the reduction of those portions of the histogram between peaks, with the peaks themselves little affected. This makes it easier to characterize the shapes of the peaks from the phases and select a consistent point between them.

Of course, this method requires setting a threshold on the gradient image to select the pixels to be bypassed. The most often used technique is simply to choose some fixed percentage of the pixels with the highest gradient value and eliminate them from the histogram of the original image. In the example shown, however, the gradient operator responds more strongly to the larger difference between the white and grey regions than to the smaller difference between the grey and dark regions. Thus, the edge-straddling pixels (and their background in the histogram) are reduced much more between the white and grey peaks than between the grey and black peaks.

Figure 48 shows another method which alleviates the problem in this image. Beginning with a range image (the difference between the darkest and brightest pixels in a 5-pixel-wide octagonal neighborhood), non-maximum suppression (also known as grey-scale thinning, skeletonization, or ridge-finding) is used to narrow the boundaries and eliminate pixels that are not actually on the

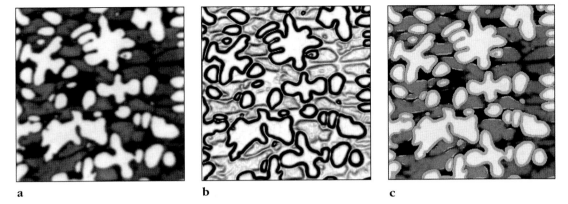

a   b   c

Figure 46. Thresholding by ignoring boundary pixels:
  (a) *original image containing three visually distinct phase regions with different mean grey levels;*
  (b) *application of a gradient operator (Sobel) to* *a;*
  (c) *The image without the 20% of the pixels having the largest gradient value, which eliminates the edge-straddling pixels in the original.*

boundary. This line is uniformly dilated to 3 pixels wide and used as a mask to remove edge-straddling pixels from the original. The plot of the resulting histogram, also in **Figure 47**, shows a much greater suppression of the valley between the grey and black peaks. All of these methods are somewhat ad hoc; the particular combination of different region brightnesses present in an image will dictate what edge-finding operation will work best and what fraction of the pixels should be removed.

Boundary lines

One of the shortcomings of thresholding is that the pixels are selected primarily by brightness, and only secondarily by location. This means that there is no requirement for regions to be continuous. Instead of defining a region as a collection of pixels with brightness values that are similar in one or more images, an alternate definition can be based on a boundary.

Manually outlining regions for measurement is one way to use this approach. Various interactive pointing devices, such as graphics tablets (also called drawing pads), touch screens, mice, or light pens, may be used. The drawing can take place while the user looks at the computer screen, at a photographic print on a tablet, or through the microscope, with the pointer device optically superimposed. None of these methods is without problems. Video displays have rather limited

Figure 47. *Brightness histograms from the original image in* *Figure 46a* *and the masked images in* *Figures 46c and 48c, showing the reduction of number of pixels with brightness in the ranges between the main peaks.*

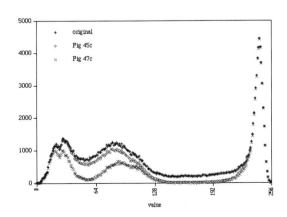

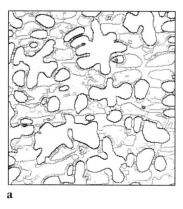 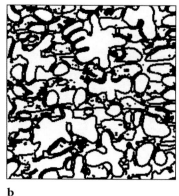 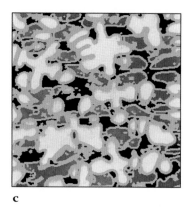

a   b   c

Figure 48. Removal of edge pixels:
   (**a**) *non-maximum suppression (grey-scale thinning) applied to* **Figure 46b***;*
   (**b**) *dilation of lines to 3 pixels wide;*
   (**c**) *removal of edges leaving uniform interior regions in the original.*

resolution. Drawing on a video representation of a live image does not provide a record of where you have been. Mice are clumsy pointing devices, light pens lose precision in dark areas of the display, touch screens have poor resolution (and your finger gets in the way), and so on.

It is beyond our purpose here to describe the operation or compare the utility of these different approaches. Regardless of what physical device is used for manual outlining, the method relies on the human visual image processor to locate boundaries and produces a result that consists of a polygonal approximation to the region outline. Most people tend to draw just outside the actual boundary of whatever features they perceive to be important, making dimensions larger than they should be, and the amount of error is a function of the contrast at the edge. (Exceptions exist, of course. Some people draw inside the boundary, but bias is commonly present in all manually drawn outlines.)

Attempts to emulate the human outlining operation with a computer algorithm require a starting point, usually provided by the human. Then the program examines each adjoining pixel to find which has the characteristics of a boundary, usually defined as a step in brightness. Whichever pixel has the highest value of local gradient is selected and added to the growing polygon, and then the procedure is repeated. Sometimes, a constraint is added to minimize sharp turns, such as weighting the pixel values according to direction.

Automatic edge-following suffers from several problems. First, the edge definition is essentially local. People have a rather adaptable capability to look ahead various distances to find pieces of edge to be connected together. Gestalt psychologists describe this as grouping. Such a response is difficult for an algorithm that looks only within a small neighborhood. Even in rather simple images, there may be places along boundaries where the local gradient or other measure of edgeness drops.

In addition, edges may touch where regions abut. The algorithm is equally likely to follow either edge, which of course gives a nonsensical result. There may also be the problem of when to end the process. If the edge is a single, simple line, then it ends when it reaches the starting point. If the line reaches another feature that already has a defined boundary (from a previous application of the routine) or if it reaches the edge of the field of view, then there is no way to complete the outline.

The major problems with edge-following are:

1. It cannot by itself complete the segmentation of the image because it has to be given each new starting point and cannot determine whether there are more outlines that need to be followed.

2. The same edge-defining criteria used for following edges can be applied more easily by processing the entire image and then thresholding.

This produces a line of pixels that may be broken and incomplete (if the edge following would have been unable to continue) or may branch (if several boundaries touch). Methods are discussed in Chapter 7, however, which apply erosion/dilation logic to deal with some of these deficiencies. The global application of the processing operation finds all of the boundaries.

Figure 49 illustrates a few of these effects. The image consists of several hand-drawn dark lines, to which a small amount of random noise is added and a ridge-following algorithm applied (Van Helden, 1994). Each of the user-selected starting points is shown with the path followed by the automatic routine. The settings used for this example instruct the algorithm to consider points out to a distance of 5 pixels in deciding which direction to move in at each point. Increasing this number produces artificially smooth boundaries, and also takes more time as more neighbors must be searched. Conversely, reducing it makes it more likely to follow false turnings. Many of the paths are successful, but a significant number are not. By comparison, thresholding the image to select dark pixels, and then skeletonizing the resulting broad outline as discussed in Chapter 7, produces good boundary lines for all of the regions at once.

The same comparison can be made with a real image. **Figure 50** shows a fluorescence image from a light microscope. In this case, the inability of the fully automatic ridge-following method to track the boundaries has been supplemented by a manually assisted technique. The user draws a line near the boundary, and the algorithm moves the points onto the nearest (within some preset maximum distance) darkest point. This method, sometimes called "active contours" or "snakes," allows the user to overcome many of the difficulties in which the automatic method may wander

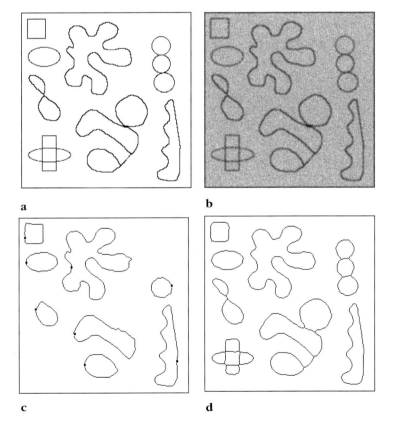

Figure 49. Test image for automatic line-following:
(a) hand-drawn lines;
(b) addition of random noise to a;
(c) lines found by automatic tracing, showing the starting points for each (notice that some portions of crossing or branching line patterns are not followed);
(d) lines found by thresholding and skeletonization.

a

b

c

d

Figure 50. Light microscope fluorescence image with three features:
   (a) original;
   (b) edge-following algorithm (blue shows fully automatic results, purple shows a feature that required manual assistance to outline);
   (c) outlines from **b** superimposed on the original;
   (d) brightness thresholding the original image;
   (e) skeletonized outlines from figure **d**;
   (f) outlines from **e** superimposed on the original.

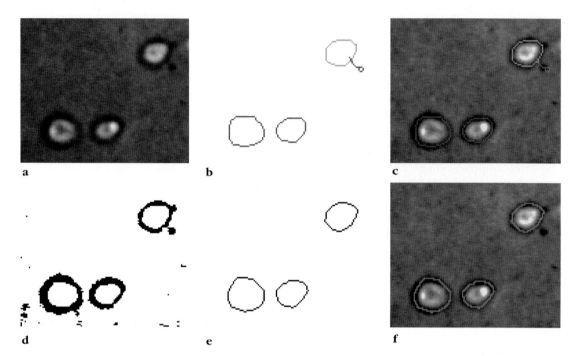

a   b   c

d   e   f

away from the correct line, never to return. It is still faster, however, to use thresholding and skeletonizing to get the boundary lines. Although the details of the lines differ, it is not evident that either method is consistently superior for delineation.

Contours

One type of line that may provide boundary information and is guaranteed to be continuous is a contour line. This is analogous to the iso-elevation contour lines drawn on topographic maps. The line marks a constant elevation or, in our case, a constant brightness in the image. These lines cannot end, although they may branch or loop back upon themselves. In a continuous image or an actual topographic surface, there is always a point through which the line can pass. For a discrete image, the brightness value of the line may not happen to correspond to any specific pixel value. Nevertheless, if there is a pair of pixels with one value brighter than and one value darker than the contour level, then the line must pass somewhere between them.

The contour line can, in principle, be fit as a polygon through the points interpolated between pixel centers for all such pairs of pixels that bracket the contour value. This actually permits measuring the locations of these lines, and the boundaries that they may represent, to less than the dimensions of one pixel, called sub-pixel sampling or measurement. This is rarely done for an entire image because of the amount of computation involved and the difficulty in representing the boundary by such a series of points, which must be assembled into a polygon.

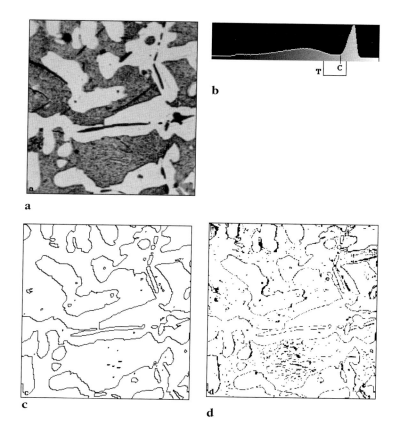

Figure 51. Cast iron (light micrograph) with ferrite (white) and graphite (dark):
(a) original image;
(b) brightness histogram showing levels used for contour (C) and threshold (T);
(c) contour lines drawn using the value shown in **b**;
(d) pixels selected by the threshold setting shown in **b**.

Instead, the most common use of contour lines is to mark the pixels that lie closest to, or closest to and above, the line. These pixels approximate the contour line to the resolution of the pixels in the original image, form a continuous band of touching pixels (touching in an eight-neighbor sense, as discussed in the following paragraph), and can be used to delineate features in many instances. Creating the line from the image is simply a matter of scanning the pixels once, comparing each pixel and its neighbors above and to the left to the contour value, and marking the pixel if the values bracket the test value.

Figure 51 shows a grey-scale image with several contour lines, drawn at arbitrarily chosen brightness values, marked on the histogram. Notice that setting a threshold range at this same brightness level, even with a fairly large range, does not produce a continuous line, because the brightness gradient in some regions is quite steep and no pixels fall within the range. The brightness gradient is very gradual in other regions, so a gradient image (**Figure 52**) obtained from the same original by applying a Sobel operator does not show all of the same boundaries, and does introduce more noise.

Drawing a series of contour lines on an image can be an effective way to show minor variations in brightness, as shown in **Figure 53**. Converting an image to a series of contour lines (**Figure 54**) is often able to delineate regions of similarity or structural meaning, even for complex three-dimensional scenes such as the figure shows. For one important class of images (range images) in which pixel brightness measures elevation, such a set of lines is the topographic map. Such images may result from radar imaging, the CSLM, interferometry, the STM or AFM, and other devices. **Figure 55** shows a scanned stylus image of a coin, with contour lines drawn to delineate the raised surfaces, and a similar image of a ball bearing. The contour lines on the ball show the roughness and out-of-roundness of the surface, and can be measured quantitatively for such a purpose.

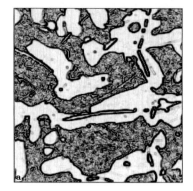
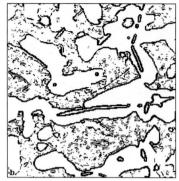

Figure 52. Gradient image obtained by applying a Sobel operator to **Figure 51a**, and the pixels selected by thresholding the 20% darkest (highest gradient) values.

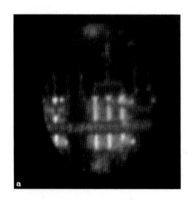
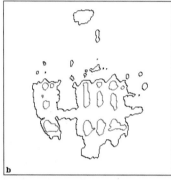

Figure 53. Ion microprobe image of boron implanted in a silicon wafer: (*a*) original image, in which brightness is proportional to concentration; (*b*) two iso-brightness or iso-concentration contour values, which make it easier to compare values in different parts of the image.

Figure 54. Real-world image (*a*) and four contour lines drawn at selected brightness values (*b*). No matter how irregular they become, the lines are always continuous and distinct.

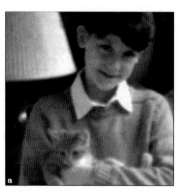
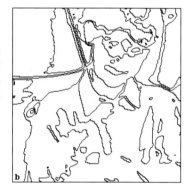

As discussed in Chapter 13, range images are often produced by surface elevation measurements, as shown in **Figure 56**. This image has elevation contours calculated from stereo pair views of a specimen in the TEM, in which the "mountains" are deposited contamination spots. The information from the contour lines can be used to generate a rendered surface as shown in the figure and discussed in Chapter 13, in order to illustrate the surface topography.

The contours drawn by selecting a brightness value on the histogram provide the same outline information as the edge pixels in regions determined by thresholding with the same value. The contour lines can be filled in to provide a pixel representation of the feature, using the logic discussed in Chapter 7. Conversely, the solid regions can be converted to an outline by another set of binary image processes. If the contour line is defined by pixel values, the information is identical to the thresholded regions. If sub-pixel interpolation has been used, then the resolution of the features may be better. The two formats for image representation are entirely complementary, although they have different advantages for storage, measurement, etc.

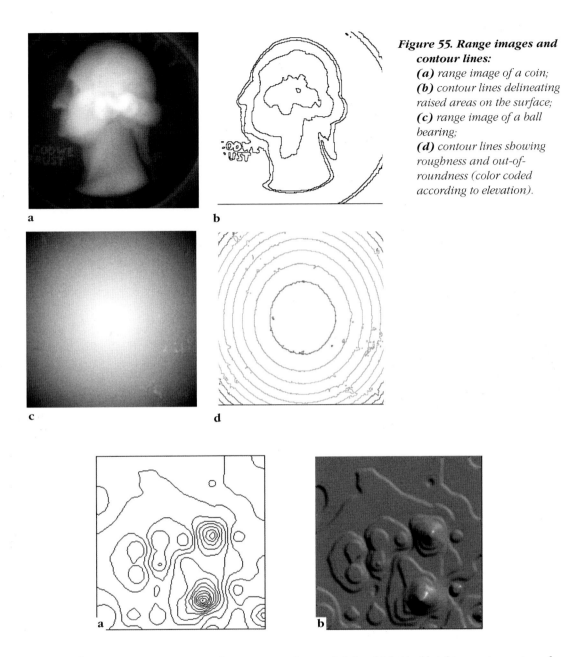

Figure 55. Range images and contour lines:
(a) range image of a coin;
(b) contour lines delineating raised areas on the surface;
(c) range image of a ball bearing;
(d) contour lines showing roughness and out-of-roundness (color coded according to elevation).

Figure 56. Elevation contour map from a range image (a) *in which pixel brightness represents surface elevation, and a reconstructed and rendered view of the surface **(b)**.*

Image representation

Different representations of the binary image are possible; some are more useful than others for specific purposes. Most measurements, such as feature area and position, can be directly calculated from a pixel-based representation by simple counting procedures. This can be stored in less space than the original array of pixels by using run-length encoding (also called chord encoding). This treats the image as a series of scan lines. For each sequential line across each region or feature, it stores the line number, start position, and length of the line. **Figure 57** illustrates this schematically.

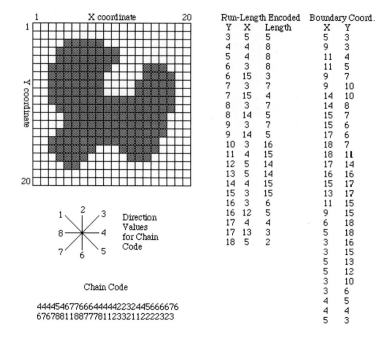

Figure 57. *Encoding the same region in a binary image by run-length encoding, boundary polygonal representation, or chain code.*

Run-Length Encoded			Boundary Coord.	
Y	X	Length	X	Y
3	5	5	5	3
4	4	8	9	3
5	4	8	11	4
6	3	8	11	5
6	15	3	9	7
7	3	7	9	10
7	15	4	14	10
8	3	7	14	8
8	14	5	15	7
9	3	7	15	6
9	14	5	17	6
10	3	16	18	7
11	4	15	18	11
12	5	14	17	14
13	5	14	16	16
14	4	15	15	17
15	3	15	13	17
16	3	6	11	15
16	12	5	9	15
17	4	4	6	18
17	13	3	5	18
18	5	2	3	16
			3	15
			5	13
			5	12
			3	10
			3	6
			4	5
			4	4
			5	3

Direction Values for Chain Code

Chain Code

4444546776664444422322445666676
676788118877781123321122222323

For typical images, the pixels are not randomly scattered, but collected together into regions or features so that the run-length encoded table is much smaller than the original image. This is the method used, for instance, to transmit fax messages over telephone lines. **Figure 58** shows how a black-and-white image is encoded for this purpose. In this example, the original image is 256 × 256 = 65,536 pixels, while the run-length table is only 1460 bytes long. The run-length table can be used directly for area and position measurements, with even less arithmetic than the pixel array. Because the chords are in the order in which the raster crosses the features, some logic is required to identify the chords with the features, but this is often done as the table is built.

The chord table is poorly suited for measuring feature perimeters or shape. Boundary representation, consisting of the coordinates of the polygon comprising the boundary, is superior for this task, although it is awkward for dealing with regions containing internal holes, because there is nothing to relate the interior boundary to the exterior. Again, logic must be used to identify the internal boundaries, keep track of which ones are exterior and which are interior, and construct a hierarchy of features within features, if needed.

A simple polygonal approximation to the boundary can be produced when it is needed from the run-length table by using the endpoints of the series of chords, as shown in **Figure 57**. A special form of this polygon can be formed from all of the boundary points, consisting of a series of short vectors from one boundary point to the next. On a square pixel array, each of these lines is either 1 or $\sqrt{2}$ pixels long and can only have 1 of 8 directions. Assigning a digit from 1 to 8 (or 0 to 7, or -3 to +4, depending on the particular implementation) to each direction and writing all of the numbers for the closed boundary in order produces chain code, also shown in **Figure 57**.

This form is particularly well suited for calculating perimeter or describing shape (Freeman, 1961, 1974; Cederberg, 1979). The perimeter is determined by counting the number of even and odd digits, multiplying the number of odd ones by $\sqrt{2}$ to correct for diagonal directions, and adding. The chain code also contains shape information, which can be used to locate corners, simplify the shape of the outline, match features independent of orientation, or calculate various shape descriptors.

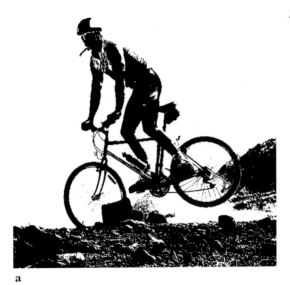

a

Figure 58. Representing a black-and-white image for fax transmission:
(a) original;
(b) run-length encoded (each horizontal line is marked with a red point at its start, just the position of the red point and the length of the line are sent);
(c) representing the same image with formed characters, a trick commonly used two decades ago.

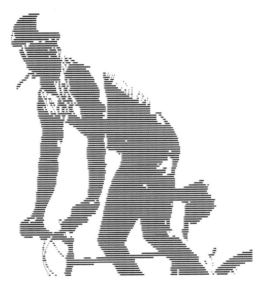

b

c

Most current-generation imaging systems use an array of square pixels, because it is well suited both to raster-scan acquisition devices and to processing images and performing measurements. If rectangular pixels are acquired by using a different pixel spacing along scan lines than between the lines, processing in either the spatial domain with neighborhood operations or in the frequency domain becomes much more difficult, because the different pixel distances as a function of orientation must be taken into account. The use of rectangular pixels also complicates measurements.

With a square pixel array, a minor problem exists, which we have already seen in the previous chapters on image processing: the four pixels diagonally adjacent to a central pixel are actually farther away than the four sharing an edge. An alternative arrangement that has been used in a few systems is to place the pixels in a hexagonal array. This has the advantage of equal spacing between all neighboring pixels, which simplifies processing and calculations. Its great disadvantage, however, is that standard cameras and other acquisition and display devices do not operate that way.

Figure 59. Ambiguous images:
(a) *If the pixels are assumed to touch at their corners, then this shows a line that separates the background pixels on either side; but those pixels also touch at their corners. If 8-connectedness or 4-connectedness is selected for feature pixels, then the opposite convention applies to background pixels;*
(b) *This shows either four separate features or one containing an internal hole, depending on the touching convention.*

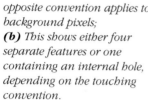

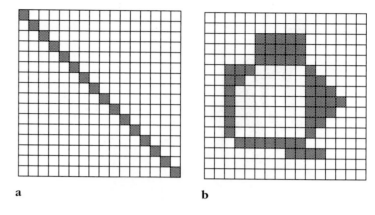

a   b

For a traditional square pixel array, it is necessary to decide whether pixels adjacent at a corner are actually touching. This will be important for the binary processing operations in Chapter 7. It is necessary in order to link pixels into features or follow the points around a boundary, as discussed previously. Although it is not evident whether one choice is superior to the other, whichever one is made, the background (the pixels which surround the features) must have the opposite relationship.

Figure 59 shows this dual situation. If pixels within a feature are assumed to touch any of their eight adjacent neighbors (called eight-connectedness), then the line of pixels in **Figure 59a** separates the background on either side, and the background pixels that are diagonally adjacent do not touch. They are therefore four-connected. Conversely, if the background pixels touch diagonally, the pixels are isolated and only touch along their faces. For the second image fragment shown, choosing an eight-connected rule for features (dark pixels) produces a single feature with an internal hole. If a four-connected rule is used, there are four features and the background, now eight-connected, is continuous.

This means that simply inverting an image (interchanging white and black) does not reverse the meaning of the features and background. **Figure 60** shows a situation in which the holes within a feature (separated from the background) become part of a single region in the reversed image. This can cause confusion in measurements and binary image processing. When feature dimensions as small as one pixel are important, there is some basic uncertainty. This is unavoidable and argues for using large arrays of small pixels to define small dimensions and feature topology accurately.

Other segmentation methods

Other methods are used for image segmentation besides the ones based on thresholding discussed previously. These are generally associated with fairly powerful computer systems and with attempts to understand images in the sense of machine vision and robotics (Ballard and Brown, 1982; Wilson and Spann, 1988). Two of the most widely described are split-and-merge and region growing, which appear to lie at opposite extremes in method.

Split-and-merge is a top-down method that begins with the entire image. Some image property is selected as a criterion to decide whether everything is uniform. This criterion is often based on the statistics from the brightness histogram. If the histogram is multimodal, or has a high standard

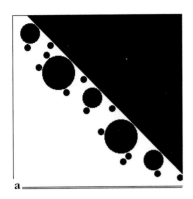
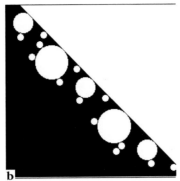

*Figure 60. Reversing an image (interchanging features and background) without changing the connectedness rules alters meaning. In image **a** the black pixels all touch at corners (8-connectedness), and so this is one feature with an irregular boundary. In image **b** the white pixels do not touch (4-connectedness), and so these are separate holes within the feature.*

deviation, etc., then the region is assumed to be nonuniform and is divided into four quadrants. Each quadrant is examined in the same way and subdivided again if necessary. The procedure continues until the individual pixel level is reached. The relationship between the parent region and the four quadrants, or children, is typically encoded in a quadtree structure, and another name is sometimes applied to this approach.

This is not the only way to subdivide the parent image and encode the resulting data structure. Thresholding can be used to divide each region into arbitrary subregions, which can be subdivided iteratively. This can produce final results having less blocky boundaries, but the data structure is much more complex, because all of the regions must be defined and the time required for the process is much greater.

Subdividing regions alone does not create a useful image segmentation. After each iteration of subdividing, each region is compared to adjacent ones that lie in different squares at a higher level in the hierarchy. If they are similar, they are merged together. The definition of "similar" may use the same tests applied to the splitting operation, or comparisons may be made only for pixels along the common edge. The latter has the advantage of tolerating gradual changes across the image.

Figure 61 shows an example in which only four iterations have been performed. A few large areas have already merged, and their edges will be refined as the iterations proceed. Other parts of the image contain individual squares that require additional subdivision before regions become visible.

An advantage of this approach is that a complete segmentation is achieved after a finite number of iterations (for instance, a 512-pixel-square image takes 9 iterations to reach individual pixels, because $2^9 = 512$). Also, the quadtree list of regions and subregions can be used for some measurements, and the segmentation identifies all of the different types of regions at one time. By comparison, thresholding methods typically isolate one type of region or feature at a time. They must be applied several times to deal with images containing more than one class of objects.

On the other hand, the split-and-merge approach depends on the quality of the test used to detect inhomogeneity in each region. Small subregions within large uniform areas can easily be missed with this method. Standard statistical tests that assume, for example, a normal distribution of pixel brightness within regions are rarely appropriate for real images, so more complicated procedures must be used (Yakimovsky, 1976). Tests used for subdividing and merging regions can also be expressed as image processing operations. A processed image can reveal the same edges and texture used for the split-and-merge tests in a way that allows direct thresholding. This is potentially less efficient, because time-consuming calculations may be applied to parts of the image that are

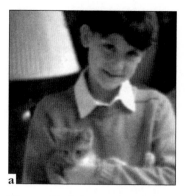 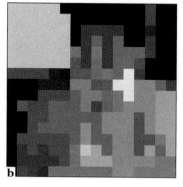 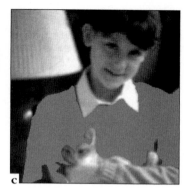

Figure 61. Other segmentation methods:
  (a) *original grey-scale image;*
  (b) *split and merge after four iterations;*
  (c) *region growing from a point in the girl's sweater.*

uniform, but the results are the same. Thresholding also has the advantage of identifying similar objects in different parts of the field of view as the same, which may not occur with split-and-merge.

Region-growing starts from the bottom, or individual pixel level, and works upward. Starting at some seed location (usually provided by the operator but in some cases located by image processing tools such as the top hat filter), neighboring pixels are examined one at a time and added to the growing region if they are sufficiently similar. Again, the comparison may be made to the entire region or just to the local pixels, with the latter method allowing gradual variations in brightness. The procedure continues until no more pixels can be added. **Figure 61c** shows an example in which one region has been identified; notice that it includes part of the cat as well as the girl's sweater. Then a new region is begun at another location. **Figure 62** shows an example of the application of this technique to a color image. The red boundary line shows the extent of the region grown from a starting point within the intestine.

If the same comparison tests are implemented to decide whether a pixel belongs to a region, the result of this procedure is the same as top-down split-and-merge. The difficulty with this approach is that the starting point for each region must be provided. Depending on the comparison tests employed, different starting points may not grow into identical regions. Also, no ideal structure is

Figure 62. Region-growing applied to a color image. The red lines show the boundaries of the region.

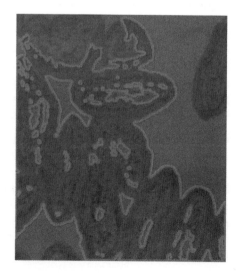

available to encode the data from this procedure, beyond keeping the entire pixel array until classification is complete. The complete classification is slow, because each pixel must be examined individually.

Region-growing also suffers from the conflicting needs to keep the test local, to see if an individual pixel should be added to the growing region, and to make it larger in scale, if not truly global, to ensure that the region has some unifying and distinct identity. If too small a test region is used, a common result is that regions leak out into adjoining areas or merge with different regions. This leaking or merging can occur if even a single pixel on the boundary can form a bridge.

Finally, there is no easy way to decide when the procedure is complete and all of the meaningful regions in the image have been found. Region-growing may be a useful method for selecting a few regions in an image, as compared to manual tracing or edge following, for example, but it is rarely the method of choice for complex images containing many regions (Zucker, 1976).

Edge following was mentioned above in terms of an algorithm that tries to mimic a human drawing operation by tracing along a boundary, and at each point selecting the next pixel to step toward based on local neighborhood values. Human vision does not restrict itself to such local decisions, but can use remote information to bridge over troublesome points. A machine vision approach that does the same constructs outlines of objects as deformable polygons. The sides of the polygon may be splines rather than straight lines, to achieve a smoother shape. These deformable boundaries are referred to as "snakes" (Kass et al., 1987). The minimum length of any side, the maximum angular change at any vertex, and other arbitrary fitting constants must reflect some independent knowledge about the region that is to be fitted. They must generally be adjusted for each application until the results are acceptable as compared to visual judgment.

Fitting is accomplished for all of the points on the boundary at once using a minimization technique, so the snakes can accommodate some missing or confusing points. They are particularly useful for tracking moving boundaries in a sequence of images, because the deformation of the snake from one moment to the next must be small. This makes them useful for tracking moving objects in robotics vision. When applied to three-dimensional arrays of voxels, as in medical imaging, they become deformable polyhedra and are called balloons.

The general classification problem

The various methods described so far have relied on human judgment to recognize the presence of regions and to define them by delineating the boundary or selecting a range of brightness values. Methods have been discussed that can start with an incomplete definition and refine the segmentation to achieve greater accuracy or consistency. Fully automatic techniques also determine how many classes of objects are present and fully subdivide the image to isolate them. They are not used very often in small computer-based systems, however, and are often much less efficient than using some human input. The task of general image segmentation can be treated as an example of a classification problem. Similar to most techniques involving elements or artificial intelligence, it may not use the same inputs or decision methods that a human employs, but it seeks to duplicate the results (and often succeeds).

One successful approach to general classification has been used with satellite imagery, in which many wavelength bands of data are available (Reeves, 1975). If each pixel in the image is plotted in a high-dimensionality space, where each axis is the measured brightness in one of the wavelength bands, it is expected that points corresponding to different classes of land use, crop type, soil or rock type, and so forth will cluster together and the clusters will be well separated from each other, as indicated in **Figure 63**. The problem then reduces to finding the clusters and fitting boundaries between them that can be used for classification. Finding clusters and boundaries between regions is discussed in a more general context in Chapter 10.

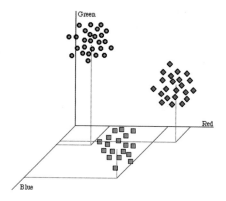

Figure 63. *Schematic illustration of pixel classification in color space. Each pixel is plotted according to its color values, and clusters identify the various regions present.*

Reduced to a single dimension (a simple grey-scale image), this classification begins with the brightness histogram. The cluster analysis looks for peaks and tries to draw thresholds between them. This is successful in a few specialized tasks, such as counting cells of one type on a microscope slide. As the number of dimensions increases, for instance using the RGB or HSI data from color imagery or adding values from a derived texture or gradient image, the separation of the clusters usually becomes more distinct. Satellite imagery with several discrete visible and infrared wavelength bands is especially well suited to this approach.

Clusters are easier to recognize when they contain many similar points, but minor regions or uncommon objects may be overlooked. Also, the number of background points surrounding the clusters (or more often lying along lines between them) confuse the automatic algorithms. These points arise from the finite size of pixels that straddle the boundaries between regions. Finding a few major clusters may be straightforward — being sure that all have been found is not.

Even after the clusters have been identified (and here, some *a priori* knowledge or input from a human can be of great assistance), different strategies can be employed to use this information to classify new points. One is to surround each cluster with a boundary, typically either a polyhedron formed by planes lying perpendicular to the lines between the cluster centers, or n-dimensional ellipsoids. Points falling inside any of these regions are immediately classified.

Particularly for the ellipsoid case, it is also possible to have a series of concentric boundaries that enclose different percentages of the points in the cluster, which can be used to give a probability of classification to new points. This is sometimes described as a "fuzzy" classification method.

A third approach is to find the nearest classified point to each new point and assign that identity to the new one. This method has several drawbacks, particularly when some densely populated clusters and others with very few members are present, or when the clusters are close or overlapping. It requires considerable time to search through a large universe of existing points to locate the closest one, as well. An extension of this technique is also used, in which a small number of nearest neighbors are identified and "vote" for the identity of the new point.

Segmentation of grey-scale images into regions for measurement or recognition is probably the most important single problem area for image analysis. Many novel techniques have been used that are rather ad hoc and narrow in their range of applicability. Review articles by Fu and Mui (1981) and Haralick and Shapiro (1988) present good guides to the literature. Most standard image analysis textbooks, such as Rosenfeld and Kak (1982), Castleman (1979), Gonzalez and Wintz (1987), Russ (1990b), and Pratt (1991) also contain sections on segmentation.

All these various methods and modifications are used extensively in other artificial intelligence situations (see, for example, Fukunaga, 1990). They may be implemented in hardware, software, or some combination of the two. Only limited application of any of these techniques has been made to the segmentation problem, although it is likely that the use of such methods will increase in the future as more color or multiband imaging is done and readily accessible computer power continues to increase.

7

Processing Binary Images

Binary images, as discussed in the preceding chapter, consist of groups of pixels selected on the basis of some property. The selection may be performed by thresholding brightness values, perhaps using several grey scale images containing different color bands, or processed to extract texture or other information. The goal of binarization is to separate features from background, so that counting, measurement, or matching operations can be performed.

As shown by the examples in Chapter 6, however, the result of the segmentation operation is rarely perfect. For images of realistic complexity, even the most elaborate segmentation routines misclassify some pixels as foreground or background. These may either be pixels along the boundaries of regions or patches of noise within regions. The major tools for working with binary images fit broadly into two groups: Boolean operations, for combining images, and morphological operations which modify individual pixels within images.

Boolean operations

In the section on thresholding color images, in Chapter 6, a Boolean operation was introduced to combine the data from individual color plane images. Setting thresholds on brightness values in each of the RGB (red, green, blue) planes allows pixels to be selected that fall into those ranges. This technique produces three binary images, which can then be combined with a logical "AND" operation. The procedure examines the three images pixel by pixel, keeping pixels for the selected regions if they are turned on in all three images.

The color thresholding example is an example of a situation in which pixel brightness values at the same location in several different images (the color channels) must be compared and combined. In some situations it is useful to compare the location and brightness value of pixels in two images. Figure 1 shows an example. Two x-ray maps of the same area on a mineral sample show the intensity distributions, and hence represent the concentration distributions for aluminum and silicon. A colocalization plot uses the pixel brightness values for each location in both images as coordinates and increments the plot. Regions in the resulting plot that have many counts represent combinations of elemental concentrations in the original sample. In the example plot, there are four phases present based on Si/Al combinations, and these can be observed in the original images. Colocalization is also used for biological samples prepared with multiple stains.

Figure 1. Colocalization: (a, b) x-ray maps showing the intensity distribution for Al and Si in a mineral; *(c)* colocalization plot.

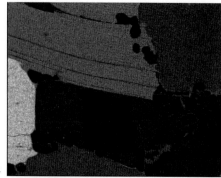
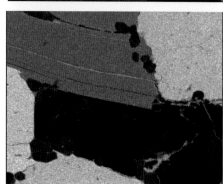

a

b

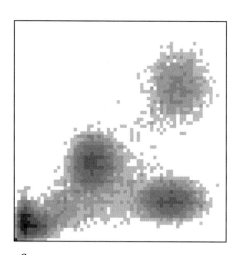

c

When a colocalization plot shows specific combinations of intensity values that are share the same location, each image can be thresholded and the two binary images combined with an AND to produce an image of the selected regions.

Note: The terminology used here will be that of "ON" (pixels that are part of the selected foreground features) and "OFF" (the remaining pixels, which are part of the background). There is no universal standard for whether the selected pixels are displayed as white, black, or some other color. In many cases, systems that portray the selected regions as white on a black background on the display screen may reverse this and print hardcopy of the same image with black features on a white background. This reversal apparently arises from the fact that in each case, the selection of foreground pixels is associated with some positive action in the display (turning on the electron beam) or printout (depositing ink on the paper). It seems to cause most users little difficulty, provided that something is known about the image. Many of the images used here are not common objects and some are made-up examples; therefore, it is important to be consistent in defining the foreground pixels (those of interest) in each case. The convention used here is that ON pixels (features) are shown as black while OFF pixels (background) are white.

Returning to our desire to combine the information from several image planes, the AND operation requires that a pixel at location *i,j* be ON in each individual plane to show up in the result. Pixels having the correct amount of blue but not of red will be omitted, and vice versa. As noted previously, this marks out a rectangle in two dimensions, or a rectangular prism in higher dimensions, for the pixel values to be included. More complicated combinations of color values can be described by delineating an irregular region in n dimensions for pixel selection. The advantage of simply ANDing discrete ranges is that it can be performed very efficiently and quickly using binary images.

Other Boolean logical rules can be employed to combine binary images. The four possibilities are AND, OR, Ex-OR (Exclusive OR) and NOT. **Figure 2** illustrates each of these basic operations. **Figure 3** shows a few of the possible combinations. All are performed pixel-by-pixel. The illustrations are based on combining two images at a time, because any logical rule involving more than two images can be broken down to a series of steps using just two at a time. The illustrations in the figures are identical to the Venn diagrams used in logic.

As described previously, AND requires that pixels be ON in both of the original images in order to be ON in the result. Pixels that are ON in only one or the other original image are OFF in the result. The OR operator turns a pixel ON in the result if it is ON in either of the original images. In the example shown in **Figure 32** of **Chapter 6**, complementary directions and thus grey-scale values, result from the Sobel direction operator as it encounters opposite sides of each striation. Thresholding each direction separately would require an OR to combine them to show the correct regions.

Ex-OR turns a pixel ON in the result if it is ON in either of the original images, but not if it is ON in both. That means that combining (with an OR) the results of ANDing together two images with those from Ex-ORing them produces the same result as an OR in the first place. There are, in fact, many ways to arrange different combinations of the four Boolean operators to produce identical results.

Figure 2. Simple Boolean operations:
    (a, b) two binary images;
    (c) A OR B;
    (d) A AND B;
    (e) A exOR B;
    (f) NOT A.

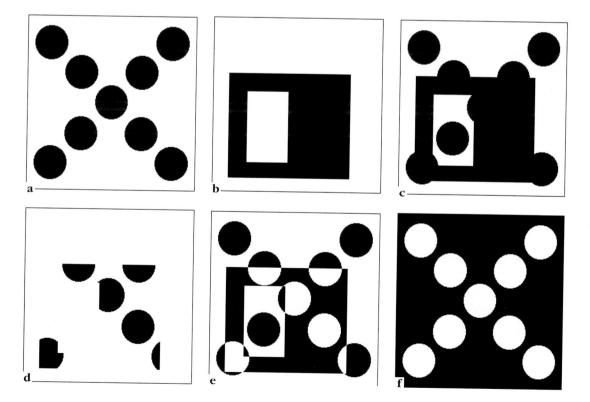

Figure 3. Combined Boolean operations:
  (a) (NOT A) AND B;
  (b) A AND (NOT B);
  (c) (NOT A) AND (NOT B);
  (d) NOT (A AND B);
  (e) (NOT A) OR B;
  (f) A OR (NOT B)

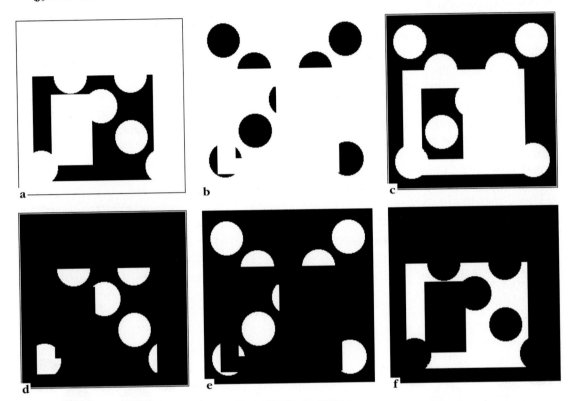

AND, OR, and Ex-OR require two original images and produce a single image as a result. NOT requires only a single image. It simply reverses each pixel, turning pixels that were ON to OFF and vice versa. Some systems implement NOT by swapping black and white values for each pixel. As long as we are dealing with pixel-level detail, this works correctly. Later, when feature-level combinations are described, the difference between an eight-connected feature and its four-connected background (discussed in Chapter 6) will have to be taken into account.

Given two binary images A and B, the combination (NOT A) AND B will produce an image containing pixels that lie within B but outside A. This is quite different from NOT (A AND B), which selects pixels that are not ON in both A and B. It is also different from A AND (NOT (B)), as shown in **Figure 3**. The order of operators is important and the liberal use of parentheses to clarify the order and scope of operations is crucial. Actually, the four operations discussed previously are redundant. Three would be enough to produce all of the same results. Consequently, some systems may omit one of them (usually Ex-OR). For simplicity, however, all four will be used in the examples that follow.

Combining Boolean operations

When multiple criteria are available for selecting the pixels to be kept as foreground, they may be combined using any of these Boolean combinations. The most common situations are multiband images, such as produced by a satellite or a scanning electron microscope (SEM). In the case of the SEM, an x-ray detector is often used to create an image (called an x-ray dot map) showing the spatial distribution of a selected element. These images may be quite noisy (Chapter 3) and difficult to threshold (Chapter 6); however, by suitable long-term integration or spatial smoothing, they can lead to useful binary images that indicate locations where the concentration of the element is above some user-selected level.

This selection is usually performed by comparing the measured x-ray intensity to some arbitrary threshold, since there is a finite level of background signal resulting from the process of slowing down the electrons in the sample. The physical background of this phenomenon is not important here. The very poor statistical characteristics of the dot map (hence the name) make it difficult to directly specify a concentration level as a threshold. The x-ray intensity in one part of the image may vary from another region for the following reasons:

1. A change in that element's concentration
2. A change in another element that selectively absorbs or fluoresces the first element's radiation
3. A change in specimen density or surface orientation. Comparison of one specimen to another is further hampered by the difficulty in exactly reproducing instrument conditions. These effects all complicate the relationship between elemental concentration and recorded intensity.

Furthermore, the very poor statistics of the images (due to the extremely low efficiency for producing x-rays with an electron beam and the low beam intensity required for good spatial resolution in SEM images) mean that these images often require processing, either as grey-scale images (e.g., smoothing) or after binarization (using the morphological tools discussed below). For our present purpose, we will assume that binary images showing the spatial distribution of some meaningful concentration level of several elements can be obtained.

As shown in **Figure** 4, the SEM also produces more conventional images using secondary or backscattered electrons. These have superior spatial resolution and better feature shape definition, but with less elemental specificity. The binary images from these sources can be combined with the x-ray or elemental information.

Figure 5 shows one example: The x-ray maps for iron (Fe) and silicon (Si) were obtained by smoothing and thresholding the grey scale image. Notice that in the grey scale images, there is a just-discernible difference in the intensity level of the Fe x-rays in two different areas. This is too small a difference for reliable thresholding. Even the larger differences in Si intensity are difficult to separate, however, Boolean logic easily combines the images to produce an image of the region containing Fe but not Si.

Figure 6 shows another example from the same data. The regions containing silver (Ag) are generally bright in the backscattered electron image, but some other areas are also bright. On the other hand, the Ag x-ray map does not have precise region boundaries because of the poor statistics. Combining the two binary images with an AND produces the desired regions. More complicated sequences of Boolean logical operations can easily be imagined (**Figure 7**).

It is straightforward to imagine a complex specimen containing many elements. Paint pigment particles with a diverse range of compositions provide one example. In order to count or measure a particular class of particles (pigments, as opposed to brighteners or extenders), it might be necessary to specify those containing iron or chromium or aluminum, but not titanium or sulfur. This would be written as

$$\text{(Fe OR Cr OR Al) AND (NOT (Ti OR S))} \tag{1}$$

The resulting image might then be combined with a higher-resolution binary produced by thresholding a secondary or backscattered electron image to delineate particle boundaries. Performing these operations can be cumbersome but is not difficult.

Most of the examples shown in earlier chapters that used multiple image planes (e.g., different colors or elements) or different processing operations (e.g., combining brightness and texture) use a Boolean AND to combine the separately thresholded binary images. The AND requires that the pixels meet all of the criteria in order to be kept. There are some cases in which the Boolean OR is more appropriate. One is illustrated in **Chapter 4, Figure 81**. This is an image of sand grains in a sandstone, viewed through polarizers. Each rotation of the analyzer causes different grains to be-

Figure 4. SEM results from a mineral:
   (a) backscattered electrons;
   (b) secondary electrons;
   (c) silicon (Si) x-ray map;
   (d) iron (Fe) x-ray map;
   (e) copper (Cu) x-ray map;
   (f) silver (Ag) x-ray map.

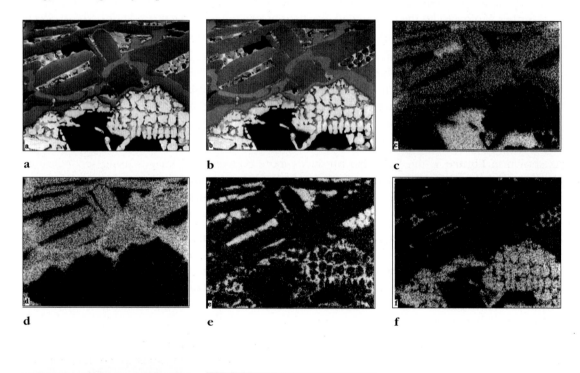

a   b   c

d   e   f

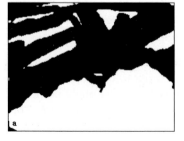
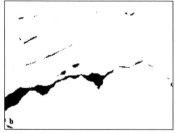

Figure 5. (a) *Iron;* ***(b)*** *iron AND NOT silicon*

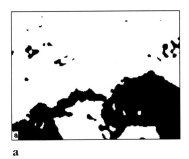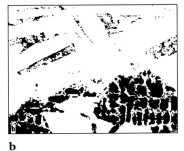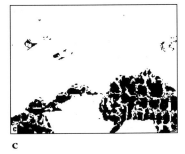

a   b   c

Figure 6. *(a)* *Silver;* *(b)* *bright levels from backscattered electron image;* *(c)* *image* *a* *AND image* *b.*

Figure 7. Further combination to delineate structure: (Cu OR Ag) AND NOT (Fe).

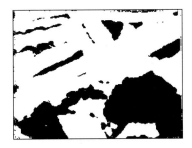

come bright or colored. In the earlier chapter, it was shown that keeping the brightest pixel value at each location as the analyzer is rotated gives an image that shows all of the grains.

Figure 8 shows an alternative approach to the same problem. Each individual image is thresholded to select those grains that are bright for that particular analyzer rotation angle. Then, all of the binary images are combined using a Boolean OR. The resulting combination delineates most of the grains, although the result is not as good as the grey-level operation for the same number of analyzer rotations.

Masks

The previous description of using Boolean logic to combine images makes the assumption that both images are binary (that is, black and white). It is also possible to use a binary image as a mask to modify a grey-scale image. This is most often done to blank out (i.e., set to background) some portion of the grey-scale image, either to create a display in which only the regions of interest are visible or to select regions whose brightness, density, and so forth are to be measured. **Figure 9** shows an example (a protein separation gel) in which the dark spots are isolated by thresholding, and then the thresholded binary image is applied as a mask to produce separated features for measurement that retain the original density values.

This operation can be performed in several physical ways. The binary mask can be used in an overlay, or alpha channel, in the display hardware to prevent pixels from being displayed. It is also possible to use the mask to modify the stored image. This can done by multiplying the grey-scale image by the binary image, with the convention that the binary image values are 0 (OFF) or 1 (ON) at each pixel. In some systems this result is implemented by combining the grey-scale and binary images to keep whichever value is darker or brighter. For instance, if the mask is white for background and black for foreground pixels then the brighter pixel values at each location will erase all background pixels and keep the grey value for the foreground pixels.

This capability has been used in earlier chapters to display the results of various processing and thresholding operations. It is easier to judge the performance of thresholding by viewing selected

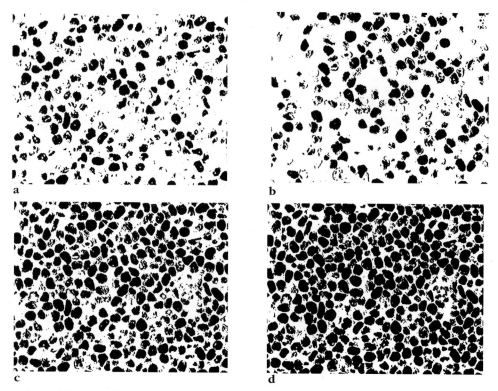

Figure 8. Combining multiple binary images.
(a, b) *binary images obtained by thresholding two of the polarized light images of a petrographic thin section of a sandstone (**Figure 81** in **Chapter 4**);*
(c) *the result of ORing together six such images from different rotations of the analyzer;*
(d) *comparison binary image produced by thresholding the grey scale image obtained by combining the same six color images to keep the brightest pixel at each location.*

pixels with the original grey-scale information, rather than just looking at the binary image. This format can be seen in the examples of texture operators in Chapter 4, for instance, as well as in Chapter 6 on Thresholding. It is also useful to use a mask obtained by thresholding one version of an image to view another version. **Figure 10** shows an example, in which values represent the orientation angle (from the Sobel derivative) of grain boundaries in the aluminum alloy are masked by thresholding the magnitude of the gradient to isolate only the boundaries.

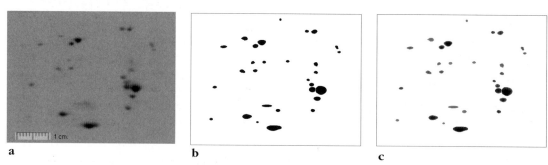

Figure 9. Preserving feature intensity values: *(a)* *original 2D gel;* *(b)* *thresholded spots;* *(c)* *masked image in which pixels within the spots retain their original brightness values.*

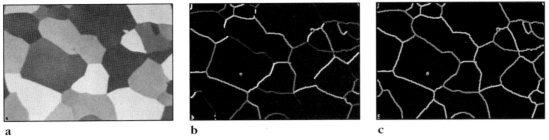

a b c

Figure 10. *Masking one image with another. The direction of a Sobel gradient applied to the light microscope image of an aluminum alloy is shown only in the regions where the magnitude of the gradient is large.*

Another use of masking and Boolean image combination is shown in **Figure 11**. An essentially cosmetic application, it is still useful and widely employed. A label superimposed on an image using either black or white may be difficult to read if the image contains a full range of brightness values. In this example, the label is used to create a mask that is one pixel larger in all directions, using dilation (discussed later in this chapter). This mask is then used to erase the pixels in the grey-scale image to white before writing in the label in black (or vice versa). The result maintains legibility for the label while obscuring a minimum amount of the image.

Finally, a binary image mask can be used to combine portions of two (or more) grey-scale images. This is shown in **Figure 12**. The composite image represents, in a very simple way, the kind of image overlays and combinations common in printing, advertising, and commercial graphic arts. Although it is rarely suitable for scientific applications, this example will perhaps serve to remind us that modifying images to create things that are not real has become relatively easy with modern computer technology. This justifies a certain skepticism in examining images, which were once considered iron-clad evidence of the truth. Detecting forgeries in digital images can be quite difficult if constructed with enough skill (Russ, 2001a).

From pixels to features

The Boolean operations described above deal with individual pixels in the image. For some purposes it is necessary to identify the pixels forming part of a connected whole. As discussed in Chapter 6, it is possible to adopt a convention for touching that is either eight-connected or

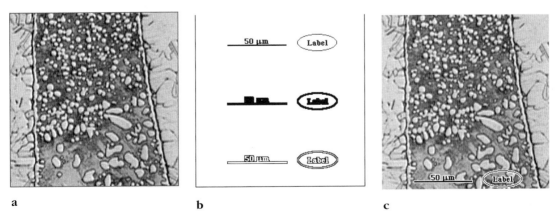

a b c

Figure 11. *Using a mask to apply a label to an image. The original image contains both white and black areas, so that simple superimposition of text will not be visible. A mask is created by dilating the label and Ex-ORing that with the original. The composite is then superimposed on the grey-scale image.*

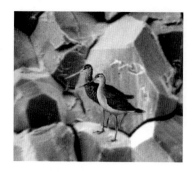

four-connected for the pixels in a single feature (sometimes referred to as a blob to indicate that no interpretation of the connected group of pixels has been inferred as representing anything specific in the image). Whichever convention is adopted, grouping pixels into features is an important step (Levialdi, 1992; Ritter, 1996).

It is possible to imagine starting with one pixel (any ON pixel, selected at random) and checking its four- or eight-neighbor positions, labeling each pixel that is ON as part of the same feature, and then iteratively repeating the operation until no neighbors remain. Then a new unlabeled pixel would be chosen and the operation repeated, continuing until every ON pixel in the image was labeled as part of some feature. The usual way of proceeding with this deeply recursive operation is to create a stack to place pixel locations as they are found to be neighbors of already labeled pixels. Pixels are removed from the stack as their neighbors are examined. The process ends when the stack is empty.

It is more efficient to deal with pixels in groups. If the image has already been run-length or chord encoded, as discussed in Chapter 6, then all of the pixels within the chord are known to touch, touching any of them is equivalent to touching all, and the only candidates for touching are those on adjacent lines. This fact makes possible a very straightforward labeling algorithm that passes one time through the image. Each chord's end points are compared to those of chords in the preceding line; if they touch or overlap (based on a simple comparison of values), the label from the preceding line is attached to this chord. If not, then a new label is used.

If a chord touches two chords in the previous line that had different labels, then the two labels are identified with each other (this handles the bottom of a letter "U" for example). All of the occurrences of one label can be changed to the other, either immediately or later. When the pass through the image or the list of chords is complete, all of the chords, and therefore all of the pixels, are identified and the total number of labels (and therefore features) is known. **Figure 13** shows this logic in the form of a flow chart.

For boundary representation (including the special case of chain code), the analysis is partially complete, since the boundary already represents a closed path around a feature. If features contained no holes and no feature could ever be surrounded by another, this would provide complete information. Unfortunately, this is not always the case. It is usually necessary to reconstruct the pixel array to identify pixels with feature labels (Kim et al., 1988).

In any case, once the individual features have been labeled, several additional Boolean operations are possible. One is to find and fill holes within features. Any pixel that is part of a hole is defined as OFF (i.e., part of the background) and is surrounded by ON pixels. For boundary representation, that means the pixel is within a boundary. For pixel representation, it means it is not connected to other pixels that eventually form a path to the edge of the field of view.

Recalling that the convention for touching (eight- or four-connectedness) must be different for the background than for the foreground, we can identify holes most easily by inverting the image

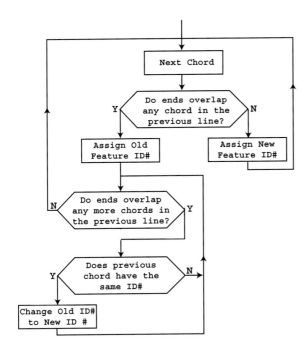

(replacing white with black and vice versa) and labeling the resulting pixels as though they were features, as shown step-by-step in **Figure 14**. Features in this inverted image that do not touch any side of the field of view are the original holes. If the pixels are added back to the original image (using a Boolean OR), the result is to fill any internal holes in the original features.

One very simple example of the application of this technique is shown in **Figure 15**. In this image of spherical particles, the center of each feature has a brightness very close to that of the substrate due to the lighting. Thresholding the brightness values gives a good delineation of the outer boundary of the particles, but the centers have holes. Filling them as described produces a corrected representation of the particles, which can be measured. This type of processing is commonly required for SEM images, whose brightness varies as a function of local surface slope so that particles frequently appear with bright edges and dark centers.

This problem is not restricted to convex surfaces nor to the SEM. **Figure 16** shows a light microscope image of spherical pores in an enamel coating. The light spots in the center of many of the pores vary in brightness, depending on the depth of the pore. They must be corrected by filling the features in a thresholded binary image.

Figure 17 shows a more complicated situation requiring several operations. The SEM image shows the boundaries of the spores clearly to a human viewer, but they cannot be directly revealed by thresholding because the shades of grey are also present in the substrate. Applying an edge-finding algorithm (in this example, a Frei and Chen operator) delineates the boundaries, and it is then possible to threshold them to obtain feature outlines, as shown. These must be filled using the method described above. Further operations are then needed before measurement: erosion, to remove the other thresholded pixels in the image, and watershed segmentation, to separate the touching objects. Both are described later in this chapter.

The use of edge-enhancement routines, discussed in Chapter 4, is often followed by thresholding the outlines of features and then filling in the interior holes. In some situations, several different methods must be used and the information combined. **Figure 18** shows a very difficult example,

Figure 14. Light microscope image of red blood cells:
　(a) original;
　(b) thresholded, which shows the thicker outer edges of the blood cells but not the thinner central regions;
　(c) image *b* inverted;
　(d) removing the edge-touching background from image *c*;
　(e) combining the features in image *d* with those in image *b* using a Boolean OR;
　(f) removing small features (dirt), edge-touching features (which cannot be measured), and separating touching features in *e*.

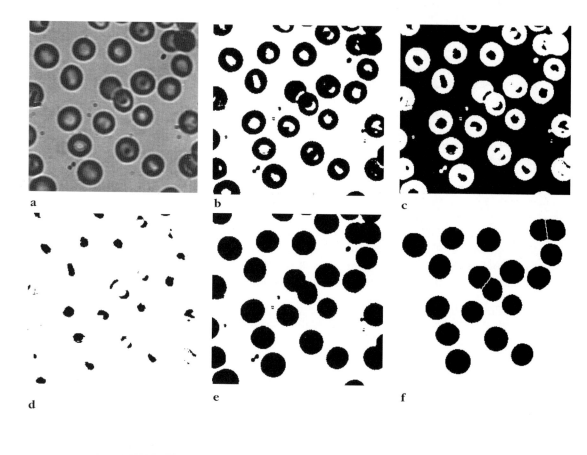

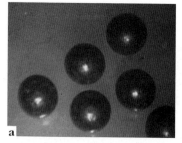

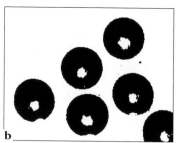

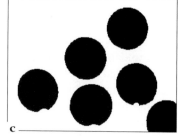

Figure 15. Image of buckshot with near-vertical incident illumination;
　(a) original grey-scale image;
　(b) brightness thresholded after leveling illumination;
　(c) internal holes filled and small regions (noise) in background removed by erosion.

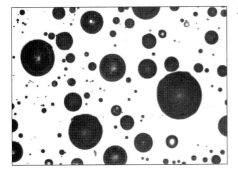

Figure 16. *Light microscope image of a polished section through an enamel coating on steel (courtesy V. Benes, Research Institute for Metals, Panenské Brezany, Czechoslovakia) shows bright spots of reflected light within many pores (depending on their depth).*

Figure 17. Segmentation of an image using multiple steps:
    (a) *original SEM image of spores on a glass slide;*
    (b) *application of a Frei and Chen edge operator to image* **a***;*
    (c) *thresholding of image* **b***;*
    (d) *filling of holes in the binary image of the edges;*
    (e) *erosion to remove the extraneous pixels; in image* **d***;*
    (f) *watershed segmentation to separate touching features in image* **e***.*

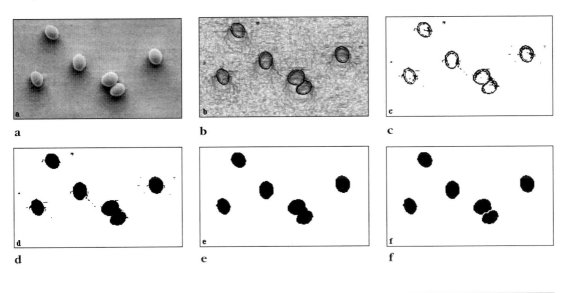

a   b   c

d   e   f

Figure 18. *Section through an epoxy resin containing bubbles. To delineate the bubbles for measurement, the bright, dark, and outlined pores must be processed in different ways and the results combined with a Boolean OR.*

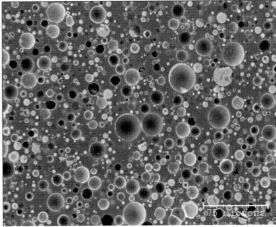

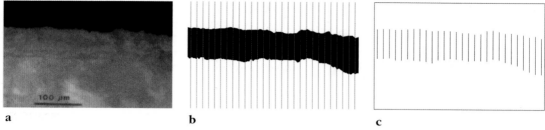

a   b   c

Figure 19. Measurement of layer thickness:
(a) paint layer viewed in cross section;
(b) thresholded layer, with superimposed grid of vertical lines; (c) AND of lines with layer producing line segments for measurement.

bubbles in epoxy resin. Some of the concave pores are dark, some light, and some bounded by a bright edge. Processing and thresholding each type of pore and then combining the results with a Boolean OR produces an image delineating all of the pores.

The Boolean AND operation is also widely used to apply measurement templates to images. For instance, consider the measurement of coating thickness on a wire or plate viewed in cross section. In the examples of **Figures 19** and **20**, the layer can be readily thresholded, but it is not uniform in thickness. In order to obtain a series of discrete thickness values for statistical interpretation, it is easy to AND the binary image of the coating with a template or grid consisting of lines normal to the coating. These lines can be easily measured. In **Figure 19**, for the case of a coating on a flat surface, the lines are vertical. For a cylindrical structure such as a similar coating on a wire, or the wall thickness of a tube, a set of radial lines can be used.

In the example of **Figure 20**, the vein is approximately circular in cross section and the lines do not perpendicularly intersect the wall, introducing a cosine error in the measurement which may or may not be acceptable. That the cross section is not round may indicate that the section plane is not perpendicular to the vein axis, which would introduce another error in the measurement. The measurement of three-dimensional structures from two-dimensional section images is dealt with by stereological techniques discussed in more detail in Chapter 8.

Figure 21 illustrates a situation in which the length of the lines give the layer thickness indirectly, requiring stereological interpretation. The image shows a section plane through coated particles

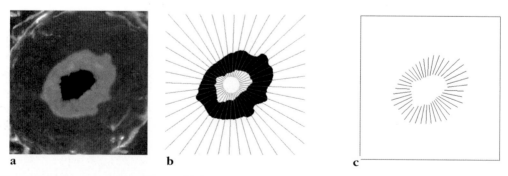

a   b   c

Figure 20. Measurement of layer thickness:
(a) cross section of vein in tissue;
(b) thresholded wall with superimposed grid of radial lines;
(c) AND of lines with layer producing line segments for measurement (note the cosine errors introduced by non-perpendicular alignment of grid lines to wall).

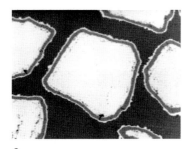 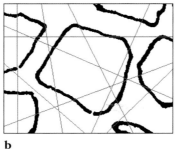 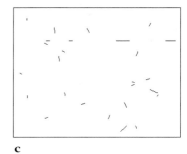

a   b   c

Figure 21. Measuring coating thickness on particles:
    (a) *original grey-scale image of a random section through embedded, coated particles;*
    (b) *thresholded binary image of the coating of interest with superimposed grid of random lines;*
    (c) *AND of the lines with the coating producing line segments for measurement.*

embedded in a metallographic mount and polished. The section plane does not go through the center of the particles, so the coating appears thicker than the actual three-dimensional thickness. This is handled by a placing a grid of random lines in the template. The distribution of line intercept lengths is related to that of the coating thickness in the normal direction. The average of the inverse intercept lengths is two-thirds the inverse of the true coating thickness, so this value can be obtained even if the image does not include a perpendicular cross section through the coating.

Selection of an appropriate grid is crucial to the success of measurements. Chapter 8 discusses the principal stereological measurements made on microstructures, to determine the volumes, surface areas, lengths, and topological properties of the components present. Many of these procedures are performed by counting the intersections made by various grids with the structures of interest. The grids typically consist of arrays of points or lines, and the lines used include regular and random grids of straight lines, circular arcs and cycloids, depending on the type of measurement desired, and the procedure used to select and prepare the specimens being imaged. In all cases, if the image can be thresholded successfully to delineate the structure, then a Boolean AND with the appropriate grid produces a result that can be measured. In some situations this requires measuring the lengths of lines, and in others simply counting the number of intersections produced.

Even for very complex or subtle images for which automatic processing and thresholding cannot delineate the structures of interest, the superimposition of grids as a mask may be important. Many stereological procedures that require only counting of intersections of various types of grids with features of interest are extremely efficient and capable of providing unbiased estimates of valuable structural parameters. Combining image capture and processing to enhance the visibility of structures with overlays of the appropriate grids — arrays of points or lines, the latter including straight lines, circles and cycloids — allows the human user to recognize the important features and intersections (Russ, 1995a). The counting may be performed manually or the computer may also assist by tallying mouse-clicks or counting marks that the user places on the image. The combination of human recognition with computer assistance provides efficient solutions to many image analysis problems.

Boolean logic with features

Having identified or labeled the pixel groupings as features, it is possible to carry out Boolean logic at the feature level, rather than at the pixel level. **Figure 22** shows the principle of a feature-based AND. Instead of simply keeping the pixels that are common to the two images, entire features are kept if any part of them touches. This preserves the entire feature, so that it can be correctly counted or measured if it is selected by the second image.

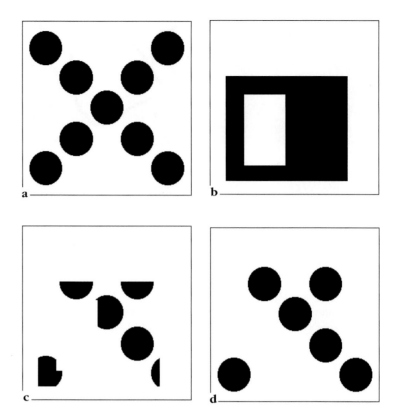

Figure 22. Schematic diagram of feature-based AND: *(a, b)* test images; *(c)* pixel-based Boolean AND of images a and b; *(d)* feature based AND of image *a* with image *b*.

Feature-AND requires a feature labeling operation to be performed on at least one of the images to be combined. Touching pixels in one image are identified as features as described previously. Then each pixel that is ON in one of those features is checked against the second image. If any of the pixels in the feature match an ON pixel in the second image, the entire feature in the first image is copied to the result. This is not the only possible implementation. It would be equally possible to check each pixel in the second image against the first, but that is less efficient. The method outlined limits the comparison to those pixels which are on, and halts the test for each feature whenever any pixel within it is matched.

Notice that unlike the more common pixel based AND, this statement does not commute; this means that (A Feature-AND B) does not produce the same result as (B Feature-AND A), as illustrated in **Figure 23**. The use of NOT with Feature-AND is straightforwardly implemented, for instance by carrying out the same procedure and erasing each feature in the first image that is matched by any pixel in the second. However, there is no need for a Feature-OR statement, since this would produce the identical result as the conventional pixel-based OR.

One use for the Feature-AND capability is to use markers within features to select them. For example, these might be cells containing a stained organelle or fibers in a composite containing a characteristic core. In any case, two binary images are produced by thresholding. In one image, the entire features are delineated, and in the second the markers are present. Applying the Feature-AND logic then selects all of the features which contain a marker.

This use of markers to select features is a particularly valuable capability in an image analysis system. **Figure 24** illustrates one way that it can be used. The original image has several red features, only some of which contain darker regions within. If one copy of the image is thresholded

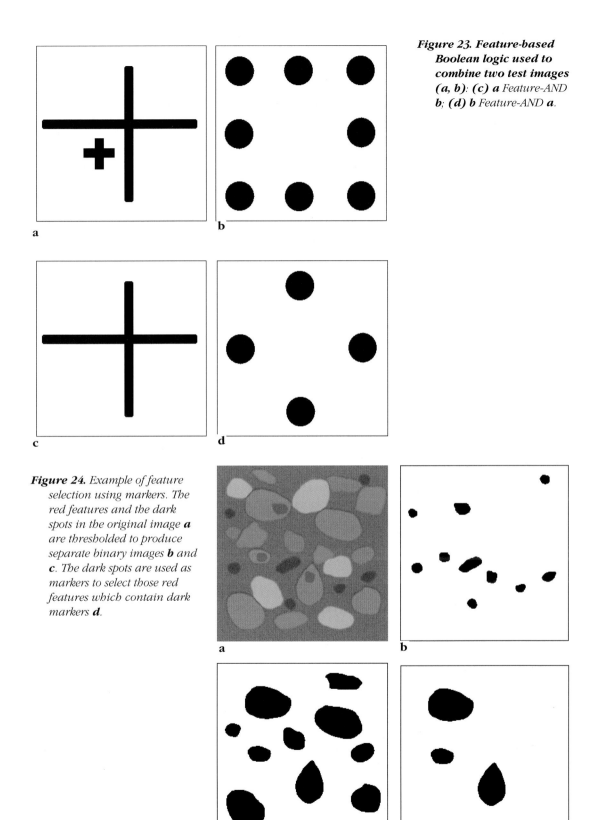

Figure 23. Feature-based Boolean logic used to combine two test images (a, b): (c) a *Feature-AND* **b; (d) b** *Feature-AND* **a.**

a

b

c

d

Figure 24. *Example of feature selection using markers. The red features and the dark spots in the original image* **a** *are thresholded to produce separate binary images* **b** *and* **c**. *The dark spots are used as markers to select those red features which contain dark markers* **d**.

a

b

c

d

Figure 25. Application of Feature-AND:
(a) original image of cells with stained nuclei;
(b) nuclei thresholded based on green intensity;
(c) cells thresholded based on red intensity;
(d) Feature-AND result showing only those cells containing green-stained nuclei;
(e) outlines of features from image *d* superimposed on original.

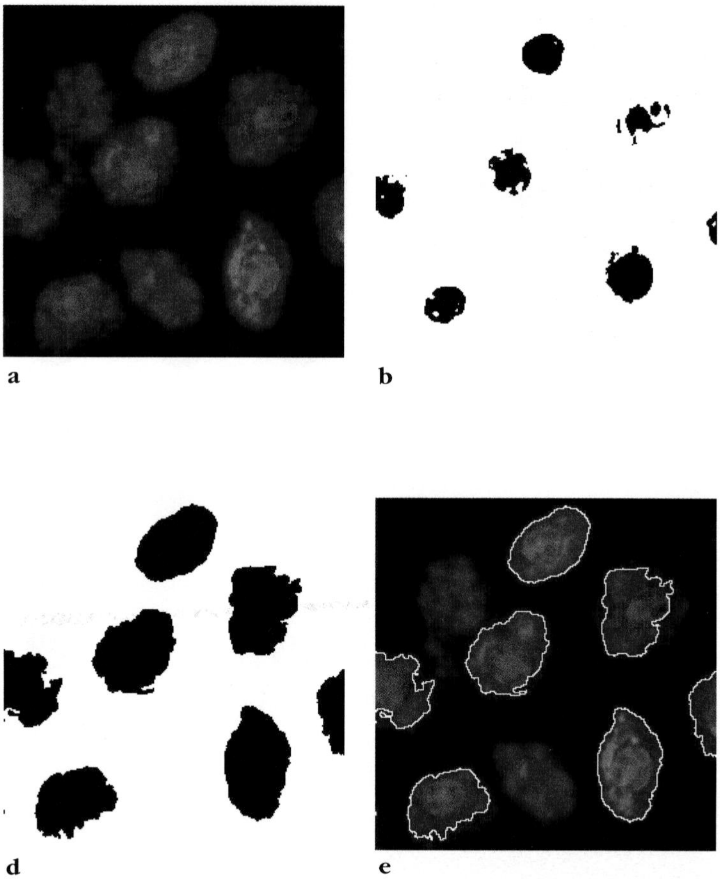

for dark spots and a second copy is thresholded for red features, then the first can be used as a set of markers to select the features of interest. A Feature-AND can be used to perform that operation.

In real applications the marker image that selects the features of interest may be obtained by separate thresholding, by processing, or by using another plane in a multiplane image. **Figure 25** shows an example. Only those cells containing green-stained nuclei are selected, but they are selected in their entirety so that they can be measured. A related procedure that uses the Feature-AND capability is the use of the nucleator (Gundersen et al., 1988), a stereological tool that counts cells in thin sections of tissue according to the presence of a unique marker within the cell such as the nucleus.

At a very different scale, the method might be used with aerial photographs to select and measure all building lots that contain any buildings, or fields that contain animals. The technique can also be used with x-ray images to select particles in SEM images, for instance, if the x-ray signal comes only from the portion of the particle which is visible to the x-ray detector. The entire particle image can be preserved if any part of it generates an identifying x-ray signal.

Feature-AND is also useful for isolating features that are partially within some region, or adjacent to it. For example, in **Figure 26** the colonies contain bacterial cells that are to be counted and measured, but some of them extend beyond the boundaries of the colony. The logic of Feature-AND allows them to be assigned to the appropriate colony and counted, and not to be counted more than once if they exit and re-enter the region. And in **Figure 27** the outline of a region has been generated (using dilation as discussed below) and used as a marker to select features that are adjacent to the substrate, so that they can be measured.

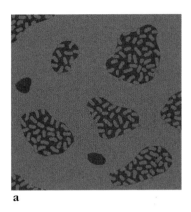
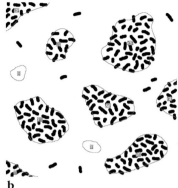

a

b

Figure 26. Colony counting:
(a) image representing colonies of bacterial cells, some of which extend beyond the stained area;
(b) counted results showing the number of cells in each colony.

Figure 27. Identifying adjacent features:
(a) image showing cross-section of a blue substrate with some orange features touching it;
(b) thresholded substrate;
(c) pixels immediately adjacent to the substrate, produced by dilating and Ex-ORing;
(d) orange features;
(e) Feature-AND of image *c* with image *d*;
(f) features identified in image *e* superimposed on the original.

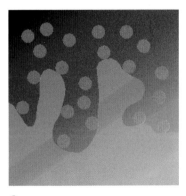
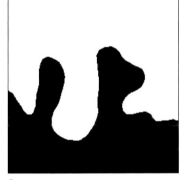
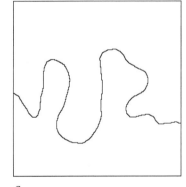

a

b

c

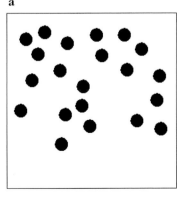
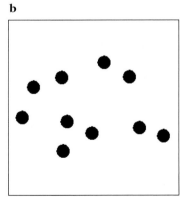
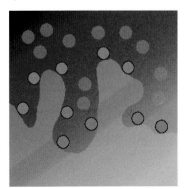

d

e

f

Selecting features by location

In a generalization of the method for identification of touching features shown in **Figure 27**, Feature-AND is also useful when applied in conjunction with images that map regions according to distance. We will see below that dilating a line, such as a grain boundary or cell wall, can produce a broad line of selected thickness. Using this line to select features that touch it selects those features which, regardless of size or shape, come within that distance of the original boundary. Counting these for different thickness lines provides a way to classify or count features as a function of distance from irregular boundaries. **Figure 28** shows an example and **Figure 29** shows an actual image of grain-boundary depletion.

Figure 30 shows a similar situation in which a pixel-based AND is appropriate. The image shows a metallurgical cross-section of a plasma-sprayed coating applied to a turbine blade. There is always a certain amount of oxide present in such coatings, which in general causes no difficulties; but if the oxide, which is a readily identifiable shade of grey, is preferentially situated at the coating-substrate interface, it can produce a region of weakness that may fracture and cause spalling of the coating. Thresholding the image to select the oxide, then ANDing this with the line representing the interface (itself obtained by thresholding the metal substrate phase, dilating, and Ex-ORing to get the custer, discussed more extensively later in this chapter) gives a direct measurement of the contaminated fraction of the interface.

An aperture or mask image can be used to restrict the analysis of a second image to only those areas within the aperture. Consider counting spots on a leaf: either the spots are due to an aerial spraying operation to assess uniformity of coverage, or perhaps they are spots of fungus or mold to assess the extent of disease. The acquired image is normally rectangular, but the leaf is not. There may well be regions outside the leaf that are similar in brightness to the spots. Creating a binary image of the leaf, then Feature-ANDing it with the total image selects those spots lying on the

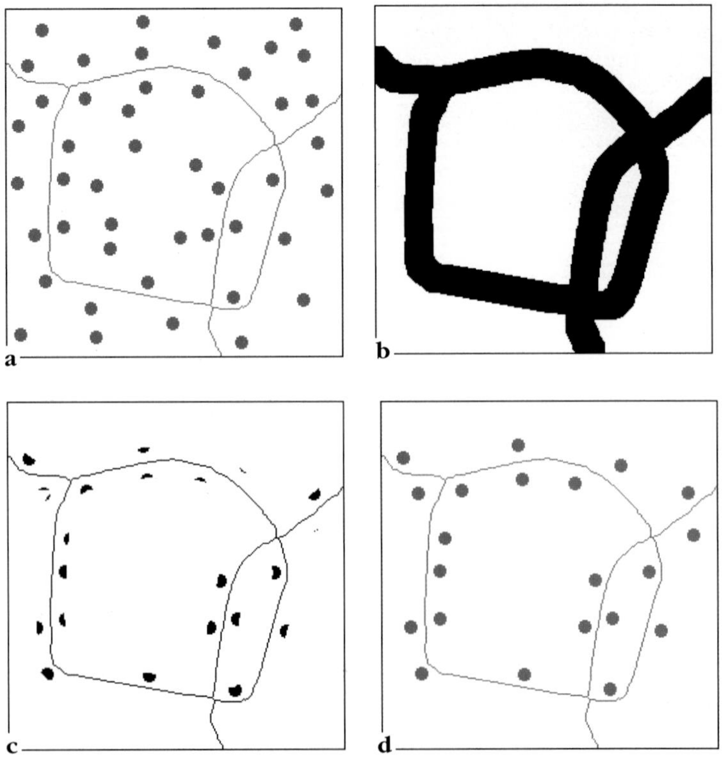

Figure 28. Comparison of pixel- and feature-AND:
(a) diagram of an image containing features and a boundary;
(b) the boundary line, made thicker by dilation;
(c) pixel-based AND of image **b** and **a** (incomplete features and one divided into two parts);
(d) feature-AND of images **b** and **a** (all features within a specified distance of the boundary).

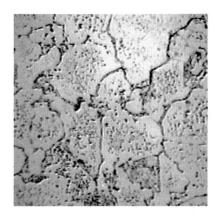

Figure 29. *Light microscope image of polished section through a steel used at high temperature in boiler tubes. Notice the depletion of carbides (black dots) in the region near grain boundaries. This effect can be measured using procedures described in the text.*

Figure 30. Isolating the oxide in a coating/substrate boundary:
  (a) *original grey-scale microscope image of a cross section of the plasma-sprayed coating on steel;*
  (b) *thresholding of the metal in the coating and the substrate;*
  (c) *applying erosion and dilation (discussed later in this chapter) to image **b** to fill holes and remove small features;*
  (d) *boundary line produced by dilating image **c** and Ex-ORing with the original;*
  (e) *thresholding the oxide in the coating, including that lying in the interface;*
  (f) *a pixel-based AND of image **d** with image **b**, showing just the fraction of the interface which is occupied by oxide.*

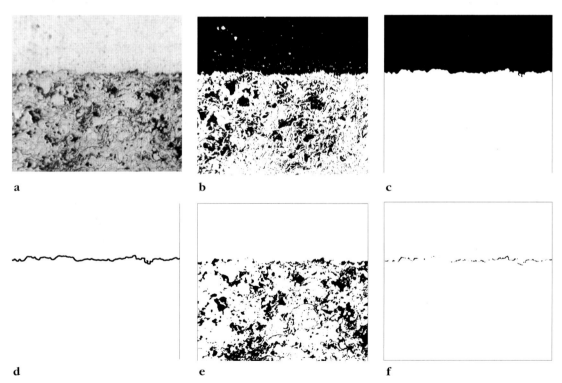

leaf itself. If the spots are small enough, this could be done as a pixel-based AND; however, if the spots can touch the edge of the leaf, the feature-based operation is safer because systems may not count or measure edge-touching features (as discussed in Chapter 9). Counting can then provide the desired information, normally expressed as number-per-unit-area where the area of the leaf forms the denominator. This procedure is similar to the colony-counting problem in **Figure 26**.

Figure 31 shows another situation, in which two different thresholding operations and a logical combination are used to select features of interest. The specimen is a polished cross section of an enamel coating on steel. The two distinct layers are different colored enamels containing different size distributions of spherical pores. Thresholding the darker layer includes several of the pores in the lighter layer, which have the same range of brightness values, but the layer can be selected by discarding features that are small or do not touch both edges of the field. This image then forms a mask that can be used to select only the pores in the layer of interest. Similar logic can be employed to select the pores in the light layer. Pores along the interface will generally be included in both sets, unless additional feature-based logic is employed.

A similar application allows identifying grains in ores that are contained within other minerals, for instance, to determine the fraction that are "locked" within a harder matrix that cannot easily be recovered by mechanical or chemical treatment, as opposed to those that are not so enclosed and are easily liberated from the matrix.

Figure 31. Selecting pores in one layer of enamel on
    steel:
    (a) original light microscope image (courtesy V.
    Benes, Research Inst. for Metals, Panenské Brezany,
    Czechoslovakia);
    (b) image a thresholded to select dark pixels;
    (c) discarding all features from image b that do not
    extend from one side to the other leaves just the layer
    of interest;
    (d) thresholding the original image to select only dark
    pores produces a binary image containing more pores
    than those in the layer;
    (e) combining images b and d with a Boolean
    Feature-AND leaves only the pores within the dark
    layer.

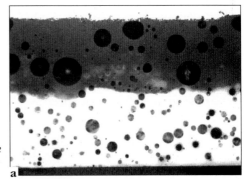

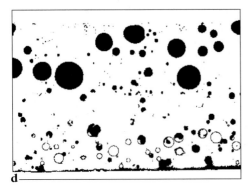

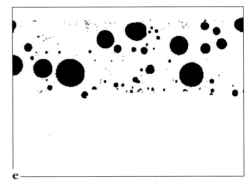

A rather different use of feature-based Boolean logic implements the disector, a stereological tool discussed in Chapter 8 that gives an unbiased and direct measure of the number of features per unit volume (Sterio, 1984). It requires matching features in two images that represent parallel planes separated by a distance T. The features represent the intersection of three-dimensional objects with those planes. Those objects which intersect both planes are ignored, but those which intersect only one plane or the other are counted. The total number of objects per unit volume is then

$$N_V = \frac{Count}{2 \cdot Area \cdot T}$$

(2)

where Area is the area of each of the images. This method has the advantage of being insensitive to the shape and size of the objects, but it requires that the planes be close enough together that no information is lost between the planes. In effect, this means that the distance T must be small compared to any important dimension of the objects.

When T is small, most objects intersect both planes. The features in those planes will not correspond exactly, but are expected to overlap at least partially. In the case of a branching three-dimensional object, both of the intersections in one plane are expected to overlap with the intersection in the second plane. Of course, since most of the objects do pass through both planes when T is small, and only the few that do not are counted, it is necessary to examine a large image area to obtain a statistically useful number of counts. That requirement makes the use of an automated method based on the Feature-AND logic attractive.

The features which overlap in the two images are those which are not counted; therefore, a candidate procedure for determining the value of N to be used in the calculation of number of objects per unit volume might be to first count the number of features in each of the two plane images (N_1 and N_2). Then, the Feature-AND can be used to determine the features which are present in both images, and a count of those features (N_{common}) obtained, giving

$$N = N_1 + N_2 - 2 \cdot N_{common}$$

(3)

However, this is correct only for the case in which each object intersects each plane exactly once. For branching objects, it will result in an error.

A preferred procedure is to directly count the features in the two planes that are not selected by the Feature-AND. The logical operation does not commute, so it is necessary to perform both operations: (#1 NOT F-AND #2) and (#2 NOT F-AND #1), and count the features remaining. This is illustrated schematically in **Figure 32**.

Figure 33 shows a typical application. The two images are separate slices reconstructed from X-ray tomography of a sintered ceramic sample. Each image is thresholded to generate a binary image of particle intersections. Each of the Feature-AND operations is performed, and the final image is the OR combination showing those features that appear in one (and only one) of the two slices. It would be appropriate to describe this image as a feature-based version of the exclusive-OR operation between the two images.

Double thresholding

Another application for Feature-AND logic arises in the thresholding of difficult images such as grain boundaries in materials or cell boundaries in tissue. It is not unusual to have nonuniform etching or staining of the cell or grain boundaries in specimen preparation. In the example of **Figure 34,** this is due to thermal etching of the interiors of the grains. The result is that direct thresholding of the image cannot produce a complete representation of the etched boundaries that does not also include "noise" within the grains.

**Figure 32. Implementation
of the Disector:**
(a) *two section images,
overlaid in different
colors to show matching
features;*
(b) *1 F-AND 2 showing
features in plane 2
matched with plane 1;*
(c) *2 F-AND 1 showing
the features matched in
the other plane;*
(d) *ORing together the 1
NOT F-AND 2 with 2
NOT F-AND 1 leaves just
the unmatched features
in both planes that area
to be counted.*

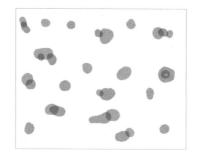

a

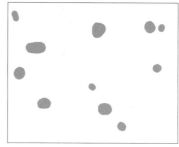

b

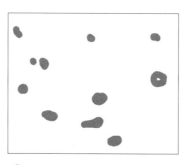

c

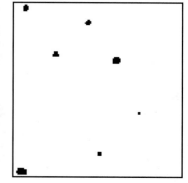

d

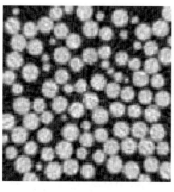

a

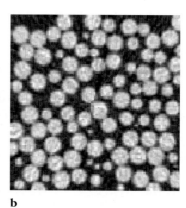

b

**Figure 33. Application of the
disector to x-ray
tomography slices through a
ceramic:**
(a) *slice 1;*
(b) *slice 2;*
(c) *binary image from slice 1;*
(d) *binary image from slice 2;*
(e) *[#1 NOT Feature-AND #2]
OR [#2 NOT Feature-AND #1].*

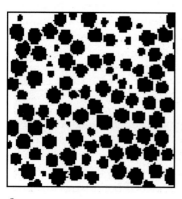

c

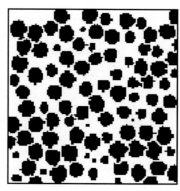

d

e

A technique for dealing with such situations has been described as "double thresholding" by Olsson (1993), but can be implemented by using Feature-AND. As illustrated in **Figure 34,** the procedure is first to threshold the image to select only the darkest pixels that are definitely within the etched boundaries, even if they do not form a complete representation of the boundaries. Then, a second binary image is produced to obtain a complete delineation of all the boundaries, accepting some noise within the grains. In the example, a variance operator was applied to a copy of the original image to increase the contrast at edges. This process allows thresholding more of the boundaries, but also some of the intra-grain structures. Then a morphological closing (discussed later in this chapter) was applied to fill in noise within the boundaries. The increase in apparent width of the boundaries is not important, because skeletonization (also discussed in the following section) is used to reduce the boundary lines to minimum width (the actual grain boundaries are only a few atoms thick).

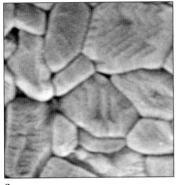

Figure 34. Double thresholding of grain boundaries in alumina:
> *(a)* original image;
> *(b)* first thresholding or dark grain boundary markers;
> *(c)* variance operator applied to original;
> *(d)* second thresholding of image **c** for all boundaries plus other marks;
> *(e)* Feature-AND of image **b** with image **d**;
> *(f)* closing applied to **e**;
> *(g)* skeletonized and pruned boundary overlaid on original.

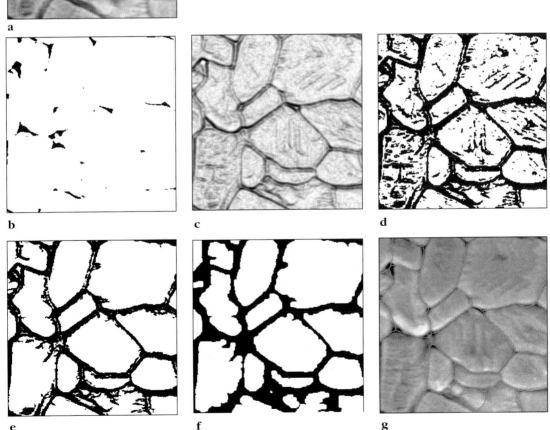

a

b   c   d

e   f   g

The two binary images are combined with a Feature-AND to keep any feature in the second image that touches one in the first. This uses the few dark pixels that definitely lie within the boundaries as markers to select the broader boundaries, while rejecting the noise within the grains. Finally, as shown in the figure, the resulting image is skeletonized and pruned to produce an image useful for stereological measurements of grain boundary area, grain size, and so forth.

In the preceding example, the grain boundary network is a continuous tesselation of the image. Hence, it could be selected by using other criteria than the double-threshold method (for instance, touching multiple edges of the field). **Figure 35** shows an example requiring the double-threshold method. The acoustic microscope image shows a cross section through a fiber-reinforced material. These images are inherently noisy, but double-thresholding (in this example selecting the bright pixels) allows the boundaries around the fibers to be selected. The fibers touch each other, so it is also necessary to separate them for measurement using a watershed segmentation as discussed in the next section.

Figure 35. Double thresholding of fiber boundaries:
    (a) original image;
    (b) first thresholding;
    (c) second thresholding;
    (d) Feature-AND;
    (e) filled boundaries;
    (f) segmented fibers.

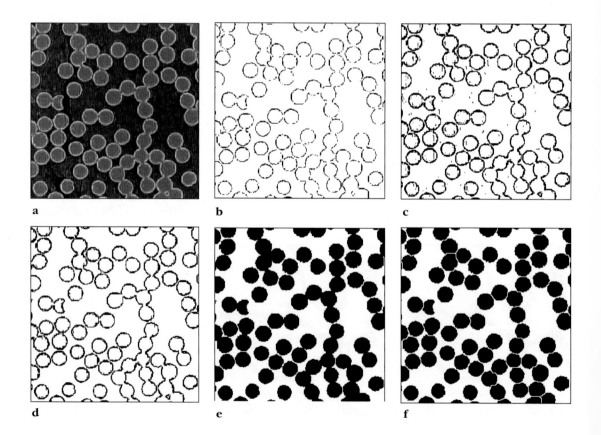

Erosion and dilation

The most extensive class of binary image processing operations is often collectively described as morphological operations (Serra, 1982; Coster and Chermant, 1985; Dougherty and Astola, 1994, 1999; Soille, 1999). These include erosion and dilation, and modifications and combinations of these operations. All are fundamentally neighbor operations, as were discussed in Chapters 3 and 4 to process grey-scale images in the spatial domain. Because the values of pixels in the binary images are restricted to 0 or 1, the operations are simpler and usually involve counting rather than sorting or weighted multiplication and addition. However, the basic ideas are the same, and it is possible to perform these procedures using the same specialized array-processor hardware sometimes employed for grey-scale kernel operations.

Rich literature, much of it French, is available in the field of mathematical morphology. It has developed a specific language and notation for the operations and is generally discussed in terms of set theory. A much simpler and more empirical approach is taken here. Operations can be described simply in terms of adding or removing pixels from the binary image according to certain rules, which depend on the pattern of neighboring pixels. Each operation is performed on each pixel in the original image, using the original pattern of pixels. In practice, it may not be necessary to create an entirely new image; the existing image can be replaced in memory by copying a few lines at a time. None of the new pixel values are used in evaluating the neighbor pattern.

Erosion removes pixels from features in an image or, equivalently, turns pixels OFF that were originally ON. The purpose is to remove pixels that should not be there. The simplest example is pixels that have been selected by thresholding because they fell into the brightness range of interest, but do not lie within large regions with that brightness. Instead, they may have that brightness value either accidentally, because of finite noise in the image, or because they happen to straddle a boundary between a lighter and darker region and thus have an averaged brightness that happens to lie in the range selected by thresholding.

Such pixels cannot be distinguished by simple thresholding because their brightness value is the same as that of the desired regions. It may be possible to ignore them by using two-parameter thresholding, for instance using the grey level as one axis and the gradient as a second one, and requiring that the pixels to be kept have the desired grey level and a low gradient. For our purposes here, however, we will assume that the binary image has already been formed and that extraneous pixels are present.

The simplest kind of erosion, sometimes referred to as classical erosion, is to remove (set to OFF) any pixel touching another pixel that is part of the background (is already OFF). This removes a layer of pixels from around the periphery of all features and regions, which will cause some shrinking of dimensions and may create other problems if it causes a feature to break up into parts. We will deal with these difficulties below. Erosion can entirely remove extraneous pixels representing point noise or line defects (e.g., scratches) because these defects are normally only a single pixel wide.

Instead of removing pixels from features, a complementary operation known as dilation (or sometimes dilatation) can be used to add pixels. The classical dilation rule, analogous to that for erosion, is to add (set to ON) any background pixel which touches another pixel that is already part of a foreground region. This will add a layer of pixels around the periphery of all features and regions, which will cause some increase in dimensions and may cause features to merge. It also fills in small holes within features.

Because erosion and dilation cause a reduction or increase in the size of regions, respectively, they are sometimes known as etching and plating or shrinking and growing. A variety of rules are followed in order to decide which pixels to add or remove and for forming combinations of erosion and dilation.

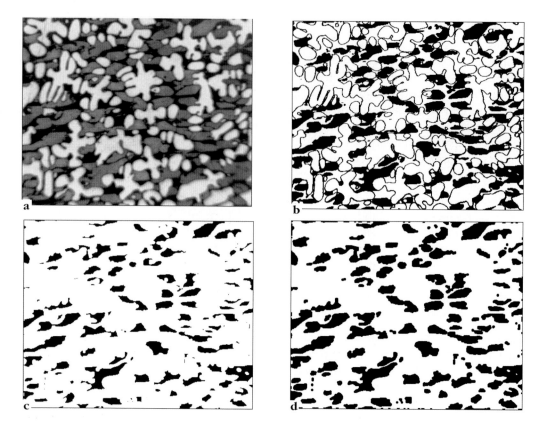

Figure 36: Removal of lines of pixels that straddle a boundary:
    (a) *original grey-scale microscope image of a three-phase metal;*
    (b) *binary image obtained by thresholding on the intermediate grey phase;*
    (c) *erosion of image **b** using two iterations;*
    (d) *dilation of image **c** using the same two iterations, restoring the feature size but without the lines.*

In the rather simple example described previously and illustrated in **Figure 36**, erosion to remove the extraneous lines of pixels between light and dark phases causes a shrinking of the features. Following the erosion with a dilation will more or less restore the pixels around the feature periphery, so that the dimensions are (approximately) restored. Isolated pixels that have been completely removed, however, do not cause any new pixels to be added. They have been permanently erased from the image.

Opening and closing

The combination of an erosion followed by a dilation is called an opening, referring to the ability of this combination to open up gaps between just-touching features, as shown in **Figure 37**. It is one of the most commonly used sequences for removing pixel noise from binary images. Performing the same operations in the opposite order (dilation followed by erosion) produces a different result. This sequence is called a closing because it can close breaks in features. Several parameters can be used to adjust erosion and dilation operations, particularly the neighbor pattern and the number of iterations, as discussed below. In most opening operations, these are kept the same for both the erosion and the dilation.

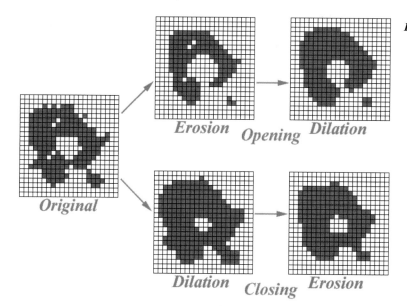

Figure 37. Combining erosion and dilation to produce an opening or a closing. The result is different depending on the order of application of the two operations.

Openings can be used in some cases to separate touching features. In the example shown in **Figure 38**, the features are all similar in size. This fact makes it possible to continue the erosion until all features have separated but none have been completely erased. After the separation is complete, dilation grows the features back toward their original size. They would merge again unless logic is used to prevent it. A rule that prevents turning a pixel ON if its neighbors belong to different features maintains the separation shown in the figure. This requires performing feature identification for the pixels, so the logic discussed previously is required at each step of the dilation. An additional rule prevents turning on any pixel that was not on in the original image, so that the features are restricted to their original sizes. If the features had different original sizes, the separation lines would not lie correctly at the junctions. The watershed segmentation technique discussed later in this chapter performs better in such cases.

If the sequence is performed in the other order, that is, a dilation followed by an erosion, the result is not the same. Instead of removing isolated pixels that are ON, the result is to fill in places where isolated pixels are OFF, missing pixels within features or narrow gaps between portions of a feature. **Figure 39** shows an example of a closing used to connect together the parts of the cracked fibers shown in cross section. The cracks are all narrow, so dilation causes the pixels from either side to spread across the gap. The increase in fiber diameter is then corrected by an erosion, but the cracks do not reappear.

The classical erosion and dilation operations illustrated above turn a pixel ON or OFF if it touches any pixel in the opposite state. Usually, touching in this context includes any of the adjacent 8 pixels, although some systems deal only with the 4 edge-sharing neighbors. These operations would also be much simpler and more isotropic on a hexagonal pixel array, because the pixel neighbor distances are all the same, but practical considerations lead to the general use of a grid of square pixels.

A wide variety of other rules are possible. One approach is to count the number of neighbor pixels in the opposite state, compare this number to some threshold value, and only change the state of the central pixel if that test coefficient is exceeded. In this method, classical erosion corresponds to a coefficient of 0. One effect of different coefficient values is to alter the rate at which features grow or shrink and to some extent to control the isotropy of the result. This will be illustrated in the next section.

Figure 38. Separation of touching features by erosion/dilation:
(**a**) *original test image;*
(**b**) *after two cycles of erosion;*
(**c**) *after four cycles;*
(**d**) *after seven cycles (features are now all fully separated);*
(**e**) *four cycles of dilation applied to image **d** (features will merge on next cycle);*
(**f**) *seven cycles of dilation using logic to prevent merging of features;*
(**g**) *nine cycles of non-merging dilation restricted to the original pixel locations, which restores the feature boundaries.*

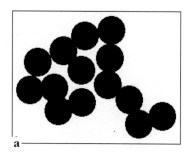
a

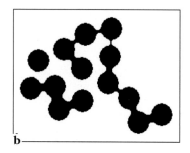
b

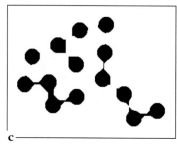
c

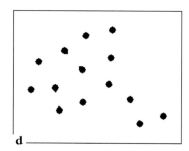
d

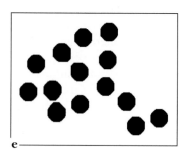
e

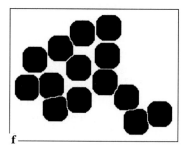
f

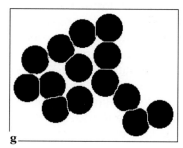
g

It is also possible to choose a large coefficient, from 5 to 7, to select only the isolated noise pixels and leave most features alone. For example, choosing a coefficient of 7 will cause only single isolated pixels to be reversed (removed or set to OFF in an erosion, and vice versa for a dilation). Coefficient values of 5 or 6 may be able to remove lines of pixels (such as those straddling a boundary) without affecting anything else.

An example of this method is shown in **Figure 40**. Thresholding the original image of the pigment cell produces a binary image showing the features of interest and creates many smaller and irregular groups of pixels. Performing a conventional opening to remove them would also cause the shapes of the larger features to change and some of them to merge. Applying erosion with a neighbor coefficient of 5 removes the small and irregular pixel groups without affecting the larger and more rounded features, as shown. The erosion is repeated until no further changes take place (the number of ON pixels in the binary image does not change). This procedure works because a corner pixel in a square has exactly five touching background neighbors and is not removed, while more irregular clusters have pixels with six or more background neighbors.

The test image in **Figure 41** shows a variety of fine lines and narrow gaps that can be removed or filled in using different neighbor coefficients and number of iterations (number of erosions followed by dilations, or vice versa).

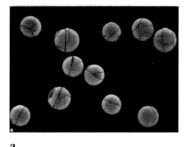 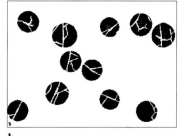 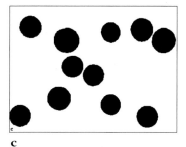

a   b   c

Figure 39. Joining parts of features with a closing:
(**a**) *original image, cross section of cracked glass fibers;*
(**b**) *brightness thresholding, showing divisions within the fibers;*
(**c**) *after application of a closing.*

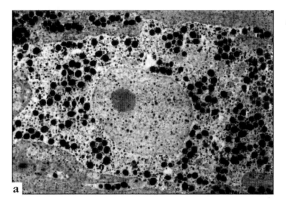

Figure 40. Removal of debris from an image:
(**a**) *original image of a pigment cell;*
(**b**) *brightness thresholding shows the pigment granules plus other, small and irregular features;*
(**c**) *erosion (neighbor coefficient = 5) leaves the large and regular granules.*

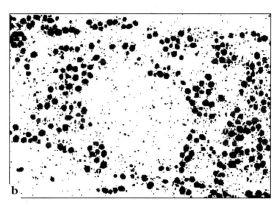 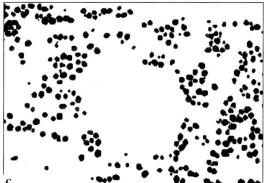

b   c

Isotropy

It is not possible for a small 3 × 3 neighborhood to define an isotropic neighbor pattern. Classic erosion applied to a circle will not shrink the circle uniformly, but will proceed at a faster rate in the 45° diagonal directions because the pixel spacing is greater in those directions. As a result, a circle will erode toward a diamond shape, as shown in **Figure 42**. Once the feature reaches this shape, it will continue to erode uniformly, preserving the shape. In most cases, however, features are not really diamond-shaped, which represents a potentially serious distortion.

Likewise, classic dilation applied to a circle also proceeds faster in the 45° diagonal directions, so that the shape dilates toward a square (also shown in **Figure 42**). Again, square shapes are stable in dilation, but the distortion of real images toward a block appearance in dilation can present a problem for further interpretation.

Figure 41. Illustration of the effect of different neighbor coefficients and number of iterations:
(a) original test image;
(b) erosion, neighbor coefficient = 3, 1 iteration, removes isolated lines and points;
(c) closing, neighbor coefficient = 2, 2 iterations, fills in gaps to connect features while removing isolated points;
(d) closing using classical operations (neighbor coefficient = 0, 1 iteration) connects most features but leaves isolated points;
(e) opening, neighbor coefficient = 7, 1 iteration, removes point noise without affecting anything else;
(f) opening, neighbor coefficient = 1, 4 iterations, removes all small features including the frame of the picture.

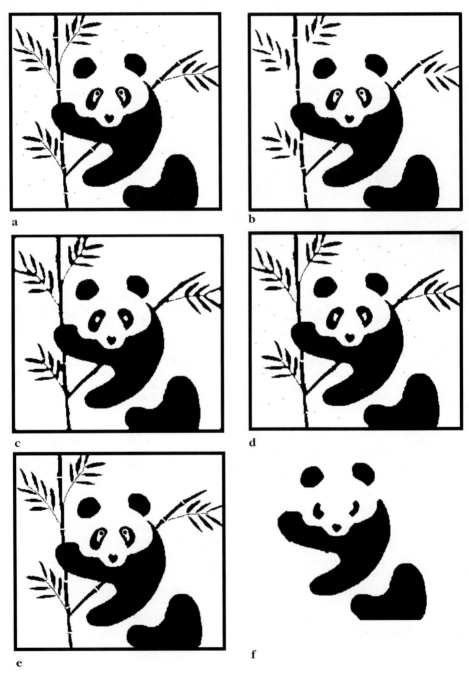

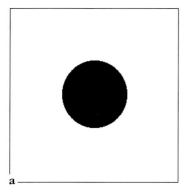
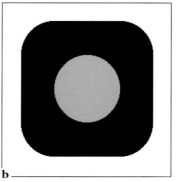
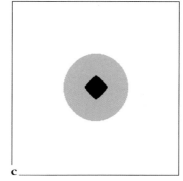

a ——— b ——— c ———

Figure 42. Testing the isotropy of classical (neighbor coefficient = 0) dilation and erosion:
(a) *original circle;*
(b) *after 50 iterations of dilation;*
(c) *after 25 iterations of erosion.*

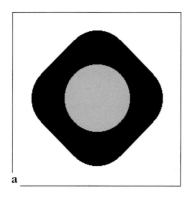
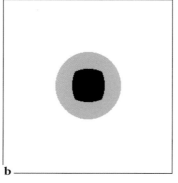

Figure 43. Isotropy tests
using a coefficient of 1:
(a) *the circle after 50*
iterations of dilation;
(b) *the circle after 25*
iterations of erosion.

a ——— b ———

A neighbor coefficient of 1 instead of 0 produces a markedly different result. For dilation, a background pixel that touches more than one foreground pixel (i.e., two or more out of the possible eight neighbor positions) will be turned ON and vice versa for erosion. Eroding a circle with this procedure tends toward a square and dilation tends toward a diamond, just the reverse of using a coefficient of 0. This is shown in **Figure 43**.

No possible intermediate value exists between 0 and 1, because the pixels are counted as either ON or OFF. If the corner pixels were counted as 2 and the edge-touching pixels as 3, it would be possible to design a coefficient that better approximated an isotropic circle. This would produce a ratio of $3/2 = 1.5$, which is a reasonable approximation to $\sqrt{2}$, the distance ratio to the pixels. In practice, this is rarely done because of the convenience of dealing with pixels in binary images as a simple 0 or 1 value with no need to take into account their neighborhood.

Another approach that is much more commonly used for achieving an intermediate result between the coefficients of 0 and 1 with their directional bias is to alternate the two tests. As shown in **Figure 44**, this alternating pattern produces a much better approximation to a circular shape in both erosion and dilation. This procedure raises the point that erosion or dilation need not be performed only once. The number of repetitions, also called the depth of the operation, corresponds roughly to the distance that boundaries will grow or shrink radially. It may be expressed in pixels or converted to the corresponding scale dimension.

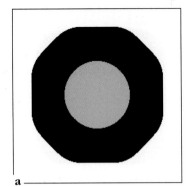
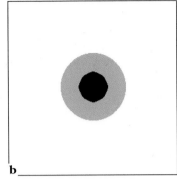

Using a larger neighborhood can also moderate the anisotropy. In **Figure 45** a 5-pixel-wide circular neighborhood is used with ten iterations of erosion and dilation. As for the alternating 0 and 1 coefficients the shapes evolve toward octagons, although the larger neighborhood provides less control over the distance used for erosion and dilation.

Each neighbor pattern or coefficient has its own characteristic anisotropy. **Figure 46** shows the rather interesting results using a neighborhood coefficient of 3. Similar to an alternating 0,1 pattern, this operation produces an 8-sided polygon; however, the rate of erosion is much lower. In dilation, the figure grows to the bounding octagon and then becomes stable, with no further pixels being added. This coefficient is sometimes used to construct bounding polygons around features.

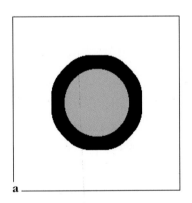
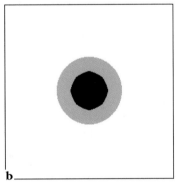

Figure 45. Classical erosion and dilation using ten iterations and a larger neighborhood size (a 5-pixel-wide approximation to a circle).

Figure 46. Octagonal shape and slow rate of addition or removal using a coefficient of 3: (a) original circle after 50 iterations of dilation (no further changes occur); *(b)* circle after 25 iterations of erosion.

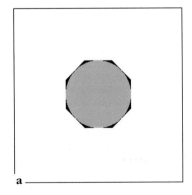
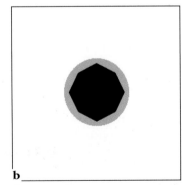

Measurements using erosion and dilation

Erosion performed n times (using either a coefficient of 0 or 1, or alternating them) will cause features to shrink radially by about n pixels (with local variations depending on the shape of the original feature). This will cause features whose smallest dimension is less than $2n$ pixels to disappear altogether. Counting the features that have disappeared (or subtracting the number that remain from the original) gives an estimate of the number of features smaller than that size. This means that erosion and counting can be used to get an estimate of size distributions without actually performing feature measurements (Ehrlich et al., 1984).

For irregularly shaped and concave features, the erosion process may cause a feature to subdivide into parts. Simply counting the number of features as a function of the number of iterations of erosion is therefore not a good way to determine the size distribution. One approach to this problem is to follow erosion by a dilation with the same coefficient(s) and number of steps. This will merge together many (but not necessarily all) of the separated parts and give a better estimate of their number, although there is still considerable sensitivity to the shape of the original features. A dumbbell-shaped object will separate into two parts when the handle between the two main parts erodes; they will not merge. This separation may be desirable, if indeed the purpose is to count the two main parts.

A second method is to use Feature-AND, discussed earlier. After each iteration of erosion, the remaining features are used to select only those original features that touch them. The count of original features then gives the correct number. This is functionally equivalent to keeping feature labels on each pixel in the image and counting the number of different labels present in the image after each cycle of erosion. This method of estimating size distributions without actually measuring features, using either of these correction techniques, has been particularly applied to measurements in geology, such as mineral particle sizes or sediments.

The opposite operation, performing dilations and counting the number of separate features as a function of the number of steps, is less common. It provides an estimate of the distribution of the nearest distances between features in the image. When this is done by conventional feature measurement, the x,y location of each feature is determined; then sorting in the resulting data file is used to determine the nearest neighbor and its distance. When the features are significantly large compared to their spacing or when their shapes are important, it can be more interesting to characterize the distances between their boundaries. This dilation method can provide that information.

Instead of counting the number of features that disappear at each iteration of erosion, it is much easier simply to count the number of ON pixels remaining, which provides some information about the shape of the boundaries. Smooth Euclidean boundaries erode at a constant rate. Irregular and especially fractal boundaries do not, since many more pixels are exposed and touch opposite neighbors. This effect has been used to estimate fractal dimensions, although several more accurate methods are available as discussed below.

Fractal dimensions and the description of a boundary as fractal based on a self-similar roughness is a fairly new idea that is finding many applications in science and art (Mandelbrot, 1982; Feder, 1988; Russ, 1994). No description of the rather interesting background and uses of the concept is included here for want of space. The basic idea behind measuring a fractal dimension by erosion and dilation comes from the Minkowski definition of a fractal boundary dimension. By dilating a region and Ex-ORing the result with another image formed by eroding the region, the pixels along the boundary are obtained. For a minimal depth of erosion and dilation, this will be called the custer and is discussed in the section titled "The custer."

To measure the fractal dimension, the operation is repeated with different depths of erosion and dilation (Flook, 1978), and the effective width (total number of pixels divided by length and number of cycles) of the boundary is plotted vs. the depth on a log-log scale. For a Euclidean boundary, this plot shows no trend; the number of pixels along the boundary selected by the Ex-OR increases linearly with the number of erosion/dilation cycles. For a rough boundary with self-similar fine detail, however, the graph shows a linear variation on log-log axes whose slope gives the fractal dimension of the boundary directly. **Figure 47** shows an example.

A variety of other methods are used to determine the boundary fractal dimension, including box-counting or mosaic amalgamation (Kaye, 1986; Russ, 1990) in which number of pixels through which the boundary passes (for boundary representation) are counted as the pixel size is increased by coarsening the image resolution, and a structured walk method (Schwarz and Exner, 1980), which requires the boundary to be represented as a polygon instead of as pixels. For a fractal boundary, these also produce straight line plots on a log-log scale, from whose slope the dimension is determined. Newer and more accurate techniques for performing the measurement are shown in Chapter 9.

Counting the number of pixels as a function of dilations also provides a rather indirect measure of feature clustering, because as nearby features merge, the amount of boundary is reduced and the region's rate of growth slows. Counting only the pixels and not the features makes it difficult to separate the effects of boundary shape and feature spacing. If all of the features are initially very small or if they are single points, this method can provide a fractal dimension (technically a Sierpinski fractal) for the clustering.

Figure 47. Measurement of Minkowski fractal dimension by erosion/dilation:
(a) test figure with upper boundary a classical Koch fractal and lower boundary a Euclidean straight line;
(b) grey pixels show difference between erosion and dilation by one iteration;
(c, d, e) differences between erosion and dilation after 2, 3, and 4 iterations;
(f) plot of log of effective width (area of grey pixels divided by length and number of iterations) vs. log of number of iterations (approximate width of grey band).

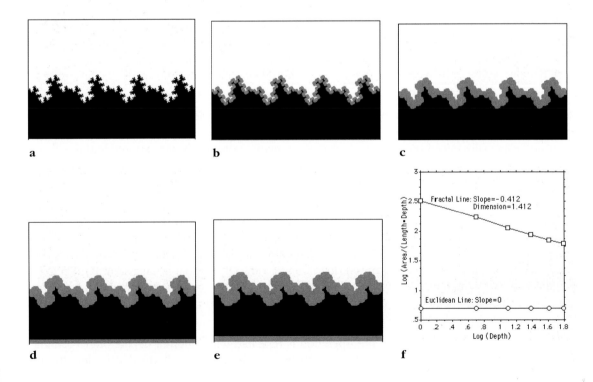

Extension to grey-scale images

In Chapter 4, one of the image processing operations described was the use of a ranking operator, which finds the brightest or darkest pixel in a neighborhood and replaces the central pixel with that value. This operation is sometimes described as a grey-scale erosion or dilation, depending on whether the use of the brightest or darkest pixel value results in a growth or shrinkage of the visible features.

Just as an estimate of the distribution of feature sizes can be obtained by eroding features in a binary image, the same technique is also possible using grey-scale erosion on a grey-scale image. **Figure 48** shows an example. The lipid spheres in this SEM image are partially piled up and obscure one another, which is normally a critical problem for conventional image-measurement techniques. Applying grey-scale erosion reduces the feature sizes, and counting the bright central points that disappear at each step of repeated erosion provides a size distribution.

The assumption in this approach is that the features ultimately separate before disappearing. This works for relatively simple images with well-rounded convex features, none of which are more than about half hidden by others. No purely two-dimensional image processing method can count the number of cannon balls in a pile if the inner ones are hidden. It is possible to estimate the volume of the pile and guess at the maximum number of balls contained, but impossible to know whether they are actually there or whether something else is underneath the topmost layer.

Figure 48. Use of grey-scale erosion to estimate size distribution of overlapped spheres:
(a) original SEM image of lipid droplets;
(b–f) result of applying repetitions of grey-scale erosion by keeping the darkest pixel value in a 5-pixel-wide octagonal neighborhood.

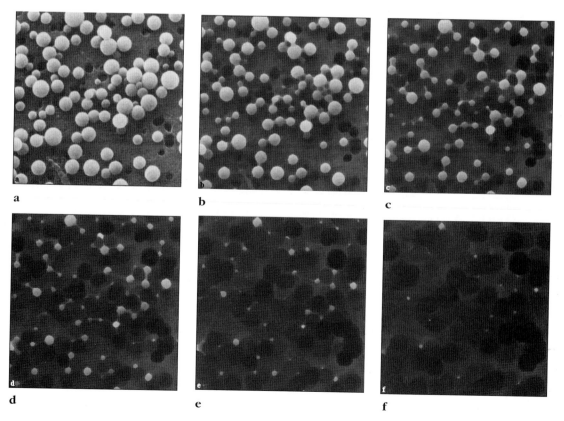

a

b

c

d

e

f

Morphology neighborhood parameters

The important parameters for erosion and dilation are the neighborhood size and shape, the comparison test that is used and the number of times the operation is repeated. The use of a simple test coefficient based on the number of neighbors, irrespective of their location in the neighborhood, provides considerable flexibility in the functioning of the operation as shown earlier. Each coefficient produces results having a characteristic shape, which distorts the original features. Also, the greater the depth, or number of iterations in the operation, the greater this effect, in addition to the changes in the number of features present.

Specific neighbor patterns can also be used for erosion and dilation operations. The most common are ones that compare the central pixel to its 4 edge-touching neighbors (usually called a "+" pattern because of the neighborhood shape) or to the 4 corner-touching neighbors (likewise called an "x" pattern), changing the central pixel if any of the 4 neighbors is of the opposite type (ON or OFF). They are rarely used alone, but can be employed in an alternating pattern to obtain greater directional uniformity than classical erosion, similar to the effects produced by alternating coefficient tests of 0 and 1.

Any specific neighbor pattern can be used, of course. It is not even required to restrict the comparison to immediately touching neighbors. As for grey-scale operations, larger neighborhoods make it possible to respond to more subtle textures and achieve greater control over directionality. **Figure 49** shows a simple example. The general case for this type of operation is called the hit-or-miss operator, which specifies any pattern of neighboring pixels divided into three classes: those that must be ON, those that must be OFF, and those that do not matter (are ignored). If the pattern is found, then the pixel is set to the specified state (Serra, 1982; Coster and Chermant, 1985).

This operation is also called template matching. The same type of operation carried out on grey-scale images is called convolution and is a way to search for specific patterns in the image. This is also true for binary images; in fact, template matching with thresholded binary images was one of the earliest methods for optical character reading and is still used for situations in which the character shape, size, and location are tightly controlled (such as the characters at the bottom of bank checks). Much more flexible methods are needed to read more general text, however. In practice, most erosion and dilation is performed using only the 8 nearest-neighbor pixels for comparison.

One method for implementing neighborhood comparison that makes it easy to use any arbitrary pattern of pixels is the fate table. The 8 neighbors each have a value of 1 or 0, depending on

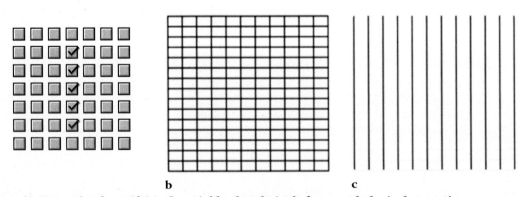

a   b   c

Figure 49. Example of specifying the neighborhood pixels for morphological operations:
   (a) a vertical neighborhood for erosion;
   (b) original pattern;
   (c) eroded result.

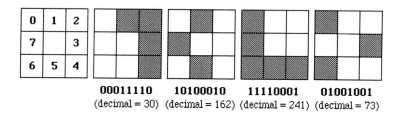

0	1	2
7		3
6	5	4

00011110   10100010   11110001   01001001

(decimal = 30)   (decimal = 162)   (decimal = 241)   (decimal = 73)

Figure 50. Constructing an address into a fate table by assigning each neighbor position to a bit value.

whether the pixel is ON or OFF. Assembling these 8 values into a number produces a single byte, which can have any of 256 possible values. This value is used as an address into a table, which provides the result (i.e., turning the central pixel ON or OFF). **Figure 50** illustrates the relationship between the neighbor pattern and the generated address.

Efficient ways to construct the address by bitwise shifting of values, which takes advantage of the machine-language idiosyncrasies of specific computer processors, makes this method very fast. The ability to create several tables of possible fates to deal with different erosion and dilation rules, perhaps saved on disk and loaded as needed, makes the method very flexible; however, it does not generalize well to larger neighborhoods or three-dimensional voxel array images because the tables become too large.

Some applications for highly specific erosion/dilation operations are not symmetrical or isotropic. These always require some independent knowledge of the image, the desired information, and the selection of operations that will selectively extract it. This is not as important a criticism or limitation as it may seem, however, because all image processing is to some extent knowledge-directed. The human observer tries to find operations to extract information he or she has some reason to know or expect to be present.

Figure 51 shows an example. The horizontal textile fibers vary in width as they weave above and below the vertical ones. Measuring this variation is important to modeling the mechanical properties of the weave, which will be embedded into a composite. The dark vertical fibers can be thresholded based on brightness, but delineating the horizontal fibers is very difficult. The procedure shown in the figure uses the known directionality of the structure.

After thresholding the dark fibers, an erosion is performed to remove only those pixels whose neighbor immediately below or above is part of the background. These pixels, shown in **Figure 51c**, can then be isolated by performing an Ex-OR with the original binary. They include the few points distinguishable between horizontal fibers and the ends of the vertical fibers where they are covered by horizontal ones.

Next, a directional dilation is performed in the horizontal direction. Any background pixel whose left or right touching neighbor is ON is itself set to ON, and this operation is repeated enough times to extend the lines across the distance between vertical fibers. Finally, the resulting horizontal lines are ORed with the original binary image to outline all of the individual fibers (**Figure 51d**). Inverting this image produces measurable features.

Examples of use

Some additional examples of erosion and dilation operations will illustrate typical applications and methods. One of the major areas of use is for x-ray maps from the SEM. These are usually so sparse that even though they are recorded as grey-scale images, they are virtually binary images even before thresholding because most pixels have zero photons and a few pixels have one.

Regions containing the element of interest are distinguished from those that do not by a difference in the spatial density of dots, which humans are able to interpret by a gestalt grouping operation. This very noisy and scattered image is difficult to use to locate feature boundaries. Dilation may be able to join points together to produce a more useful representation.

Figure 51. Using directional erosion and dilation to segment an image:
(**a**) original grey-scale image of a woven textile;
(**b**) brightness thresholding of image **a**;
(**c**) end pixels isolated by performing a vertical erosion and ExORing with the original;
(**d**) completed operation by repeated horizontal dilation of image **c** and then ORing with the original.

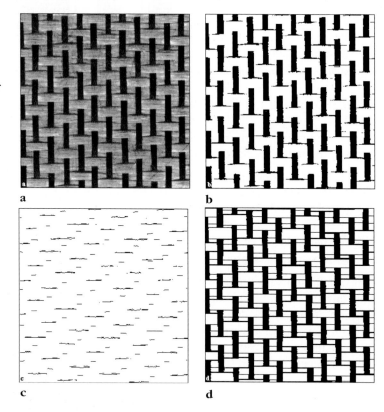

a

b

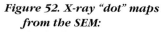

c

d

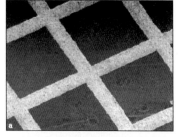

a

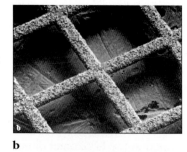

b

Figure 52. X-ray "dot" maps from the SEM:
(**a**) backscattered electron image of a gold grid above an aluminum stub;
(**b**) secondary electron image;
(**c**) gold x-ray dot image;
(**d**) aluminum x-ray image (notice the shadows of grid).

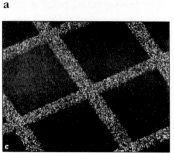

c

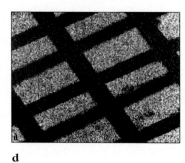

d

Figure 52 shows a representative x-ray map from an SEM. Notice that the dark bands in the aluminum dot map represent the shadows where the gold grid blocks the incident electron beam or the emitted x-rays en route to the detector. **Figure 53** shows the result of thresholding the gold map and applying a closing to merge the individual dots. **Figure 54** illustrates the results for the aluminum map. Because it has more dots, it produces a somewhat better definition of the region edges.

Other images from the light and electron microscope sometimes have the same essentially binary image as well. Examples include ultrathin biological tissue sections stained with heavy metals and viewed in the TEM, and chemically etched metallographic specimens. The dark regions are frequently small, corresponding to barely resolved individual particles whose distribution and clustering reveal the desired microstructure (membranes in tissue, eutectic lamellae in metals, etc.) to the eye. As for the case of x-ray dot maps, it is sometimes possible to utilize dilation operations to join such dots to form a well-defined image.

In **Figure 55**, iron carbide particles in a steel specimen are etched to distinguish the regions with and without such structures. The islands of lamellar structure are important, but not completely defined by the individual dark carbide particles. Dilation followed by erosion (a closing) merges together the individual lamellae, dark regions are also found within the essentially white grains because of the presence of a few dark points in the original image. Following the closing with an opening (for a total sequence of dilation, erosion, erosion, dilation) produces a useful result.

In the example, the closing used a neighborhood coefficient of 1 and 6 iterations, and the opening used a neighborhood coefficient of 0 and 4 iterations. The number of iterations is based on the size of the gap to be filled or feature to be removed. The presence of 45- and 90-degree edges in the processed binary images reveals the anisotropic effects of the erosion/dilation operations.

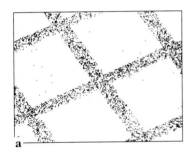
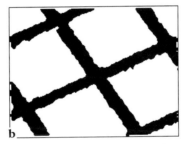
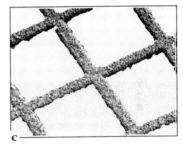

Figure 53. Delineating the gold grid:
   (a) *thresholded x-ray map;*
   (b) *image **a** after two repetitions of closing;*
   (c) *the backscattered electron image masked to show the boundaries from image **b** (notice the approximate location of edges).*

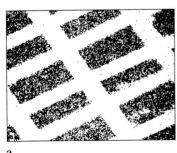
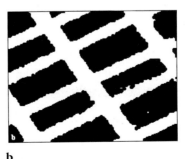

Figure 54. Delineating the aluminum map:
(a) *thresholding (notice the isolated continuum x-rays recorded within the grids);* *(b)* *after erosion with a neighborhood coefficient of 7 to remove the isolated pixels and dilation (two cycles) to fill the regions.*

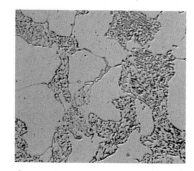

a

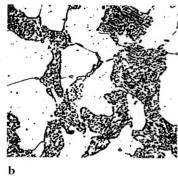

b

Figure 55. Combined closing and opening to delineate a region:
(a) *original grey-scale image of chemically etched metallographic specimen (dark regions are iron carbide);*
(b) *brightness threshold applied to image* **a**;
(c) *closing applied to fill in gaps between lamellae;*
(d) *opening applied to remove small isolated features;*
(e) *region boundaries superimposed on original image.*

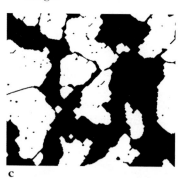

c

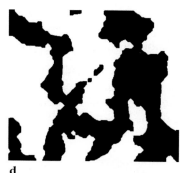

d

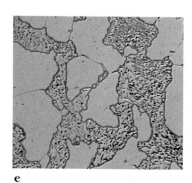

e

Using different coefficients in the various operations sometimes lessens the obvious geometric bias. The choice of appropriate parameters is largely a matter of experience with a particular type of image and human judgment of the correctness of the final result.

There is a basic similarity between using these morphological operations on a thresholded binary image and some of the texture operators used in Chapter 4 on grey-scale images. In most cases, similar (but not identical) results can be obtained with either approach (provided the software offers both sets of tools). For instance, **Figure 56** shows the same image of curds and whey used earlier to compare several grey-scale texture processing operations. Background leveling and thresholding the smooth, white areas (the curds) produces the result shown. Clearly, many regions in the textured whey protein portion of the image are just as bright as the curds. In grey-scale texture processing, these were eliminated based on some consideration of the local variation in pixel brightness. In this image, that variation produces narrow and irregular thresholded regions. An opening, consisting of an erosion to remove edge-touching pixels and a dilation to restore pixels smoothly to boundaries that still exist, effectively removes the background clutter as shown in the figure. Small features are shaded grey and would normally be removed based on size to permit analysis of the larger curds. The erosion/dilation approach to defining the structure in this image amounts to making some assumptions about the characteristic dimensions of the features, their boundary irregularities, and their spacings.

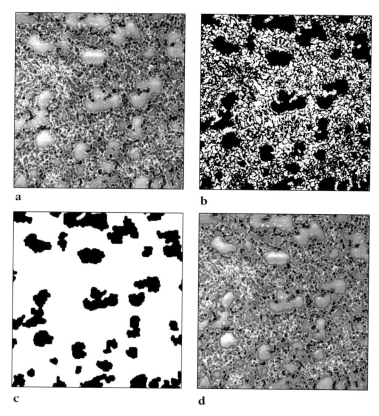

Figure 56. Segmenting the curds and whey image by erosion/dilation:
(a) *original image;*
(b) *thresholded;*
(c) *morphological opening;*
(d) *outlines superimposed on original image.*

a

b

c

d

The custer

Erosion/dilation procedures are often used along with Boolean combinations. In the examples of **Figures 27** through **30** the lines used to test for adjacency were obtained by dilating the binary image and then Ex-ORing the result with the original. Also, the outlines shown in many of the figures to compare the results of processing to the original image can be produced by performing an erosion followed by an Ex-OR with the original binary image. This leaves the outlines which were then applied as a mask to the original grey-scale image. Whether obtained by erosion or dilation, or doing both and Ex-ORing the results, the outline is called the custer of a feature, apparently in reference to George Herbert Armstrong Custer, who was also surrounded.

The custer can be used to determine neighbor relationships between features or regions. As an example, **Figure 57** shows a three-phase metal alloy imaged in the light microscope. Each of the individual phases can be readily delineated by thresholding (and in the case of the medium grey image, applying an opening to remove lines of pixels straddling the white-black boundary). Then the custer of each phase can be formed as described previously.

Combining the custer of each phase with the other phases using an AND keeps only the portion of the custer that is common to the two phases. The result is to mark the boundaries as white-grey, grey-black, or black-white, so that the extent of each type can be determined by simple counting. In other cases, Feature-AND can be used to select the entire features that are adjacent to one region (and thus touch its custer), as illustrated previously.

Euclidean distance map

The directional bias present in morphological operations because of their restriction to pixels on a square grid can be largely overcome by performing equivalent operations using a different

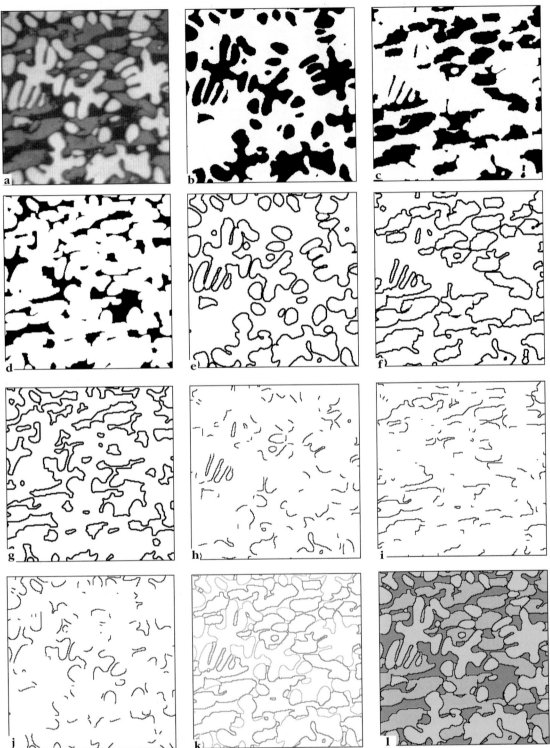

Figure 57. Use of Boolean logic to measure neighbor relationships: (a) *an original light microscope image of a three-phase metal;* **(b–d)** *thresholded white, grey, and black phases;* **(e–g)** *surrounding outlines of each phase produced by dilation and ExOR with original;* **(h–j)** *AND of outlines of pairs of phases;* **(k)** *OR of all ANDed outlines using different colors to identify each phase/phase interface;* **(l)** *outlines filled to show idealized phase regions.*

technique. It makes use of a grey-scale image, produced from the original binary, in which every pixel within a feature is assigned a value that is its distance from the nearest background pixel. This is called the Euclidean distance map, or EDM.

Most of the image processing functions discussed in this and preceding chapters operate either on grey-scale images (to produce other grey-scale images) or on binary images (to produce other binary images). The Euclidean distance map is a tool that works on a binary image to produce a grey-scale image. The definition is simple enough: each pixel in the foreground is assigned a brightness value equal to its straight line (thus, "Euclidean") distance from the nearest point in the background. In a continuous image, as opposed to a digitized one containing finite pixels, this is unambiguous. In most pixel images, the distance is taken from each pixel in the feature to the nearest pixel in the background.

Searching through all of the background pixels to find the nearest one to each pixel in a feature and calculating the distance in a Pythagorean sense would be an extremely inefficient and time-consuming process for constructing the EDM. Some researchers have implemented a different type of distance map in which distance measured in only a few directions. For a lattice of square pixels, this may either be restricted to the 90° directions, or it may also include the 45° directions (Rosenfeld and Kak, 1982). This measuring convention is equivalent to deciding to use a 4-neighbor or 8-neighbor convention for considering whether pixels are touching. In either case, the distance from each pixel to one of its 4 or 8 neighbors is taken as 1, regardless of the direction. Consequently, as shown in **Figure 58**, the distance map from a point gives rise to either square or diamond-shaped artefacts and is quite distorted, as compared to the Pythagorean distance. These measuring conventions are sometimes described as city-block models (connections in 4 directions) or chessboard models (8 directions), because of the limited moves available in those situations.

A conceptually straightforward, iterative technique for constructing such a distance map can be programmed as follows:

1. Assign a brightness value of 0 to each pixel in the background.
2. Set a variable N equal to 0.
3. For each pixel that touches (in either the 4- or 8-neighbor sense, as described previously) a pixel whose brightness value is N, assign a brightness value of N + 1.
4. Increment N and repeat step 3, until all pixels in the image have been assigned.

The time required for this iteration depends on the size of the features (the maximum distance from the background). A more efficient method is available that gives the same result with two passes through the image (Danielsson, 1980). This technique uses the same comparisons, but propagates the values through the image more rapidly. It can be programmed as follows:

6	5	4	3	4	5	6
5	4	3	2	3	4	5
4	3	2	1	2	3	4
3	2	1	0	1	2	3
4	3	2	1	2	3	4
5	4	3	2	3	4	5
6	5	4	3	4	5	6

3	3	3	3	3	3	3
3	2	2	2	2	2	3
3	2	1	1	1	2	3
3	2	1	0	1	2	3
3	2	1	1	1	2	3
3	2	2	2	2	2	3
3	3	3	3	3	3	3

$\sqrt{18}$	$\sqrt{13}$	$\sqrt{10}$	3.0	3.2	3.6	4.2
$\sqrt{13}$	$\sqrt{8}$	$\sqrt{5}$	2.0	2.2	2.8	3.6
$\sqrt{10}$	$\sqrt{5}$	$\sqrt{2}$	1.0	1.4	2.2	3.2
$\sqrt{9}$	$\sqrt{4}$	$\sqrt{1}$	0	1.0	2.0	3.0
$\sqrt{10}$	$\sqrt{5}$	$\sqrt{2}$	1.0	1.4	2.2	3.2
$\sqrt{13}$	$\sqrt{8}$	$\sqrt{5}$	2.0	2.2	2.8	3.6
$\sqrt{18}$	$\sqrt{13}$	$\sqrt{10}$	3.0	3.2	3.6	4.2

Figure 58. *Arrays of pixels with their distances from the center pixel shown (from left to right) for the cases of 4- and 8-neighbor paths, and in Pythagorean units.*

1. Assign the brightness value of 0 to each pixel in the background and a large positive value (greater than the maximum feature width) to each pixel in a feature.
2. Proceeding from left to right and top to bottom, assign each pixel within a feature a brightness value one greater than the smallest value of any of its neighbors.
3. Repeat step 2, proceeding from right to left and bottom to top.

A further modification provides a better approximation to the Pythagorean distances between pixels (Russ and Russ, 1988b). The diagonally adjacent pixels are neither a distance 1 (8-neighbor rules) or $\sqrt{2} = 1.414$ (4-neighbor rules) away. The latter value is an irrational number, but closer approximations than 1.00 or 2.00 are available. For instance, modifying the above rules so that a pixel brightness value must be larger than its 90° neighbors by 2 and greater than its 45° neighbors by 3 is equivalent to using an approximation of 1.5 for the square root of 2.

The disadvantage of this method is that all of the pixel distances are now multiplied by two, increasing the maximum brightness of the EDM image by this factor. For images capable of storing a maximum grey level of 255, this represents a limitation on the largest features that can be processed in this way. If the EDM image is 16 bits deep (and can hold values up to 65,535), however, this is not a practical limitation. It also opens the way to selecting larger ratios of numbers to approximate $\sqrt{2}$, getting a correspondingly improved set of values for the distance map. For instance, $7/5 = 1.400$ and $58/41 = 1.415$.

It takes no longer to compare or add these values than it does any others, and the ratio $58/41$ allows dimensions larger than 1024 pixels. Because this dimension is the half-width, features or background up to 2048 pixels wide can be processed ($1024 \times 41 = 41,984$, which is less than $2^{16} - 1 = 65,535$). Of course, the final image can be divided down by the scaling factor (41 in this example) to obtain a result in which pixel brightness values are the actual distance to the boundary (rounded or truncated to integers) and the total brightness range is within the 0 to 255 range that most displays are capable of showing.

The accuracy of an EDM constructed with these rules can be judged by counting the pixels whose brightness values place them within a distance s. This is just the same as constructing a cumulative histogram of pixel brightness in the image. **Figure 59** plots the error in the number of pixels vs. integer brightness for a distance map of a circle 99 pixels in diameter; the overall errors are not large. Even better accuracy for the EDM can be obtained by performing additional comparisons to pixels beyond the first 8 nearest neighbors. Adding a comparison to the 8 neighbors in the 5×5 neighborhood whose Pythagorean distance is $\sqrt{5}$ produces values having even less directional sensitivity and more accuracy for large distances. If the integer values 58 and 41 mentioned above are used to approximate $\sqrt{2}$, then the path to these pixels consisting of a "knight's move" of one 90°- and one 45°-pixel step would produce a value of $58 + 41 = 99$. Substituting a value of 92 gives a close approximation to the Pythagorean distance ($92/41 = 2.243$; $\sqrt{5} = 2.236$) and produces more isotropic results.

Figure 59. Difference between theoretical area value (πr^2) and the actual area covered by the EDM as a function of brightness (distance from boundary) shows increasing but still small errors for very large distances.

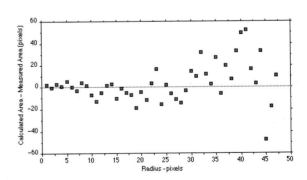

There is another algorithm that produces a Euclidean distance map with real number values. During the passes through the image, the X and Y distances from the nearest background point are accumulated separately for each pixel within the features, and then the actual Pythagorean distance is calculated as the square root of the sum of squares. Of course, it is still necessary to convert to an integer representation for display purposes. In general, the better the quality of the EDM values the better the results obtained using the EDM for erosion, dilation, and watershed segmentation as described in the next section.

Comparison of the pixel-by-pixel erosion and dilation described earlier with the circular pattern provided thresholding by the EDM of either the foreground (erosion) or background (dilation) to select pixels that are farther from the edge than any desired extent of erosion shows that the EDM method is much more isotropic (**Figure 60**). Furthermore, the distance map is constructed quickly and the thresholding requires no iteration, so the execution time of the method does not increase with feature size (as do classical erosion methods) and is preferred for large features or depths.

When more irregular shapes are subjected to erosion and dilation, the difference between the iterative methods and thresholding the EDM is also apparent, with EDM methods avoiding the 90- and 45-degree boundaries present with the traditional morphological tools. **Figure 61** shows the same example of closing and opening applied to the image in **Figure 55**. The distance used for both closing and opening was 5.5 pixels (note that with the EDM it is possible to specify distances are real numbers rather than being restricted to integers), and the final outlines trace the edges of the structures with much greater fidelity.

Watershed segmentation

A common difficulty in measuring images occurs when features touch, and therefore cannot be separately identified, counted, or measured. This situation may arise when examining an image of

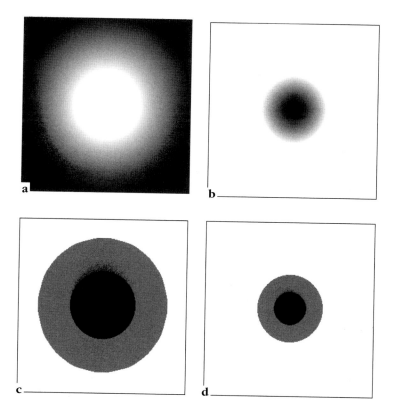

Figure 60. Isotropic erosion and dilation achieved by using the Euclidean distance map for dilation and erosion (compare to Figures 42–46):
(a) the EDM of the background around the circle;
(b) the EDM of the circle;
(c) dilation achieved by thresholding the background EDM at a value of 50;
(d) erosion achieved by thresholding the circle EDM at a value of 25.

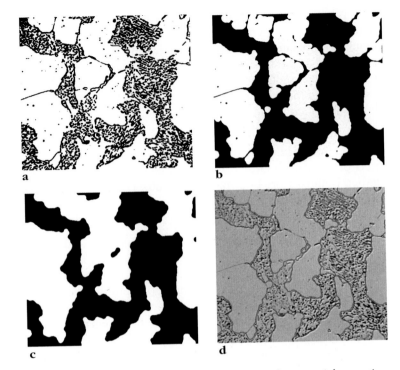

Figure 61. Closing and opening using the EDM:
(a) thresholded original image (same as **Figure 55**);
(b) closing, distance of 5.5 pixels;
(c) opening; distance of 5.5 pixels;
(d) outlines superimposed on original image.

a

b

c

d

a thick section in transmission, where actual feature overlap may occur, or when particles resting on a surface tend to agglomerate and touch each other. One method for separating touching, but mostly convex, features in an image is known as watershed segmentation (Beucher and Lantejoul, 1979; Lantejoul and Beucher, 1981). It relies on the fact that eroding the binary image will usually cause touching features to separate before they disappear.

The classical method for accomplishing this separation (Jernot, 1982) is an iterative one. The image is repetitively eroded, and at each step those separate features that disappeared from the previous step are designated ultimate eroded points (UEPs) and saved as an image, along with the iteration number. Saving these is necessary because the features will in general be of different sizes and would not all disappear in the same number of iterations, as mentioned earlier in connection with **Figure 38**. The process continues until the image is erased.

Then, beginning with the final image of UEPs, the image is dilated using classical dilation, but with the added logical constraint that no new pixel may be turned ON if it causes a connection to form between previously separate features or if it was not ON in the original image. At each stage of the dilation, the image of UEPs that corresponds to the equivalent level of erosion is added to the image using a logical OR. This process causes the features to grow back to their original boundaries, except that lines of separation appear between the touching features.

The method just described has two practical drawbacks: the iterative process is slow, requiring each pixel in the image to be processed many times, and the amount of storage required for all of the intermediate images is quite large. The same result can be obtained more efficiently using an EDM. Indeed, the name "watershed" comes directly from the EDM. Imagine that the brightness values of each pixel within features in an EDM correspond to a physical elevation. The features then appear as a mountain peak. **Figure 62** illustrates this for a circular feature.

If two features touch or overlap slightly, the EDM shows two peaks, as shown in **Figure 63**. The slope of the mountainside is constant, so the larger the feature the higher the peak. The ultimate eroded points are the peaks of the mountains, and where features touch, the flanks of the mountains intersect. The saddles between these mountains are the lines selected as boundaries by the

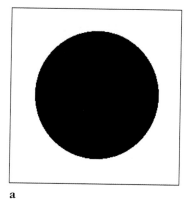 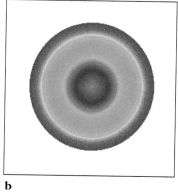 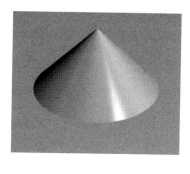

a **b** **c**

Figure 62. Interpreting the Euclidean distance map as the height of pixels:
   (a) binary image of a circular feature;
   (b) Euclidean distance map with pixels color coded to show distance from boundary;
   (c) rendered display showing pixel heights.

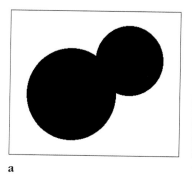 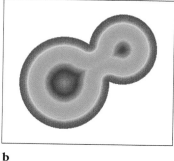 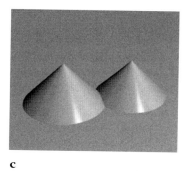

a **b** **c**

Figure 63: EDM for touching features:
   (a) binary image of two touching circular features;
   (b) Euclidean distance map with pixels color coded to show distance from boundary;
   (c) rendered display showing pixel heights. Note the boundary between the two cones.

segmentation method. They are locations where water running down from the mountains arrives from two different peaks, and thus are generally called watershed lines. The placement of these lines according to the relative height of the mountains (size of the features) gives the best estimate of the separation lines between features, which are divided according the regions that belong to each mountain top.

Implementing the segmentation process using an EDM approach (Russ and Russ, 1988b) is very efficient, both in terms of speed and storage. The distance map image required is constructed without iteration. The ultimate eroded points are located as a special case of local maxima (A further discussion of UEPs is included in the next section), and the brightness value of each directly corresponds to the iteration number at which it would disappear in the iterative method. Dilating these features is fast, because the distance map supplies a constraint. Starting at the brightest value and "walking down the mountain" covers all of the brightness levels. At each one, only those pixels at the current brightness level in the distance map need to be considered. Those that do not produce a join between feature pixels are added to the image. The process continues until all of the pixels in the features, except for those along the separation lines, have been restored.

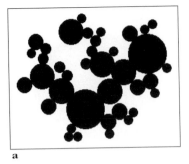
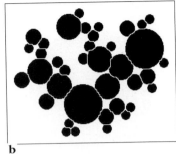

Figure 64. Watershed segmentation on an image of touching circles of different sizes.

a   b

Figure 64 shows an example of this method, applied to an image consisting of touching circles. Since these are of different sizes, the method described earlier in **Figure 38** does not work, but watershed segmentation separates the features. For a image of real particles, as shown in **Figure 65**, the method works subject to the assumption that the features are sufficiently convex that the EDM does not produce multiple peaks within each feature.

Of course, this method is not perfect. Watershed segmentation cannot handle concave and irregular particles, nor does it not separate particles whose overlap is so great that there is no minimum in the EDM between them. Depending on the quality of the original distance map, watershed segmentation may subdivide lines of constant width into many fragments because of the apparent minima produced by aliasing along the line edges. In most cases, the effort needed to correct such defects is much less than would have been required to perform manual separation of the original features.

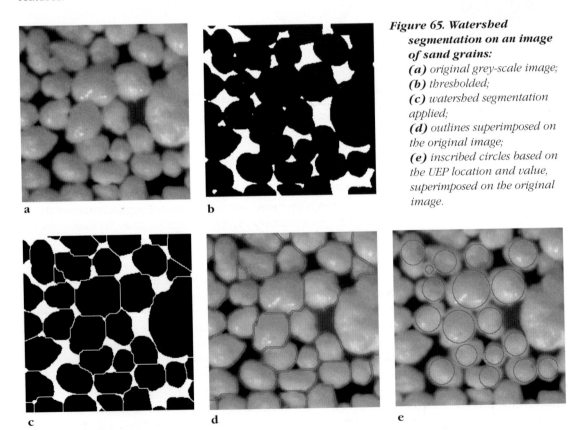

Figure 65. Watershed segmentation on an image of sand grains:
(a) original grey-scale image;
(b) thresholded;
(c) watershed segmentation applied;
(d) outlines superimposed on the original image;
(e) inscribed circles based on the UEP location and value, superimposed on the original image.

a   b

c   d   e

The presence of holes within features confuses the watershed algorithm and breaks the features up into many fragments. It is therefore necessary to fill holes before applying the watershed, although there may also be holes in the image between features as well as those within them. Normal hole filling would fill them in since any region of background not connected to the edge of the image is considered a hole. This difficulty can be overcome if some difference in hole size or shape can be identified to permit filling only the holes within features and not those between them (Russ, 1995f). In the example shown in **Figure 66**, the holes within features (organelles within the cells) are much rounder than spaces between the touching cells. Isolating these holes by measurement, and ORing them with the original image, allows watershed segmentation to separate the cells.

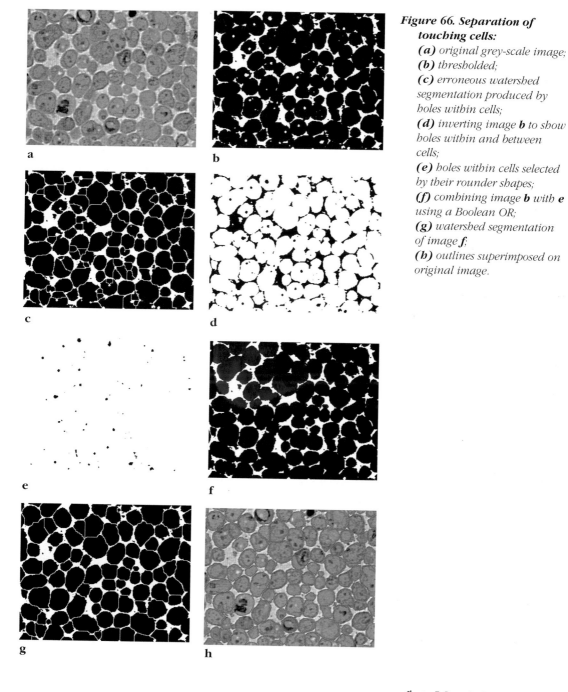

Figure 66. Separation of touching cells:
(a) original grey-scale image;
(b) thresholded;
(c) erroneous watershed segmentation produced by holes within cells;
(d) inverting image **b** to show holes within and between cells;
(e) holes within cells selected by their rounder shapes;
(f) combining image **b** with **e** using a Boolean OR;
(g) watershed segmentation of image **f**;
(h) outlines superimposed on original image.

Ultimate eroded points

The ultimate eroded points (UEPs) described previously in the watershed segmentation technique can be used as a measurement tool in their own right. The number of points gives the number of separable features in the image, while the brightness of each point gives a measure of their sizes (the inscribed radius, shown in **Figure 65e**). In addition, the location of each point can be used as a location for the feature if clustering or gradients are to be investigated.

The formal definition of a UEP in a continuous, rather than pixel-based, image is simply a local maximum of brightness in the EDM image. Since the image is subdivided into finite pixels, the definition must take into account the possibility that more than one pixel may have equal brightness, forming a plateau. The operating definition for finding these pixels is recursive.

$$\{U: \quad \forall \ U_j \text{ neighbors of } U_i, |U_j| \le |U_i| \tag{5}$$
$$\text{AND}$$
$$\forall \ U_j \text{ neighbors of } U_i \text{ such that } |U_j| = |U_i|, U_i \in U\}$$

In other words, the set of pixels which are UEPs must be as bright or brighter than all neighbors; if the neighbors are equal in brightness, then they must also be part of the set.

The brightness of each pixel in the distance map is the distance to the nearest boundary. For a UEP, this must be a point that is equidistant from at least three boundary locations. Consequently, the brightness is the radius of the feature's inscribed circle. **Figure 67** shows the UEPs for the touching circles from **Figure 64**. A histogram of the brightness values of the UEP pixels gives an immediate measure of the size distribution of the features. This is much faster than convex segmentation, because the iterative dilation is bypassed, and much faster than measurement, since no feature identification or pixel counting is required. Even for separate features, the maximum point of the EDM provides a measurement of the radius of an inscribed circle, a useful size parameter.

Other EDM-based measurements

The Euclidean distance map provides values that can be effectively used for many types of measurements. For example, the method described above for determining a fractal dimension from successive erosion and dilation operations has two shortcomings: it is slow and has an orientational bias because of the anisotropy of the operations. The EDM offers a simple way to obtain the same information (Russ, 1988) as will be discussed in detail in Chapter 9.

Because the distance map encodes each pixel with the straight line distance to the nearest background point, it can also be used to measure the distance of many points or features from irregular boundaries. In the example shown in **Figure 68** the image is thresholded to define the boundary lines (which might represent grain boundaries, cell membranes, etc.) and points (particles, organelles, etc.). The image of the thresholded features is applied as a mask to the Euclidean distance map of the interior so that all pixels in the features have the distance values. Measuring the brightness of the features gives the distance of each feature from the boundary.

Figure 67. The ultimate points for the touching features from Figure 64.

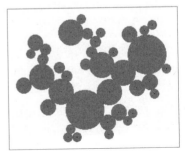

Figure 68. *Measurement of distance from a boundary:*

(a) example image;
(b) thresholded interior region;
(c) thresholded features;
(d) Euclidean distance map of the interior (color coded);
(e) distance value assigned to features;
(f) histogram of distances for features.

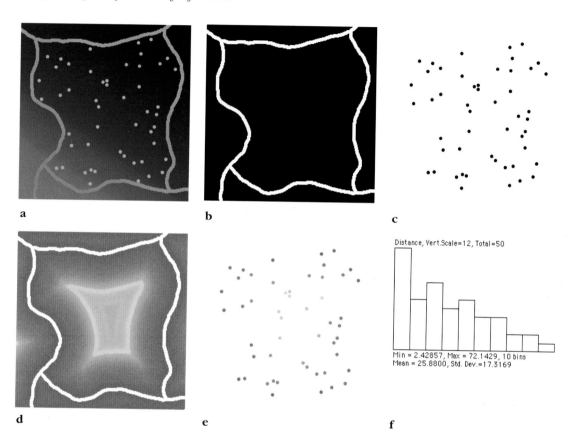

a   b   c

d   e   f

EDM values can also be combined with the skeleton of features or of the background, as discussed in the next section.

Skeletonization

Erosion can be performed with special rules that remove pixels, except when doing so would cause a separation of one region into two. The rule for this is to examine the touching neighbors; if they do not form a continuous group, then the central pixel cannot be removed (Pavlidis, 1980; Nevatia and Babu, 1980; Davidson, 1991; Lan et al., 1992; Ritter and Wilson, 1996). The definition of this condition is dependent on whether four- or eight-connectedness is used. In either case, the selected patterns can be used in a fate table to conduct the erosion (Russ, 1984). The more common convention is that features, and thus skeletons, are eight-connected while background is four-connected, and that is the convention used in the following examples.

Skeletonization by erosion is an iterative procedure, and the number of iterations required is proportional to the largest dimension of any feature in the image. An alternative method for constructing the skeleton uses the Euclidean distance map. The ridge of locally brightest values in the

EDM contains those points that are equidistant from at least two points on the boundaries of the feature. This ridge constitutes the medial axis transform (MAT). As for the UEPs, the MAT is precisely defined for a continuous image but only approximately defined for an image composed of finite pixels (Mott-Smith, 1970).

In most cases, the MAT corresponds rather closely to the skeleton obtained by sequential erosion. Since it is less directionally sensitive than any erosion pattern and because of the pixel limitations in representing a line, it may differ slightly in some cases. The uses of the MAT are the same as the skeleton, and in many cases, the MAT procedure is used but the result is still described as a skeleton.

Figure 69 shows several features with their (eight-connected) skeletons. The skeleton is a powerful shape factor for feature recognition, containing both topological and metric information. The topological values include the number of end points, the number of nodes where branches meet, and the number of internal holes in the feature. The metric values are the mean length of branches (both those internal to the feature and those having a free end) and the angles of the branches. These parameters seem to correspond closely to what human observers see as the significant characteristics of features. **Figure 70** shows the nomenclature used.

The numbers of each type of feature are related by Euler's equation:

$$\text{\# Loops} = \text{\# Branches} - \text{\# Ends} - \text{\# Nodes} + 1 \tag{4}$$

A few specific cases appear to violate this basic rule of topology, requiring careful interpretation of the digitized skeleton. **Figure 71** shows two of them. The ring skeletonizes to a single circular branch that has one loop, a single branch, and no apparent node, however, the rules of topology

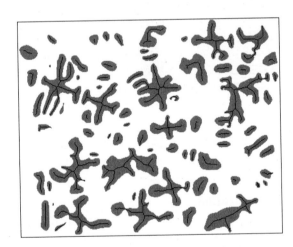

Figure 69. A binary image containing multiple features, with their skeletons superimposed.

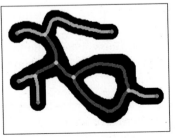

Figure 70. The skeleton of a feature with five end points, five nodes, five external branches, five internal branches, and one loop (skeleton has been dilated for visibility).

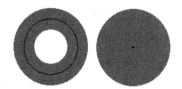

Figure 71. *Skeletons for a ring and a circle, as discussed in the text.*

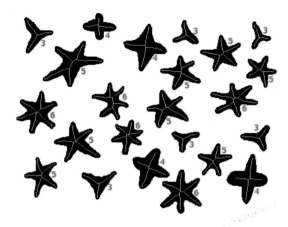

Figure 72. *Labeling star-shaped features according to the number of end points in the skeleton.*

require that there be a "virtual" node someplace on the ring where the two ends of the linear branch are joined. Likewise, the symmetrical circle figure skeletonizes to a single point. which, having fewer than two neighbors, would be classified as an end. In reality, this point represents a short branch with two ends. Special rules can correctly handle these special cases.

Locating the nodes and end points in a skeleton is simply a matter of counting neighbors. Points along the skeleton branches have exactly two neighbors. End points have a single neighbor, while nodes have more than two. The topology of features is an instantly recognizable shape descriptor that can be determined quickly from the feature skeleton. For example, in **Figure 72** the number of points in each star is something that humans identify easily as a defining shape parameter. Counting the number of skeleton pixels that have just one neighbor allows labeling them with this topological property. Similarly, an easy distinction between the letters A, B, and C is the number of loops (1, 2, and 0, respectively). As topological properties, these do not depend on size, position, or any distortion of the letters (for example by the use of different fonts).

Segment lengths are important measures of feature size, as will be discussed in Chapter 9. These can also be determined by counting, keeping track of the number of pixel pairs that are diagonally or orthogonally connected, or by fitting smoothed curves through the points and to measure the length, which gives more accurate results. Counting the number of nodes, ends, loops, and branches defines the topology of features. These topological events simplify the original image and assist in characterizing structure, as illustrated in **Figure 73**.

Skeletons are very useful for dealing with images of crossed fibers. **Figure 74** shows a diagrammatic example in which several fibers cross each other. In a few situations, it is necessary to actually follow individual fibers in such a tangle. This can be done (generally using rather specialized software and some prior knowledge about the nature of the fibers) by skeletonizing the image. The regions around each nodes where the skeletons cross are then examined, and the branches identified that represent the continuation of a single fiber (Talbot et al., 2000). The criteria are typically that the local direction change be small, and perhaps that the width, color or density of the fiber be consistent. When fibers cross at a shallow angle, the skeleton often shows two nodes with a segment that belongs to both fibers. Images of straight fibers are much easier to disentangle than curved ones.

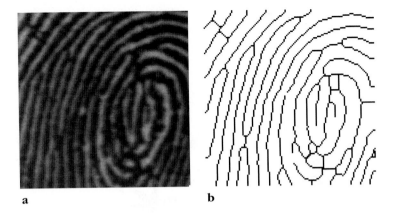

a   b

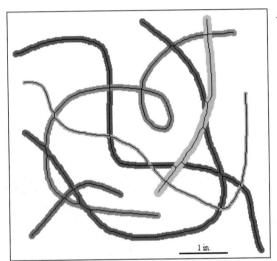

Figure 74. Example of crossing fibers, as discussed in the text, with superimposed skeleton lines.

A much simpler result is possible if the required information is just the total number and average length of the fibers. Regardless of the number of nodes or fiber crossings, the number of fibers is just half the number of end points, which can be counted directly (with a small error introduced by the probability that an end of one fiber will lie on a second fiber). Measuring the total length of the skeleton (with a correction for the end points as discussed below) and dividing by the number gives the average value. In **Figure 74**, there are 12 ends, thus 6 fibers, and a total of 40.33 inches of skeleton length, for an average length of 6.72 inches.

In other situations, such as the example shown in **Figure 75**, it may be useful to separate the branches of the skeleton for individual measurements of parameters such as length or orientation angle. Removing the exact node pixels is not sufficient to accomplish this, because the remaining branches may still be connected. This arises from the nature of eight-connected logic. **Figure 76** shows an enlargement of a portion of the skeleton network from **Figure 75** in which the node points for topological counting and near-node points that must also be removed to separate the branches are color coded for illustration. This technique is particularly appropriate for branched structures such as the roots of plants, provided that they can be spread out to produce a two-dimensional image. A stereological method is also used for measuring the total length of three-dimensional structures from projections discussed in Chapter 8.

Just as the skeleton of features may be determined in an image, it is also possible to skeletonize the background. This is often called the "skiz" of the features. **Figure 77** shows an example.

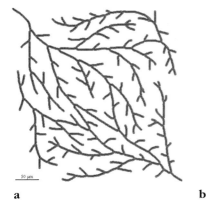

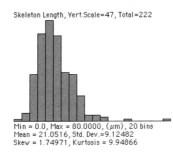

Skeleton Length, Vert.Scale=47, Total=222

Min = 0.0, Max = 80.0000, (μm), 20 bins
Mean = 21.0516, Std. Dev.=9.12482
Skew = 1.74971, Kurtosis = 9.94866

Figure 75. *Separating the branches of the skeleton of a network for measurement of their lengths.*

a   **b**

Figure 76. *Detail of the skeleton from* **Figure 75** *showing nodes. Removing the red node points does not disconnect all of the branches; the green "near-node" points must also be deleted to assure that no eight-connections remain between different branches. In the figure, end points are shown as blue.*

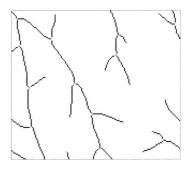

Figure 77. The skiz of the same image shown in Figure 69: *(a) complete skeleton of the background; (b) pruned skeleton.*

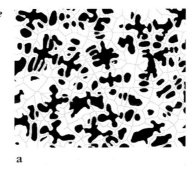
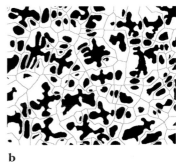

a   b

Consisting of points equidistant from feature boundaries, it effectively divides the image into regions of influence around each feature (Serra, 1982). It may be desirable to eliminate from the skiz those lines that are equidistant from two portions of the boundary of the same feature. This elimination is easily accomplished, since branches have an end; other lines in the skiz are continuous and have no ends except at the image boundaries. Pruning branches from a skeleton (or skiz) simply requires starting at each end point (points with a single neighbor) and eliminating touching pixels until a node (a point with more than two neighbors) is reached.

Boundary lines and thickening

Another use for skeletonization is to thin down boundaries that may appear broad or of variable thickness in images. This phenomenon is particularly common in light microscope images of metals whose grain boundaries are revealed by chemical etching. Such etching preferentially attacks the boundaries, but in order to produce continuous dark lines, it also broadens them. In order to measure the actual size of grains, the adjacency of different phases, or the length of boundary lines, it is preferable to thin the lines by skeletonization.

Figure 78. Skeletonization of grain boundaries:
(a) metallographic image of etched 1040 steel;
(b) thresholded image showing boundaries and dark patches of iron carbide (and pearlite);
(c) skeletonized from image *b*;
(d) pruned from image *c*;
(e) enlarged to show eight-connected line;
(f) converted to four-connected line;
(g) grains separated by thickened lines;
(h) identification of individual grains.

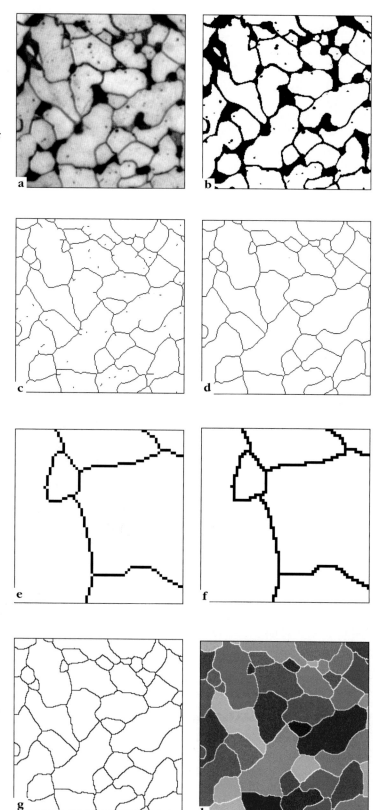

Figure 78 shows an example. The original polished and etched metal sample has dark and wide grain boundaries, as well as dark patches corresponding to carbides and pearlite. Thresholding the image produces broad lines, which can be skeletonized to reduce them to single-pixel width. Since this is properly a continuous tesselation, it can be cleaned up by pruning all branches with end points.

The resulting lines delineate the grain boundaries, but because they are eight-connected, they do not separate the grains for individual measurement. Converting the lines to four-connected, called thickening, can be accomplished with a dilation that adds pixels only for a few neighbor patterns corresponding to eight-connected corners (or the skeleton could have been produced using four-connected rules to begin with). The resulting lines separate the grains, which can be identified and measured as shown.

Figure 79 shows how this approach can be used to simplify an image and isolate the basic structure for measurement. The original image is a light micrograph of cells. It might be used to measure the variation in cell size with the distance from the two stomata (openings). This process is greatly simplified by reducing the cell walls to single lines. Leveling the background brightness of the original image and then thresholding leaves boundary lines of variable width. Skeletonizing them produces a network of single-pixel-wide lines that delineate the basic cell arrangement.

Unfortunately, the grain boundary tesselation produced by simple thresholding and skeletonization is incomplete in many cases. Some of the boundaries may fail to etch because the crystallographic mismatch across the boundary is small or the concentration of defects or impurities is low. The result is a tesselation with some missing lines, which would bias subsequent analysis. **Figure 80** shows one of the simplest approaches to dealing with this situation. Skeletonizing the incomplete network is used to identify the end points (points with a single neighbor). It is reasoned that these points should occur in pairs, so each is dilated by some arbitrarily selected distance which, it is hoped, will span half of the gap in the network.

The resulting dilated circles are ORed with the original network and the result is again skeletonized. Wherever the dilation has caused the circles to touch, the result is a line segment that joins the corresponding end points. This method is imperfect, however. Some of the points may be too far apart for the circles to touch, while in other places, the circles may obscure details by touching several existing lines, oversimplifying the resulting network. It is not easy to select an appropriate dilation radius, because the gaps are not all the same size (and not all of the grains are either). In addition, unmatched ends, or points due to dirt or particulates within the grains, can cause difficulties.

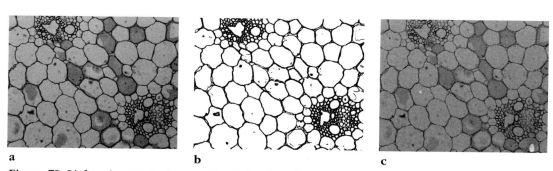

a   b   c

Figure 79. Light microscope image of cells in plant tissue:
   (a) original;
   (b) thresholded;
   (c) skeleton superimposed on original (image courtesy Data Translations, Inc.)

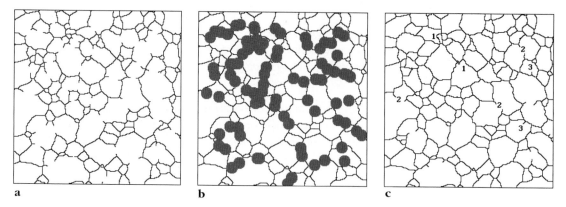

a   b   c

Figure 80. Dilation method for completing grain boundary tesselation:
   (a) incomplete network;
   (b) dilation of end point by arbitrary radius, shown as circles overlaid on the original;
   *(c) re-skeletonization of network, showing typical errors such as removal of small grains (**1**), large gaps still not joined (**2**), and dangling single ends (**3**).*

Other methods are also available. A computationally intensive approach locates all of the end points and uses a relaxation method to pair them up, so that line direction is maintained, lines are not allowed to cross, and closer points are matched first. This method suffers some of the same problems as dilation if unmatched end points or noise are present, but at least it deals well with gaps of different sizes. A third approach, the use of watershed segmentation based on the EDM, is perhaps the most efficient and reasonably accurate method. As shown in **Figure 81**, it correctly draws in most of the missing lines, but erroneously segments grains with concave shapes (which are fortunately rare in real microstructures).

Combining skeleton and EDM

The skeleton and the EDM are both important measurement tools for images, and by combining them in various ways it is possible to efficiently extract quite a variety of numeric values to quantify image data. A few examples will illustrate the variety of techniques available.

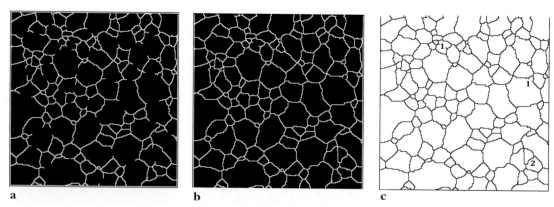

a   b   c

Figure 81. Watershed segmentation applied to the same image as Figure 80:
   (a) the image is inverted to deal with the grains rather than the boundaries;
   (b) watershed lines are drawn in, connecting most of the broken boundaries;
   (c) in the re-inverted result typical errors appear such as large gaps not joined (1) and false segmentation of irregular shaped grains (2).

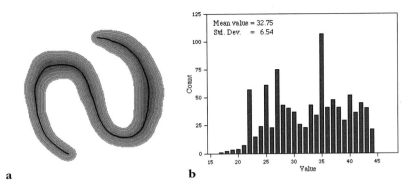

Figure 82. An irregular feature shown with its skeleton superimposed on the EDM (using pseudo-color), and the histogram of the EDM values selected by the skeleton.

a   b

The Euclidean distance map discussed previously provides values that measure the distance of every pixel from the background. For features of irregular shape or width, the pixels along the center line correspond to the centers of inscribed circles, and their EDM values can be used to measure the width and its variation. The skeleton provides a way to sample these pixels, for example by using the skeleton as a mask and then examining the histogram as shown in **Figure 82**.

The skeleton provides a basic tool for measuring the length of such irregular features, but in general is too short. The EDM values for the pixels at the end points of the skeleton give the radii of the inscribed circles at the ends. Adding these values to the skeleton length corrects for the shortness of the skeleton and provides a more accurate measure of the length of the irregular feature.

The skeleton of the background (the skiz) can be combined with the EDM of the background to determine the minimum separation distance between features. Minimum EDM values along the pruned skiz correspond to the centers of circles that touch two features, and twice those values correspond to the separation distances.

The example in **Figure 83** shows a diagram of a neuron with neurites that branch. Thresholding the central cell body, inverting the image, and creating the EDM produces a measurement of the

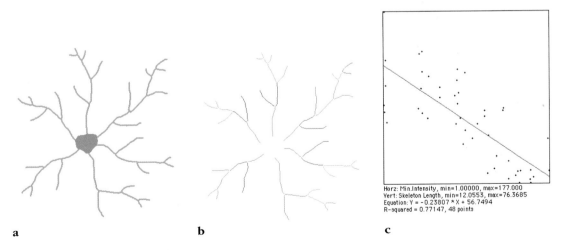

a   b   c

Figure 83. Relating distance to length:
(a) diagram of a neural cell;
(b) skeleton segments of the neurites, color coded according to distance from the cell body (values obtained from the EDM as described in the text);
(c) plot of distance vs. length.

distance of points from the cell body. The skeleton of the neurites can be separated into its component branches by removing the nodes, and the resulting segments applied as a mask to the EDM. This assigns numeric values to the pixels in the branches that determine the distance from the cell body. It may be desirable to use either the minimum or the mean value as an effective distance measurement. Plotting the skeleton length for each branch against the EDM values shows that the lengths are correlated with distance.

Measuring the distance of each feature in an image from the nearest point on the skiz (using the method shown in **Figure 68**) provides a measure of clustering in images. Many other combinations can be devised to solve measurement problems in images that combine distance and topological information.

8

Global Image Measurements

The distinction between image processing, which has occupied most of the preceding chapters, and image analysis lies in the extraction of information from the image. As mentioned several times previously, image processing, like word processing (or food processing) is the science of rearrangement. Pixel values may be altered according to neighboring pixel brightnesses, or shifted to another place in the array by image warping, but the sheer quantity of pixels is unchanged. So in word processing it is possible to cut and paste paragraphs, perform spell-checking, or alter type styles without reducing the volume of text. And food processing is also an effort at rearrangement of ingredients to produce a more palatable mixture, not to boil it down to the essence of the ingredients. Image analysis, by contrast, attempts to find those descriptive parameters, usually numeric, that succinctly represent the information of importance in the image.

The processing steps considered in earlier chapters are in many cases quite essential to carrying out this task. Defining the features to be measured frequently requires image processing to correct acquisition defects, enhance the visibility of particular structures, threshold them from the background, and perform further steps to separate touching objects or select those to be measured. And we have seen in several of the earlier chapters opportunities to use these processing methods themselves to obtain numeric information.

Global measurements and stereology

There are two major classes of image measurements: ones performed on the entire image field (sometimes called the "scene"), and ones performed on each of the separate features present. The latter feature-specific measurements are covered in the next chapter. The first group of measurements are most typically involved in the characterization of three-dimensional structures viewed as section planes in the microscope, although the methods are completely general and some of the relationships have been discovered and are routinely applied by workers in earth sciences and astronomy. The science of stereology relates the measurements that can be performed on two-dimensional images to the three-dimensional structures that are represented and sampled by those images. It is primarily a geometrical science, whose most widely used rules and calculations have a deceptive simplicity. Reviews of modern stereological methods can be found in (Russ and De-hoff, 2001; Howard and Reed, 1998; Kurzydlowski and Ralph, 1995), while classical methods are described in (Dehoff and Rhines, 1968; Underwood, 1970; Weibel, 1979; Russ, 1986).

The simplest and perhaps most frequently used stereological procedure is the measurement of the volume fraction that some structure occupies in a solid. This could be the volume of nuclei in cells, a particular phase in a metal, porosity in ceramic, mineral in an ore, etc. Stereologists often use the word "phase" to refer to the structure in which they are interested, even if it is not a phase in the chemical or thermodynamic sense. If a structure or phase can be identified in an image, and that image is representative of the whole, then the area fraction which the phase occupies in the image is a measure of the volume fraction that it occupies in the solid. This relationship is, in fact, one of the oldest known relationships in stereology, used in mineral analysis 150 years ago.

Of course, this requires some explanation and clarification of the assumptions. The image must be representative in the sense that every part of the solid has an equal chance of being examined, so the sections must be uniformly and randomly placed in the solid. Trying to measure the volume fraction of bone in the human body requires that head, torso, arms, and legs all have an equal chance of being viewed; that is the "uniform" part of the assumption. Random means, simply, that nothing is done to bias the measurements by including or excluding particular areas in the images. For example, choosing to measure only those images in which at least some bone was visible would obviously bias the measurements. More subtle, in many cases, is the tendency of micro-scopists to select areas for imaging that have some aesthetic quality (collecting pretty pictures). Al-most certainly this will tend to bias the results. A proper random stereological sampling procedure does not allow the human to select or shift the view.

Many published papers in all fields of science that use microscopy include images with the cap-tion "representative microstructure" or "typical microstructure," and in no case is this likely to be true. Either the particular image selected has been chosen because it shows most clearly some feature of the structure that the author believes is important, or it displays the best qualities of specimen preparation and image contrast, or some other characteristic that makes it (almost by de-finition) non-typical. In most real structures, there is no such thing as one typical field of view in a true statistical sense. That is why it is important to collect many images from multiple fields of view, spread throughout the specimen in an unbiased way. Data are collected from many fields and combined to represent the entire structure.

Assuming that one image could be a uniform, random sample of the structure, then the "expected value" of the area fraction of the structure is equal to the volume fraction. Of course, in any given image that may not be the result. In some images, the phase or structure of interest may not even be present, while in others it may occupy the entire field of view. In general it is necessary to se-lect an appropriate magnification so that the structures are visible, and to examine multiple fields of view and to average the measurements. The average then approaches the true value as more measurements are included.

One way to measure the area fraction of a structure is, of course, to use the image histogram. If the phase has a unique grey scale or color value, then the area of peak in the histogram provides a di-rect measure of the number of pixels covered, and hence the total area, regardless of whether it occupies one large or many small regions in the image. As shown in previous chapters, however, it is common to require image processing before thresholding can selectively delineate a structure, and to require editing of the binary image after thresholding. These steps also affect the area mea-surement, so in most cases the determination of area fraction must be made from the final binary image. All that is required is to count the black and white pixels.

Although this is a simple procedure, it is difficult to assess the accuracy of the measurement. Pix-els along the boundaries of features or regions present a challenge because thresholding and sub-sequent morphological processing may include or exclude them from the total. An image consist-ing of a single large, compact region has many fewer edge pixels (and thus less potential

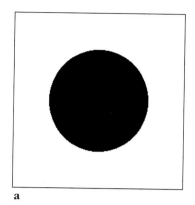

Figure 1. Two images with the same area fraction (26%) of black pixels:
(a) *one large compact region;*
(b) *many small irregular features. The measurement precision depends on the total periphery of the black-white boundary. It is also interesting to note that most human observers do not estimate area fractions very accurately, nor judge that these two images have the same area of black pixels.*

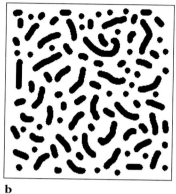

a   b

measurement error) than an image in which the same total area is distributed as many small or irregular features (**Figure 1**).

There is a preferred way to determine area fraction (and hence volume fraction) that is very efficient and does allow an estimation of the measurement precision. Traditionally, this method has been performed manually, but it is also easy to accomplish using a computer. A grid of points is superimposed on the image, and the fraction of the points that fall on the structure of interest is counted. The expected value of this point fraction is also the volume fraction. Often, the number of points in the grid is very small so that manual counting can be done at a glance. The grid may be on an eyepiece reticule in the microscope, or overlaid on a video screen or photograph, or generated within the computer. The points should be far enough apart that they provide independent measures of the structure (in other words, at the image magnification being used, two points should rarely fall into the same feature). If the structure is random, then any grid of points can be used and a regular square grid is convenient. If the structure is highly regular, then the grid itself should be randomized to prevent bias as discussed above.

When a grid is superimposed on the original grey-scale or color image (with whatever enhancement has been provided by processing), the human viewer can use independent knowledge and judgment to decide whether each point is within the region of interest. People are very good at this. But they are not very good at counting, so it may still be useful to have the human mark the points and the computer perform the counting operation as shown in **Figure 2**.

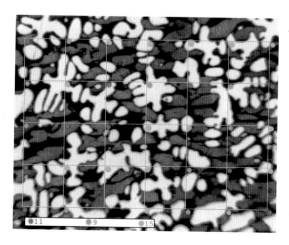

Figure 2. *Computer counting of marks. A human has placed color marks near the grid points (intersection of the lines) that fall on each phase of interest, and the computer has counted them. For the white phase, the estimated volume fraction is 15/35 = 42.8%.*

The points become a probe into the three-dimensional microstructure, and the number of points that "hit" the phase of interest allows an estimate of the measurement precision, since for independent events the standard deviation is just the square root of the count. This permits making a quick estimate of the number of images (multiple fields of view on multiple sections) that will be needed to achieve the desired final measurement precision. For example, if a grid of 25 points is used (a 5 × 5 array), and about 5 points, on average, lie on the phase of interest, that corresponds to a volume fraction of 20%. To determine the actual value with a relative precision of (say) 5% (in other words 20±1% volume fraction) it is only necessary to apply the grid to multiple fields of view until a total of 400 hits have been tallied (the square root of 400 is 20, or 5%). This would require about 80 fields of view (400/5).

A grid of points can also be efficiently applied to a thresholded and processed binary image using Boolean logic as shown in Chapter 7. If the grid is combined with the binary image using a Boolean "AND," and the surviving points are counted, the result is just those points that fell onto the phase of interest as shown in **Figure 3**. The accepted notation for these relationships is

$$V_V = A_A = P_P \tag{1}$$

meaning that the volume of the phase of interest per unit volume of material, V_V, equals (or more precisely is measured by) the area fraction A_A or the point fraction P_P.

Volume fraction is a dimensionless ratio, so the magnification of the image need not be known exactly. However, it is also possible to measure the volume of a specific structure by cutting a series of sections through it and measuring the area in each section (Gundersen, 1986). As shown in **Figure 4**, the volume of the sampled space is defined by the size and spacing of the sections, and the number of "hits" made by the grid points provides an absolute measure of the feature volume. Each grid point samples the structure and represents a volume in space equal to the area of a grid square times the section spacing. In this case, of course, the magnification must be calibrated.

In many cases, as shown in **Figure 5**, it is necessary to measure two volumes, that of the structure of interest and of an enclosing structure. In the example, a sectioned rat lung, the area of lung

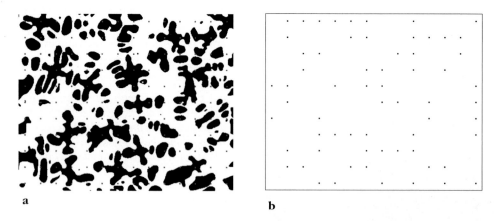

a   b

Figure 3. *Binary image of the white phase in the metal structure from **Figure 2**, with a superimposed point grid (points enlarged for visibility). A Boolean AND of the two images leaves just the points that lie on the phase **(b)**, which the computer then counts to determine P_P = 64/154 = 41.5%. The density of points illustrated in this image is somewhat too high for optimum precision estimation, because cases occur in which multiple points fall on the same feature.*

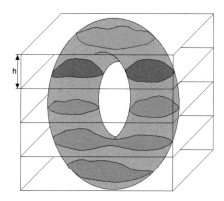

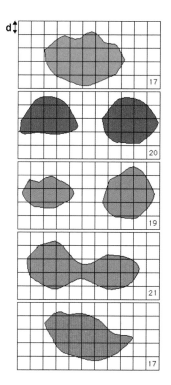

Figure 4. *Cavalieri's method for measuring the volume of an object. The grids on each section plane divide the object into cells. Counting the grid points that fall on the structure of interest provides a measure of the number of cells within the structure, and hence a measure of the volume. In the example, if the plane spacing (b) is 5 μm and the grid spacing (d) is 2 μm, then each cell has a volume of 5 × 2 × 2 = 20 μm³, and the total number of hits (17 + 20 + 19 + 21 + 17 = 94) estimates the total volume as 1880 μm3. Measuring the area of each intersection and integrating the volume with Simpson's rule gives an estimate of 1814 μm³.*

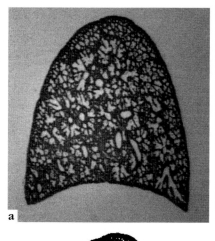

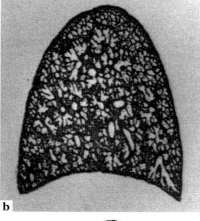

Figure 5. One section of rat lung tissue: *(a) original image; (b) leveled; (c) thresholded; (d) internal gaps filled. The areas of images c and d are used to determine the void volume within the lung.*

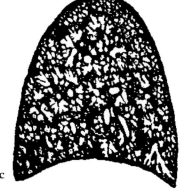

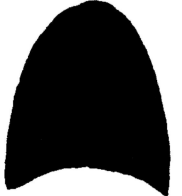

tissue in each section is added including internal voids, and the net area is also summed. The void area within the lung is then calculated as

$$Volume = \frac{\sum Filled\ Area - \sum Net\ Area}{\sum Filled\ Area}$$
(2)

Surface area

Another global parameter that is easily measured stereologically is the surface area. Surfaces can be the boundary between two structures, such as the surface area of the nucleus, the total area of cell wall in plant tissue, the total grain boundary area in a metal, or the surface of porosity in a ceramic. Note that in some of these examples the surface separates two different phases or structures, while in others it separates different regions (cells or grains) that are the same in structure and composition. Surfaces are usually very important in structures, because they are the interfaces where chemistry and diffusion take place, and control many properties such as strength, fracture, light scattering, etc.

In a two-dimensional section image through a three-dimensional structure, boundaries and surfaces are seen as lines. The total length of these lines is proportional to the amount of surface area present in the three-dimensional solid. The surface may not intersect the section plane perpendicularly, in fact in general it will not. If the surfaces are isotropic (have an equal probability of being oriented in any direction), then the relationship between total surface area per unit volume of sample and the total length of line per unit area of image is

$$S_V = \tfrac{4}{\pi} B_A$$
(3)

where S_V is the accepted notation for the surface area per unit volume, and B_A denotes the total length of boundary per unit area of image. Notice that both terms have dimensions of 1/length, and that it is consequently important to know the image magnification. **Figure 6** shows an example. The boundary lines (colored) have a total length of 9886 μm, and the image area is 15,270 μm^2. This gives a calculated surface area per unit volume of 0.0824 $\mu m^2/\mu m^3$, or 82.4 mm^2/mm^3.

Once again, it is difficult to specify the precision of such a measurement. Measuring the length of a boundary line in a digitized image is one of the most error-prone tasks in image measurement because of the pixellation of the image and the common observation that as magnification is increased, more irregularities in the boundary become visible and the measured boundary length increases. The preferred method for determining surface area is consequently to place a grid of lines on the image and to count the number of intersection points which they make with the line representing the surface of interest. The relationship between the surface area per unit volume (S_V, square micrometers per cubic micrometer) and the number of intersections (P_L, number per micrometer) is just

$$S_V = 2 \cdot P_L$$
(4)

where the factor 2 compensates for the various angles at which the grid lines can intersect the boundary. Again, because this is now a counting experiment, the measurement precision can be estimated from the square root of the number of intersection points, provided that the lines (which are the probes into the microstructure in this measurement) are far enough apart that the intersections are independent events.

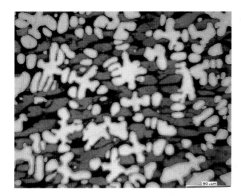

Figure 6. The boundary lines around the white phase in the same image as Figures 2 and 3 can be isolated using the techniques from Chapter 7, and measured to determine the surface area as described in the text.

Generating a grid of lines on the same image as in **Figure 6** and counting intersections (**Figure 7**) produces a similar measurement result as the boundary line technique. The total length of the grid lines is 4646 μm. Performing a Boolean AND and counting the intersections gives 197 hits (some are a single pixel and some more than one, depending on the angle between the boundary and the line). Using **Equation 4**, this corresponds to a surface area per unit volume of 0.0848 $\mu m^2/\mu m^3$. Based on the number of counts, the estimated relative precision is ±7.2% (0.0848 ± 0.0061 $\mu m^2/\mu m^3$).

Placing grid lines on images and counting intersections can be performed in all of the same ways (manually, manual marking with computer counting, or automatically using Boolean logic) as discussed above for point counting. The problem with this method as described is that it relies on the assumption that the surfaces being measured are isotropic. In real structures this criterion is rarely met. Consequently, if the structure is not isotropic, then it is necessary to construct a grid of lines that does sample the structure isotropically (in addition to the requirements of uniform and random sampling noted above). Many of the developments in modern stereology are aimed at finding practical ways to meet this isotropic, uniform, random (IUR) requirement. To visualize the meaning of isotropic directions, consider a hemisphere as shown in **Figure 8**. Each direction in space is represented by a point on the sphere. Points should be distributed evenly across the spherical surface.

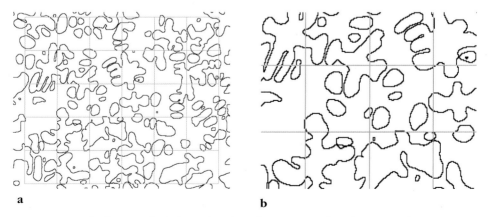

a   b

Figure 7. ANDing a grid of lines with the boundary lines from Figure 6 and counting the intersections also measures the surface area, as described in the text.

Figure 8. *A hemisphere showing a direction in three-dimensional space represented by a point on the sphere.*

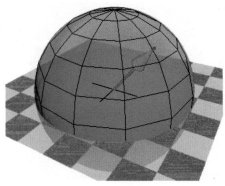

The most successful approach to generating isotropic, uniform and random lines to probe the surfaces in a three dimensional structure is called "vertical sectioning" (Baddeley et al., 1986). It requires selecting some direction in the structure that can always be identified. This might be the axis of the backbone in an animal, or the normal to a surface in a rolled metal sheet, or the direction of gravity for sedimentary layers of rock. Then all sections are cut parallel to this direction, but rotated uniformly and randomly about it, as shown in **Figure 9**. Note that this is emphatically not the way most sections are cut when biological tissue is embedded and microtomed (those sections are all perpendicular to the same direction). It would also be possible to cut the vertical sections as a pie is normally cut, with radial slices, but these would oversample the center of the pie compared to the periphery.

The vertical axis direction is present on all sections, so these cut planes are directionally biased. If lines were drawn on these sections with uniform directions in the plane, as shown in **Figure 10**, they would cluster near the north pole on the hemisphere. Directions near the equator would be undersampled. That bias can be compensated by drawing lines that are sine-weighted, as shown in **Figure 11**. Instead of drawing lines in uniform angle steps, they are drawn with uniform steps in the sine of the angle. This produces more directions around the equator and spreads out the directions near the north pole so that the points are uniformly distributed on the sphere. While a set of radial lines as shown in the figure is isotropic, it is not uniform (the center is oversampled and the corners undersampled).

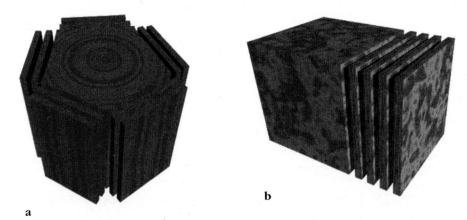

a b

Figure 9. Method for cutting vertical sections:
   (a) *correct — all sections are parallel to and rotated uniformly about a single selected axis;*
   (b) *incorrect — sections are all perpendicular to a common direction.*

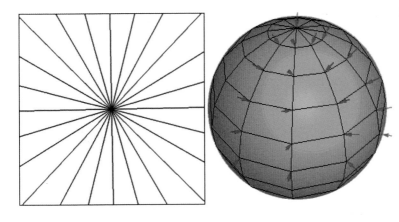

Figure 10. Drawing lines with uniform angles on each plane, and the resultant clustering of directions near the north pole of the hemisphere of orientations.

Figure 11. Drawing lines with sine-weighted angles on each plane, and the resultant uniform distribution of orientations in three-dimensional space.

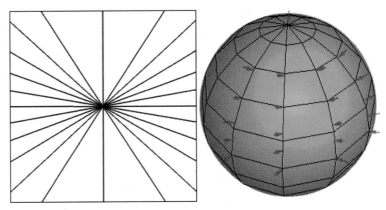

The most convenient way to draw sine-weighted lines that uniformly sample the area is to generate cycloids as shown in **Figure 12**. The cycloid is the path followed by a point on the circumference of a rolling circle. It is sine-weighted and when drawn on vertical sections has exactly the correct set of orientations to provide isotropic sampling of directions in the three-dimensional solid from which the sections were cut. Counting the intersections made by the cycloid grid with the boundary lines in the image provides the P_L value needed to calculate the surface area per unit volume. The length of each quarter arc of the cycloid line is just twice its height.

If the specimen is actually isotropic, the method of cutting vertical sections and counting intersections using a grid of cycloids will produce the correct answer, at the expense of doing a bit more work (mostly in sample preparation) than would have been needed if the isotropy was known beforehand. But if the specimen has any anisotropy, the easy method of cutting parallel sections and drawing straight line grids would produce an incorrect answer with an unknown amount of bias, while the vertical section method gives the true answer.

ASTM Grain Size

More than 100 years ago, when naval gunnery was introducing larger and larger guns onto battleships, brass cartridge casings were used to hold the gunpowder and projectile, essentially an enlarged version of a modern rifle cartridge. It was observed that after firing it was sometimes difficult to extract the used brass cartridge from the gun chamber, because the material fractured when it was pulled from the rear rim. The metal flowed and thinned when the charge was detonated, and clearly some difference in material structure was related to the tendency to tearing.

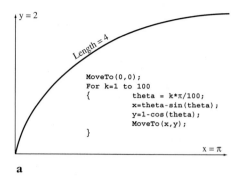

```
MoveTo(0,0);
For k=1 to 100
{
        theta = k*π/100;
        x=theta-sin(theta);
        y=1-cos(theta);
        MoveTo(x,y);
}
```

y = 2

Length = 4

x = π

a

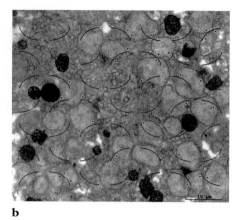

b

*Figure 12. Procedure for drawing an arc of the cycloid (**a**), and a cycloid grid superimposed on a vertical section image (**b**). The intersections (marked in color) of the cycloid lines with the membranes provide an unbiased measure of the total surface area per unit volume, $S_V = 2 P_L = 2 \cdot 39 / 331.5 \mu m = 0.235$ $\mu m^2/\mu m^3$.*

From that observation, a method for measuring a microstructural parameter known as the ASTM (American Society for Testing and Materials) "grain size" was developed, and used for quality control of naval brass, and later many other metals and nonmetals. In fact, several different standard techniques are used, which have been adjusted with appropriate constants so that they agree approximately with each other's numeric values; but, in fact, the methods measure two entirely different characteristics of microstructure (neither of which is the "size" of the grains).

The first method proposed was to count the number of visible grains per square inch on a polished section at 100x magnification. The number of grains N is then related to the "grain size number" G by

$$N = 2^{(G-1)}$$

(5)

where the value G is never reported with a precision better than 0.5. An equivalent version adjusted to metric dimensions is also in use.

A second method for determining the value G is based on drawing a grid of lines on the image. Because many metals are anisotropic due to the forming processes, the grains are elongated in one direction. In order to avoid directional bias in the measurement, a circular grid is used. The number of intersections made by the line with the grain boundaries per unit length of the line (N_L where length is in millimeters) can is used to calculate

$$G = 6.6457 \cdot \log_{10} N_L - 3.298$$

(6)

The constants are needed to convert the metric units and to make the results approximately agree with the grain count method. Again, the results are rounded to the nearest 0.5; **Figure 13** shows an example.

There are also other methods that are part of the ASTM standard (E112), such as counting the number of triple points (places where three grains meet at a point) per unit area, and most of these methods may be implemented either by hand count or by computer.

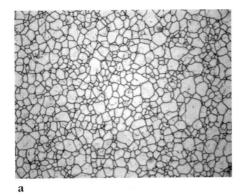
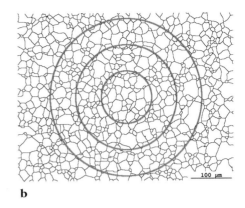

a   b

Figure 13. Light microscope image of a low carbon steel (a), which is prepared by leveling, thresholding and skeletonizing to delineate the grain boundaries (b). Counting the number of grains inside the largest circle (445, counting each one that intersects the circle as 1/2) gives a grain size number G = 8.7. Counting the intercepts with the concentric circle grids (147 with a grid length of 2300 µm) gives a grain size number G = 9.1. Both values would normally be reported as a grain size number of 9.

The intercept count method (**Equation 6**) in reality measures the total surface area of grain boundary. Note the use of N_L which, similar to the P_L value in **Equation 4**, is proportional to the surface area per unit volume. The importance of grain boundary area makes sense from a mechanical property standpoint since creep in materials occurs due to grain boundary sliding and grain rotation, and grain deformation occurs by motion of dislocations which start and end at these same boundaries. The grain count and triple-point count methods actually measure the total length per unit volume of the edges of grains, which is a parameter related primarily to diffusion. Measurement of the length of structures is discussed in the following paragraphs.

The fact that one of these parameters can be even approximately tied to the other is due to the limited application of the method to metals that have been heat-treated so that they are fully recrystallized. In this condition, the distribution of actual three-dimensional grain sizes approaches a constant, more-or-less log-normal state in which the structure may coarsen with time (large grains grow and small ones vanish) but the structure remains self similar. Hence there is an approximately consistent relationship between the length of edges and the area of surfaces.

The same relationship does not apply to metals without this heat treatment, and so the notion of a single numerical value that can characterize the microstructure is flawed, even for quality control purposes, and the measurement method used does matter. But 100 years of use have sanctified the technique and most practitioners are not aware of what their procedure actually measures in the microstructure.

Actually measuring the "size" (usually the volume) of individual grains or cells in a three-dimensional solid is quite difficult. It has been done in a few cases by literally taking the material apart (e.g., by chemically dissolving a thin layer along the boundaries so the grains are separated), and measuring each one. Other researchers have used an exhaustive serial sectioning technique that produces a complete three-dimensional volumetric image of the structure, from which measurements can be made. Both of these approaches are far too laborious for routine practical use. Determining the mean volume of cells can be done using the Disector method described below. This actually measures the number per unit volume, but the inverse of that quantity is the mean volume per feature. This method relies heavily on computer-based image processing to deal with the large number of images. **Figure 14**, below, will show an example.

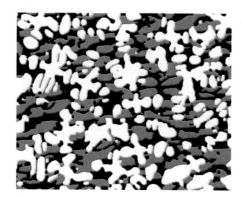

Figure 14. The three-phase aluminum-zinc alloy from Figure 2, with the phase boundaries shown in color.

It is also possible to measure the variance of the size distribution of the features using a point-sampled intercept method applied to IUR section planes, described below. But if the actual size distribution of the three-dimensional features is needed, then the more intensive methods must be undertaken.

Multiple types of surfaces

In most kinds of real samples, there are several different phases or structures present, and consequently many different types of boundary surfaces. In a three-phase material, containing regions which for convenience can be identified as types α, β and γ, there are six possible interfaces (α-α, α-β, α-γ, β-β, β-γ, and γ-γ) and the number goes up rapidly in more complex structures. Some of the possible interface types may be absent, meaning that those two phase regions never touch (e.g., nuclei in separate cells do not touch each other, it makes no sense to consider a surface between two pores, etc.). Measuring the amounts of each different type of interface can be very useful in characterizing the overall three-dimensional structure.

Figure 14 shows a three-phase metal structure. Notice that no white dendritic region touches another one, for example. Chapter 7 showed how Boolean logic with the dilated region outlines can be used to delineate each type of interface. Once the image of the boundaries has been isolated, counting intersections with a grid provides the measurement of surface area per unit volume.

Figure 15 shows a simpler, idealized, two-phase microstructure. By thresholding each phase, using morphological operations such as a closing, and Boolean logic to combine two derived images, each of the three distinct boundary types can be isolated (in the image, they have been combined

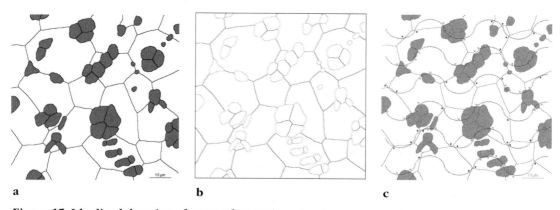

a   b   c

Figure 15. Idealized drawing of a two-phase microstructure
   (a) *the three different types of interface boundaries present*
   (b) *and the result of counting the intersections of these boundaries with a cycloid grid*
   (c). *The measurements and calculated results are detailed in the text.*

as color channels for visualization purposes). Assuming this is a vertical section, a cycloid grid such as the one shown can be used to estimate the surface area per unit volume as shown in the figure, using **Equation 4**.

It may be instructive to illustrate and compare the various measurement procedures described above for volume surface area measurement, and using the magnification calibration shown on the image in **Figure 15**. Counting pixels estimates the area fraction, and hence the volume fraction of the grey phase at 17.3%. Placing a square grid of 90 points produces 14 hits, for an volume fraction estimate using **Equation 1** of 15.6%. Measuring the length of the boundary lines for each type of interface and applying equation 3 produces the results listed below. Counting intersections of the grid lines with each type of boundary and applying equation 4 gives another estimate of surface area, also shown in the table. The image area is 5453.6 μm^2 and the grid used had a total length of 614 μm.

Boundary	Length (μm)	$S_V = (4/\pi) \cdot$ Length/Area	Grid counts	$S_V = 2\,P_L$
White-white	441.96	103.2 mm²/mm³	28	101.8 mm²/mm³
Grey-white	551.24	128.7	37	134.5
Grey-grey	123.30	28.8	8	29.1

The agreement between these different methods is quite satisfying, but only the counting methods allow a simple estimate of the measuring precision be made. Note that it is possible to squeeze a considerable amount of surface area into a small volume.

Length

Length measurement is usually applied to structures that are elongated in one direction, such as neurons or blood vessels in tissue, fibers in composites, or dislocations in metals. It is also possible, however, to measure the total length of edges, such as the edges of polyhedral grains in a metal (as mentioned earlier in connection with the ASTM grain size measurement), or any other line that represents the intersection of surfaces.

When a linear structure intersects the sampling plane, the result is a point. The number of such points is proportional to the total length of the line. If the linear structures in the three-dimensional solid are isotropic, then the relationship between the total length of line per unit volume L_V (with units of micrometers per cubic micrometer or length^{-2}) and the total number of points per unit area P_A (with units of number per square micrometer or length^{-2}) is

$$L_V = 2 \cdot P_A \qquad (7)$$

where the constant 2 arises, as it did in the case of surface area measurements, from considering all of the angles at which the plane and line can intersect. In some cases a direct count of points can be made on a polished surface. For example, fibers in a composite are visible, and dislocations can be made so by chemical etching.

In the example of **Figure 13**, the triple points where three grains meet represent the triple lines in space that are the edges of the grains. These are paths along which diffusion is most rapid. To isolate them for counting, the skeleton of the grain boundaries can be obtained as shown in Chapter 7. The branch points in this tesselation can be counted as shown in **Figure 16** because they are points in the skeleton that have more than two neighbors. Counting them is another way (less commonly used) to calculate a "grain size" number.

Figure 16. *The image from*
   Figure 13, *thresholded and*
   skeletonized with the 1732
   branch points in the skeleton
   color coded (with an enlarged
   portion for visibility).

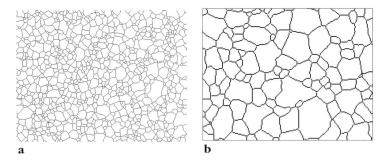

a   b

One convenient way to measure the length of a structure, independent of its complexity or connectedness, is to image a thick section (considerably thicker than the width of the linear portions of the structure). In this projected image, the length of the features is not truly represented because they may incline upwards or downwards through the section. Any line drawn on the image represents a surface through the section, with area equal to the product of its length and the section thickness. Counting the number of intersections made by the linear structure with the grid line, and then calculating the total length using the relationship in **Equation 7**, provides a direct measurement of the total length per unit volume.

If the sample is isotropic, any grid line can be used. If not, then if the sections have been taken with isotropic sectioning, a circle grid can be used since that samples all orientations in the plane. But the most practical way to perform the measurement without the tedium of isotropic section orientation or the danger of assuming that the sample is isotropic is to cut the sections parallel to a known direction (vertical sectioning) and then use cycloidal grid lines, as shown in **Figure 17**. In this case, since it is the normal to the surface represented by the lines that must be made isotropic in three-dimensional space, the generated cycloids must be rotated by 90° to the "vertical" direction.

In the example of **Figure 17**, the intersections of the grid lines with the projections of the microtubules allow the calculation of the total length per unit volume using **Equation 7**. There are 41 marked intersections; of course, these could also be counted by thresholding the image and ANDing it with the grid, as shown previously in this chapter and in Chapter 7. For an image area of 12,293 μm^2, an assumed section thickness of 3 μm, and a total length of grid lines of 331.2 μm, the length calculation from **Equation 7** gives:

Figure 17. *Application of a cycloid grid to a TEM image of*
   a section containing filamentous microtubules.
   Counting the number of intersections made with the
   grid allows calculation of the total length per unit
   volume, as discussed in the text.

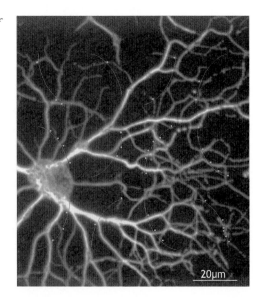

$$L_V = 2 \cdot 41 / (12293 * 3) \; \mu m/\mu m^3 = 2.22 \; mm / mm^3$$

It is rare to find a real three-dimensional structure that is isotropic. If the structure is (or may be) anisotropic, it may be necessary to generate section planes that are isotropic. Procedures for doing so have been published, but in general they are tedious, wasteful of sample material, and hard to make uniform (that is, they tend to oversample the center of the object as compared to the periphery).

Another way to generate isotropic samples of a solid, either for surface area or length measurement, is to subdivide the three-dimensional material into many small pieces, randomly orient each one, and then make convenient sections for examination. This is perhaps the most common approach that people really use. With such isotropic section planes, it is not necessary to use a cycloid grid. Any convenient line grid will do. If there is preferred directionality in the plane, circular line grids can be used to avoid bias. If not, then a square grid of lines can be used. If the structure is highly regular, then it is necessary to use randomly generated lines (which can be conveniently performed by the computer). **Figure 18** shows examples of a few such grids. Much of the art of modern stereology lies in performing appropriate sample sectioning and choosing the appropriate grid to measure the desired structural parameter.

Sampling strategies

Several of the examples shown thus far have represented the common situation of transmission microscopy in which views are taken through thin slices, generally using the light or electron microscope. The requirement is that the sections be much thinner than the dimensions of any

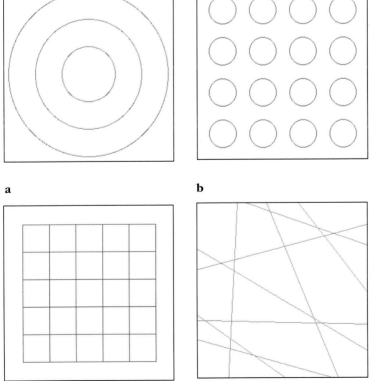

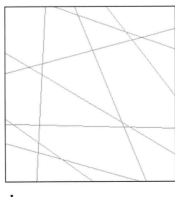

Figure 18. Examples of line grids:
(**a**) concentric circles;
(**b**) array of circles;
(**c**) square line grid;
(**d**) random lines.

a

b

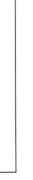

c

d

structures of interest, except for the case above of thick sections used for length measurement. For opaque materials, the same strategies are used for sectioning but the images are obtained by reflected light, or by scanning electron microscopy, or any other form of imaging that shows just the surface. Many imaging techniques in fact represent the structure to some finite depth beneath the surface, and most preparation methods such as polishing produce finite surface relief in which the software structures are lower than the harder ones. Again, the criterion is that the depth of information (e.g., the depth from which electrons are emitted in the scanning electron microscope, or the depth of polishing relief) is much less than the dimensions of any structures of interest. Corrections to the equations above for measuring volume, area and length can be made for the case of finite section thickness or surface relief, but they are complicated and require exact measurement of the thickness.

Although the procedures for obtaining isotropic sampling have been outlined, little has been said thus far about how to achieve uniform, random sampling of structures. It is of course possible to cut the entire specimen up into many small pieces, select some of them by blind random sampling, cut each one in randomly oriented planes, and achieve the desired result. However, that is not the most efficient method (Gundersen and Jensen, 1987). A systematic or structured random sample can be designed that will produce the desired unbiased result with the fewest samples and the least work. The method works at every level through a hierarchical sampling strategy, from the selection of a few test animals from a population (or cells from a petri dish, etc.) to the selection of tissue blocks, the choice of rotation angles for vertical sectioning, the selection of microtomed slices for viewing, the location of areas for imaging, and the placement of grids for measurement.

To illustrate the procedure, consider the problem of determining the volume fraction of bone in the human body. Clearly, there is no single section location that can be considered representative of such a diverse structure: a section through the head would show proportionately much more bone than one at the waist. Let us suppose that, in order to obtain sufficient precision, we have decided that eight sections are sufficient for each body. For volume fraction, it is not necessary to have isotropic sections so we could use transverse sections. In practice, these could be obtained non-destructively using a computerized tomography (CT) scanner or magnetic resonance imaging (MRI). If the section planes were placed at random, there would be some portions of the body that were not viewed while some planes would lie close together and oversample other regions. The most efficient sampling would space the planes uniformly apart, but it is necessary to avoid the danger of bias in their placement, always striking certain structures and avoiding others.

Systematic random sampling would proceed by generating a random number to decide the placement of the first plane somewhere in the top one-eighth of the body. Then position the remaining planes with uniform spacing, so that each has the same offset within its one-eighth of the body height. These planes constitute a systematic random sample. A different random number placement would be used on the next body, and the set of planes would be shifted as a unit. This procedure guarantees that every part of the body has an equal chance of being measured, which is the requirement for random sampling.

When applied to the placement of a grid on each image, two random numbers are generated which specify the position of the first point (the upper left corner) of the grid. The other grid points then shift as a unit with uniform spacing. The same logic applies to selecting measurement positions on a slide in the microscope. If for adequate statistical sampling it has been decided to acquire images from, for example, 8 fields of view on slide, then the area is divided into 8 equal areas as shown in **Figure 19**, two random numbers are generated to position the first field of view in the first rectangle, and the subsequent images are acquired at the same relative position in each of the other areas.

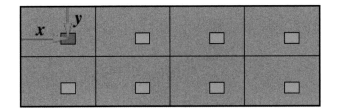

For rotations of vertical sections, if it is decided to use five orientations as shown earlier in **Figure 9**, then a random number is used to select an angle between 0 and 72° for the first cut, and then the remaining orientations are placed systematically at 72-degree intervals. For selection of animals from a population, if 7 animals are to be examined from a group of 100, a random number selects one of the first 14, and then each fourteenth animal after that is selected.

The method can obviously be generalized to any situation. It is uniform and random because every part of the sampled population has an equal probability of being selected. Of all of the possible slices and lines that could be used to probe the structure, each one has an equal probability of being used.

The mantra of the stereologist in designing an experiment is to achieve IUR sampling of the structure. For some types of probes the requirement of isotropy can be relaxed because the probe itself has no directionality, and thus is not sensitive to any anisotropy in the specimen. Using a grid of points, for example, to determine the volume fraction of a structure of interest, does not require the vertical sectioning strategy described previously because the point probe has no orientation. Any convenient set of planes that uniformly and randomly sample the structure can be probed with a uniformly and randomly placed grid to obtain an unbiased result.

The disector, described in the next section, is a volume probe and hence also has no directionality associated with it. Pairs of section planes can be distributed (uniformly and randomly) through the structure without regard to orientation. Being able to avoid the complexity of isotropic sectioning is a definite advantage in experimental design.

As noted previously, for measurement of length or surface area the probes (surfaces and lines) have orientation, so they must be placed isotropically, as well as uniformly and randomly. It is in these cases that a strategy such as vertical sectioning and the use of cycloidal grids becomes necessary. Using a systematic random sampling approach reduces the number of such sections that need to be examined, as compared to a fully random sampling, but it does not alleviate the need to guarantee that all orientations have an equal probability of being selected. It bears repetition that unless it can be proven that the sample itself is isotropic (and uniform and random), then unless an appropriate IUR sampling strategy is employed the results will be biased and the amount of the bias cannot be determined.

Determining number

Figure 20 shows several sections through a three-dimensional structure. Subject to the caveat that the sections must be IUR, it is straightforward from the areas of the intersections or by using a point count with a grid to determine the total volume of the tubular structure (**Equation 1**). From the length of the boundary line, or by using intercept counts of the boundary with a suitable line grid, the total surface area of the structure can be determined (**Equations 3** and **4**). From the number of separate features produced by the intersection of the object with the planes, the length of the

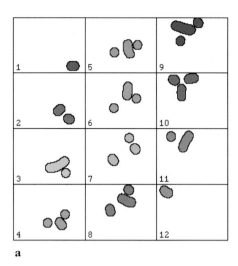

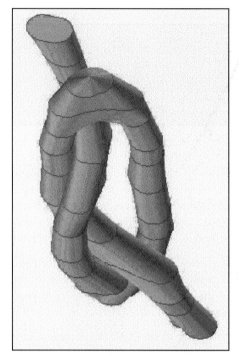

Figure 20.
(**a**) Multiple sections through a tubular structure, from which the volume, surface area and length can be determined. Only by arranging them in order, aligning them, and reconstructing the volume
(**b**) can the presence of a single string arranged in a right-handed knot be recognized.

tube can be estimated (**Equation 7**). But there is nothing in the individual section planes that reveals whether this is one object or many, and if it is one object whether the tube is branched or not. The fact that the single tube is actually tied into a knot is of course entirely hidden. It is only by connecting the information in the planes together, by interpolating surfaces between closely spaced planes and creating a reconstruction of the three dimensional object, that these topological properties can be assessed.

Volume, surface area, and length are metric properties. The plane surfaces cut through the structure and the grids of lines and points placed on them represent probes that sample the structure and provide numerical information that can be used to calculated these metric properties, subject to the precision of the measurement and to the need for uniform, random and (except for volume measurement) isotropic sampling. Topological properties of number and connectedness can not be measured using plane, line or point probes. It is necessary to actually examine a volume of the sample.

In the limit, of course, this could be a complete volumetric imaging of the entire structure. Nondestructive techniques such as confocal light microscopy, medical CT, MRI or sonic scans, or stereoscopic viewing through transparent volumes, can be used in some instances. They produce dramatic visual results when coupled with computer graphics techniques (which are shown in Chapters 11 and 12); however, these are costly and time consuming methods that cannot easily be applied to many types of samples. Serial sectioning methods in which many sequential thin sections are cut, or many sequential planes of polish are prepared and examined, are much more difficult and costly because of the problems of aligning the images and compensating for distortion or variation in spacing or lack of parallel orientation.

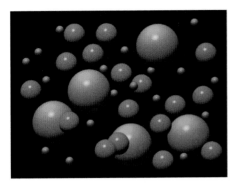

a

Figure 21.
> *(a)* A volume containing large (green), medium (orange) and small (purple) objects;
> *(b)* an arbitrary section through the volume;
> *(c)* the appearance of the objects in the plane. The sizes of the intersections are not the size of the objects, and the number of intersections with each does not correspond to the number per unit volume because large objects are more likely to be intersected by the plane.

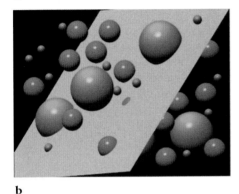

b

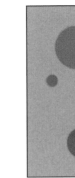

c

It is a very common mistake to count the number of features visible on a section plane and from that try to infer the number of objects in the three-dimensional volume. The fact that the units are wrong is an early indication of trouble. The number of features imaged per unit area does not correspond to the number per unit volume. In fact, the section plane is more likely to strike a large object than a small one so the size of the objects strongly influences the number that are observed to intersect the sectioning plane, as shown in **Figure 21**.

There is a relationship between number per unit area and number per unit volume based on the concept of a mean diameter for the features. For spheres, the mean diameter has a simple meaning. The number per unit volume N_V can be determined from the number per unit area N_A as

$$N_V = \frac{N_A}{D_{mean}} \qquad (8)$$

More precisely, the expected value of N_A is the product of $N_V \cdot D_{mean}$. For convex but not spherical shapes, the mean diameter is the mean caliper or tangent diameter averaged over all orientations. This can be calculated for various regular or known shapes, but is not something that is known *a priori* for most structures. So determining something like the number of grains or cells or nuclei per unit volume (whose inverse would give the mean volume of each object) is in fact rarely practical.

For objects that are not convex, have protrusions or internal void, or holes and bridges (multiple connected shapes), the concept of a mean diameter becomes even more nebulous and less useful. It turns out that the integral of the mean surface curvature over the entire surface of the object is related to this mean diameter. As noted below, the surface curvature is defined by two principal radii. Defining the mean local curvature as

$$H = \frac{1}{2}\left(\frac{1}{r_1} + \frac{1}{r_2}\right) \qquad (9)$$

and integrating over the entire surface gives a value called the integral mean curvature M, which equals $2\pi \cdot D_{mean}$. In other words, the feature count N_A on a section plane is actually a measure of the mean curvature of the particles and hence the mean diameter as it has been defined previously. If the number per unit volume can be independently determined, for instance using the disector method described in the next section, it can be combined with N_A to calculate the mean diameter.

Curvature, connectivity, and the disector

Surfaces and lines in three-dimensional structures are rarely flat or straight, and in addition to the relationship to mean diameter introduced above, their curvature may hold important information about the evolution of the structure, or chemical and pressure gradients. For grain structures in equilibrium, the contact surfaces are ideally flat but the edges still represent localized curvature. This curvature can be measured by stereology.

Surface curvature is defined by two radii (maximum and minimum). If both are positive as viewed from "inside" the object bounded by the surface, the surface is convex. If both are negative the surface is concave, and if they have opposite signs, the surface has saddle curvature (**Figure 22**). The total integrated curvature for any closed surface around a simply connected object (no holes, bridges, etc.) is always 4π. For more complicated shapes, the total curvature is $4\pi(N - C)$ where N is the number of separate objects and C is the connectivity.

For a simple array of separate objects, regardless of the details of their shape, C is zero (they are not connected) and the total integrated curvature of the structure gives a measure of how many objects are present. To measure this topological quantity, a simple plane surface is not adequate as explained above. The total curvature can be measured by considering a sweeping plane probe moving through the sample (this can be physically realized by moving the plane of focus of a confocal microscope through the sample, or by using a medical imaging device) and counting the events when the plane probe is tangent to the surface of interest. Convex and concave tangent points (T^{++} and T^{--}, respectively) are counted separately from saddle tangencies (T^{+-}). Then the

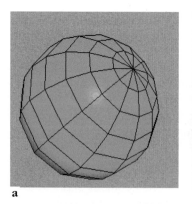
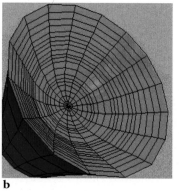
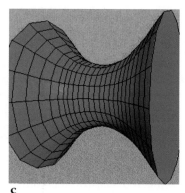

a   b   c

Figure 22. Surface curvature: (a) convex; (b) concave; (c) saddle

net tangent count is $(T^{++} + T^{--} - T^{+-})$ gives the quantity $(N - C)$, also called the Euler characteristic of the structure, as

$$(N-C) = \tfrac{1}{2}\left(T^{++} + T^{--} - T^{+-}\right) = \tfrac{1}{2}T_{net} \tag{10}$$

There are two extreme cases in which this is useful. One is the case of separate (but arbitrarily and complexly shaped) objects, in which C is 0 and N is one-half the net tangent count. This provides a straightforward way to determine the number of objects in the measured volume. The other situation of interest is the case of a single object, typically an extended complex network with many branchings such as neurons, capillaries, textiles used as reinforcement in composites, etc. In this case, N is 1 and the connectivity can be measured. Connectivity is the minimum number of cuts that would be needed to separate the network. For flow or communication through a network, it is the number of alternate paths, or the number of blockages that would be required to stop the flow or transmission.

In many situations, such as the case of an opaque matrix, it is not practical to implement a sweeping tangent plane. The simplest practical implementation of a volume probe that can reveal the important topological properties of the structure is the disector (Sterio, 1984). This consists of two parallel planes of examination, which can be two sequential or closely spaced thin sections examined in transmission. For many materials samples, it is implemented by polishing an examination plane which is imaged and recorded, polishing down a small distance (usually using hardness indentations or scratches to gauge the distance and also to facilitate aligning the images), and acquiring a second image.

The disector logic compares the images in the two parallel planes and ignores any feature that continues through both planes, even if the position and shape have changed somewhat. The planes must of course be close enough together that this determination can be made unequivocally. Usually this means that the spacing must be significantly less than any characteristic dimension of the features or structure of interest, and so most features that intersect one plane will intersect both. **Figure 23** shows the possible combinations of events that may be found. Any features that are present in one plane and not the other imply that the three-dimensional structure had a end point somewhere between the two planes. This represents a convex curvature and is counted as a T^{++} event.

Typically, much more rare is the case in which a hollow feature in one plane becomes solid in the other plane. This represents the end of a void or, more generally, a hollow with concave curvature, and is counted as a T^{--} event. Any branching in the structure, in which one feature in one of the two planes can be presumed to connect to two features in the other, represents a saddle surface and is counted as a T^{+-} event. The tangent events from the disector are summed in the same way shown in **Equation 10** to determine the net tangent count and the Euler characteristic of the structure.

Figure 23. *Possible combinations of features in the two planes of the disector. Features that continue through with no topological change are ignored. Feature ends are counted as convex (T^{++}) events and void ends are counted as concave (T^{--}) ones. Branching indicates the presence of saddle surface with T^{+-} curvature.*

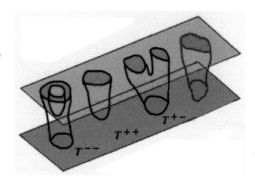

Because most of the features seen in the disector images continue through both sections and so contribute no information, it is necessary to examine many pairs of sections, which of course must be aligned to compare intersections with the features. When the matrix is transparent and viewed in a confocal microscope, examining and comparing the parallel section planes is straightforward. When conventional serial sections are used, it is attractive to use computer processing to align and compare the images. The Feature-AND logic described in Chapter 7 is particularly useful in this regard, to find features that continue through both sections. It is also necessary to sample a large image area, well distributed to meet the usual criteria of random, uniform sampling (since the disector is a volume probe, isotropy is not an issue).

For opaque matrices, the problems are more severe. Generally it is necessary to prepare a polished section, image it, place some fiducial marks on it for reference, and then polish down to some greater depth in the sample and repeat the process. If the fiducial marks are small pyramidal hardness indentations (commonly used to measure hardness of materials), the reduction in their size provides a measure of the distance between the two planes. Aligning and comparing the two images to locate new features can be quite tedious.

Figure 24 shows an example. The specimen is a titanium alloy in which the size of colonies of Widmanstatten laths is of interest. Each colony is identified by its lath orientation. After one set of images was acquired on a metallographically polished plane, the material was polished down a further 5 μm (as measured from the size change of a microhardness indentation) and additional corresponding images acquired. In the example, another colony (identified by the red arrow) has appeared. From the total number of positive tangent events and the volume sampled by the disector, the mean colony volume was determined.

Anisotropy and gradients

There is much emphasis above on methods for performing sectioning and applying grids that eliminate bias in those structures that may not be IUR. Of course, when the specimen meets those criteria then any sampling method and grid can be used, but in most cases it is not possible to assume

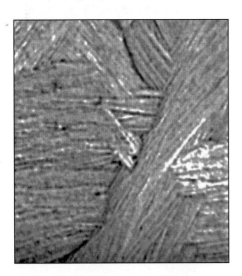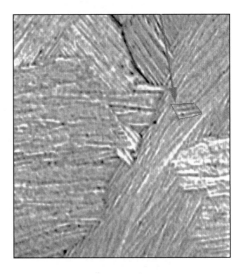

Figure 24. Scanning electron micrographs of colonies of laths in a titanium alloy (images courtesy Dr. H. Fraser, Dept. of Materials Science and Engineering, Ohio State University, Columbus, OH). The two images represent parallel planes with a measured spacing of 5 μm. A new colony (red arrow and outline) appears in one image, producing a single positive tangent count (T^{++}).

an IUR structure. Thus, techniques such as vertical sectioning and cycloid grids are used, since they will provide unbiased results whether the specimen is IUR or not, at the cost of somewhat more effort in preparation and measurement.

In some situations, it may be important to actually measure the anisotropy (preferred orientation) in the specimen, or to characterize the nonuniformity (gradients) present in the structure. This requires more effort. First, it is usually very important to decide beforehand what kind of anisotropy or gradient is of interest. Sometimes this is known *a priori* based on the physics of the situation. Deformation of materials in fabrication and the growth of plants typically produce grains or cells that are elongated in a known direction, for example. Many physical materials and biological tissues have structures that vary markedly near surfaces and outer boundaries, so a gradient in that direction may be anticipated. Anisotropy can be qualitatively determined visually, by examining images of planes cut in orthogonal directions, as shown in **Figures 25** and **26**. It is usually necessary to examine at least two planes to distinguish the nature of the anisotropy as shown in **Figure 27**.

Figure 25. Anisotropy in muscle tissue, visible as a difference in structure in transverse (b,d) and longitudinal (a,c) sections.

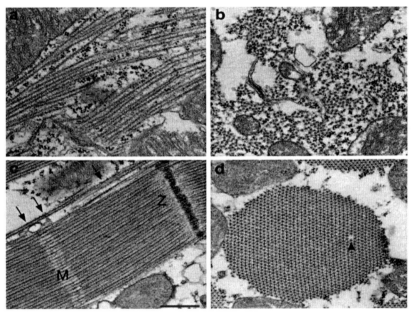

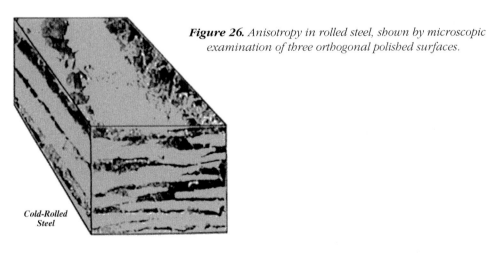

Figure 26. Anisotropy in rolled steel, shown by microscopic examination of three orthogonal polished surfaces.

Cold-Rolled Steel

Figure 27. *The need to examine at least two orthogonal surfaces to reveal the nature of anisotropy. In the example, the same appearance on one face can result from different three-dimensional structures.*

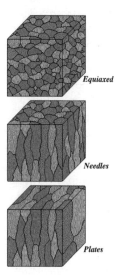

Equiaxed

Needles

Plates

When there is expectation that directionality is present in the structure, the classic approach is to use grids to measure selectively in different directions. For example, in the case shown in **Figure 28**, the number of intercepts per unit line length (which measures the surface area per unit volume) can be measured in different directions by using a rotated grid of parallel lines. Since each set of lines measures the projected surface area normal to the line direction, the result shows the anisotropy of surface orientation. Plotting the reciprocal of number of intersections/line length (called the intercept length) as a function of orientation produces a polar (or rose) plot as shown in the figure, which characterizes the mean shape of the grains or cells.

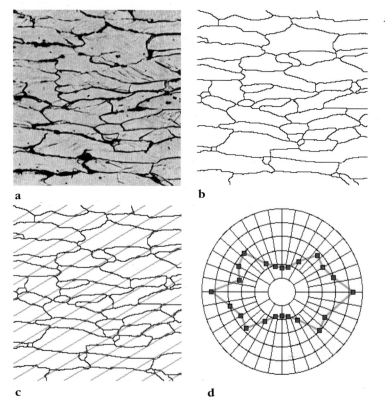

a

b

c

d

Figure 28. Characterizing anisotropy:
(a) an anisotropic metal grain structure;
(b) the idealized grain boundaries produced by thresholding and skeletonization;
(c) measuring the number of intercepts per unit line length in different orientations by rotating a grid of parallel lines;
(d) the results shown as a polar plot of mean intercept length.

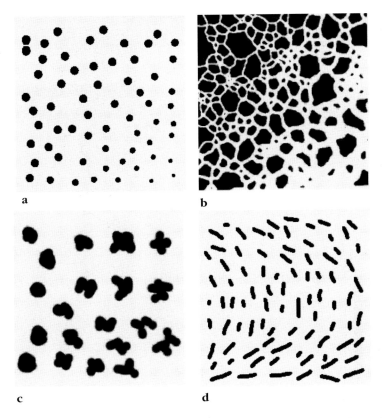

Figure 29. Schematic examples of gradients in:
(a) size;
(b) area fraction;
(c) shape;
(d) orientation.

a   b

c   d

Gradients can sometimes be observed by comparing images from different parts of a specimen, but because visual judgment of metric properties such as length of boundary lines and area fraction of a phase is not very reliable it is usually safest to actually perform measurements and compare the data statistically to find variations. The major problem with characterizing gradients is that they are rarely simple. An apparent change in the number of features per unit area or volume may hide a more significant change in feature size or shape, for example. **Figure 29** shows some examples in which gradients in size, number, shape and orientation are present. A secondary problem is that once the suspected gradient has been identified, a great many samples and fields of view may be required to obtain adequate statistical precision to properly characterize it.

Figure 30 shows a simple example of the distribution of cell colonies in a petri dish. Are they preferentially clustered near the center, or uniformly distributed across the area? By using the method shown in Chapter 7 to assign a value from the Euclidean distance map (of the area inside the petri dish) to each feature, and then plotting the number of features as a function of that value, the plot of count vs. radial distance shown in **Figure 31** is obtained. This would appear to show a decrease in the number of features toward the center of the dish; but this is does not correctly represent the actual situation, because it is not the number but the number per unit area that is important, and there is much more area near the periphery of the dish than near the center. If the distribution of number of features as a function of radius is divided by the number of pixels as a function of radius (which is simply the histogram of the Euclidean distance map), the true variation of number per unit area is obtained as shown in the figure.

Size distributions

Much of the contemporary effort in stereological development and research has been concerned with improved sampling strategies to eliminate bias in cases of non-IUR specimens. There have also

Figure 30. Distribution of features within an area (e.g., cell colonies in a petri dish), with each one labeled according to distance from the periphery.

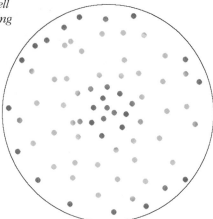

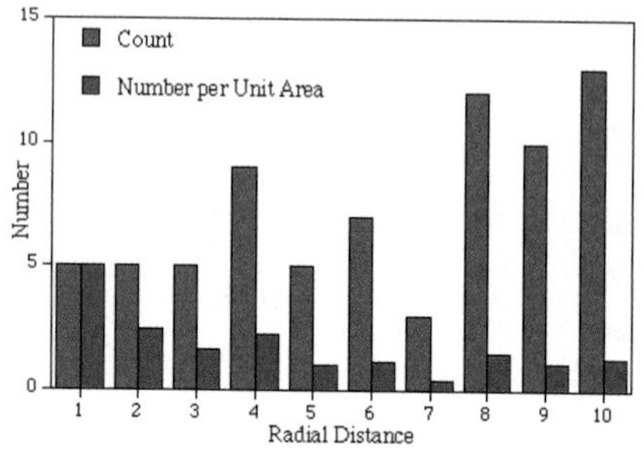

Figure 31. Data from *Figure 30.* Plot of number and number per unit area as a function of distance.

been interesting developments in so-called second order stereology that combine results from different types of measurements, such as using two different types of grids to probe a structure or two different and independent measurements. One example is to use a point grid to select features for measurement in proportion to their volume (points are more likely to hit large than small particles). For each particle that is thus selected, a line is drawn (in a random direction) through the selection point to measure the radius from that point to the boundary of the particle.

Figure 32 shows this procedure applied to the white dendritic phase in the image used earlier. The grid of points selects locations. For each point that falls onto the phase of interest, a radial line in uniformly randomized directions is drawn to the feature boundary. For convex shapes, the length of this line may consist of multiple segments which must be added together. For isotropic structures or isotropic section planes, the line angles uniformly sample directions. For vertical sections through potentially anisotropic structures, a set of sine-weighted angles should be used.

The length of each line gives an estimate of particle volume:

$$V = \tfrac{4}{3}\pi r^3 \tag{11}$$

which is independent of particle shape. Averaging this measurement over a surprisingly small number of particles and radius measurements gives an estimate of the volume-weighted mean volume (in other words, the volume-weighted average counts large particles more often than small ones, in proportion to their volume).

A more common way to define a mean volume is on a number-weighted basis, where each particle counts equally. This can be determined by dividing the total volume of the phase by the number of particles. We have already seen how to determine the total volume fraction using a point

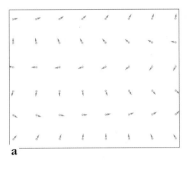

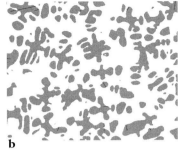

Figure 32. Measuring point-sampled intercepts: (a) an array of grid points, each having a direction associated with it; (b) applying the grid to the image from Figure 2 and measuring the radial distance from those grid points that fall on the phase of interest to the boundary in the chosen direction. Note that, for convex shapes, the radial distance is the sum of all portions of the intercept line.

count, and the number of particles per unit volume using the disector. Dividing the total by the number gives the number-weighted mean volume.

Once both the mean volumes have been determined, they can be combined to determine the standard deviation of the distribution of particle sizes, independent of particle shape, since for the conventional number-weighted distribution the variance is given by the difference between the square of the volume-weighted mean volume and the square of the number-weighted mean volume

$$\sigma^2 = V_V^2 - V_N^2 \tag{12}$$

Although this may appear to be a rather esoteric measurement, in fact it gives an important characterization of the size distribution of particles or other features that may be present in a solid, which as we have seen are not directly measurable from the size distribution of their intersections with a plane section.

Classical stereology (unfolding)

Historically, much of classical stereology was concerned with exactly that problem, determining the size distribution of three-dimensional features when only two-dimensional sections through them were measurable (Weibel, 1979; Cruz-Orive, 1976, 1983). The classical method used was to assume a shape for the particles (i.e., that all of the particles were the same shape, which did not vary with size). The most convenient shape to assume is (of course) a sphere. The distribution of the sizes of circles produced by random sectioning of a sphere can be calculated as shown in **Figure 33**. Knowing the sizes of circles that should be produced if all of the spheres were of the same size makes it possible to calculate a matrix of α values that enable solving for the distribution of sphere sizes that must have been present in the three-dimensional structure to produce the observed distribution of circle sizes, as shown in **Figure 34**.

$$N_{V_{sphere,i}} = \sum \alpha_{i,j} \cdot N_{A_{circle,j}} \tag{13}$$

Other shapes have also been proposed, as a compromise between mathematical ease of calculation and possible realistic modeling of real world shapes. These have included ellipsoids of revolution (both oblate and prolate), disks, cylinders, and a wide variety of polyhedra, some of which can be assembled to fill space (as real cells and grains do). Tables of alpha coefficients for all

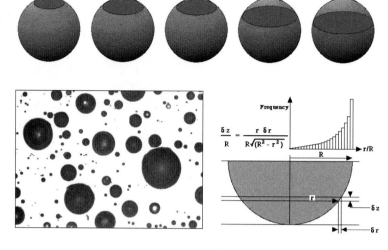

Figure 33. *Sectioning a sphere at random produces a distribution of circle sizes.*

$$\frac{\delta z}{R} = \frac{r\,\delta r}{R\sqrt{(R^2 - r^2)}}$$

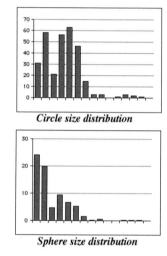

Graphite nodules in cast iron

Circle size distribution

Sphere size distribution

Figure 34. *Unfolding the size distribution of spheres that must have been present to produce an observed distribution of circle sizes. The sample is a cast iron containing graphite nodules; note that the features are not perfectly circular, even though a sphere model has been used in the unfolding.*

these exist and can be rather straightforwardly applied to a measured distribution of the size of two-dimensional features viewed on the section plane.

However, there are several critical drawbacks to this approach. First, the ideal shapes do not usually exist. Nuclei are not ideal spheres, cells and grains are not all the same polyhedral shape (in fact, the larger ones usually have more faces and edges than smaller ones), precipitate particles in metals are rarely disks or rods, etc. Knowledge of the shape of the three-dimensional object is critical to the success of the unfolding method, since the distribution of intersection sizes varies considerably with shape (**Figure 35** shows an example of cubes vs. spheres). It is very common to find that size varies with shape, which strongly biases the results. Small errors in the shape assumption produce very large errors in the results. For example, the presence of a few irregularities or protrusions on spheres results in many smaller intersection features, which are mis-interpreted as many small spherical particles.

The second problem is that from a mathematical point of view, the unfolding calculation is ill-posed and unstable. Variations in the distribution of the number of two-dimensional features as a function of size result from counting statistics. The variations are typically greatest at the end of the

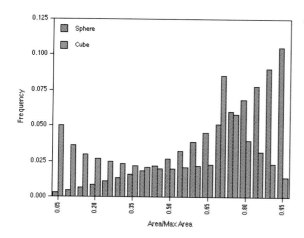

Figure 35. Size distribution of intercept areas produced by random sectioning of a sphere and a cube.

distribution, for the few largest features which are rarely encountered. But in the unfolding process these errors are magnified and propagated down to smaller sizes, often resulting in negative numbers of features in some size classes, and greatly amplifying the statistical uncertainty.

For these reasons, although unfolding was a widely used classical stereological method for decades, it has fallen out of favor in the last 15–20 years. Instead there has been increased emphasis on finding unbiased ways to measure structural parameters using more robust tools. Nevertheless, in spite of these limitations (or perhaps because their magnitude and effect are not sufficiently appreciated), unfolding of size distributions is commonly performed. When the shape of the three-dimensional objects is not known, it is common to assume they are simple spheres, even when the observed features are clearly not circles. The argument that this gives some data that can be compared from one sample to another, even if it is not really accurate, is actually quite wrong and simply betrays the general level of ignorance about the rules and application of stereological procedures.

9

Feature-Specific Measurements

Measurements that can be performed on each of the individual features in images can be grouped into four classes: brightness (including color values and parameters such as density that are related to brightness), location (both absolute position and relative to other features present), size, and shape. For each class, quite a variety of different specific measurements can be made, and there are a variety of different ways to perform the operations. Most image analysis systems offer at least a few measures in each class. Users find themselves at some time or another having to deal with several different measurement parameters. The problem is frequently to decide which of the measured parameters is most useful or appropriate for solving a particular problem.

Most of these techniques produce a numeric output suitable for statistical analysis or presentation graphics. Frequently, the interpretation of the data is left to a separate program, either a simple spreadsheet relying on the user's programming ability, or a dedicated statistics package. In a few cases, the numbers are converted to go/no go decisions or become the basis for classification, discussed in the next chapter. Examples might include quality control testing of the size and placement of holes in a part, medical pathology decisions based on the identification of the presence of cancerous cells, or recognition of different objects in the field of view.

Brightness measurements

Normally, in the kinds of images we have been discussing here, each pixel records a numeric value that is often the brightness of the corresponding point in the original scene. Several such values can be combined to represent color information. The most typical range of brightness values is from 0 to 255 (8-bit range), but depending on the type of camera, scanner or other acquisition device a large range of 10 or more bits, up to perhaps 16 (0 to 65,535) may be encountered. Most programs that accept images from sources such as cooled cameras and scanners having more than 8 bits of depth store them as 16 bit images (occupying two bytes per pixel for grey-scale images, or 6 bytes per pixel of red, green, and blue [RGB] values for color images), even if the actual grey-scale or tonal resolution is less than 16 bits. Some systems use the 0–255 value range for all bit depths but report decimal values for images having more than 8 bits of depth. This has the advantage of permitting easy comparisons between images acquired with different depths. Rarely, the stored values may be real numbers rather than integers (for instance, elevation data). In most cases, however, these images are still stored with a set of discrete integer "grey" values because it is easier to manipulate such arrays and convert them to displays. In such cases, a calibration table or function is maintained to convert the pixel values to meaningful real numbers when needed.

The process of creating such a calibration function for a particular imaging device, or indeed for a particular image, is far from trivial (Inoue, 1986; Chieco et al., 1994; Swing, 1997; Boddeke, 1998). Many of the cameras and other devices that have been mentioned for acquiring images are neither perfectly linear nor exactly logarithmic, nor completely consistent in the relationship between the pixel's numeric value and the input signal (e.g., photon intensity). Many video cameras have an output function that varies with the overall illumination level. The presence of automatic gain circuits, or user-adjustable gamma controls, make it more difficult to establish and maintain any kind of calibration. In general, any kind of automatic gain or dark level circuitry, automatic color balancing, etc., will serve to frustrate calibration of the camera. With consumer-level video and still cameras, it is not always possible to turn such "features" off.

For color imaging, cameras may incorporate automatic white balance adjustments (which are intended for a type of scene much different than the majority of scientific images). Control of the color temperature of the light source and maintaining consistency of the camera response to perform meaningful color measurement is rarely possible with video type cameras. Chapter 1 showed examples of correcting color values using measured RGB intensities from a standard color chart. It is important to note that the typical color camera has RGB sensors that respond to a relatively broad range of wavelengths, and that many different combinations of actual photon colors can produce identical stored RGB values. In general, it is not practical to attempt to perform colorimetry (the detailed measurement of color) using such cameras, and of course complications arising from light sources, viewing geometry, optics, etc., make the problem even more difficult.

Even when the use of a stable light source and consistent camera settings can be assured, the problem of grey scale calibration remains. Some standards are reasonably accessible, for example, density standards in the form of a step-wedge of film. Measurement of the brightness of regions in such a standard can be performed as often as needed to keep a system in calibration. In scanning large area samples such as electrophoresis gels or x-ray films, it is practical to incorporate some density standards into every sample so that calibration can be performed directly. In other cases, separate standard samples can be introduced periodically to check calibration.

Optical density is defined as

$$O.D. = -\log_{10}\left(\frac{I}{I_0}\right) \tag{1}$$

where I/I_0 is the fraction of the incident light that penetrates through the sample without being absorbed or scattered. If a camera or scanner and its light source are carefully adjusted so that the full range of linear brightness values covers the range of optical density from 0.1 (a typical value for the fog level of unexposed film) to 2.5 (a moderately dense exposed film), the resulting calibration of brightness vs. optical density would be as shown in **Figure 1**. The shape of the curve is logarithmic.

At relatively low-density/bright pixel values the sensitivity is quite good. A difference of 1 pixel brightness value at the bright end of the scale is only about 0.002. At the high-density/dark-pixel end of the scale, however, a difference of one pixel brightness value corresponds to an optical density change of 0.3, which is very large. This is an indication that when trying to apply a linear camera or scanner to optical density reading, more than 8 bits of grey scale are needed. An input device with more precision can be used with a lookup table that converts the values to the logarithmic optical density scale and then stores that in an 8-bit image. This problem becomes more severe as higher density values are encountered. Films containing high amounts of silver can easily reach densities of 3.5. Satisfactorily digitized such films requires using scanners with at least 12, and preferably 14 bits per channel precision.

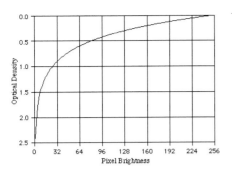

Figure 1. *Calibration of optical density vs. pixel brightness if the latter is adjusted linearly to span the range from 0.1 (fog level) to 2.5 (typical exposed film).*

It is not uncommon to include a grey wedge in a film to be scanned for one- or two-dimensional separation of organic molecules. **Figure 2** shows an example. The grey wedge of known density values allows the construction of a calibration scale (**Figure 3**) that can then be used to measure the optical density of each object (**Figure 4**). In this application, the total amount of protein in each spot is proportional to the integrated optical density, which is the product of the average density and the area.

Figure 2. *Scanned image of a 2D electrophoresis gel with a grey-scale calibration wedge.*

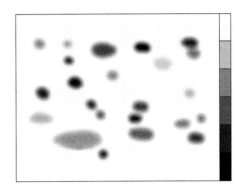

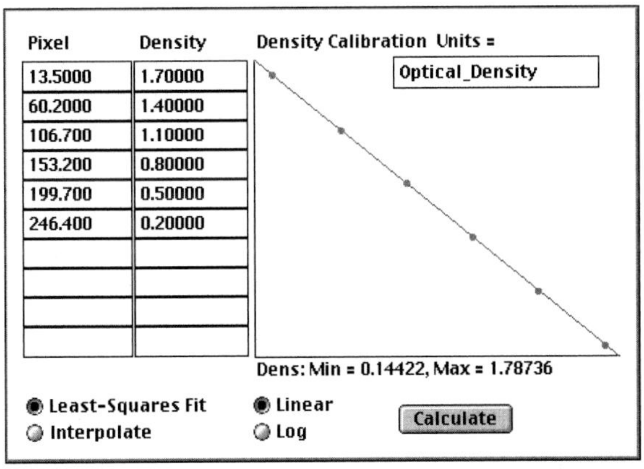

Pixel	Density
13.5000	1.70000
60.2000	1.40000
106.700	1.10000
153.200	0.80000
199.700	0.50000
246.400	0.20000

Density Calibration Units =
Optical_Density

Dens: Min = 0.14422, Max = 1.78736

● Least-Squares Fit ● Linear
○ Interpolate   ○ Log   [Calculate]

Figure 3. *Calibration plot from the grey-scale wedge in **Figure 2**, showing the relationship between optical density and pixel brightness for this particular scanner.*

Figure 4. *Measured data from **Figure 2**, using the calibration plot from **Figure 3** to compute the integrated optical density of each spot.*

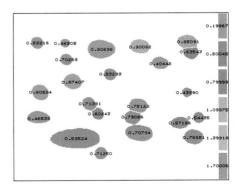

The use of a calibration scale raises another point. It is common for features to contain some variation in pixel brightness. The average density (or whatever other quantity is calibrated against pixel brightness) is not usually recorded linearly. It thus becomes important to take this into account when determining an average value for the density, or an integrated total dose, or any other calibrated quantity. If all of the pixels within the feature are simply averaged in brightness, and then that value is converted using the calibration scale, the wrong answer will be obtained. It is instead necessary to convert the value from each pixel to the calibrated values, and then sum or average those. It is also important not to include adjacent background pixels that are not part of the feature, which means that the delineation should be exact and not some arbitrary shape (a circle or square) drawn around the features. Reliance on manual outlining in not usually acceptable, since humans usually draw outlines larger than the boundaries around features. The solution is to use the same routines that threshold and segment the image into discrete features. The pixels in that binary image define the features and can be used as a mask to locate the corresponding pixels in the grey-scale array.

For one-dimensional measurements of density, the procedure is the same. **Figure 5** shows an example of a film exposed in a Debye–Scherer x-ray camera. The total density of each line, and its position, are used to measure the crystal structure of materials. Knowing that the lines extend vertically, it is reasonable to average the values in the vertical direction to reduce noise and obtain a more precise plot of the density variations along the film (**Figure 6**). Converting the individual pixel values to density before summing them is the correct procedure that gives the proper values for the relative line intensities. The linear plots of intensity values may be subtracted to find differences or used with statistical routines to detect peaks.

Figure 7 shows a similar procedure for tracks or columns in an electrophoresis separation. Using the brightness profile measured between the tracks allows a simple correction to be made for background variations due to nonuniformities in thickness or illumination. The brightness values

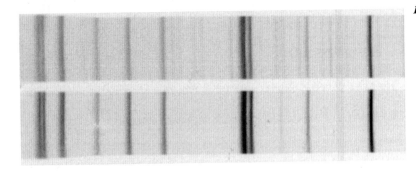

Figure 5. Two Debye–Scherer x-ray films. The vertical lines occur at angles that are related to the atomic spacing in the lattice structure of the target material. Small differences in intensity and the presence of additional lines indicate the presence of trace amounts of additional compounds.

Figure 6. Integrated intensity plots along the films from Figure 5, with the difference between them.

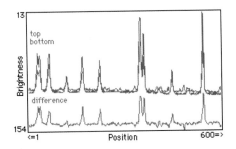

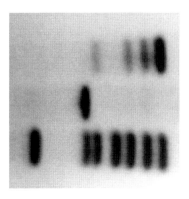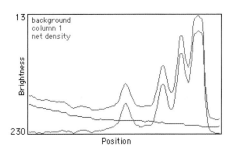

Figure 7. *A 1D electrophoresis separation. Intensity scans along the center of each track are leveled by subtracting scans between the tracks (the example shows the top track).*

are averaged across the center of the columns, avoiding the edges. Calibration of the position of bands within the columns is usually done with respect to markers of known molecular weight that are placed in adjacent columns. This is necessary because the distance scale is generally not very linear or constant in such specimens.

Of course, not all images have this convenient relationship between intensity and a property of the sample being imaged, such as density. In microscope images, phase differences can also produce contrast, and diffraction effects or polarization effects may also be present. In real-world images, the surface orientation and characteristics of objects influence the brightness, as does the interplay between the light source color and the surface color. In most of these cases, the brightness cannot be measured to provide information about the sample. It is difficult enough to use the relative brightness values to delineate regions that are to be grouped together or separated from each other.

When color images are digitized, the problem of having enough bits to give enough precision for each of the color planes is amplified. Many of the higher-end scanners acquire more than 8 bits, often as many as 12, for each of the RGB planes, use these to determine the color information, and then may create an optimized 8-bit representation to send to the computer. Even with this increase in precision, it is difficult to achieve accurate color representation. As pointed out in Chapter 1, the digitization of color requires far greater control of camera settings and lighting than can normally be achieved with a video camera. Even a flat bed scanner, which offers greater consistency of illumination and typically uses a single charge coupled device (CCD) linear array with various filters to obtain the RGB information, is not a good choice for measurement of actual color information, however, such scanners can be calibrated to reproduce colors adequately on particular printers.

The pixel brightness value need not be optical density or color component information, of course. Images are so useful to communicate information to humans that they are used for all kinds of data. Even within the most conventional expression of the idea of imaging, pixel values can be related to the concentration of dyes and stains introduced into a specimen. In an x-ray image from the scanning electron microscope (SEM), the brightness values are approximately proportional to elemental concentration. These relationships are not necessarily linear nor easy to calibrate. x-ray emission intensities are affected by the presence of other elements. Fluorescence intensities depend not only on staining techniques and tissue characteristics, but also on time, since bleaching is a common phenomenon.

In infrared imaging, brightness is a measure of temperature. Backscattered electron images from the scanning electron microscope have brightness values that increase with the average atomic number, so that they can be used to determine chemical composition of small regions on the sample. In a range image, the pixel brightness values represent the elevation of points on the surface and can be calibrated in appropriate units.

To support this range of applications, it is generally useful to be able to measure the mean intensity or a calibrated "density" value, as well as finding the brightest or darkest pixel values in each region or feature, and perhaps the standard deviation of the brightness values as a measure of variation or texture. For color images, it may be useful to report the RGB components (usually as values ranging from 0 to 255), but in most cases the hue, saturation and intensity are more directly useful. The saturation and intensity are generally measured on either the 0–255 scale or reported as percentages, but the hue may be reported as an angle from 0 to 360°, as is shown in **Figure 8**. Note that several different hue, saturation and intensity (HIS) spaces are shown, as discussed in Chapter 1, and it is important to know which one is being used to convert the stored RGB pixel values, particularly for the saturation values.

These examples are at best a tiny sample of the possible uses of pixel values, but the measurement of the stored values and conversion to some calibrated scale is a broadly useful technique. Statistical analysis of the data provides mean values and standard deviations, trends with position, comparisons between locations, within or between images, and so forth. For such procedures to work, it is important to establish useful calibration curves, which requires standards or fundamental knowledge and is a subject beyond the scope of this text.

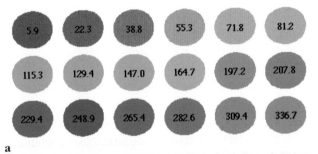

a

Figure 8. Mean color values for a series of color spots:
(a) Hue, reported as angles from 0 to 360°, for features with full saturation;
(b) saturation, reported as percent, for features with constant hue and intensity;
(c) intensity, reported as percent, for features with constant hue and saturation.

b

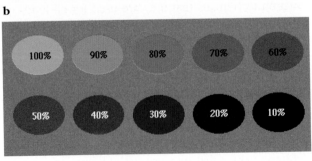

c

Determining location

In several of the examples for measuring brightness values, the location of features was also needed for interpretation of the results. For a typical irregular feature extending over several pixels, there can be several different definitions of location, some easier to calculate than others. For instance, the x, y coordinates of the midpoint of a feature may be determined simply as halfway between the minimum and maximum limits of the pixels comprising the feature. Normally, the pixel addresses themselves are just integer counts of position, most often starting from the top left corner of the array. This convention arises from the way that most computer displays work, using a raster scan from the top left corner. There may be some global coordinate system of which the individual image is just a part, and these values may also be integers, or real number values that calibrate the pixel dimensions to some real world units such as latitude and longitude, or millimeters from the edge of a microscope sample.

Establishing a real-world calibration for pixel dimensions is often quite difficult, and maintaining them while shifting the specimen or the camera (by moving the microscope stage or the satellite, for instance) presents a variety of challenges. Often, locating a few known features in the image itself can serve to establish fiduciary marks that allow this sort of calibration, so that all of the other features in the image can be accurately located. Shifting the sample, stage or camera so that successive viewing frames overlap allows position calibration to be transferred from one field to the next, but the errors are cumulative and may grow rapidly due to the difficulty of accurately locating the same feature(s) in each field to a fraction of a pixel. This also assumes that there are no distortions or scan nonlinearities in the images. Relying on the stage motion for position information depends upon the precision of that mechanism (which may be much worse if directions are reversed due to backlash), and the fidelity with which the sample motion corresponds to that of the stage.

The feature's minimum and maximum limits are easy to determine by finding the pixels with the largest and smallest coordinates in the horizontal and vertical directions. These limiting coordinates define a bounding rectangle around the feature, and the midpoint of the box is then taken as a location for the feature. The midpoint is not usually the preferred representation of location, however, because it is too easily biased by just a few pixels (for instance a whisker sticking out from the rest of the feature). One application in which these box coordinates are used, however, is in computer drawing programs. Many such programs allow the user to select a number of drawn objects and then move them into alignment automatically. The options are typically to align the objects vertically by their top, center, or bottom, and horizontally by their left, center, or right edges. These are exactly the box coordinates and midpoint.

The center of the so-called bounding box is useful in a few situations such as the gel scan, because the x and y coordinates have meaning in terms of how the sample was created. For most real images, this is not the case. When the x-y axes are arbitrary, the bounding box is very biased and sensitive to object orientation, as shown in **Figure 9**. More representative of the geometric center of a feature is the location of the center of a bounding or circumscribed circle. Fitting such a circle to the points on the object periphery is straightforward, and made more efficient by using only those points that represent the vertices of a bounding polygon, fitted as described later in this chapter by rotating axes to a limited number of directions (typically about every 10°) and finding the bounding box limits for each orientation. Of course, the size and center location of the bounding circle is not sensitive to changes in the orientation of the axes or the feature.

For a non-convex feature or one containing internal holes, the geometric center may not even lie within the feature bounds. Nor is it sensitive to the actual feature shape. For irregularly shaped features, it is usually preferable to take into account the feature shape and location of all the pixels present. This approach defines the centroid of the feature, a unique x, y point that would serve to

Figure 9. *Rotation of a figure and the changes in the size and shape of the bounding box.*

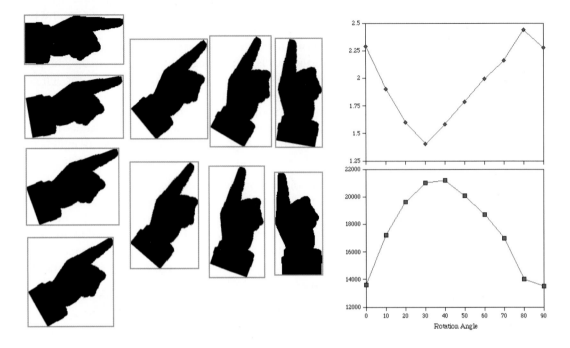

balance the feature on a pinpoint if it were cut out of a rigid, uniform sheet of cardboard. The co-ordinates of this point can be determined by averaging the coordinates of each pixel in the object.

$$C.G._x = \frac{\sum_i x_i}{Area}$$

$$C.G._y = \frac{\sum_i y_i}{Area}$$

(2)

where the *Area* is just the total number of pixels present. Notice that this equation provides a set of coordinates that are not, in general, integers. The center of gravity or centroid of an object can be determined to sub-pixel accuracy, which can be very important for locating features accurately in a scene. **Figure 10** compares the geometric center and the centroid for an irregular feature.

If the centroid is calculated according to **Equation 2** using only the boundary pixels, as is some-times done (especially if features are encoded with boundary representation as described in Chapter 7), the result is quite wrong. The calculated point will be biased toward whichever part of the boundary is most complex and contains the most pixels (**Figure 11**). This bias can even vary with the orientation of the boundary with respect to the pixel array because square pixels are larger in the diagonal direction than in their horizontal and vertical dimension.

The centroid location can be calculated correctly from a boundary representation such as chain code. The correct calculation uses the pairs of coordinates x_i, y_i for each point in the boundary,

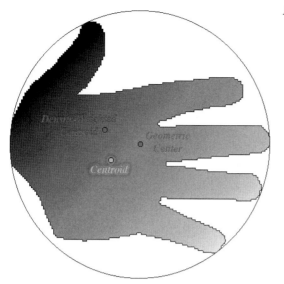

Figure 10. *Centroid (green), density weighted centroid (red) using the pixel density values, and geometric center (blue) determined as the center of the bounding circle, for an irregular feature.*

Figure 11. *Effect of boundary irregularities on centroid determination. The right hand side of the circle is irregular while the left hand side is smooth. The centroid location determined by using just the boundary pixels (magenta) is shifted to the right, as compared to the location determined using all of the pixels in the feature.*

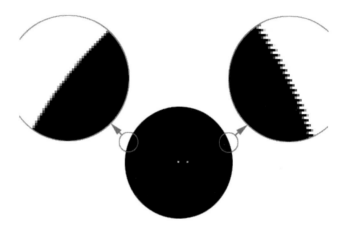

where x_0, y_0, x_n, and y_n are the same point (i.e., the boundary representation is a closed loop with the two ends at the same place).

$$C.G._x = \frac{\sum_i \left(x_i + x_{i-1}\right)^2 \cdot \left(y_i - y_{i-1}\right)}{Area} \qquad (3)$$

$$C.G._y = \frac{\sum_i \left(y_i + y_{i-1}\right)^2 \cdot \left(x_i - x_{i-1}\right)}{Area}$$

and it is now necessary to calculate the area as

$$Area = \frac{\sum_i \left(x_i + x_{i-1}\right) \cdot \left(y_i - y_{i-1}\right)}{2} \qquad (4)$$

Parenthetically, it is worth noting here that some of the attractiveness of chain code or boundary representation as a compact way to describe a feature is lost when you try to use that data to calculate things like the area or centroid of the feature.

The definition of centroid or center of gravity just given treats each pixel within the feature equally. For some purposes, the pixel brightness, or a value calculated from it using a calibration curve, makes some pixels more important than others. For example, the accurate location of the spots and lines in the densitometric examples shown earlier would benefit from this kind of weighting. That modification is quite easy to introduce by including the brightness-derived value in the summations in **Equation 2**. **Figure 10** shows the density-weighted centroid in comparison to the conventional centroid in which all pixels are treated as equal.

$$C.G._x = \frac{\sum_i Value_i \cdot x_i}{\sum_i Value_i}$$

$$C.G._y = \frac{\sum_i Value_i \cdot y_i}{\sum_i Value_i}$$

(5)

The denominator is now the integrated density (or whatever the parameter related to brightness may be). Of course, this kind of calculation requires access to the individual pixel brightness values, and so cannot be used with a boundary representation of the feature.

For a convex shape, the centroid may not lie within the bounds of the feature. When a unique representative point that always lies within the bounds of a potentially irregular shape is required, the ultimate eroded point or (UEP) determined from the EDM is the center of the largest inscribed circle in the feature and can often be used.

Orientation

Closely related to the location of the centroid of a feature is the idea of determining its orientation. There are a number of different parameters that are used, including the orientation of the longest dimension in the feature (the line between the two points on the periphery that are farthest apart, also known as the maximum Feret's diameter), and the orientation of the major axis of an ellipse fitted to the feature boundary. Just as the centroid is a more robust descriptor of the feature's location than is the midpoint, however, an orientation defined by all of the pixels in the image is often better than any of these. This is due to the fact that it is less influenced by the presence or absence of a single pixel around the periphery, where accidents of acquisition or noise may make slight alterations in the boundary.

The moment axis of a feature is the line around which the feature, if it were cut from rigid, uniform cardboard, would have the lowest moment of rotation. It can also be described as the axis which best fits all of the pixels in the sense that the sum of the squares of their individual distances from the axis is minimized. This is the same criterion used to fit lines to data points when constructing graphs. Determining this axis and its orientation angle is straightforward, and just involves summing pixel coordinates and the products of pixel coordinates for all of the pixels in the image. As for the example in **Equation 5**, it is possible to weight each pixel with some value such as the density, instead of letting each one vote equally. The most convenient procedure for the calculation is to add up a set of summations as listed in **Equation 6**.

$$S_x = \sum x_i$$

$$S_y = \sum y_i$$

$$S_{xx} = \sum x_i^2 \tag{6}$$

$$S_{yy} = \sum y_i^2$$

$$S_{xy} = \sum x_i y_i$$

Once these sums have been accumulated for the feature, the net moments about the x and y axes, and the angle of the minimum moment are calculated as shown in **Equation 7**.

$$M_x = S_{xx} - \frac{S_x^2}{Area}$$

$$M_y = S_{yy} - \frac{S_y^2}{Area}$$

$$M_{xy} = S_{xy} - \frac{S_x \cdot S_y}{Area} \tag{7}$$

$$\Theta = \tan^{-1}\left\{ \frac{M_{xx} - M_{yy} + \sqrt{(M_{xx} - M_{yy})^2 + 4 \cdot M_{xy}^2}}{2 \cdot M_{xy}} \right\}$$

Figure 12 shows an example of the measurement of orientation angle on features. Notice that features that intersect the edges of the image field are not measured as will be discussed in the next section. The measurement can also be applied to lines, as shown in **Figure 13**. In this case the axons were thresholded and skeletonized, and the nodes removed leaving line segments. To characterize the distribution of orientations for the axons, it is more meaningful to plot the total length of segments as a function of angle rather than the number. **Figure 14** shows an example combining position and angle. The orientation of the cells in the tissue varies with vertical position. This is an example of a gradient as discussed in Chapter 8.

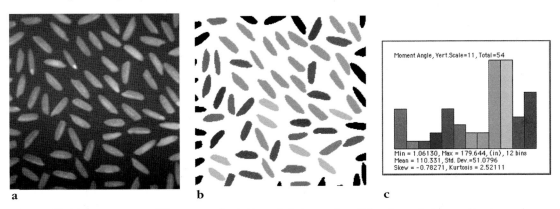

a   b   c

Figure 12. Measurement of feature orientation: (a) rice grains; (b) color coded according to angle; (c) distribution of grains according to angle.

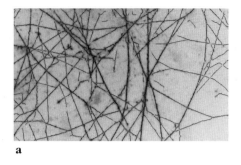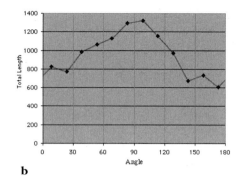

a

b

Figure 13. Measurement of fiber orientation:
(a) image of axons, with skeleton segments superimposed (nodes removed as described in Chapter 7);
(b) cumulative length of fibers as a function of their angles, showing preferred orientation.

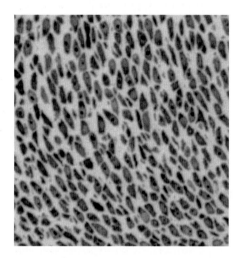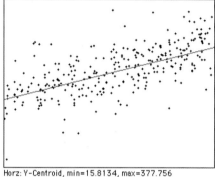

Horz: Y-Centroid, min=15.8134, max=377.756
Vert: Moment Angle, min=0.0, max=180.0
Equation: Y = 0.11408 * X + 90.9333
R-squared = 0.595, 303 points

Figure 14. Cells in tissue, showing a gradient of moment angle with vertical position.

Neighbor relationships

The location of individual features may be less important in some applications than the relationships between neighboring features. For instance, **Figure 15** shows several distributions of features. How can such distributions be compactly described to reveal the extent to which they are random, regularly spaced, or clustered?

Schwarz and Exner (1983) showed that a histogram of the distribution of the distances between nearest neighbors can provide an answer. Actually, the distance between any pair of neighbors, second nearest, etc., can be used as well, but in most cases the nearest-neighbor pairs are the easiest to identify. Once the coordinates of the centroid points representing each feature have been determined, sorting through the resulting table to locate the nearest neighbor for each point is a straightforward task (best left to the computer). The straight line distances between these points are calculated and used to construct the histogram. This in turn can be characterized by the mean and variance (or standard deviation) of the distribution. A word of caution is needed in dealing with feature points located adjacent to the edge of the field of view (Reed and Howard, 1997): if the distance to the edge is less than the distance found to the nearest neighbor within the field of view, the distance should not be used in the distribution, because it may cause bias. It is possible that

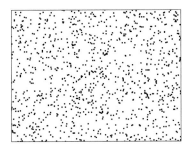 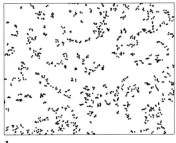 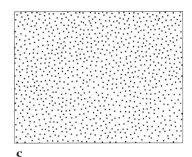

a   b   c

Figure 15. Feature distributions illustrating:
   (a) *random;*
   (b) *clustered;*
   (c) *spaced or self-avoiding arrangements.*

another feature outside the field of view would actually be closer. For large images (fields of view) containing many features, this problem is only a minor concern. The nearest-neighbor distance method also generalizes to three dimensions, in the case of three-dimensional (3D) imaging; the method has been used with a confocal microscope (Baddeley et al., 1987; Russ et al., 1989; Reed et al., 1997). A related statistical test on all neighbor pairs can also be used (Shapiro et al., 1985).

Consider now the particular distributions shown in **Figure 15**. The image in **Figure 15a** is actually a random distribution of points, often called a Poisson random distribution because the histogram of nearest-neighbor distances is in fact a Poisson distribution. This is the sort of point distribution you might observe if you just sprinkled salt on the table. Each point is entirely independent of the others, thus "random." For such a distribution, the mean distance between nearest neighbors is just

$$Mean = \frac{0.5}{\sqrt{\frac{N}{Area}}} \tag{8}$$

where N is the number of points within the area of the field of view. For a Poisson distribution, the variance is equal to the mean (the standard deviation is equal to the square root of the mean). The consequence is that for a random distribution of points, the number of points per unit area of the surface is all that is needed to determine the mean and variance of the histogram of nearest-neighbor distances.

When clustering is present in the point distribution, most points have at least one neighbor that is quite close by. Consequently, the mean nearest-neighbor distance is greatly reduced. In most cases, the variance also becomes less, as a measure of the uniformity of the spacing between the clustered points. As shown in the image in **Figure 15b**, this clustering produces a histogram (**Figure 16**) that is much narrower and has a much smaller mean value than the Poisson distribution obtained for the random case. Examination of stars in the heavens indicates that they strongly cluster (into galaxies and clusters of galaxies). People also cluster, gathering together in towns and cities.

When the points are self-avoiding as shown in **Figure 15c**, the nearest-neighbor distances are also affected. The mean value of the histogram increases to a larger value than for the random case. The variance also usually drops, as a measure of the uniformity of the spacings between points. Self-avoiding or regular distributions are common in nature, whether you look at the arrangement of mitochondria in muscle tissue or precipitate particles in metals, because the physics of diffusion plays a role in determining the arrangement. The mitochondria are distributed to provide energy as uniformly as practical to the fibers. Forming one precipitate particle

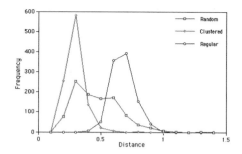

Figure 16. *Histogram of nearest-neighbor distances for each of the point distributions in* **Figure 15**. *The mean value of the clustered distribution is less than, and that for the self-avoiding distribution is greater than that for the random one.*

depletes the surrounding matrix of that element. The same effect occurs in the growth of cacti in the desert. Even the location of shopping centers is to some degree self-avoiding, in order to attract a fresh market of customers.

The ratio of the mean value of the nearest-neighbor distance distribution to that which would be obtained if the same number of points were randomly distributed in the same area provides a useful measure of the tendency toward clustering or self-avoidance for the features, and the variance of the distribution provides a measure of the uniformity of the tendency. Finding nearest-neighbor pairs using the centroid coordinates of features can also be used to characterize anisotropy in feature distributions. Instead of the distance between nearest neighbors, we can measure the direction from each feature to its nearest neighbor. For an isotropic arrangement of features, the nearest-neighbor directions should be a uniform function of angle. Plotting the histogram as a rose plot shows any deviations from this uniform function and indicates the degree of anisotropy.

For instance, if the regularly spaced distribution of feature points in **Figure 15c** is measured, the rose plot is reasonably circular and indicates that the distribution is isotropic. If the image is stretched 10% in the horizontal direction and shrunk 10% in the vertical direction, the total number of features per unit area is unchanged. The visual appearance of the image (**Figure 17**) does not reveal the anisotropy to a casual observer, but a plot of the rose of nearest-neighbor directions (**Figure 18**) shows that most of the features now have a nearest neighbor that is situated above or below. The elongation of the rose plot is a sensitive indicator of this type of anisotropy.

Measuring nearest-neighbor distances using the feature centroids is fine when the features are small compared to the distances between them. When features are large compared to the distances that separate them, and particularly when they are irregular in shape, vary in size, and have different orientations, it may be more appropriate to measure the distance from edge to edge rather than between centroids (Yang et al., 2001, suggest that it is the variance of the distribution of these distances that is most sensitive to inhomogeneity and to anisotropic clustering). The minimum separation distance is the shortest edge-to-edge distance between a point on one feature and that on its neighbor. As shown in **Figure 19**, this may be much different from the centroid-to-centroid distance, and in fact may involve a different neighbor.

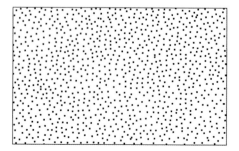

Figure 17. *Stretching the point distribution in* **Figure 15c** *horizontally and compressing it vertically introduces nonuniformity in the nearest-neighbor directions.*

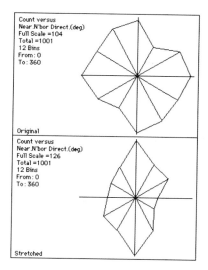

Count versus
Near.N'bor Direct.(deg)
Full Scale =104
Total =1001
12 Bins
From: 0
To: 360

Original

Count versus
Near.N'bor Direct.(deg)
Full Scale =126
Total =1001
12 Bins
From: 0
To: 360

Stretched

Figure 18. Rose plot of nearest-neighbor directions for the point distributions in *Figures 15c* and *17*.

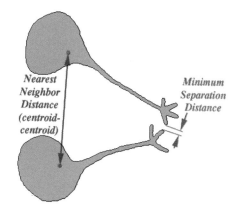

Nearest
Neighbor
Distance
(centroid-
centroid)

Minimum
Separation
Distance

Figure 19. Centroid-to-centroid distance and minimum separation distance for two features.

The Euclidean distance map (EDM) introduced in Chapter 7 on binary images can be used to determine those edge-to-edge distances as shown in **Figure 20**. The skiz, or skeleton of the background between features, is a Voronoi tesselation of the image with one feature in each cell. The EDM of the cells in this tesselation measures the distance of every pixel from the lines. Assigning these EDM values to the features (the Boolean masking operation used in Chapter 7) gives each feature a minimum brightness of distance value that is exactly half the distance to the feature with the closest boundary point, because the skiz passes halfway between features.

A second method for measuring minimum separation distance is to construct the EDM of the background and find the local minima along the points in the skiz. These are midway between points of closest approach, and provide another measurement of minimum separation distance between features. With this technique, it is possible to measure multiple minimum separations between different points on one feature and those on one or several neighbors.

In the case of a space-filling structure such as cells in tissue, grains in a metal, or fields in an aerial survey, the number of adjacent neighbors is also of interest. The features are separate, so there must be a line of background pixels that separate them. In many cases, this line is produced by skeletonizing the original thresholded image of the boundaries and then inverting it to define the pixels. Counting the number of neighbors for each feature can be accomplished by checking the feature identification number of pixels that touch each of the background pixels in the boundaries. Building a table of the features that abut each other feature allows counting the number of such neighbors.

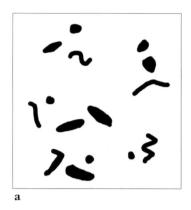 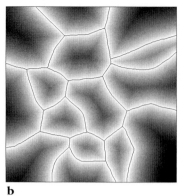 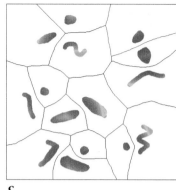

a
b
c

Figure 20. Determining minimum separation distance:
(a) features;
(b) the skiz of the features and the EDM of the cells in the resulting Voronoi tessellation;
(c) EDM values assigned to pixels in the features (shown in false color). The minimum value for each feature is half the distance to its nearest neighbor.

Labeling the features according to the number of neighbors can reveal some interesting properties of the structure. **Figure 21** shows the labeling of the number of neighbors in a diatom, an essentially two-dimensional (2D) structure. The pairing of the five- and seven-neighbor cells is apparent in the colored image, but might go unnoticed in the original. **Figure 22** shows a similar labeling for grains in a 3D metal structure, as revealed on a 2D section. For an equilibrium structure such as a fully recrystallized metal, the distribution of nearest neighbors should be log normal (as it is for the example shown).

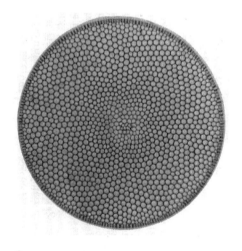 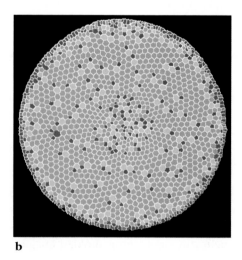

a
b

Figure 21. An image of a diatom
(a) with the holes in the structure color-coded according to the number of sides
(b) The predominant shape is six-sided, but some five- and seven-sided holes generally lie adjacent to each other.

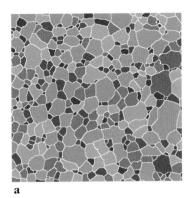

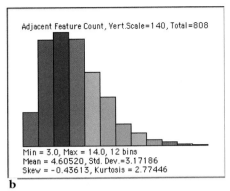

Adjacent Feature Count, Vert.Scale=140, Total=808

Min = 3.0, Max = 14.0, 12 bins
Mean = 4.60520, Std. Dev.=3.17186
Skew = -0.43613, Kurtosis = 2.77446

a   b

Figure 22. Grains in a steel alloy, color coded according to the number of nearest neighbors. The plot of the frequency distribution of number of neighbors is log-normal in both two and three dimensions for an equilibrium grain structure.

Alignment

One thing that people are very good at seeing in images that requires a special computer algorithm is the alignment and arrangement of features. We are so good at it that we sometimes find such alignments and arrangements when they do not really exist. Constellations in the sky are a good example of this tendency to bring order to disorder.

Many image analysis situations include an algorithmic procedure for determining if an alignment or arrangement is needed. One of the most common is completing broken lines, especially straight lines. Such a procedure is useful at all magnifications, from trying to locate electric transmission lines in reconnaissance photos (which show the towers but not the wires) to trying to delineate atomic lattices in transmission electron microscopy. In general, the points along the line are not spaced with perfect regularity and may not lie precisely on the line. This irregularity, and the sensitivity to noise in the form of other points of features near but not part of the line, make frequency-domain techniques difficult to apply and poor in resulting precision.

Transforming the image into a different space provides the key. The use of Fourier space was shown in Chapter 5, but many alternative spaces are less common. Transformation into Hough space can be used to find alignments (Hough, 1962; Duda and Hart, 1972; Ballard, 1981). Different Hough spaces are used to fit different kinds of shapes, and it is necessary in most cases to have a pretty good idea of the type of line or other arrangement that is to be fit to the data. We will start with the straight line, because it is the simplest case. The conventional way to fit a line to data points on a graph is the so-called "least-squares" method where the sum of the squares of the vertical deviations of each point from the line is minimized. The Hough method is superior to this because it minimizes the deviations of points from the line in a direction perpendicular to the line, and it deals correctly with the case of the points not being uniformly distributed along the line.

Two parameters are required to define a straight line. In Cartesian coordinates, the equation of a straight line is

$$y = m \cdot x + b \tag{9}$$

where m is the slope and b the intercept. Because m becomes infinitely large for lines that are nearly parallel to the y-axis, this representation is not usually used in the Hough transform. Instead, the polar coordinate representation of a line is used. This consists of a radius ρ and angle φ (the length and angle of a normal to the line from the origin). These define the line as shown schematically in **Figure 23**. It is possible either to allow the angle to vary from 0 to 2π and to keep ρ

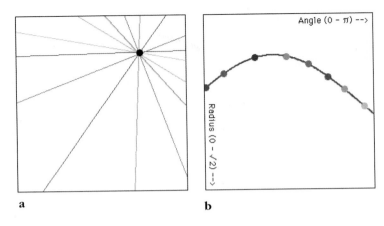

positive, or to allow ρ to be either positive or negative and to restrict the angle φ to a range of 0 to π. The latter convention is used in the examples that follow. The black point shown in **Figure 23a** generates the sinusoid in Hough space shown in **Figure 23b**. Each point along this sinusoid corresponds to the ρ-φ values for a single line passing through the original point. Several of these are shown in color, where the color of the point in Hough space matches the corresponding line in real space.

Hough space is an accumulator space. This means that it sums up the votes of many pixels in the image, and points in Hough space that have a large total vote are then interpreted as indicating the corresponding alignment in the real-space image. For the linear Hough transform, used to fit straight lines to data, the space is an array of cells (pixels, since this is another image) with coordinates of angle and radius. Every point in Hough space defines a single straight line with the corresponding angle φ and radius ρ that can be drawn in the real-space image.

To construct the Hough transform, every point present in the real-space image casts its votes into the Hough space for each of the lines that can possibly pass through it. As shown in **Figure 23**, this means that each point in the real-space image generates a sinusoid in Hough space. Each point along the sinusoid in Hough space gets one vote added to it for each point in the real-space image, or perhaps a fractional vote based on the density of the point in real space. The superposition of the sinusoids from several points in real space causes the votes to add together where they cross. These crossing points, as shown in **Figure 24**, occur at values of ρ and φ that identify the lines that go through the points in the real-space image.

In this example, the duality of lines and points in real and Hough space is emphasized. Each of the five original points (labeled A–E) in real space produces a sinusoid (similarly labeled) in Hough space. Where these sinusoids cross, they identify points in Hough space (labeled 1–6). These points correspond to lines back in real space (similarly labeled) that pass through the same points. Notice for instance that three lines pass through point A in real space, and that the sinusoid labeled A in Hough space passes through the points for each of those three lines.

If several such alignments of points in the real-space image exist, then there will be several locations in the Hough transform that receive numerous votes. It is possible to find these points either by thresholding (which is equivalent to finding lines that pass through a selected minimum number of points) or by looking for local maxima (peaks in the Hough transform), for example by using a top-hat filter.

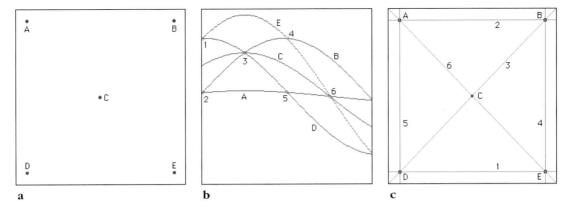

a   b   c

Figure 24. Duality of lines and points in Hough and real space. *Each of the labeled points in* **(a)** *generates a sinusoidal line in the Hough space shown in* **(b)**. *The numbered crossing points in this space generate the lines in the real-space image shown in* **(c)**.

If the original real-space image contains a step in brightness, and an image-processing operation such as a gradient (e.g., Sobel filter) has been applied, then an improved detection and fit of a line to the edge can be achieved by letting each point in the image vote according to the magnitude of the gradient. This means that some points have more votes than others, according to how probable it is that they lie on the line. The only drawback to this approach is that the accumulator space must be able to handle much larger values or real numbers when this type of voting is used, than in the simpler case where pixels in a binary image of feature points either have one vote or none. **Figure 25** shows an example of fitting a line to a noisy edge using an gradient operator and

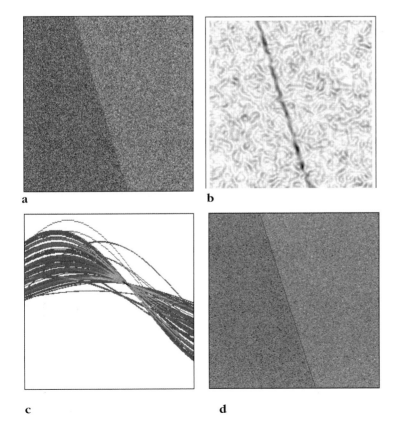

a   b

c   d

Figure 25. Fitting a line to a noisy edge using the Hough transform:
(a) *the original noisy image;*
(b) *smoothing to reduce the noise and application of a Sobel gradient filter;*
(c) *Hough transform produced from the gradient image;*
(d) *line defined by the maximum point in the Hough transform.*

the Hough transform. Notice that the location of the maximum point in Hough space involves the same requirements for using the pixel values to interpolate a location to sub-pixel dimensions as discussed at the start of this chapter.

For measurement of the spacings of parallel lines, Hough spaces reduce the problem to measuring the vertical distance between peaks in the transform. As shown in **Figure 26**, the application of a derivative to an SEM image of a line on an integrated circuit produces peaks at the same φ value, and measuring the distance in ρ provides direct measures of the width and spacing of the lines. Similarly, to measure the angular orientation of lines it is straightforward to determine the φ values in the transform.

This proportional voting system is useful when there are many points to be fit, with some points being more important than others. Summing the votes according to brightness (or some value obtained from brightness) allows some points to be weighted more and produces an improved fit.

Figure 26. Measuring line width
on an integrated circuit:
(a) original SEM image;
(b) horizontal derivative applied;
(c) Hough transform, showing peaks corresponding to line edges and the distances that measure width and spacing.

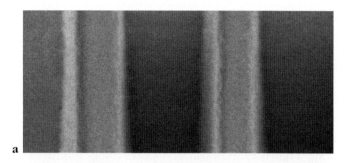

a

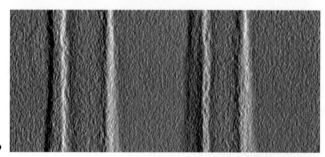

b

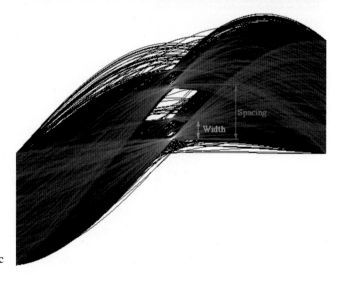

c

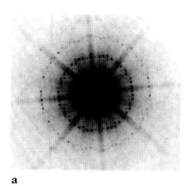
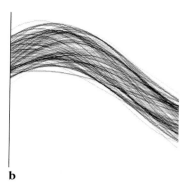

a
b

Figure 27. Convergent beam electron diffraction pattern

(a) and its Hough transform **(b)** Each peak in the transform space identifies an alignment of points in the original pattern.

Figure 27 shows a Hough transform of a convergent beam electron diffraction pattern. The most intense spots in the Hough transform identify each of the spot alignments in the pattern.

The Hough transform can be adapted straightforwardly to other shapes, but the size and dimensionality of the Hough space used to accumulate the votes increases with the complexity of the shape. Fitting a circle to a series of points is used to measure electron diffraction patterns and to locate holes in machined parts. A generalized circular Hough transform requires a three-dimensional space, because three parameters are required to define a circle (the x,y coordinates of the center and the radius). Each point in the real-space image produces a cone of votes into the Hough space, corresponding to all of the circles of various radii and center positions that could be drawn through the point.

If one or two of these values are known (for instance, the center of the electron diffraction pattern is known, or the radius of the drilled hole) or at least can vary over only a small range of possible values, then the dimensionality or size of the Hough space is reduced and the entire procedure becomes quite rapid. Accurately fitting a circle to an irregularly spaced set of points of varying brightness is a good example of the power that the Hough approach brings to image measurement. Because the brightness of the point in Hough space that defines the circle is also the summation of the votes from all of the points on the corresponding circle in real space, this approach offers a useful way to integrate the total brightness of points in the electron diffraction pattern as well.

Figure 28 shows an example of using a circular Hough transform to locate the "best fit" circles in a selected area diffraction pattern. The pattern itself has bright spots with irregular locations around each circle. A human has little difficulty in estimating where the circles lie, but this is generally a difficult thing for computer algorithms that examine only local pixel regions to accomplish. The Hough transform locates the circles and also provides a measure of the integrated brightness around each circle. This approach has been used to identify asbestos fibers from the very spotty electron diffraction patterns obtained from a few fibers (Russ et al., 1989).

Figure 29 shows an example from machine vision used to locate edges and holes accurately for quality control purposes or robotics guidance. Despite overall noise in the image, the fit is quite rapid and robust. A separate region of interest (ROI) is set up covering the area where each feature is expected. In each ROI, a gradient operator is applied to identify pixels on the edge. These are then used to perform a Hough transform, one for a straight line and one for a circle. The resulting feature boundaries are shown, along with the measured distance between them. Many pixels have contributed to each feature, so the accuracy of location is much better than the pixel dimensions.

The Hough transform approach can be used to fit other alignment models to data as well. The limitation is that as the algebraic form of the model changes, each of the adjustable constants requires another dimension in Hough space. Constructing the transform and then finding the maximum points becomes both memory-intensive and time-consuming.

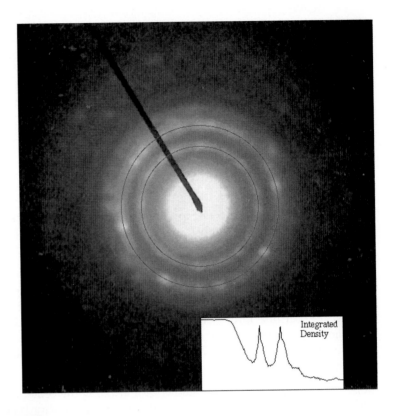

Figure 28. Selected area electron diffraction pattern with principal circles located by a circular Hough transform, and the integrated circular density of the pattern.

Integrated
Density

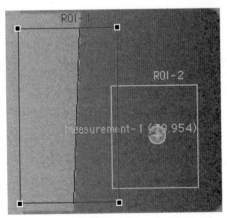

Figure 29. Use of the Hough transform to locate an edge and a circle in a machined part, in order to measure the distance between them to sub-pixel accuracy.

Counting features

Counting the number of features present in an image or field of view is one of the most common procedures in image analysis. The concept seems entirely straightforward, and it is surprising how many systems get it wrong. The problem has to do with the finite bounds of the field of view. In the case in which the entire field of interest is within the image, there is little difficulty. Each feature has simply to be defined by some unique point and those points counted. Depending on how features are recognized, some algorithms may ignore features that are entirely contained within holes in other features. This problem most often arises when boundary representation is used to define the feature boundaries in the binary image. Determining whether it is appropriate to count features that lie inside other features is a function of the application, and consequently must be left up to the user.

When the field of view is a sample of the entire structure or universe to be counted, the result for the number of features is generally given as number-per-unit-area. When features intersect the edge of the field of view, it is not proper to count all features that can be seen. The most common solution to produce an unbiased result is to count those features that touch two adjacent edges, for instance the top and left, and to ignore those that touch the other two edges, for instance the right and bottom. This is equivalent to counting each feature by its lower right corner. Each feature has one and only one lower right corner, therefore, counting those points is equivalent to counting the features. (**Figure 30**).

This method is the same as determining the number of people in a room by counting noses. Since each person has one nose, the nose count is the same as the people count. If a smaller region was marked within the room, so that people might happen to straddle the boundary, counting the noses would still work. Anyone whose nose was inside the region would be counted, regardless of how much of the person lay outside the region. Conversely, any person whose nose was outside would not be counted, no matter how much of the person lay inside the region. It is important to note that in this example, we can see the portions of the people that are outside the region, but in the case of the features in the image, we can usually cannot (unless the counting is performed within a reduced area inside the full image, another possible solution). Any part of the feature outside the field of view is by definition not visible, and we cannot know anything about the amount or shape of the feature outside the field of view. That is why it is important to define a unique point for each feature to use in counting.

The convention of counting features that touch two edges only is not implemented in all systems. Some software packages offer a choice of counting all features regardless of edge touching, or counting only those features that do not touch any edge. Note that when measuring features, as opposed to counting them, a more complicated procedure will be needed. A feature that intersects any edge cannot be measured, because it is not all imaged and therefore no size, shape or position information can be correctly obtained. If only the features in **Figure 31** that did not touch any edge were counted, the proportions of large and small features would be wrong. It is more likely that a large feature will touch an edge, and so a disproportionate fraction of the large features intersect an edge of the field of view and cannot be measured.

This bias can be corrected in two ways. The methods produce the same result, but are implemented differently. The older method is to set up a "guard frame" within the image, as shown in **Figure 32**. In this case, features that touch the lower and right edges of the field of view are not counted or measured, as before. Features that cross the top and left edges of the guard frame are counted and measured in their entirety. Features that lie only within the guard frame are not counted, whether they touch the actual edge of the field of view or not. The number of features counted is then an accurate and unbiased measure of the number per unit area, but the area

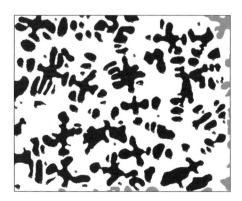

Figure 30. Counting features by a unique point. The red dots mark the right end of the lowest line of pixels in each feature. Features that touch the upper and left boundaries are counted, but those that touch the bottom and right edges are not.

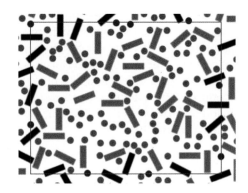

Figure 31. When an image area (shown by the green frame) lies within a larger field of objects to be measured, some will be intersected by the edge. These cannot be measured because their extent outside the image area is unknown. In the example shown, although it includes three times as many small red features as long blue ones, the frame intersects (and removes from the measurement) twice as many blue ones, biasing the result.

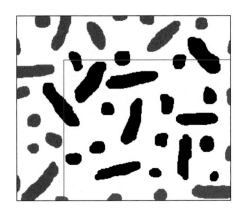

Figure 32. Measurement using a guard frame. Features that lie partially or entirely within the inner region are counted. Features that touch the outer edge of the image or lie entirely in the guard frame are not. The width of the guard frame must be large enough that no feature can span it.

reported for the measurement is the area within the guard frame, not the entire area of the image. It is necessary for the guard region to be wide enough that no feature can extend from within the active region across the guard region to the edge of the field, so the active region may be reduced to a fraction of the total image area.

The second method uses the entire image area and measures all of those features that do not touch any of the edges. In order to compensate for the bias arising from the fact that larger features are more likely to touch the edge and be bypassed in the measurement process, features are counted in proportion to the likelihood that a feature of that particular size and shape would be likely to touch the edge of a randomly placed image frame. The so-called adjusted count for each feature is calculated as shown in **Figure 33** as:

$$Count = \frac{W_x \cdot W_y}{(W_x - F_x) \cdot (W_y - F_y)} \qquad (10)$$

where W_x and W_y are the dimensions of the image in the x and y directions (in pixels), and F_x and F_y are the maximum projected dimensions of the feature in those directions. These are simply the same bounding-box coordinates as discussed previously in connection with finding a feature's location. When the feature dimensions are small compared to the dimensions of the field of view, the fraction is nearly 1.0 and simple counting is unaffected. This is the case for counting small features. When the feature extends across a larger fraction of the field of view in either direction, it is more likely that a random placement of the field of view on the sample will cause it to intersect an edge; thus the features that can be measured must be counted as more than one to correct for those that have been overlooked. The adjusted count factor makes that compensation.

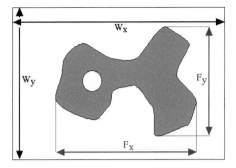

Figure 33. Dimensions of the image and the feature used to adjust the count for correct results.

Figure 34. Example of the adjusted count for features that vary in size:
(a) *adjusted count for each feature;*
(b) *size distribution data with no adjusted count to correct for bias due to features intersecting the edge;*
(c) *using the adjusted count — note the difference in the total number of features and mean feature size.*

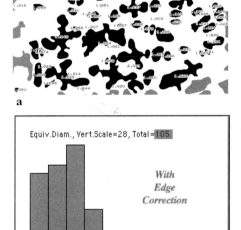

a

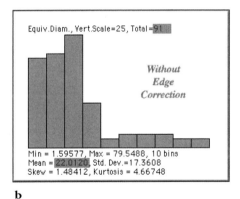

Equiv.Diam., Vert.Scale=25, Total = 91

Without Edge Correction

Min = 1.59577, Max = 79.5488, 10 bins
Mean = 22.0120, Std. Dev.=17.3608
Skew = 1.48412, Kurtosis = 4.66748

b

Equiv.Diam., Vert.Scale=28, Total = 105

With Edge Correction

Min = 1.59577, Max = 79.5488, 10 bins
Mean = 24.6932, Std. Dev.=19.4177
Skew = 1.24410, Kurtosis = 3.62359

c

Figure 34 shows an example of an image containing features of varying sizes and shapes, with the adjusted count for each. A plot of the size distribution shows that using the adjusted count significantly affects the mean size, the shape of the distribution, and the total number of features.

Special counting procedures

The examples of counting in the previous section make the tacit assumption that the features are separate and distinct. In earlier chapters, procedures for processing images in either the grey-scale or binary format were shown whose goal was to accomplish the separate delineation of features to permit counting and measurement; however, these methods are not successful in numerous situations, or they are, at least, very difficult. Sometimes, if there is enough separate knowledge about the specimen, counting can be accomplished even in these difficult cases.

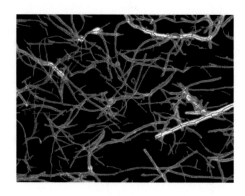

Figure 35. *Image of crossing fibers, with the skeleton superimposed, and a total of 222 end points.*

As an example, **Figure 35** shows a collection of crossing fibers. Such structures are common in biological samples, wood fibers used in paper production, food technology, textiles, and many more situations. Because the fibers cross, from the point of view of the image analysis algorithms, there is only a single feature present, and it touches all sides of the field of view. It is possible, however to estimate the number of fibers per unit area, and the average fiber length. By thresholding the fibers and skeletonizing the resulting binary image, a series of crossing midlines is revealed. As discussed in Chapter 7, the end points of fibers can be counted as those pixels in the skeleton that have exactly one touching neighbor. This is not a perfect method, as there may be some ends of real fibers that are hidden because they lie exactly on another fiber, but in principle it is possible to detect these occurrences as well because they produce pixels with exactly three neighbors, and one of the angles at the junction will be about 180°. Even without this refinement, however, half of the end point count gives a useful approximation for the number of fibers.

Recall that, in the preceding section, we decided to count each feature by one unique point. Counting the end points of fibers uses two unique points per fiber. It is a little like the old joke about how to count the number of cows in a field ("Count the number of hooves and divide by four."). In this case, we count the number of end points and divide by two, to get the number of fibers. If a fiber has one end in the field of view and the other end out, it is counted (correctly) as ½ fiber, because the other end would be counted in a different field of view. Dividing by the image area gives the number of fibers per unit area. If the total length of fiber (the total length of the skeletonized midline) is divided by the number of fibers (one half the number of ends), the result is the average fiber length. If the fibers are much longer than the field of view so that there are no end points present in most fields of view, it then becomes necessary to combine the data from many fields of view to obtain a statistically meaningful result.

In the earlier chapter on binary image processing, several techniques for separating touching features were discussed. One of the more powerful, known as watershed segmentation, utilizes the EDM. This operation assigns a grey-scale value to each pixel within a feature proportional to the distance from that pixel to the nearest background point. The valleys, or points that lie between two higher pixels in this distance map, are then used to locate boundaries that are ultimately drawn between features in order to separate them. Because there is a built-in assumption in this method that any indentation around the periphery of the feature cluster indicates a separation point, this technique is also known as convex segmentation.

If the purpose of the processing and segmentation is to count the features, a short-cut method saves much of the computation. In the EDM, every local maximum point (pixels equal to or greater than all eight of their neighbors) is a unique point that represents one feature that will eventually be separated from its touching companions. Finding these so-called ultimate eroded points provides another rapid way to count the features present. In addition, the grey-scale value of that point in the EDM is a measure of the size of the feature, since it corresponds to the radius of the

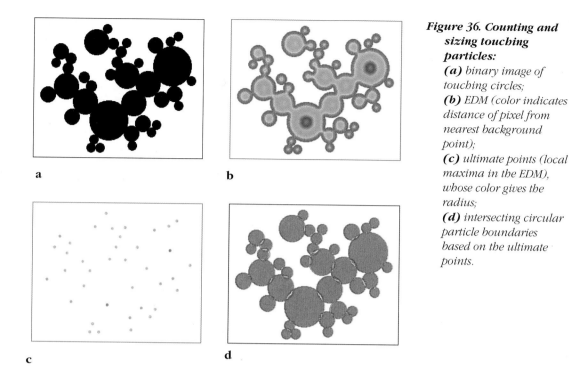

Figure 36. Counting and sizing touching particles:
(**a**) *binary image of touching circles;*
(**b**) *EDM (color indicates distance of pixel from nearest background point);*
(**c**) *ultimate points (local maxima in the EDM), whose color gives the radius;*
(**d**) *intersecting circular particle boundaries based on the ultimate points.*

circle that can be inscribed within it. **Figure 36** shows a simple example of some touching circles, with the ultimate points found from the EDM.

Counting touching particles presents many difficulties for image analysis algorithms. If the particles are not simple convex shapes that lie in a single plane and happen to touch at their boundaries, watershed segmentation is not usually able to separate them successfully. A typical example of a more difficult problem is shown in **Figure 37**. The clay particles that coat this paper sample form

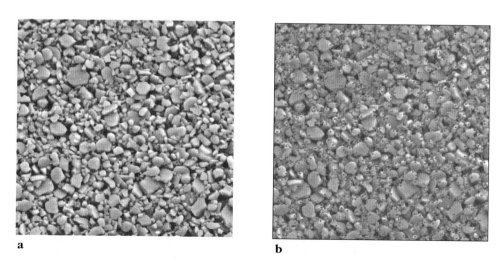

Figure 37. Counting overlapping particles:
(**a**) *SEM image of clay particles on paper;*
(**b**) *superimposed points from a top-hat filter used to locate a local brightest point, which can be used to estimate the number of particles.*

a layer that is essentially one particle thick, but the overlaps are quite extensive. In order to obtain a useful estimate of the number of particles per unit area of the paper, it is again necessary to use the idea of finding one unique point per particle.

In this case, the way the image is formed by the scanning electron microscope provides an answer. Most of the particles are somewhat angular and have a single highest point that appears bright in the secondary electron image. These points (shown in the figure) can be isolated using a top hat filter, as discussed in Chapter 4. In the example, the top-hat filter finds one unique point with a local maximum in brightness for most of the clay particles. A few are missed altogether because they have a shape or orientation that does not produce a characteristic bright point, and a few particles have sufficiently irregular shapes that they produce more than a single characteristic point. This means that counting the points gives only an estimate of the particle density on the paper, but for many quality control purposes this sort of estimate is sufficient to spot changes.

The top-hat filter used in the preceding example is a specific case of a feature-matching or template operation, that looks throughout the image for a particular pattern of bright and dark pixels. A more general case uses cross correlation, as discussed in Chapter 5. The example in **Figure 38** shows an aerial photograph of trees in the forests on Mount Mitchell, North Carolina. It is desired to count the trees to monitor damage from acid rain. A useful short-cut method is to use the image of the pointed top of one tree as a target, cross correlate with the entire image, and count the resulting spots. Of course, this method is only approximate; it does a good job of finding trees that are partially hidden or in front of another tree, but will miss trees that do not have the characteristic pointed top of the target example.

Another approach to counting particles in clusters is shown in **Figure 39**. This is a transmission electron microscope (TEM) image of carbon black particles, which are present in the form of clusters of varying sizes. If it can be assumed that the particles in the clusters are similar in size and density to the isolated one, then it becomes possible to estimate the number of particles in a cluster from the integrated density of the cluster. Measuring the average value of the integrated optical density of a isolated particles, and dividing that value into the integrated density of each cluster, provides a number that is an estimate of the number of particles present.

Feature size

The most basic measure of the size of features in images is simply the area. For a pixel-based representation, this is the number of pixels within the feature, which is straightforwardly determined by counting. For boundary representation, the area can be calculated as discussed earlier (**Equation 4**). Of course, it must be remembered that the size of a feature in a 2D image may be related to the size of the corresponding object in 3D space in various ways depending on how the image

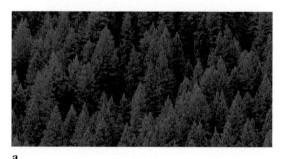
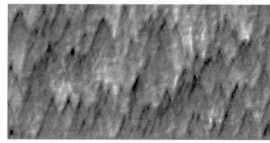

a   b

Figure 38. Counting with cross-correlation:
   (a) aerial photograph of trees — the red outline marks the tree top selected as the target for matching;
   (b) cross-correlation result, with identified tree tops marked.

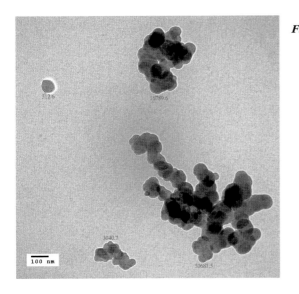

Figure 39. Clusters of carbon black particles viewed in the transmission electron microscope. Dividing the integrated optical density of each cluster by the integrated density for the single particle provides an estimate of the number of particles in each cluster (10, 54, and 162 particles in the clusters shown).

was obtained. The most common type of images are projections, in which the features show the outer dimensions of the objects, or planar sections, in which the features are slices across the objects. In the latter case, it is possible to estimate the volume of the objects using stereological methods as discussed in the preceding chapter. In this chapter, we will assume that the feature size is directly represented in the image.

Figure 40 shows a projected image of spherical particles dispersed on a flat substrate. The diameters can be measured straightforwardly from such an image subject to the usual restriction that there must be enough pixels in each feature to give a precise measure of its size. When the particles cover a large size range, as they do in this image, this creates a problem. With the resolution of a typical video camera, the smallest features are only one or a few pixels in size, and are not well defined (in fact many are not even thresholded). A high-resolution digital camera provides superior results. The alternative would be to increase the optical magnification to enlarge the small particles, but then the large ones would be likely to intersect the edges of the screen and could not be measured. Multiple sets of data taken at several magnifications would be required, unless a high-resolution camera can be used.

Even for such a simple idea as counting pixels to determine feature area, some decisions must be made. For instance, consider the feature shown in **Figure 41**. Should the pixels within internal holes be included in the area or not? Of course, this depends on the intended use of the data. If the hole is a section through an internal void in an object, then it should be included if the area of the feature is to be related to the object volume; but it is hard to know whether the hole may be a section through a surface indentation in that object, in which case it would be more consistent to also include in the area those pixels in fjords around the feature boundary. As shown in the figure, this produces three different possible area measurements, the net area, the filled area, and the convex area.

Measuring the first two can be accomplished as a simple counting exercise. In the process of labeling the pixels that touch each other and comprise the feature, the presence of internal holes can be detected and the pixels within them counted. These pixels can be added back to the original image to fill in the holes, if desired. Determining whether to include those pixels in the area then becomes a user decision based on other knowledge.

The convex area is a slightly more difficult proposition. In some cases, a combination of dilation and erosion steps can be used to construct a convex hull for the feature and fill any boundary

Figure 40. Effect of resolution on feature measurement:
(a) *image of spherical particles dispersed on a flat surface;*
(b) *enlarged portions of images obtained at video camera resolution and digital camera resolution;*
(c) *same regions after thresholding, hole filling, and watershed segmentation.*

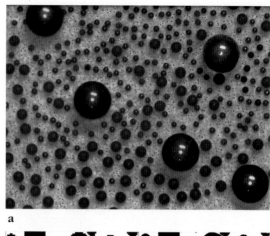

a

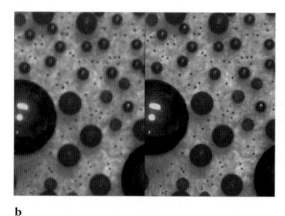

b

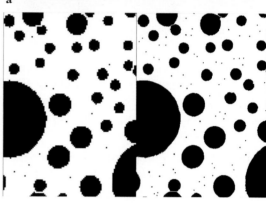

c

Net Area=8529   Filled Area=9376   Convex Area=11227

Figure 41. *Three possible measures for feature area: net, filled, and convex.*

irregularities, so that pixel counting can be used to determine the area. On a square pixel grid, however, these methods can cause some other distortions of the feature shape, as was shown in Chapter 7. Another approach that constructs an *n*-sided polygon around the feature is sometimes called the taut-string or rubber-band boundary of the feature, because it effectively defines the minimum area for a convex shape that will cover the original feature pixels.

By rotating the coordinate axes, it is similarly possible to locate the minimum and maximum points in any direction. The procedure of rotating the coordinate system, calculating new x',y' values for the points along the feature boundary, and searching for the minimum and maximum values, is simple and efficient. For any particular angle of rotation α, the sine and cosine values are needed. In most cases these are simply stored in a short table corresponding to the specific angles used in the program. Then the new coordinates are calculated as

$$x' = x \cdot \cos\alpha + y \cdot \sin\alpha$$
$$y' = y \cdot \sin\alpha - x \cdot \cos\alpha$$

(11)

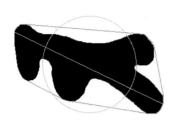

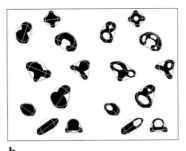

a
b

Figure 42. Comparison of the bounding polygon (red), the longest chord (yellow) and equivalent circle (green — the circle centered at the feature centroid having the same area) for an irregular feature, and an assortment of features.

When this process is carried out at a series of rotational angles, the points with the largest difference in each rotated coordinate system form the vertices of the bounding polygon discussed above. For purposes of constructing the convex or taut string outline, using a modest number of rotation steps will produce a useful result. For instance, with 18 steps (rotating the axes in 10-degree steps) a bounding polygon with 36 vertices and sides is obtained. **Figure 42** shows an example, comparing the bounding polygon to the equivalent circle and longest dimension for various feature shapes. It is only for extremely long and narrow features that more sides might be required to produce a bounding polygon that is a good approximation to the outer boundary.

No matter how the area is defined and determined, it of course requires that a conversion factor between the size of the pixels and the dimensions of the real-world structures be established. Calibration of dimension is usually done by capturing an image of a known standard feature and measuring it with the same algorithms as later used for unknown features. For macroscopic or microscopic images, a measurement scale may be used. Of course, it is assumed that the imaging geometry and optics will not vary; this is a good assumption for glass lenses in light microscopes, but not necessarily for electron lenses used in electron microscopes. For some remote sensing operations, the position and characteristics of the camera are known and the magnification is calculated geometrically.

Most modern systems use square pixels that have the same vertical and horizontal dimensions, but for distances to be the same in any direction on the image, it is also necessary that the viewing direction be normal to the surface. If it is not, then image warping as discussed in Chapter 3 is required. Some systems, particularly those that do not have square pixels, allow different spatial calibrations to be established for the horizontal and vertical directions. For area measurements based on pixel counting, this does not matter; but for length measurements and the shape parameters discussed in the next section, this discrepancy creates serious difficulties.

Circles and ellipses

Once the area has been determined, it is often convenient to express it as the equivalent circular diameter. This is linear size measure, calculated simply from the area as

$$Eq.Diam. = \sqrt{\tfrac{4}{\pi} Area} \qquad (12)$$

Figure 42b shows several features of different sizes and shapes with the equivalent circle diameter shown based on the net feature area (pixel count). Features of different shape or orientation can fool the eye and make it difficult to judge relative size. The equivalent diameter values offer a simple and easily compared parameter to characterize size.

Circles are widely used as size measures. Besides the equivalent circle with the same area as the feature, the inscribed and circumscribed circle can be used (**Figure 43**). The circumscribed circle is determined by using the corners of the bounding polygon, sorting through them to find the two

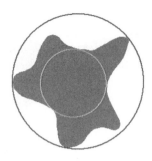

Figure 43. *Circumscribed and inscribed circles for an irregular feature. The centers of these circles do not generally coincide with each other or with the feature centroid.*

or three that define the circle that encloses all of the others (a concise algorithm for finding the circle is in Arvo, 1991). The inscribed circle is easily found as the maximum value of the EDM of the feature; the maximum pixel marks the center and its value gives the radius.

Because most real features have quite irregular shapes, it is not easy to find size measures that compactly and robustly describe them and allow for their classification and comparison. The use of equivalent circular diameter is one attempt. Recognizing that not all features are equiaxed or evenly approximately round, some systems also provide for the use of an ellipse to describe the feature. The fact that the ellipse has two axes seems to allow describing both a size, a degree of departure from circularity, and even an orientation.

The major and minor axes of the ellipse may be determined in several different ways, however. These actually represent some quite different aspects of the feature size and shape, and may be more misleading than helpful unless the user is fully aware of (and careful with) their various biases.

One definition of the ellipse axes can be taken from the minimum and maximum caliper dimensions of the feature, discussed previously. The maximum caliper dimension does a good job of representing a maximum dimension, and indicates the feature orientation at least within the step size of the search (e.g. 10°). If this is taken as the major dimension of the ellipse, then the minor axis could assigned to the minimum caliper dimension. This approach can lead to several difficulties. First, as pointed out previously, this value may seriously overestimate the actual minimum dimension for a long, narrow feature. Second, the direction of the minimum dimension is not, in general, perpendicular to the maximum dimension. Third, the resulting ellipse area is not the same as the area of the feature.

Basing the ellipse breadth on the minimum caliper dimension is suspect. As a result, a modification of this approach uses the maximum caliper dimension as the ellipse major axis, and determines the minor axis in order to make the ellipse area agree with the feature area. The area of an ellipse is $(\pi/4)\cdot a\cdot b$ where a and b are the axes; therefore, once the major axis has been determined, the minor axis can be adjusted to agree with the feature area. The orientation angle can be either the approximate value determined from the steps used in the maximum caliper dimension search, or the orientation angle determined from the moment calculation shown earlier (**Equation 7**). This tends to produce ellipses that have a longer and narrower shape than our visual perception of the feature.

The moments from **Equation 7** can also be used to produce a fitted ellipse. This is perhaps the most robust measure, although it requires the most calculation. Surprisingly, it seems to be little used. Instead, many systems fit an ellipse not to all of the pixels in the feature area, but instead to the pixels along the feature boundary. This procedure is computationally simple but very hard to justify analytically, and irregularities along any portion of the feature's boundary will significantly bias the ellipse.

Caliper dimensions

Caliper dimensions represent another description of feature size. The maximum caliper or maximum Feret's diameter is sometimes called the feature length, because it is the longest distance between any two points on the periphery. A projected or shadow dimension in the horizontal or vertical direction can be determined simply by sorting through the pixels or the boundary points to find the smallest and largest coordinates, and then taking the difference. These dimensions were introduced above in terms of the bounding box around the feature, used to correct for its probability of intersecting the edge of a randomly placed image field.

The extreme points determined in a variety of directions were used to construct the bounding polygon described above. With such a polygon, the minimum and maximum caliper diameters can be found simply by sorting through the pairs of corner points. The pair of vertices with the greatest separation distance is a close approximation to the actual maximum dimension of the feature. The worst-case error occurs when the actual maximum chord is exactly halfway between the angle steps, and in that case the measured length is short by

$$Meas.Value = True\ Value \cdot \cos\left(\frac{\alpha}{2}\right) \tag{13}$$

For the example mentioned previously of 10-degree steps, the cosine of 5° is 0.996. This means that the measurement is less than one-half percent low. For a feature whose actual maximum dimension is 250 pixels, the value obtained by the rotation of coordinate axes would be one pixel short in the worst-case orientation.

If the same method is used to determine a minimum caliper dimension for the feature (sometimes called the breadth), this is equivalent to finding the pair of opposite vertices on the bounding polygon that are closest together. The error here can be much greater than for the maximum caliper dimension, because it depends on the sine of the angle and on the length of the feature rather than its actual breadth. A narrow feature of length L and actual width W oriented at an angle the same 5° away from the nearest rotation step would have its breadth estimated as $L \cdot \sin(5) = 0.087 \cdot L$. This does not even depend on the width W, and if the actual length L is large and the width W is small, the potential error is very great.

Of course, it is also possible to search directly for the maximum chord by sorting through the points to find the two with maximum separation. There are various ways to speed up this search, which would otherwise have to calculate the sum of squares of the x- and y- coordinate differences between all pairs of boundary points. One is to consider only those points that lie outside the equivalent circle. Determining the area by pixel counting (in this case, the area including any internal holes) and converting it to the equivalent diameter with **Equation 12**, provides a circle size. Locating that circle with its center on the feature centroid will cover any points inside the circle, and leave just those points that lie farther away. These are candidates for the most widely separated pair.

An even more restrictive selection of the points to be searched can be obtained from the dimensions of the bounding rectangle. As shown in **Figure 44**, arcs drawn tangent to each side with their center in the middle of the opposite side will enclose most of the boundary of the feature. Only points that lie on or outside the arcs need to be used in the search, and points lying outside one arc need only to be combined with those that lie outside the opposite arc. For a reasonably complex feature whose boundary may contain thousands of points, these selection algorithms offer enough advantage to be worth their computational overhead when the actual maximum dimension is needed.

Consider a feature shaped like the letter "S" shown in **Figure 45**. If this is a rigid body, say a cast-iron hook for use in a chain, the length and breadth as defined by the minimum and maximum caliper dimensions may have a useful meaning. On the other hand, if the object is really a worm

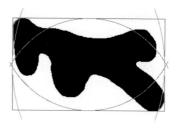

Figure 44. *Construction used to limit the search for boundary points giving the maximum chord. The blue arcs are drawn with centers in the middle of the horizontal edges of the bounding box, and the green arcs are drawn with centers in the middle of the vertical edges. Only the red points along the perimeter, which lie outside those arcs, are candidates for endpoints of the longest chord.*

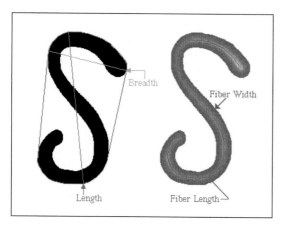

Figure 45. *Comparison of caliper dimensions (length and breadth) with values determined from the skeleton and the EDM (fiber length and fiber width)*

or fiber that is flexible, and the overall shape is an accident of placement, it would be much more meaningful to measure the length along the fiber axis and the width across it. To distinguish these from the maximum and minimum caliper dimensions, often called length and breadth, these are sometimes called the fiber length and fiber width.

Two quite different approaches are used to measure these dimensions. Of course, it is still up to the user to determine which set of parameters offers the most useful values for describing the features in a particular situation. One approach goes back to the binary image processing discussed in Chapter 7. If the feature is skeletonized, the length of the skeleton offers a measure of the length of the fiber. The skeleton is shorter than the actual length of the fiber, but this can be corrected by adding the value of the Euclidean distance map at each end point of the skeleton.

The length of the skeleton itself can be estimated by counting the pixel pairs that are present, keeping track of those that touch along their edges and their corners (because on a square pixel grid the distance between pixels that touch diagonally is greater by $\sqrt{2}$ than the distance orthogonally). This produces a slight overestimate of the length. Instead of using the strictly geometric distances of 1.0 and 1.414, Smeulders (1989) has shown that calculating the length as

$$Length = 0.948 \cdot (num.orthogonal\ nbors)$$
$$+ 1.340 \cdot (num.diagonal\ nbors)$$

(14)

gives a mean error of only 2.5% for lines that run in all directions across the square pixel grid, but, of course, larger errors can be encountered for specific worst-case orientations.

A more accurate measurement can be performed by fitting a smooth curve to the pixels. Several ways are used to accomplish this, including polynomial and Bezier curves. The most efficient method is to use the same technique described below for perimeter measurement, in which the image is smoothed and a super-resolution line interpolated through the pixels.

As described in Chapter 7, combining the skeleton with the EDM also provides a tool to measure the fiber width. Assigning the grey-scale values from the EDM to the skeleton pixels along the midline represents the radius of the inscribed circle centered at each point. Averaging these values for all of the points in the midline gives the mean fiber width, and it is also possible to measure the variation in width.

An older and less accurate (but still used) approach to estimating values for the length and width of a fiber is based on making a geometric assumption about the fiber shape. If the feature is assumed to be a uniform-width ribbon of dimensions F (fiber length) and W (fiber width), then the area (A) and perimeter (P) of the feature will be $A = F \cdot W$ and $P = 2 \cdot (F + W)$. The area and perimeter parameters can both be measured directly. As we will see in the next section, the perimeter is one of the more troublesome values to determine. For a ribbon with smooth boundaries as assumed here, however, the perimeter can be measured with reasonable accuracy. Then the fiber length and width can be calculated from the measured perimeter and area as

$$F = \frac{P - \sqrt{P^2 - 16 \cdot A}}{4}$$

(15)

$$W = \frac{A}{F}$$

Minor modifications to this model can be made, for example by assuming that the ends of the ribbon are rounded instead of square, but the principle remains the same. The difficulty with this approach is its sensitivity to the shape model used. If the feature is not of uniform width or is branched, for instance, the average width obtained from the skeleton and EDM still produces a consistent and meaningful result, while the calculation in **Equation 15** may not.

Perimeter

The perimeter of a feature seems to be a well-defined and familiar geometrical parameter. Measuring a numerical value that really describes the object turns out to be less than simple, however. Some systems estimate the length of the boundary around the object by counting the pixels that touch the background. Of course, this underestimates the actual perimeter because, as noted earlier for the measurement of skeleton length, the distance between corner-touching pixels is greater than it is for edge-touching pixels. Furthermore, this error depends on orientation, and the perimeter of a simple object like a square will change as it is rotated under the camera. **Figure 46** compares the variation in perimeter that is obtained by counting the edges of pixels to the more accurate value obtained from the chain code, as a square is rotated. The sensitivity of measurement values to orientation is often used as a test of system performance.

Figure 46. Comparison of perimeter estimation by chain code vs. summation of pixel edge lengths, as a function of orientation.

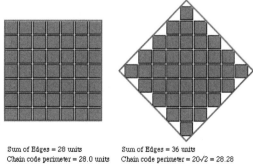

Sum of Edges = 28 units
Chain code perimeter = 28.0 units

Sum of Edges = 36 units
Chain code perimeter = 20√2 = 28.28

If boundary representation is used to represent the feature, then the Pythagorean distance between successive points can be summed to estimate the perimeter, as

$$Perim. = \sum_i \sqrt{\left(x_i - x_{i-1}\right)^2 + \left(y_i - y_{i-1}\right)^2} \qquad (16)$$

In the limiting case of chain code, the links in the chain used for boundary representation are either 1.0 or 1.4142 pixels long, and can be used to estimate the perimeter. It is only necessary to count the number of odd chain code values and the number of even chain code values, since these distinguish the orthogonal or diagonal directions. The same argument as used above for the irregularity of the pixel representation of the midline applies to the boundary line, and using the modified values from **Equation 14** may be applied to reduce this source of error.

The most accurate perimeter measurements, with the least sensitivity to the orientation of feature edges, are obtained by fitting smooth curves to the feature boundaries. The easiest way to do this is by antialiasing the edge so that the pixels near the edge have grey values that fill in the steps (Neal et al., 1998), as shown in **Figure 47**. The process uses the Laplacian of a Gaussian (LoG) filter, which is also used in operators such as the Canny edge locator discussed in Chapter 4 to most accurately define the location of feature boundaries.

The actual boundary is constructed by drawing and measuring straight line segments across the antialiased pixels. These line segments are drawn between points along the pixel edges that are linearly interpolated based on the grey scale values. The points correspond to the location where the midpoint value would lie, treating the pixels as spaced points. This is functionally equivalent to enlarging the image using super resolution and bilinear interpolation to fill in the new, tiny pixels, as shown in **Figure 48**.

Although the super-resolution boundary measurement technique is very accurate and extremely robust to feature rotation, the basic difficulty with perimeter measurements is that for most objects the perimeter itself is very magnification-dependent. Higher-image magnification reveals more boundary irregularities and hence a larger value for the perimeter. This is not the case for area, length, or the other size dimensions discussed previously. As the imaging scale is changed so that the size of individual pixels becomes smaller compared to the size of the features, measurement of these other parameters will of course change, but the results will tend to converge toward a single best estimate. For perimeter, the value usually increases.

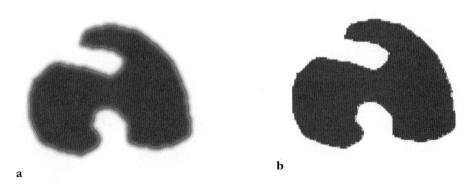

a

b

Figure 47. Fitting a smooth boundary for perimeter measurement:
   (a) contour line on a smoothed (antialiased) feature;
   (b) the contour line superimposed on the original pixels.

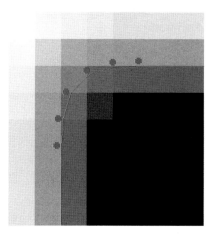

In many cases, plotting the measured perimeter against the size of the pixels, or a similar index of the resolution of the measurement, produces a plot that is linear on logarithmic axes. This kind of self-similarity is an indication of fractal behavior, and the slope of the line gives the fractal dimension of the boundary. This will be used below as a measure of feature shape.

Even if the feature boundary is not strictly fractal (implying the self-similarity expressed by the linear log-log plot of perimeter vs. measurement scale), there is still often some increase in measured perimeter with increased imaging magnification. The only exceptions are smooth (Euclidean) objects such as membranes or surfaces in which tension or an energy term enforces local smoothness for physical reasons. This dependency on magnification makes the perimeter values suspect as real descriptors of the object, and at least partially an artefact of the imaging method and scale used. Further, any noise in the image may be expected to cause a roughening of the boundary and increase the apparent perimeter.

Figure 49 shows a simple example. Random grey-scale noise is superimposed on six circles. The original circles were drawn with a diameter of 80 pixels, and had a measured area of 5024 pixels and perimeter of 254 pixels. Measuring a series of noisy images will produce a value for the area that averages to the correct mean, as pixels are added to or removed from the feature, but the perimeter is always increased as shown by the results in **Table 1**. The variation in area measurements is only 0.5%, while that for the perimeter measurements is 8%, and the mean value is far too high. This bias introduced by noise in the imaging procedure is another cause for concern in perimeter measurements.

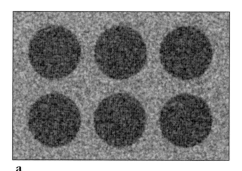

a

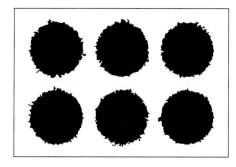

b

Figure 49. Six identical circles superimposed on grey scale noise
  (a), *then thresholded, internal holes filled*
  (b) *and measured. The results are shown in Table 1.*

Table 1. Results from circle measurements in Figure 49

Circle			Area	Perimeter
1	5027	358		
2	5042	338		
3	4988	343		
4	5065	391		
5	5020	372		
6	5030	313		
average	5028.7	352.5		
Standard deviation.			25.4 (0.5%)	27.4 (8%)
original	5024	254		

If perimeter is measured, there is still the need to choose among the same three alternatives discussed for area measurements. The total perimeter includes the length of boundaries around any internal holes in the feature. The net or filled perimeter excludes internal holes and just measures the exterior perimeter. The convex perimeter is the length of the convex hull or bounding polygon and bridges over indentations around the periphery of the feature. The same considerations as mentioned in connection with area measurement apply to selecting whichever of these measures describes the aspect of the feature that is important in any particular application.

Describing shape

Shape is not something that human languages are well equipped to deal with. We have few adjectives that describe shape, even in an approximate way (e.g., rough vs. smooth, or fat vs. skinny). In most conversational discussion of shapes, it is common to use a prototypical object instead ("shaped like a . . ."). Of course, this assumes we all agree about the important aspects of shape found in the selected prototype. Finding numerical descriptors of shape is difficult because the correspondence between them and our everyday experience is slight, and the parameters all have a "made-up" character.

The oldest class of shape descriptors are simply combinations of size parameters, arranged so that the dimensions cancel out. Length/breadth, for example, gives us an "aspect ratio," and changing the size of the feature does not change the numerical value of aspect ratio. Of course, this assumes we have correctly measured a meaningful value for length and breadth, as discussed earlier.

Dozens of size parameters are possible; therefore, they can be combined in hundreds of ways into a formally dimensionless expression that might be used as a shape descriptor. In fact, only a few relatively common combinations are possible, but even these are plagued by total inconsistency in naming conventions. **Table 2** summarizes some of the most widely used shape parameters calculated as combinations of size measurements. Note that in any particular system the same parameter may be called by some quite different name, or the name shown for a different parameter in the table. Also, some systems define the parameters as the inverse of the formula shown, or may omit constant multipliers such as π.

The burden placed on the user, of course, is to be sure that the meaning of any particular shape descriptor is clearly understood and that it is selected because it bears some relationship to the observed changes in the shape of features, because it is presumably being measured in order to facilitate or quantify some comparison. **Figures 50** through **53** illustrate several of these parameters which distinguish between features. In general, each of them captures some aspect of shape, but of course none of them is unique. An unlimited number of visually quite different shapes can be created with identical values for any of these dimensionless shape parameters.

Table 2. Representative shape descriptors

$$Formfactor = \frac{4\pi \cdot Area}{Perimeter^2}$$

$$Roundness = \frac{4 \cdot Area}{\pi \cdot Maximum\ Diameter^2}$$

$$Aspect\ Ratio = \frac{Maximum\ Diameter}{Minimum\ Diameter}$$

$$Elongation = \frac{Fiber\ Length}{Fiber\ Width}$$

$$Curl = \frac{Length}{Fiber\ Length}$$

$$Convexity = \frac{Convex\ Perimeter}{Perimeter}$$

$$Solidity = \frac{Area}{Convex\ Area}$$

$$Compactness = \frac{\sqrt{\left(\frac{4}{\pi}\right)Area}}{Maximum\ Diameter}$$

$$Modification\ Ratio = \frac{Inscribed\ Diameter}{Maximum\ Diameter}$$

$$Extent = \frac{Net\ Area}{Bounding\ Rectangle}$$

Figure 50 shows four variations on one basic shape, which is stretched and smoothed by erosion and dilation. Notice that *formfactor* varies with surface irregularities, but not with overall elongation, while *aspect ratio* has the opposite behavior. **Figure 51** shows four variations on one basic shape with the values of several shape parameters. Examination of the values shows that the parameters vary quite differently from one shape to another. **Figure 52** shows several shapes with the values of their *curl*.

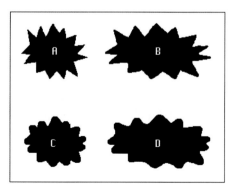

Figure 50. *Variations on a shape produced by erosion/dilation and by horizontal stretching. The numeric values for formfactor and aspect ratio (listed below) show that stretching changes the aspect ratio and not the formfactor, and vice versa for smoothing the boundary.*

Shape	Formfactor	Aspect ratio
A	0.257	1.339
B	0.256	2.005
C	0.459	1.294
D	0.457	2.017

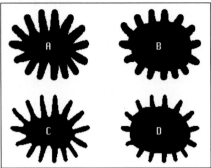

Figure 51. *Another set of four related shapes, with the numeric values for their measured shape parameters.*

Shape	Roundness	Convexity	Solidity	Compactness
A	0.587	0.351	0.731	0.766
B	0.584	0.483	0.782	0.764
C	0.447	0.349	0.592	0.668
D	0.589	0.497	0.714	0.768

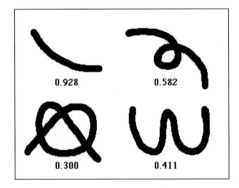

Figure 52. *Four features with different values of curl, indicating the degree to which they are "curled up."*

Figure 53 illustrates the differences between these parameters in a different way. The "features" are simply the 26 capital letters, printed in a font with a serif (Times New Roman). In each horizontal row, the colors code the value of a different measured shape parameter. The variation in each set is from red (largest numeric value) to magenta (smallest numeric value). The independent variation of each of the shape factors is remarkable. This suggests on the one hand that shape factors are a powerful tool for feature identification; however, the large variety of such factors, and the inability of human vision to categorize or estimate them, reminds us that people do not use these parameters to recognize letters.

Another group of simple dimensionless shape parameters can be calculated based on the various definitions of location introduced above. For a perfectly symmetrical feature, such as a circle, the

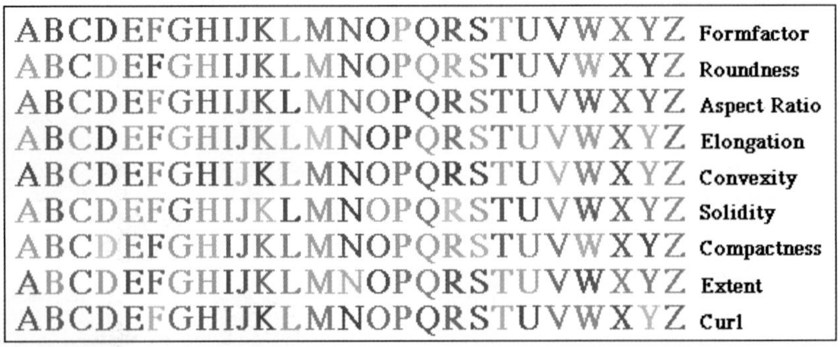

ABCDEFGHIJKLMNOPQRSTUVWXYZ	Formfactor
ABCDEFGHIJKLMNOPQRSTUVWXYZ	Roundness
ABCDEFGHIJKLMNOPQRSTUVWXYZ	Aspect Ratio
ABCDEFGHIJKLMNOPQRSTUVWXYZ	Elongation
ABCDEFGHIJKLMNOPQRSTUVWXYZ	Convexity
ABCDEFGHIJKLMNOPQRSTUVWXYZ	Solidity
ABCDEFGHIJKLMNOPQRSTUVWXYZ	Compactness
ABCDEFGHIJKLMNOPQRSTUVWXYZ	Extent
ABCDEFGHIJKLMNOPQRSTUVWXYZ	Curl

Figure 53. *Measurement of a series of shapes (letters of the alphabet). In each row, the colors of the features code the relative numeric value (red = high, magenta = low) of a different shape parameter, corresponding to the labels.*

centroid and geometric center (the center of the bounding circle) will coincide. If the feature is not symmetric, the distance between these two points, normalized by dividing by the radius of the bounding circle, produces a value between 0 and 1 that measures the asymmetry. The distance between the unweighted centroid (in which all pixels in the feature are counted equally) and the weighted centroid (in which pixels are counted according to some calibrated density function) can be used in the same way.

Similar ratios using other location measures are less useful. For example, the center determined as an average of the location of perimeter pixels is very resolution sensitive. As shown earlier in **Figure 11**, the roughness on the right side of the circle becomes visible only at high magnification, but would shift the apparent center of this visually symmetrical feature.

Likewise, the center of the largest inscribed circle in the feature also creates difficulties. Many non-convex features have more than one maximum in their EDM. Each local maximum is the center of an inscribed circle (tangent to at least three points on the feature boundary). Using the largest as a measure of size is meaningful in some circumstances, but the location is rarely useful. As shown in **Figure 54**, the inscribed circle center is undefined when the feature has more than one equal maximum in the EDM, and even when it does not, the location is insensitive to many aspects of feature shape.

Fractal dimension

Quite a few of the shape parameters discussed previously and summarized in **Table 2** include the perimeter of the feature. As pointed out, this is often a problematic size parameter to measure, with a value that is an artefact of image magnification. In fact, the concept of perimeter may be fundamentally flawed when it is applied to many real objects. If a real-world object is actually fractal in shape, the perimeter is undefined. Measuring the object boundary at higher magnification will always produce a larger value of perimeter. Consider a cloud, for example. What is the length of the boundary around the projected image of the cloud? Measurements covering many orders of magnitude, from a single small cloud in the sky observed by visible light, up to entire storm systems viewed by radar or from weather satellites, show that the perimeter of clouds obeys fractal geometry. Presumably this trend would continue at smaller and smaller scales, at least down to the dimensions of the water molecules. What, then, does the perimeter really mean?

Objects that are fractal seem to be the norm rather than the exception in nature. Euclidean geometry with its well-defined and mathematically tractable planes and surfaces is usually only found as an approximation over a narrow range of dimensions where mankind has imposed it, or in limited situations where a single energy or force term dominates (e.g., surface tension). Roads, buildings,

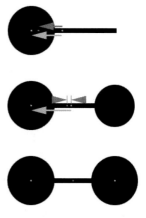

Figure 54. Location of the geometric center (magenta), center of the inscribed circle (green), and centroid (red), showing the effects of asymmetry and shape.

and the surface of the paper on which this book is printed are flat, straight and Euclidean, but only in the dimension or scale where humans perceive and control. Magnify the paper surface and it becomes rough. Look at the roads from space and they cease to be straight. The use of fractal dimensions to describe these departures from Euclidean lines and planes is a relatively recent conceptual breakthrough that promises a new tool for describing roughness.

Briefly, the fractal dimension is the rate at which the perimeter (or surface area) of an object increases as the measurement scale is reduced. A variety of ways are used to measure it. Some are physical, such as the number of gas molecules that can adhere to the surface in a monolayer, as a function of the size of the molecule (smaller molecules probe more of the small surface irregularities and indicate a larger surface area). Some are most easily applied in frequency space, by examining the power spectrum from a two-dimensional Fourier transform as discussed in Chapter 13. Others are relatively easily measured on a thresholded binary image of features.

Perhaps the most widely used fractal measurement tool is the so-called Richardson plot. This was originally introduced as a procedure applied manually to the measurement of maps. Setting a pair of dividers to a known distance, the user starts at some point on the boundary and strides around the perimeter. The number of steps multiplied by the stride length produces a perimeter measurement. As the stride length is reduced, the path follows more of the local irregularities of the boundary and the measured perimeter increases. The result, plotted on log-log axes, is a straight line whose slope gives the fractal dimension. Deviations from linearity occur at each end: at long stride lengths, the step may miss the boundary altogether, while at short stride lengths the finite resolution of the map limits the measurement.

When boundary representation is used for a feature, a Richardson plot can be constructed from the points by calculating the perimeter using the expression in **Equation 16**, and then repeating the same procedure using every second point in the list, every third point, and so forth. As points are skipped, the average stride length increases and the perimeter decreases, and a Richardson plot can be constructed. When every nth point in the list is used to estimate the perimeter, there are n possible starting positions. Calculating the perimeter using each of them, and averaging the result, gives the best estimate. The stride length for a particular value of n is usually obtained by dividing the total perimeter length by the number of strides. In all these procedures, it is recognized that there may be a partial stride needed at the end of the circuit, and this is included in the process.

When the x,y coordinates of the boundary points are digitized in a grid, a variability in the stride length is required. Unlike the manual process of walking along a map boundary, there may not be a point recorded at the location one stride length away from the last point, and so it is necessary either to interpolate from the actual data or to use some other point and alter the stride length. Interpolation makes the tacit assumption that the boundary is locally straight, which is in conflict with the entire fractal model. Altering the stride length may bias the plot. Combined with the general difficulties inherent in the perimeter measurement procedure, the classical stride length method is usually a poor choice for measuring digitized pixel images.

Using the super-resolution perimeter measurement, however, which naturally interpolates points as needed, another Richardson method can be employed. By applying smoothing kernels with progressively larger Gaussian standard deviations to blur the boundary, small irregularities are removed and the perimeter decreases. Plotting the measured perimeter vs. the standard deviation of the smoothing kernel, on log-log axes, produces a straight line whose slope gives the feature fractal dimension as shown in **Figure 55**. The dimension is a value greater than 1 (the topological or Euclidean dimension of a line) and 2 (the dimension of a plane), and may be thought of as the degree to which the line spreads out into the plane.

A second measurement technique was shown in the chapter on binary image processing. Dilating the boundary line by various amounts is equivalent to sweeping a circle along it. The area of the

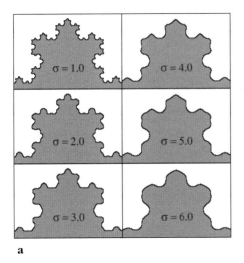

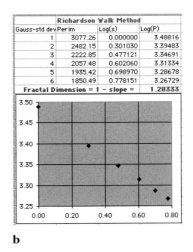

Richardson Walk Method			
Gauss-std dev Perim	Log(s)	Log(P)	
1	3077.26	0.000000	3.48816
2	2482.15	0.301030	3.39483
3	2222.85	0.477121	3.34691
4	2057.48	0.602060	3.31334
5	1935.42	0.698970	3.28678
6	1850.49	0.778151	3.26729
Fractal Dimension = 1 – slope =			1.28333

a   b

Figure 55. Progressive Gaussian smoothing of the outline of a Koch snowflake (theoretical fractal dimension = 1.262) and perimeter measurement produces a Richardson measurement of the fractal dimension.

band swept over by the circle does not increase directly with the radius, because of the irregularities of the boundary. Plotting the area swept out by the circle (sometimes called the sausage) vs. the radius (again on log-log axes) produces a line whose slope gives the fractal dimension. This Minkowski technique is actually older than the Richardson method. It works well on pixel-based images, particularly when the EDM is used to perform the dilation. Using the cumulative histogram of the EDM of the region on either side of the feature outline to construct the log-log plot is the least sensitive to feature orientation, and much faster than iterative dilation, since it assigns to each pixel a grey scale value equal to the distance from the boundary. Examples of this method were shown in Chapter 7; **Figure 56** shows the measurement of the same Koch snowflake.

The Minkowski method produces a dimension that is not identical to the Richardson method (or to other fractal dimension procedures), and so it is important when comparing values obtained from different specimens to use only one of these methods. Neither method gives the exact result expected theoretically for the Koch snowflake fractal, due to the finite resolution available in the pixel image, but both are reasonably close.

A third approach to fractal dimension measurement produces another dimension, similar in meaning but generally quite different in value from the others discussed. The Kolmogorov dimension is determined manually by grid counting. A mesh of lines is drawn on the image and the number of grid squares through which the boundary passes is counted. When this number is plotted on log-log axes vs. the size of the grid, the slope of the line again gives a dimension, as shown in **Figure 57**. Automatic implementation and application to a pixel image can be performed by progressively coarsening the image into 2 × 2, 3 × 3, etc. blocks of pixels, and is sometimes called mosaic amalgamation. This is perhaps the fastest method but has the least numeric precision because it has the fewest possible steps and hence the fewest points to establish the line.

No matter how it is determined, the fractal dimension produces a single numeric value that summarizes the irregularity of "roughness" of the feature boundary. **Figure 58** shows examples of several natural fractals. The relationship between this boundary and what it may represent in three dimensions is not simple. For the case of a section through an isotropic surface, the boundary fractal dimension is smaller than the surface fractal dimension by exactly 1.0, the difference between the topological dimension of the sectioning plane and the volume in which the object resides. Few real

Figure 56. *The cumulative histogram of the Euclidean distance map around the outline of the Koch snowflake produces a Minkowski measurement of the fractal dimension.*

Minkowski Sausage Method				
EDM Value	Pixel Count	Cumulative	Log(R)	Log(A)
1	9330	9330	0.00000	3.96988
2	5956	15286	0.30103	4.18429
3	5198	20484	0.47712	4.31141
4	4052	24536	0.60206	4.38980
5	4448	28984	0.69897	4.46216
6	4008	32992	0.77815	4.51841
7	4070	37062	0.84510	4.56893
8	3416	40478	0.90309	4.60722
9	3580	44058	0.95424	4.64402
10	3620	47678	1.00000	4.67832
11	3640	51318	1.04139	4.71027
12	3796	55114	1.07918	4.74126
13	3096	58210	1.11394	4.76500
14	3260	61470	1.14613	4.78866
15	3074	64544	1.17609	4.80986
16	3114	67658	1.20412	4.83032
17	2978	70636	1.23045	4.84903
18	3082	73718	1.25527	4.86757
19	3072	76790	1.27875	4.88530
20	3000	79790	1.30103	4.90195
Fractal Dimension = 2 − slope =			1.28257	

a

b

Figure 57. *Counting the boxes of increasing size through which the boundary of the Koch snowflake passes and the log-log plot. The plot is a straight line but the slope does not give an accurate fractal dimension for the shape.*

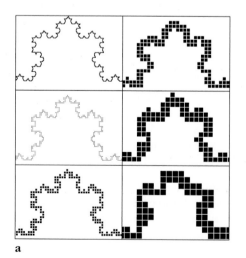

Kolmogorov Box Count Method			
cell width	count	Log(w)	Log(N)
1	4020	0	3.60422605
2	1985	0.30103	3.29776051
3	1294	0.47712125	3.11193428
4	928	0.60205999	2.96754798
5	713	0.69897	2.85308953
6	603	0.77815125	2.78031731
7	521	0.84509804	2.71683772
8	432	0.90308999	2.63548375
9	363	0.95424251	2.55990663
10	322	1	2.50785587
Fractal dimension = − slope =			1.093811

a

b

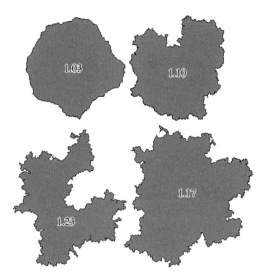

Figure 58. Several fractal outlines with varying fractal dimensions.

surfaces are perfectly isotropic, however, and in the presence of preferred orientations this simple relationship breaks down. Even more serious, if the boundary measured is a projected outline of a particle, the boundary irregularities will be partially hidden by other surface protrusions, and the measured fractal dimension will be too small by an amount that depends on the size of the particle and on its roughness. There is no general correction for this, and despite the fact that this procedure is very commonly used, the data obtained (and their subsequent interpretation) remain very open to question. Chapter 13 discusses the meaning and method of measurement for fractal surfaces, which have dimensions between 2 and 3.

Harmonic analysis

The fractal dimension attempts to condense all of the details of the boundary shape into a single number that describes the roughness in one particular way. There can, of course, be an unlimited number of visually different boundary shapes with the same fractal dimension or local roughness. At the other extreme it is possible to use a few numbers to preserve all of the boundary information in enough detail to effectively reconstruct the details of its appearance.

Harmonic analysis is also known as spectral analysis, Fourier descriptors, or shape unrolling (Schwartz and Shane, 1969; Ehrlich and Weinberg, 1970; Zahn and Roskies, 1972; Granlund, 1972; Beddow et al., 1977; Persoon, 1977; Flook, 1982; Kuhl and Giardina, 1982; Kaye et al., 1983; Rohlf and Archie, 1984; Barth and Sun, 1985; Ferson et al., 1985; Bird et al., 1986; Diaz et al., 1989; Rohlf, 1990; Diaz et al., 1990; Verscheulen et al., 1993; Lestrel, 1997). It begins by converting the boundary to a function of the form radius (angle) or $\rho(\varphi)$. As shown in **Figure 59**, a radius drawn from the feature centroid is drawn as a function of angle, and plotted to unroll the shape. This plot obviously repeats every 2π, and as a periodic or repeating function is straightforwardly subjected to Fourier analysis. This allows the determination of the a and b terms in the series expansion

$$\rho(\varphi) = a_0 + a_1 \cos(\varphi) + b_1 \sin(\varphi) + a_2 \cos(2\varphi) + b_2 \sin(2\varphi) + \ldots \tag{17}$$

It is often more convenient to represent the values as amplitude c and phase δ for each sinusoid:

$$c_i = \sqrt{a_i^2 + b_i^2} \tag{18}$$

$$\rho(\varphi) = \sum c_i \cdot \sin(2\pi i \varphi - \delta_i)$$

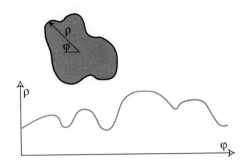

Figure 59. *Illustration of the procedure for unrolling a feature profile.*

This series continues up to an *n*th term equal to half the number of points along the periphery, although it is a characteristic of Fourier analysis that only the first few terms are needed to preserve most of the details of feature shape. As shown in **Figure 60**, with only one or two dozen terms in the series, the original shape can be redrawn to as good a precision as the original pixel representation. In many cases, the phase information δ_i for each term in the series can be discarded without much effect on the shape characterization, and a single coefficient c_i used for each frequency. The first few values of c in the harmonic or Fourier expansion of the unrolled boundary thus contain a great deal of information about the feature shape.

Of course, this method has serious problems if the shape is reentrant so that the radial vector is multivalued. In order to avoid that problem, an alternative approach to shape unrolling plots the slope of the line as a function of the distance along the line. This plot is also a repeating function, and can be analyzed in exactly the same way.

The chain code boundary representation of a feature already contains the slope vs. position information along the boundary, but with the problem that the data are not uniformly spaced (the diagonal links being longer than the horizontal and vertical ones). An effective way to deal with

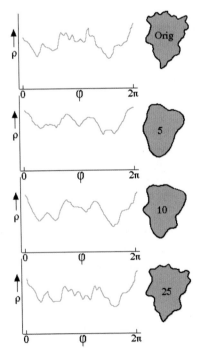

Figure 60. *Reconstruction of a real feature outline (an extraterrestrial dust particle) from the first 5, 10, and 25 terms in the Fourier expansion (from Kaye, 1983).*

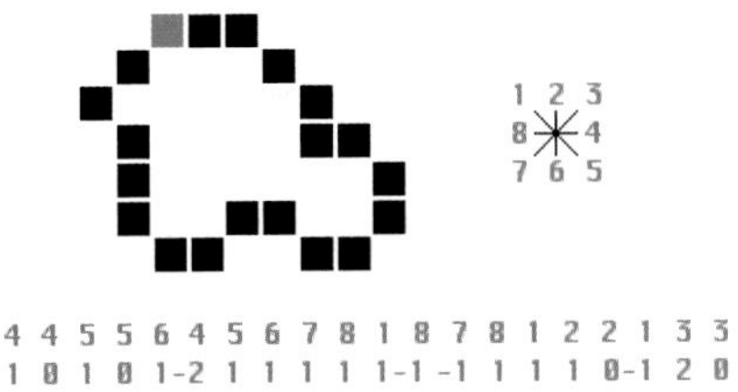

Figure 61. Chain code representations for a feature outline, showing the conventional direction codes and below them the differential chain code.

```
1 2 3
8 ✳ 4
7 6 5
```

```
4 4 5 5 6 4 5 6 7 8 1 8 7 8 1 2 2 1 3 3
1 0 1 0 1-2 1 1 1 1 1-1 -1 1 1 1 0-1 2 0
```

this is to replace each horizontal link with five shorter conceptual sublinks, each in the same direction, and each diagonal line with seven shorter sublinks. The ratio of 7:5 is close enough to $\sqrt{2}$ for practical purposes, and the total number of sublinks along the boundary is still reasonably short. A plot of the link value (which indicated direction) vs. position now gives the unrolled feature shape. Performing a Fourier analysis of the sequence of values along the chain code for the feature produces a list of c_i values that contain the shape information. The interpretation of these values is hampered because of the discontinuity in the direction numbers.

Chain code need not be recorded as a set of values corresponding to each of the eight possible pixel neighbor directions. The difficulty in analysis that results from the discontinuity between directions eight and one can be overcome by converting to the "first difference chain code" as shown in **Figure 61**. This is just the differences between values using modulo arithmetic, so that a zero indicates the edge proceeding straight ahead in whatever direction it was already, positive values indicate bends of increasing angle in one direction and negative values indicate the opposite direction. In this form, the shape is rotation-invariant (at least in 45-degree steps), except for the fact that the links in the original chain were not all of the same length. It is also easier to find corners, by defining them as a minimum net change in value over some distance (Freeman and Davis, 1977).

The most successful of the harmonic analysis techniques is to plot the x- and y- projections of the feature outline, treat them as real and imaginary parts of a complex number, and perform a Fourier transform on the resulting values as a function of position along the boundary, as shown in **Figure 62**. Again, this results in a set of c_i values that summarize the feature shape.

These can be compared between classes of objects using standard statistical tests such as stepwise regression or principal components analysis, to determine which of the terms may be useful for feature classification or recognition. In a surprising number of cases, this approach proves to be successful. The identification of particles in sediments with the rivers that deposited them, the correlation of the shape of foraminifera with the water temperature in which they grew, distinguishing the seeds from various closely related plant species, and the discrimination of healthy from cancerous cells in Pap smears, are but a few of the successes of this approach.

Despite its successes, the harmonic analysis approach has been little used outside of the field of sedimentation studies. In part, this neglect is due to the rather significant amount of computing needed to determine the parameters, and the need to apply extensive statistical analysis to interpret them. As computer power has continued to increase and cost to decrease, however, this cannot be the major reason any longer. The probable cause is that the frequency terms have no obvious counterpart in human vision. The shape information that we extract visually from images does not reveal these numeric factors. The distinction between two sediments based on the seventh harmonic coefficient can be understood intellectually to somehow represent the presence or amplitude of that frequency in the boundary irregularities of the object, but to a human observer that is masked by other variables. The success of the approach illustrates the power of computer-based measurement algorithms to surpass human skills not only quantitatively (in terms of accuracy and precision) but even qualitatively (in terms of the types of things that can be measured). But that doesn't mean that humans feel comfortable using such tools.

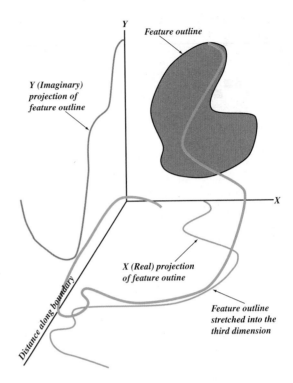

Figure 62. *Unrolling a feature shape by plotting the x- and y- coordinates of boundary points as a function of position along the boundary, and combining them as real and imaginary parts of complex numbers.*

Feature outline

Y (Imaginary) projection of feature outline

X (Real) projection of feature outine

Feature outline stretched into the third dimension

Distance along boundary

Topology

Harmonic analysis uses characteristics of feature shape that are quite different from those that human vision selects. On the other hand, topological parameters are those which seem most obvious to most observers. When asked to differentiate the stars on the U.S., Australian, and Israeli flags we do not use color, dimension or angles, but the number of points. The most obvious difference between a disk and the letter "O" is not the slight ellipticity of the latter, but the presence of the central hole. Topological properties are quite different from metric ones. If the feature were drawn onto a sheet of rubber, stretching it to any size and with any distortion will not change the topology. Smoothing an irregular outline does not alter the topological information.

Some topological properties of features can be determined directly from the pixel array, such as the number of internal holes. Other properties, such as the number of points on the stars mentioned previously, are most readily determined using the skeleton. As discussed in Chapter 7, the skeleton consists of pixels along the midline of the features. Pixels with only a single touching neighbor are end points, while those with more than two neighbors are branch points. Counting the branch and end points, and the number of loops (holes), provides a compact topological representation of feature characteristics. **Figure 63** shows an example of using the end points to characterize shape.

These characteristics of features are important to visual classification and recognition, as can be easily shown by considering our ability to recognize the printed letters in the alphabet regardless of size and modest changes in font or style. Many character recognition programs that convert images of text to letters stored in a file make heavy use of topological rules.

Another topological property of a feature is its number of sides. In the case of a space-filling structure such as cells in tissue, grains in a metal, or fields in an aerial survey, the number of sides each feature has is the number of other features it adjoins. This was discussed previously in its relation to relative feature position. Labeling the features according to the number of neighbors can reveal some interesting properties of the structure, as was shown earlier in **Figures 21** and **22**.

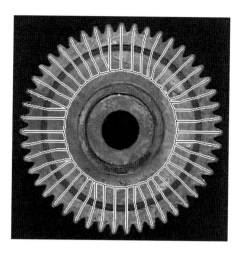

Figure 63. *Skeleton of an image of a gear used for topological characterization. The 47 end points efficiently count the number of teeth, and, of course, there is one hole.*

The number of sides that a feature has can also be described in another way. If corner points are defined as arbitrarily abrupt changes in boundary direction, then counting the number of sides can be accomplished directly from the chain code. A second approach that is less sensitive to minor irregularities in the boundary pixels uses the convex or bounding polygon. As described earlier, this polygon is usually constructed with some fixed and relatively large number of sides. For instance, performing rotation of axes in 10-degree steps would form a 36-sided polygon. Many of the vertices in this polygon may be close together if the feature shape has a relatively sharp corner. Setting an arbitrary limit on the distance between vertices that can be merged (usually expressed as a percentage of the total polygon perimeter) allows collecting nearby vertices together. Of course, counting the vertices is equivalent to counting the sides. Setting a threshold for the minimum length of the polygon side (again, usually as a percentage of the total perimeter) to consider it as a representation of a side of the feature can be used to count sides.

None of the four types of shape characterization (dimensionless ratios, fractal dimension, harmonic analysis, and topology) is completely satisfactory. One (harmonic analysis) is too unfamiliar and different from the human interpretation of shape. One (dimensionless ratios) is convenient for calculation but not very specific. One (fractal dimension) corresponds well with the human idea of boundary roughness but does not capture more macroscopic aspects of shape. Also, one (topology) is just the opposite in that it represents the gross aspects of feature shape but not the fine details. In real situations, several complementary techniques may be needed.

Three-dimensional measurements

Many of the measurement procedures discussed above for 2D images generalize directly into three dimensions. Images acquired by confocal light microscopy, seismic imaging, medical or industrial tomography, and even, in some cases, serial sectioning can be represented in many different ways, as discussed in Chapter 12. For image processing and measurement purposes, however, an array of cubic voxels (volume elements, the 3D analog to pixels or picture elements) is the most useful. Image processing in these arrays uses neighborhoods just as in two dimensions, although these contain many more neighbors and consequently take longer to apply (in addition to the fact that there are many more voxels present in the image).

Image measurements still require identifying those pixels that are connected to each other. In two dimensions, it is necessary to decide between an 8-connected and a 4-connected interpretation of touching pixels. In three dimensions, voxels can touch on a face, edge, or corner (6-, 18- or 26-connectedness); again, the rules for features and background cannot be the same. It is more difficult to identify internal holes in features because the entire array must be tested to see if there is any connection to the outside, but the logic remains the same.

This consistency of principle applies to most of the measurements discussed in this chapter. Summing up the numeric values of voxels (or something calculated from them) to obtain the total density, or water content, or whatever property has been calibrated, is straightforward. So are location measurements using the voxel moments. Orientations in 3D space require two angles instead of one. Neighbor relationships (distance and direction) have the same meaning and interpretation as in two dimensions.

The 3D analog to feature area is feature volume, obtained by counting voxels. The caliper dimensions in many directions and the bounding polyhedron can be determined by rotation of coordinate axes and searching for minimum and maximum points. Of course, getting enough rotations in three dimensions to fit the polyhedron adequately to the sample is much more work than in two dimensions. In fact, everything done in 3D voxel arrays taxes the current limits of small computers: their speed, memory (to hold all of the voxels), displays (to present the data using volumetric or surface rendering), and the human interface. For instance, with a mouse, trackball, or other pointing device it is easy to select a location in a 2D image. How do you accomplish this in three dimensions? Various schemes have been tried (some requiring a real-time stereo display), none with wide acceptance.

It was noted earlier that perimeter is a somewhat troublesome concept and a difficult measurement in two dimensions. The analog to perimeter in three dimensions is the surface area of the feature, and it has all of the problems of perimeter plus some more. The idea that the surface area may be an artefact of voxel resolution remains and is exacerbated by the somewhat coarser resolution usually available in 3D images. Measuring the length of the perimeter accurately is difficult in two dimensions. For a 3D surface, the boundary representation is the list of coordinates of vertices of a polyhedron with triangular facets. Calculating the area of a triangle from its three corners is straightforward, but knowing which three points to use for any particular triangle is not. As a very simple example, consider four points as shown in **Figure 64**. The surface can be constructed between them two different ways, with different surface areas (usually both are calculated and the average used).

Boundary representation in two dimensions relies on the fact that there is only one path around any feature, no matter how complicated. This is not true in three dimensions. There is no unique order in which triangular facets between boundary voxels must or can be followed. In fact, for objects that are topologically shaped like a torus (have at least one open hole through them), there is no guarantee that a continuous surface path will completely cover the surface and reach all points on it. This means that there is no convenient analog to chain code, and many of the 2D measurements that were based on it become difficult to perform in three dimensions.

Figure 64. *Tiling a surface with triangular facets has two different solutions. In this simple example, the elevation of the four corners of a square are shown. Triangles can be constructed using either diagonal as the common line. As shown, this produces a surface that is either convex or concave, with a surface area of either 1.366 or 1.414 square units.*

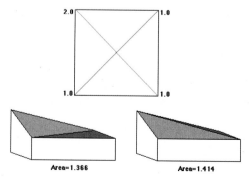

Likewise, the 3D skeleton is harder to obtain. Actually, two "kinds" of skeleton can be calculated for voxel arrays. One is the set of midlines, and the other is a set of planes. The latter is formed by connecting the skeleton lines in each plane section, while the former is a connection between the junction points of the skeletons in each plane section. This set of midlines can also be obtained as a medial axis transform, by using the 3D analog of the EDM to find the centers of inscribed spheres. Neither type of skeleton by itself captures all of the topological properties of the feature. The planes can show twists and protrusions not visible in the line skeleton, for example.

Measuring the length of a voxel line is similar to a pixel line. The voxels can touch in three different ways; therefore, the rule shown earlier in **Equation 14** must be extended to become:

$$Length = 0.877 \cdot (num.\,of\ face\ touching\ neighbors)$$
$$+ 1.342 \cdot (num.\,of\ edge\ touching\ neighbors) \qquad (19)$$
$$+ 1.647 \cdot (num.\,of\ corner\ touching\ neighbors)$$

although deciding what voxel patterns to count to identify the important topological properties of the structure is not entirely clear.

Most of the shape parameters calculated as ratios of dimensions have simple (although equally limited) generalizations to three dimensions. Harmonic analysis can also be performed in three dimensions, by expressing the radius as a function of two angles and performing the Fourier expansion in two dimensions. There is no analog to chain code or the description of slope as a function of position, so the method is restricted to shapes that are not re-entrant or otherwise multiple-valued (only one radius value at each angle). Fractal dimensions are very important for dealing with 3D surfaces and networks, although in most cases it remains easier to measure them in two dimensions.

In fact, this generalization holds for most image measurement tasks. The practical difficulties of working with 3D voxel arrays are considerable. The size of the array and the amount of computing needed to obtain results are significant. Because of memory restriction, or limitations in the resolution of the 3D-imaging techniques, the voxel resolution is usually much poorer than the available pixel resolution in a 2D image of the structure. Consequently, to the extent that the needed information can be obtained from 2D images and related by stereology to the 3D structure, that is the preferred technique. It is faster and often more precise.

This approach does not work for all purposes. Strongly anisotropic materials require so much effort to section in enough carefully controlled orientations, and are still so difficult to describe quantitatively, that 3D imaging may be preferred. Above all, topological properties of the structure such as the number of objects per unit volume, or the connectivity of a network, are simply not accessible on 2D sections (although a technique using two such parallel planes to sample 3D topology was presented in Chapter 8). Many aspects of 3D topology can only be studied in three dimensions, and consequently require 3D imaging, processing, and measurement.

The discussion of 2D images was based on an array of pixels, and so far all of the discussion of 3D images has assumed they consist of voxels. As will be discussed in Chapter 10, many 3D structures are studied by obtaining a set of parallel section planes that are relatively widely spaced. This is generally described as a "serial section" technique, although physical sectioning is not always required. Constructing the object(s) from the sections is discussed in Chapter 12.

Measuring the features from the sections is computationally straightforward. The volume is estimated as the summation of section area times section spacing, and the surface area can be estimated as the summation of the section perimeter times section spacing, but few objects have perfectly smooth surfaces. The section perimeter will reveal the roughness in the plane of the section,

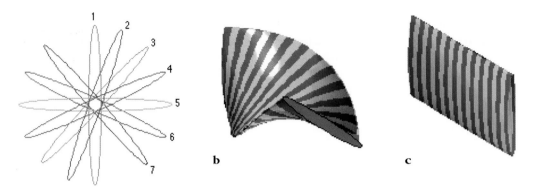

a **b** **c**

Figure 65. Reconstruction of a spiral structure:
 (a) *the individual section outlines;*
 (b) *the correct reconstruction of the surfaces;*
 (c) *the incorrect reconstruction that results if the outlines are rotated for a "best fit."*

but the reconstruction technique generally connects the section profiles together with planes that are perfectly smooth, which underestimates the surface area. Even if the surface is smooth, the volume and surface area will be underestimated if it is curved.

Aligning the sections correctly is vital both to correctly understand the topology of the structure, and to measure the volume and surface. In the simple example shown in **Figure 65**, the actual structure is a spiral. If the serial sections are rotated to achieve a "best fit" from one section to the next, the result is a straight, untwisted structure with less volume and surface area than the actual structure.

Only when the sections are very closely spaced do these problems go away. In the limit when the section spacing is the same as the resolution within the individual section images, it is equivalent to a cubic voxel array. This is generally preferred for measurement purposes.

10

Feature Recognition and Classification

Template matching and cross-correlation

Recognition and classification are essentially complementary functions that lie at the "high end" (i.e., require the most complicated algorithms) in the field of image analysis (Duda and Hart, 1973). Classification is concerned with establishing criteria that can be used to identify or distinguish different populations of objects that may appear in images. These criteria can vary widely in form and sophistication, ranging from example images of representatives of each class to numeric parameters for measurement, to syntactical descriptions of key features. Recognition is the process by which these tools are subsequently used to find a particular feature within an image. It functions at very different levels, including such different processes as finding a face in an image, or matching that face to a specific individual.

Generally, computers tend to be better than humans at classification because they are not distracted by random variations in noncritical parameters and can extract useful statistical behavior to isolate groups. Sometimes these groups are meaningful. On the other hand, people are generally much better (or at least faster) at recognition than are computers, because they can detect the few critical factors that provide identification of familiar objects. But humans do not fare as well with unfamiliar objects or even with unfamiliar views of common ones.

Various recognition and classification techniques involve an extremely broad range of complexities. At the low end, operations such as scanning UPC bar codes (Universal Product Code) on supermarket packaging or automatic sorting and routing mail to the proper zip code, are based on careful design of the target to facilitate the reading function. These are normally detected by linear scans instead of acquiring full images as used elsewhere in this text, and UPC codes are symmetric (with black-and-white reversal) so that the scan can be used in either direction.

The basic statistics behind classification is independent of image analysis, since the parameters used for classification and identification can come from any source. A good introduction to the statistics can be found in textbooks such as (Divijver and Kittler, 1980; Schalkoff, 1992; Haykin, 1993; Stefik, 1995; Hand, 1981, Pao, 1989).

Probably the lowest level functionality that utilizes two-dimensional pixel images is the restricted optical character recognition (OCR) of the type applied to processing checks. The characters

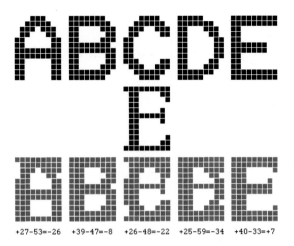

Figure 1. *Matching each of the five letter templates with a target letter produces a net score (sum of red matched pixels minus blue unmatched pixels) that is greatest for the correct match.*

+27-53=-26   +39-47=-8   +26-48=-22   +25-59=-34   +40-33=+7

printed on bank checks are restricted to numerals 0–9 and a few punctuation marks. Furthermore, the characters are in a fixed size, location and orientation, and in a special fixed font designed to make them easily distinguishable. In such highly constrained situations, a technique known as template matching provides fast results with minimum computation.

The example in **Figure 1** shows the application of template matching to the letters A through E. A template consisting of black pixels that cover the shape of each target character is stored in memory. Each letter to be recognized is combined with all of the stored templates using an exclusive-OR function to count the number of pixels that match and the number which do not. The template that gives the highest net score (number of matches minus number of misses) is selected as the identification of the character. In some implementations, the net score may be normalized by dividing by the number of black pixels in the template, if this varies substantially for the various characters.

In the example, the templates are not exact and have enough width and extra pixels to cover a modest range of variation in the target character, but obviously cannot handle widely divergent fonts or styles. The similarities in shape between the various letters (e.g., B and E) do not create a serious problem and the error rate for this approach is very low, provided that the characters meet the assumptions of size, orientation, font, etc., that are built into the templates. The presence of small amounts of noise due to dirt, etc., is tolerated as well.

This type of template matching is a rather specialized and restricted case of cross correlation, which can be used for grey scale or color images as well as binary pixel arrays. Chapter 5, on image processing in Fourier space, introduced the cross-correlation procedure as a technique for matching a target image with a second image to locate brightness patterns. This method can be applied to images of text or any other features, provided that a set of representative target images can be established.

It is not necessary to perform cross correlation using a Fourier transform. When the target is very small, it may be efficient to perform the mathematics in the spatial domain. The target pattern is moved to every possible position in the image and at each location i,j the cross-correlation value is summed according to **Equation 1**, to produce a result as shown in **Figure 2**.

$$\frac{\displaystyle\sum_{x=0}^{s}\sum_{y=0}^{s}B_{x+i,y+j}\cdot T_{x,y}}{\sqrt{\displaystyle\sum_{x=0}^{s}\sum_{y=0}^{s}B_{x+i,y+j}^{2}\cdot\sum_{x=0}^{s}\sum_{y=0}^{s}T_{x,y}^{2}}} \tag{1}$$

```
2 7 3 9 8 8 9 9 9 3 4 7 7 7 7
1 6 9 7 7 7 2 2 6 8 6 3 7 8 8                    5 8 6 6 5 3 3 2 5 7 6 7 7
8 8 4 3 4 4 9 2 4 7 7 6 5 3 3                    7 6 4 6 3 4 3 6 6 3 7 6 4
5 9 5 6 5 4 8 7 9 1 6 9 4 8 4                    6 4 6 3 6 6 5 7 2 5 8 3 3
9 4 7 1 7 8 6 8 3 4 9 5 1 4 8                    5 4 3 5 8 7 7 1 1 8 4 3 4
5 5 5 8 5 9 5 6 3 9 8 7 9 3 1     3 5 7          4 3 5 6 6 6 6 2 7 7 2 5 3
2 5 1 7 2 5 6 3 4 7 2 6 4 9 4     5 9 5          5 3 5 2 5 6 5 3 5 4 6 3 4
8 3 6 3 6 9 4 2 2 7 8 3 7 4 6     7 5 3          3 5 3 5 9 1 0 4 5 7 5 5 5
4 5 5 8 8 4 1 9 9 7 8 3 6 8 6                    6 6 7 7 1 0 4 7 7 6 3 5 6
7 5 5 4 1 5 6 7 6 8 2 3 2 3 3                    7 6 4 2 3 6 6 5 6 3 3 5 4
5 3 3 5 6 6 2 6 7 9 9 5 8 3 1                    4 5 5 7 4 3 6 7 6 5 4 7 3
5 9 6 5 2 3 9 9 9 5 8 3 6 2 4                    7 6 7 5 1 6 7 6 6 6 5 4 0
8 8 4 7 4 5 8 1 7 7 6 6 5 9 5                    7 4 5 5 7 5 1 5 7 6 5 3 6
4 5 4 8 6 4 2 7 9 7 2 4 5 9 7                    4 4 7 5 6 1 3 8 5 4 5 6 7
7 3 7 4 8 8 2 9 3 7 3 5 5 7 1
```

| Image | Target | Result |

Figure 2. Cross correlation using pixels with single digit values. The best match is marked in red (note that it is not an exact match).

where **B** and **T** are the pixel brightness values for the image and target, respectively, and the summations are carried out over the size **s** of the target. This value is very high where bright pixels in the target and image align, and the denominator normalizes the result for variations in overall brightness of the target or the image. In addition to providing a quantitative measure of the degree of match, the correlation score can be scaled appropriately to produce another grey-scale image in which brightness is a measure of how well the target matches each location in the image, and can be processed with a top hat filter, or thresholded, to detect matches that are present.

Figure 3 shows an example image from Chapter 5, in which several different fonts have been used for the letters A through E. Each of the letters in the first set (which is repeated in sets 6 and 9) was used as the target. The cross-correlation results are marked with red dots showing the maximum values of cross-correlation. The letter is found where it recurs in the same font, but most of the other fonts are not matched at all. The exception, font number 4, shows that the characters are similar enough to be matched but that they also generate false matches.

Cross-correlation looks for very specific details of feature shape and brightness, and while it is reasonably robust when a feature is partially obscured (by noise or camouflage), it is not very tolerant of changes in size or orientation. **Figure 4** shows an example of one of the major uses of the technique, the identification of military targets. The target image (an F-15 aircraft) produces a cross-correlation value that drops to 84% with a 10-degree rotation, and 80% for a 20-degree rotation. Both values are still higher than the correlation with different aircraft, which are 72% for an F-14 and 47% for a B-1. Of course, the images must be scaled to the same approximate size before the calculation is performed. In practice, it would be necessary to have target images at many different orientations. Views in other directions (from the side, front, oblique views, etc.) would also be required.

Parametric description

Recognition of features in images covers an extremely wide range of applications. In some cases the targets are fully known and can be completely represented by one or several images, so that cross-correlation is an appropriate method. In others, the goal is to have the computer "understand" natural three-dimensional scenes in which objects may appear in a wide variety of presentations. Applications such as automatic navigation or robotics require that the computer be able to extract surfaces and connect them hierarchically to construct three-dimensional objects, which are then recognized (see, for example, Roberts, 1982; Ballard and Brown, 1982; Ballard et al., 1984). The topics and goals discussed here are much more limited: for the image analysis system to be able to recognize discrete features in essentially two dimensional scenes. If the objects are three dimensional and can appear in different orientations, then each different two-dimensional view may be considered as a different target object.

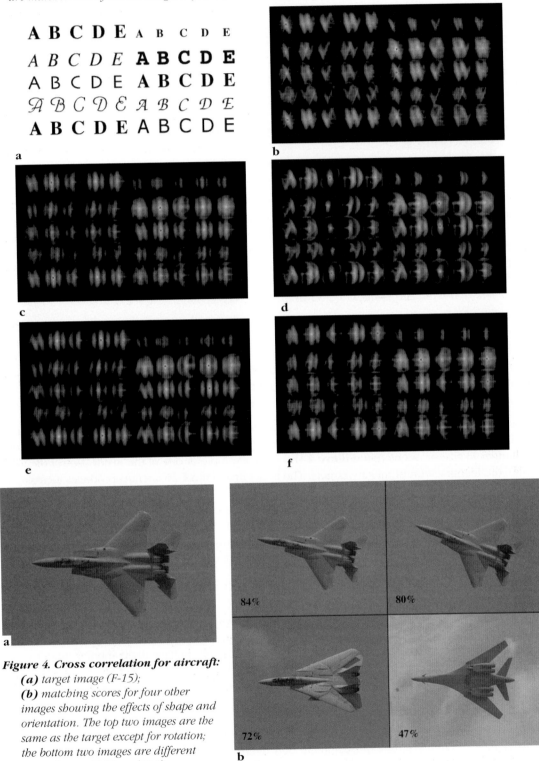

Figure 3. *Cross correlation with letters in different fonts. The letters in the first set (repeated in set 6 and 9) are matched one by one in images b–f as discussed in the text.*

Figure 4. Cross correlation for aircraft:
(a) target image (F-15);
(b) matching scores for four other images showing the effects of shape and orientation. The top two images are the same as the target except for rotation; the bottom two images are different aircraft types (F-14 and B-1).

The simplest situation, but one that satisfies a very large percentage of practical applications, uses the feature-specific measurement parameters introduced in the previous chapter. These methods are called parametric descriptions. **Figure 5** shows a simple example, in which the features can be grouped into two classes based on their shape. Several of the shape descriptors introduced before can be used here; the example shows the formfactor (4π area/perimeter^2). A distribution of form-factor values for the features in the image shows two well separated populations. Setting a limit between the two groups can separate them into the respective classes. In the figure, the "round" features have been identified with a red mark.

Note that other measurement parameters such as area (**Figure 5c**) do not distinguish between the groups. Finding a single parameter that can be successfully used to separate classes is not usually possible, and when it is, selecting the best one from the many possible candidates by trial and error can be a time-consuming process.

In most cases, a combination of parameters is needed for successful classification, and statistical methods are used to find the best ones. As a simple thought experiment (from Castleman, 1996), consider a system to sort fruit, where the target classes are apples, lemons, grapefruit, and cherries. Apples and cherries can be distinguished on the basis of size (e.g., diameter), as can lemons and grapefruit. But apples have a range of sizes that overlap lemons and grapefruit, so a second para-meter is needed to distinguish them, for instance the average hue, distinguishing between red and yellow (at least, this will work if green apples are excluded from the process). This can best be shown as a two-dimensional plot of parameter space, as shown in **Figure 6**.

Note that the various classes are still distinct in this example, so that drawing "decision lines" between them is straightforward once the range of values for the different classes has been estab-lished. This is most typically done by measuring actual samples. Rather than just measuring "typical" specimens, it would be most efficient in this case to intentionally select examples of each fruit that are considered to be extremes (largest, smallest, reddest, yellowest) to map out the boundaries.

The goals in deciding upon the measurement parameters to use are:

1. The ability to discriminate the various classes, preferably with no overlap at all but at least with minimum overlap (handling of situations in which there is overlap is described in the following paragraphs)

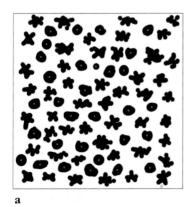

a

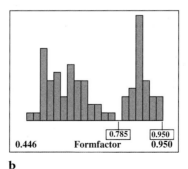

| 0.785 | 0.950 |

0.446   Formfactor   0.950

b

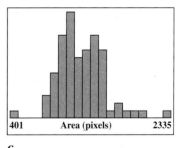

401   Area (pixels)   2335

c

Figure 5. Some hand-drawn features, with their histograms for formfactor (b) and area (c). The formfactor histogram shows two separate classes; the features with values greater than 0.785 are marked with red dots and are visually "rounder" than the others. The area histogram shows only a single class and does not distinguish the two types of features.

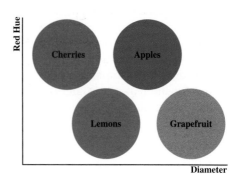

Figure 6. Classes for fruit sorting discussed in the text.

2. To have the smallest practical number of parameters, which simplifies the training process in which extremes in all combinations of parameters are desired
3. To be independent of each other, so that each one measures a very different characteristic of the objects
4. To be reliable, so that the parameter values will not vary over time or due to uncontrolled variables, and they can be measured consistently if system hardware is modified or replaced

Sometimes, these goals conflict with one another. For example, adding more parameters often provides less overlap of classes, but it may complicate the training process. Finding multiple parameters that are truly independent can be difficult. In the case of the apples, one parameter is a measure of size and the other of color, so we may expect them to be independent. But shape parameters, which are often very important for classification, may be quite interrelated to each other and to the size parameters from which they are calculated. It usually requires a statistical procedure to determine which function best in any particular situation (an example is shown in the following).

Reliability is difficult to predict when a classification scheme is initially established. By definition, changes in object appearance due to unexpected variations cannot be excluded. For instance, if color is being used to distinguish fabricated components and the pigmentation used in the ink being applied is changed by the supplier, or incandescent lights are replaced by fluorescent ones, or a different camera is substituted for one that has failed, the RGB values and whatever hue or other information is derived from them will change. It may or may not be practical to introduce a calibration step that will adjust the new values to match the old. The alternative is to remeasure a training population using the new ink, lights or camera, and reestablish class limits.

Three situations are encountered in general classification. Each situation will be described in this chapter:

1. *Imposed criteria (the classical expert system)* — A human expert supplies rules. Software may optimize the order in which they are applied and search for relevant rules, but does not derive them
2. *Supervised classification* — This is a training set of examples that are supposed to be prototypes of the range of classes and class variations are presented to the system, which then develops a strategy for identifying them. The number of classes and examples identified for each class are specified by a human.
3. *Unsupervised classification* — The system is presented with a set of examples as described previously, but not told which class each belongs to, or perhaps even the number of classes. The system attempts to define the class regions in order to maximize the similarity of objects within each cluster and the differences between groups.

There are other situations in which classification of images is not based on the statistics of individual feature measurement parameters, but on characteristics of the entire scene. The most often cited example of this type of discrimination uses the Brodatz (Brodatz, 1966) texture images representing various kinds of natural and man-made surfaces. A few are shown in **Figure 7**. The Fourier transform power spectra of these images (**Figure 8**) reveal characteristic frequencies and orientations, or ratios of amplitudes at specific frequencies, which can be used to distinguish them. This same logic can be implemented in hardware using a set of filter banks to select the various frequencies, and performing identification in real time.

Figure 7. A few of the Brodatz textures:
   (a) *bark;*   *(b)* *wool cloth;*
   (c) *wood grain;*   *(d)* *bricks;*
   (e) *straw;*   *(f)* *herringbone cloth;*
   (g) *sand;*   *(h)* *bubbles;*
   (i) *pigskin.*

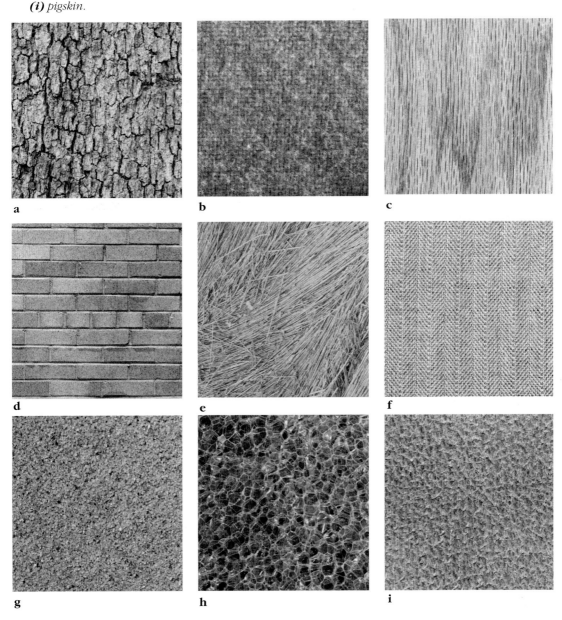

Figure 8. The Fourier transform power spectra for each of the images in Figure 7.

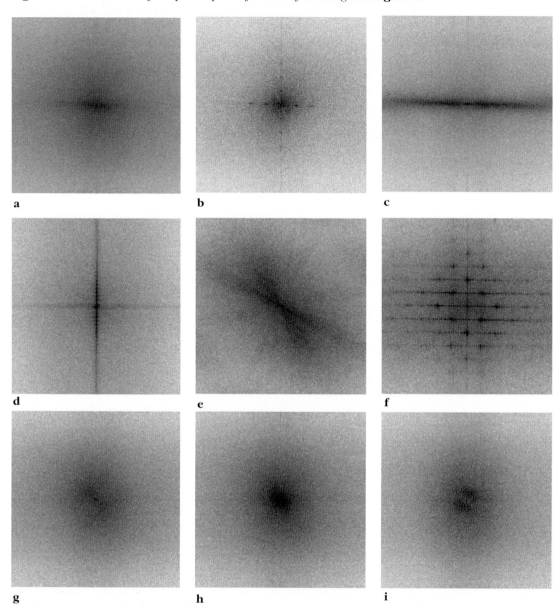

a b c

d e f

g h i

The principal use of this technology seems to be in classification of remote sensing (satellite and aerial photographs). When combined with multiband spectral intensity ratios as discussed below, the textures can be used to identify various types of crops, rocks, and other land use patterns. Although they apply to the entire scene rather than a single feature, the various numeric values, such as ratios of amplitudes at various frequencies and orientations, are used in the same way as feature-specific measurements in the classification processes described in this chapter.

Decision points

In many practical cases, the classes are not as completely distinct as the example shown in **Figure 5**. Commonly, when training populations are measured, the histograms of parameter values may

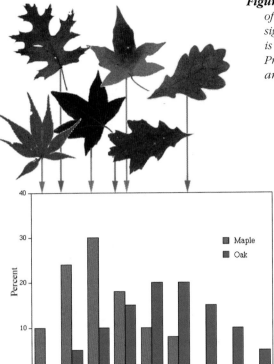

Figure 9. *Values of formfactor measured on a variety of maple and oak leaves. The histograms are significantly overlapped, indicating that formfactor is not the best parameter to use for identification. Probably a method using the skeleton end points and external branches would be more successful.*

overlap as shown in **Figure 9**. Such overlaps usually indicate the need to find other parameters that offer better discrimination, but it is not always possible to avoid some degree of overlap, and in that case it is necessary to establish a decision threshold that produces an acceptable probability of error.

As shown in **Figure 10**, the decision threshold combines with the probability distribution function for the measurement parameter to establish the expected error rate. The area of the tail of the distribution function (as a percentage of the total) gives the probability of identifying a member of one population as being in the other class. Sometimes the decision threshold is set to make the two errors (wrongly identifying A as B, or B as A) equal, which minimizes the total error.

In other cases, economic factors must be taken into account. For example, consider the case of two different "O" rings used in engines, one in a tractor engine and the other in a helicopter engine, which are distinguished by an imaging operation that measures thickness. The economic cost of occasionally shipping a part intended for a helicopter to be used in a tractor is probably very small. The part will likely function there, in which case the only extra cost is perhaps the use of a more costly polymer or the loss of the more valuable part. But shipping a tractor part for use in a helicopter would produce much greater liability if the engine failed, and probably a greater likelihood of failure in a more demanding environment. In such a case it would be desirable to set the error rate for mistakenly identifying a tractor part as a helicopter one to something very low (one in 1 million or less) and accepting a much higher rate (perhaps one in 1000) for the opposite error.

Similar considerations arise in biomedical imaging. There is much concern about automated diagnosis, such as the identification using image analysis of cancer cells in Pap smears, or lesions in mammograms (Karssemeijer, 1998), because of liability issues. The most widely accepted course of action has been to set the decision thresholds for identifying suspicious features very

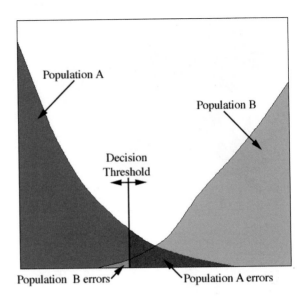

Figure 10. *Setting a decision point when distributions overlap, as discussed in the text. The probability of misclassifying a feature is measured by the area in the tail of each distribution past the decision threshold.*

low, accepting many false positives which can subsequently be screened again by an experienced human, but hopefully minimizing false negatives in which disease might be missed.

Multidimensional classification

In the examples shown earlier, the histogram or probability distribution function has been plotted as a function of a single measurement parameter. In the example of **Figure 6**, two parameters (size and color) were used. In such cases, it is often possible to reduce the problem to a single derived parameter by fitting a new axis line through the data, usually called either a linear discriminant line or a context line. As shown in **Figure 11**, a distribution of data points measured on a training population and plotted on two parameter axes may have values that overlap in both individual parameters, but be much better separated when projected onto another derived axis which is a linear combination of the two. This line can be fit by linear regression through the points, or by using principal components analysis.

Curved lines can be used in principle, but in practice it is difficult to perform robust nonlinear regression unless the form of the functional dependence is known ***a priori***, and in that case it is usually better to transform the measurement variables beforehand. For instance, instead of area, it might be better to use equivalent diameter (which varies as the square root of area) to obtain a plot for which a linear regression line provides a better fit, as illustrated in **Figure 12**.

Once the new axis has been fit to the data points, a histogram of values projected along the new derived parameter (shown in **Figure 11**) can be used for classification just as discussed previously for a directly measured parameter. In fact, the formfactor used previously is actually itself a combination of area and perimeter measurements, so this process is simply one more step toward obtaining a derived parameter that most directly distinguishes the classes of interest.

Using a decision point determined along the best-fit line between two populations generates a decision line (or in higher dimension spaces when more than two parameters are used, a decision plane) that separates the two populations. This works well when the populations are reasonably compact and equiaxed, but, as shown in **Figure 13**, does not separate populations that have irregular shapes. Techniques that can locate an optimum decision plane (the Bayes classifier) for such cases are much more computationally intensive. It is also possible to distinguish multiple populations by piecewise-linear decision boundaries, or by quadratic or higher power boundaries.

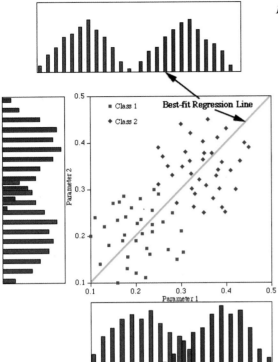

Figure 11. Two populations of points that overlap on both parameter axes, with a linear discriminant or context line along which they are best separated.

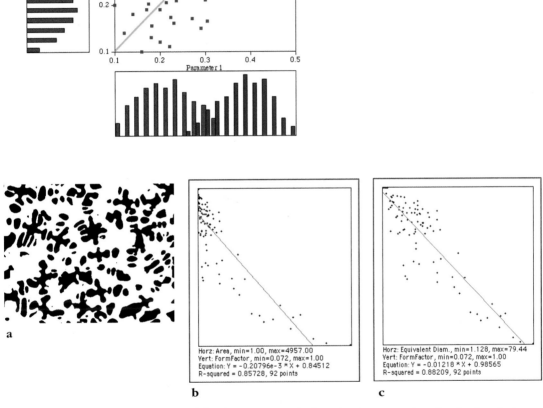

| Horz: Area, min=1.00, max=4957.00 |
| Vert: FormFactor, min=0.072, max=1.00 |
| Equation: Y = -0.20796e-3 * X + 0.84512 |
| R-squared = 0.85728, 92 points |

| Horz: Equivalent Diam., min=1.128, max=79.44 |
| Vert: FormFactor, min=0.072, max=1.00 |
| Equation: Y = -0.01218 * X + 0.98565 |
| R-squared = 0.88209, 92 points |

b   **c**

Figure 12. Features from an image of dendrites in a metal alloy, showing regression plots for formfactor vs. area (b) and formfactor vs. equivalent diameter (c).

Fortunately, in most such cases the addition of additional parameters separates the various population classes well enough that simple linear methods can be used.

Population classes like those shown in **Figure 13b**, which are elongated and oriented at an angle to the axes defined by the measurement parameters, have a some correlation between the parameters.

Figure 13. Classification examples in two dimensions:
(a) separable classes showing the decision boundary perpendicular to the linear discriminant or regression line;
(b) classes that are not separable by the boundary in figure a, with an optimal Bayes classifier (blue line) that does separate them;
(c) multiple classes separated by piecewise linear decision boundaries;
(d) multiple classes separated by quadratic decision boundaries.

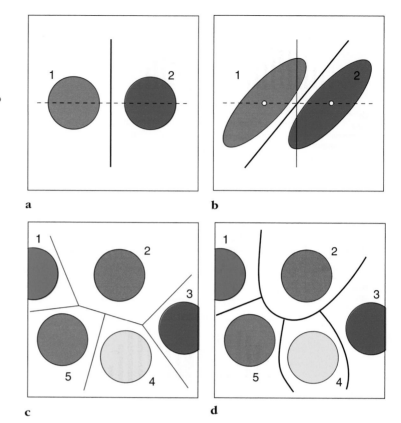

This creates problems for classification, as noted above, so it is desirable to make the population area more equiaxed, and preferably circular. The covariance of the data set is defined as

$$c(i,j) = \frac{\sum_{k=1}^{n}\left(x_{k,i} - \mu_i\right)\cdot\left(x_{k,j} - \mu_j\right)}{n-1} \tag{2}$$

where x is the measurement value, i and j identify the two parameters, μ are the mean values for each parameter, and k runs through the n features in the population. The covariance can vary between $+\sigma_i\sigma_j$ and $-\sigma_i\sigma_j$ where σ are the standard deviation values for each parameter. A value of zero for $c(i,j)$ indicates no correlation and the minimum or maximum value indicates perfect correlation as shown in **Figure 14**.

The previous examples showed only two measured parameters, but in general there may be N axes for a high-dimensionality space. In that case, all of the covariances $c(i,j)$ for the various parameters measured can be collected into a covariance matrix **C**. This matrix can be used to transform an irregular population cluster to an equiaxed, circular one. For each measurement vector x (defined by all of the n measurement parameters), the quantity r calculated as

$$r^2 = (x-\mu)'C^{-1}(x-\mu) \tag{3}$$

is called the Mahalanobis distance from the point representing the feature measurement parameters to the mean of the population μ. This is a generalization of the usual concept of distance,

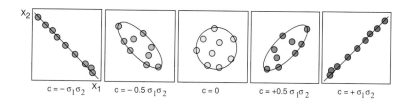

$c = -\sigma_1\sigma_2$ $c = -0.5\,\sigma_1\sigma_2$ $c = 0$ $c = +0.5\,\sigma_1\sigma_2$ $c = +\sigma_1\sigma_2$

appropriate for measurements in which the axes have different meanings and scales. In the case of an equiaxed population cluster (zero covariance), the Mahalanobis distance is the same as the usual Euclidean distance.

It is helpful in measuring distances along the various axes to compensate for the different scales of the various measurement parameters by normalizing the distance measurements. This is done by dividing each one by an appropriate scaling constant, ideally the standard deviation of the parameter values. This is called the "standardized Euclidean distance."

Of course, the classification methods can be generalized to more than two dimensions (it just becomes harder to illustrate with simple graphics). **Figure 15** shows an example from remote imaging, in which the intensities of reflected light detected in different Landsat Thematic Mapper wavelength bands are used to classify terrain types (Grasselli, 1969; Sabins, 1986). Patterns of spectral

Figure 15. Land use classification using Thematic Mapper images:
  (a) one image showing reflectivity in a single wavelength range;
  (b) reflectance vs. wavelength plots and cluster diagram for reflectivity values from different terrain types;
  (c) classification of land use using these data.

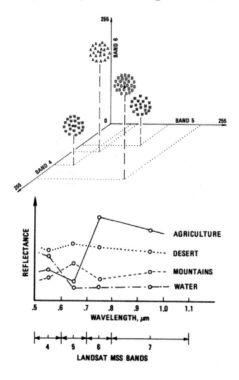

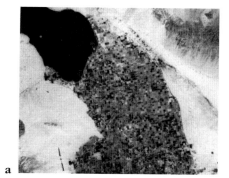

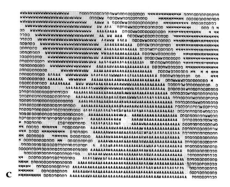

intensity are associated with particular types of vegetation, minerals, etc. A supervised training program is used in which an operator marks locations and the image analysis system plots the point in terms of the measured intensities in each wavelength band. The clusters of points (which are shown schematically) then mark the various classes, which are used to label the images pixel by pixel.

There is no reason to expect the clusters of points corresponding to each class to form a regular spherical shape in the N-dimensional parameter space, of course, and examples below will show alternative ways of establishing these regions. One of the simplest methods is to establish maximum and minimum limit values for each parameter. This corresponds to a set of rectangular boxes in parameter space (**Figure 16**) that define each class. Training such a system is simplified because it is not necessary to find a representative population, but rather to find or predict extreme values.

Another method for establishing region boundaries is to measure a representative training population for each class, and to characterize the distribution of values by the mean and standard deviation for each parameter. Using the mean values as the coordinates of the center, and a multiple of each parameter's standard deviation as the lengths of the axes, this generates ellipsoids as shown in **Figure 17**. The surfaces of these ellipsoids may be used as absolute class boundaries, but it is more useful to measure the distance of each new feature's parameter coordinates from the various classes in terms of the standard deviation.

Figure 16. *Range limits for class regions in parameter space (illustrating three independent parameters)*

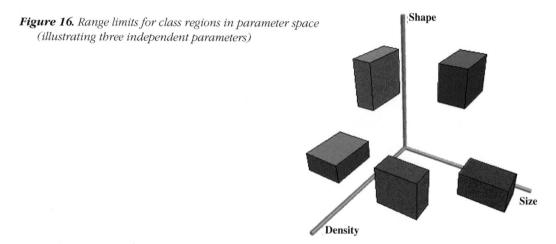

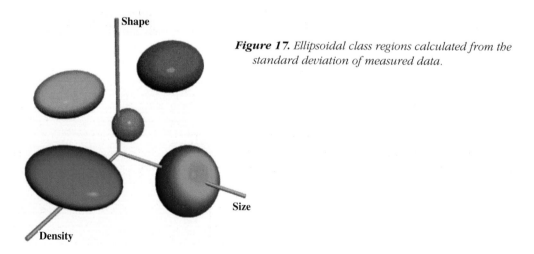

Figure 17. *Ellipsoidal class regions calculated from the standard deviation of measured data.*

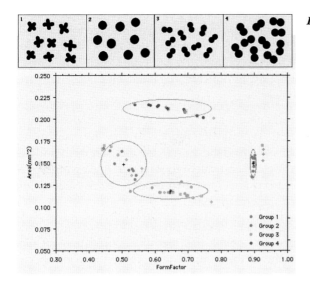

Figure 18. *Two-dimensional example of statistical limits. Note that some points lie outside the 2-sigma boundaries. Solid points indicate the training populations shown at the top; shaded points represent identification of additional features. Points are identified with the nearest cluster measured as discussed in the text.*

Figure 18 shows a two-dimensional example for simplicity. The training populations are shown at the top, along with the plots of the points and the two-sigma ellipses for each class. Note that for the training population and for additional features measured subsequently, some of the points lie outside the two-sigma limit, as would be expected. Note also that some of the classes are much larger (more variation in the parameter values) than others, and that the ellipses may be elongated in some cases because one parameter varies more than another. The standard deviation, shown as the length of each ellipse axis, becomes a scale with which to interpret the rather confusing distances of parameter space. Using the standard deviation normalizes the various axis units as discussed above. The concept of a "distance" in parameter space is not well defined and may be distorted in different directions or regions of the plot. Unfortunately, this is often the case when shape factors are used for identification since they are often not all independent (so the axes are not orthogonal) and are certainly not linear (a change in aspect ratio from 1.1 to 1.5 is far different from a change from 4.1 to 4.5, for instance).

If a new feature is measured, and its parameter coordinates do not place it inside one of the class boundaries, it may still be identified as being "most like" one class by measuring the distance in parameter space from the feature coordinates to the center of each class (the mean values), and scaling this number by dividing by the standard deviation. Because of the different cluster sizes, this means that a point could actually be closer to one class on the plot but more "like" a different one. In the example, a point close to the blue class might be fewer standard deviations away from the magenta one, and would be identified accordingly.

Learning systems

It can be very difficult to collect a truly representative set of features with which to establish training populations that produce classes that can be applied without alteration to many new features and situations. In particular, the extreme-valued features that lie near the end of the distributions are usually rare. Furthermore, an approach using mean and standard deviation rather than the actual shape of the distribution may oversimplify the measurements, which in many image analysis situations do not produce Gaussian distributions.

Figure 11, in the previous section, illustrated the ability to estimate the probability of classification error from the shape of the distribution histogram. Using the actual histogram thus extends traditional "hard" classification in which a feature is assigned to one class or excluded from it, to the "fuzzy" logic situation in which shades of probability are admitted. Fuzzy logic is an important extension of classical logic in which the various classification rules in the knowledge base contain probabilities. An example would be "If **A** can fly, there is a 70% chance that it is a bird; if **A** cannot fly, there is a 5% chance that it is a bird," which accommodates butterflies, which fly but are not birds, and penguins, which are birds but do not fly. In our case, the parameter histogram gives a direct way to measure the conditional probabilities.

Fuzzy logic has been applied to expert systems and neural nets (both discussed below as engines for assigning classifications based on multiple rules). Typically the result is to slow the convergence process because it is necessary to evaluate all paths and find the most likely, not simply to find one path through the rules. In a formal sense, fuzzy logic is equivalent to Bayesian logic with leveled classic sets. For comprehensive information on fuzzy logic, refer to (Zadeh, 1965; Negoita and Ralescu, 1975, 1987; Sanchez and Zadeh, 1987; Zimmerman, 1987).

As an illustration of a learning system that uses histograms to establish decision points, and works in multi-parameter space using linear discriminant or context line methods, populations of nine kinds of natural nuts were used (**Figure 19**). Some of these represented more than one species (e.g., one class included both white and red oak acorns, both with and without their caps, and another included several kinds of pecans) so that histograms were generally not Gaussian and sometimes were multimodal (**Figure 20**). Images from a training population of about 20 of each variety of nut were captured with a monochrome video camera (this work was done in the 1980s, so much of the hardware was primitive by current standards), and the features measured to obtain a total of 40 parameters for each feature.

Some parameters such as location and orientation were discarded based on human expectation that they were not meaningful. Others were discarded by subsequent statistical analysis, leaving a net of 17 that were actually used, so discrimination was performed in a 17-dimensional space. Not all of the dimensions are truly independent (orthogonal), however, because many of the shape parameters are based on size measures used in various combinations. Linear discriminant lines were

Figure 19. A few of the nuts used in the learning example discussed in the text.

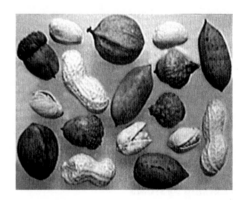

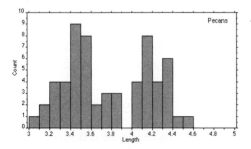

Figure 20. A bimodal length distribution for two species of pecans.

constructed in this space between each pair of nut classes, using stepwise regression (Draper and Smith, 1981). Parameters were added to or removed from the equation of the context line based on the F-value (an arbitrary cutoff value of 4.0 was used), eliminating variables that did not improve the ability to distinguish particular population groups.

This elimination helps toward the goal of using independent parameters, as well as simplifying the total problem and reducing the number of training examples required. Many of the shape parameters, for example, use some of the same size information. For example, the convexity and form-factor defined in Chapter 8 both use the perimeter. If one of them shows a high correlation with category discrimination, there is a good chance that others that incorporate perimeter will also show a correlation. Stepwise regression will select the one that has the highest correlation and predictive power, and discard the others.

The resulting context lines used as few as two or as many as eight terms. Some parameters were used in many cases (e.g., average brightness), while others appeared in only one or two equations but were then often the most important single parameter (e.g., convex area was highly important in distinguishing pistachios from almonds). On the average, each of the 17 parameters was used 11 times in the total of 55 pairwise context lines, and each context line equation included an average of 5 parameters. **Figure 21** shows several examples. The coefficients in the equations for the linear discriminant or context lines are derived by regression, and represent the angles between the line and each of the parameter axes in N-space.

Discrimination of hickory nuts from almonds, and acorns from peanuts, is easy because the distributions are entirely separate, even though the distributions are somewhat irregular in shape. The acorn–pecan distribution (**Figure 22**) shows a slight overlap, which was the case in about 16% of the pairwise discriminant plots. Using the logic shown earlier in **Figure 11**, the decision point was located to make the probability of misclassification errors equal for both classes. In the acorn–pecan case, this amounted to about 1% and arose when a large acorn was viewed from the side without its end cap, as shown in **Figure 23**. The most likely error was confusion of an acorn with a filbert.

Once the discriminant functions (the equations of the context lines) have been established and distributions of derived parameter values along those lines set up, the system can go to work

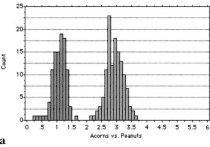

a

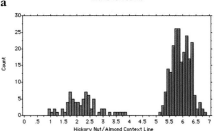

b

Figure 21. Context lines and frequency distributions for hickory nuts–almonds and acorns–peanuts, examples of entirely separated classes. The regression equations are:

Acorns (type 1) vs. Peanuts (type 3) = 3.928 + 0.773 · Aspect Ratio - 5.007 · Fractal Dimension + 0.068 · Brightness

Hickory Nuts (type 2) vs. Almonds (type 6) = −2.266 − 2.372 · Breadth + 2.184 · Width + 0.226 · Brightness +0.318 · Contrast +2.374 · Texture

Figure 22. *Context line and frequency distribution for acorns-pecans, showing overlap. The regression equation is:*

Acorns (type 1) vs. Pecans (type 4) = 1.457 + 6.141 · Formfactor - 2.153 · Convex Perimeter + 1.768 · Convex Area + 2.926 · Length - 1.575 · Breadth - 1.131 · Extent

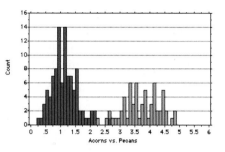

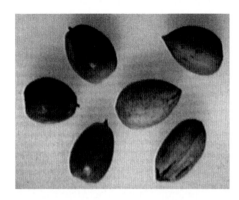

Figure 23. *View of several large acorns without their end caps and pecans, showing a situation in which confusion between the two classes may arise.*

identifying nuts. The decision points along each context line position planes (perpendicular to the lines) in the high-dimensionality space which form polyhedra around each class. The problem is that with a training population of only 20 nuts from each class, the positions of those decision points are imperfect.

As the system examines more images (eventually a total of about 1000 nuts), the derived parameter values (positions along each context line) are calculated and the histograms are updated. This does not require any additional computer memory, since the histograms have already been established. Identification of nut types proceeds on the basis of the stored decision points. But whenever a value is added to the end of a histogram (within the last 5% of its area), the program asked the operator to confirm the identification and then reestablished the decision threshold using the then current histogram. In this way the system learned from the additional specimens to which it has been exposed, which gradually increased the number of observations near the important limits of each distribution.

Figure 24 shows a table with the final results. A total of 3.7% of the nuts were misidentified, but most of these errors occurred very early in the learning process; there was only one error in the last 200 nuts. The system started out with an approximate idea of the limits of each class, and refined these limits with more information. It should be noted that many of the parameters used for each identification were not familiar to the human operators, and almost certainly did not represent the logic they used to identify the nuts. But the system quickly became as proficient as the humans.

In other examples, an automated system based on this same logic has surpassed the humans who trained it (Russ and Rovner, 1987). In the study of archaeological sites in the American southwest and much of central America, a subject of considerable interest is the process of domestication of corn, *Zea mays*. It is widely believed, although not proven, that corn is a domesticated offshoot of the wild grass teosinte, of which there are many varieties. Little remains of corn in an archaeological context that can be dated, but it happens that corn, like all grasses (and many other plants), produces small silica bodies called opal phytoliths in and between the cells on the stalk, leaves, and

| | | | | | Identified Type | | | | |
Actual Type		1	2	3	4	5	6	7	8	9
Acorns	1	91	0	0	1	0	0	0	10	0
Hickory Nuts	2	0	70	0	1	0	0	1	0	0
Peanuts	3	0	0	126	0	0	1	0	0	0
Pecans	4	2	1	0	54	0	0	3	0	0
Pistachios	5	0	0	0	0	126	0	0	0	0
Almonds	6	0	0	0	0	0	224	0	0	0
Brazil Nuts	7	0	3	0	6	0	0	115	0	0
Filberts	8	8	0	0	0	0	0	0	67	0
Walnuts	9	0	0	0	0	0	0	0	0	107

Figure 24. *"Confusion matrix" showing errors in nut identification.*

other parts of the plant. They are generally a few micrometers in size, and act to stiffen the plant tissue. They are also selectively produced at any site of injury (including cropping by animals).

From an anthropological point of view, phytoliths are of interest for two reasons. First, they survive in the soil for long periods of time and can be recovered from layers that are datable and show other signs of human habitation. Second, they have shapes that are distinctive. Research over several decades has shown that phytoliths can be used taxonomically to identify species of grasses, including corn and its precursors (Twiss et al., 1969; Rovner, 1971; Pearsall, 1978; Piperno, 1984). Most of this identification has been carried out by humans, who have accumulated photographs (mostly using the scanning electron microscope since the particles are only a few micrometers in size and have significant three-dimensional structure so that they cannot be studied satisfactorily with the light microscope) and built catalogs from which matching comparison to unknowns can be performed. The success rate for skilled observers in blind tests is generally better than 95%. This has been at the cost of a very substantial amount of effort, however, and the knowledge and experience are not readily transferred to other researchers. The human eye does not deal too well with the need to characterize variation, and the individual phytoliths vary widely in shape. Such a situation is ripe for the use of computer image analysis methods.

Slides were prepared with phytoliths extracted from a training suite of five known species of maize and teosinte and SEM images analyzed to determine several size and shape parameters, which were used as described above to establish discriminant classes. On the original set of objects, this produced a better than 99% correct identification. After applying the results to a total of 300 objects from 5 additional species of plants (three maize and two teosinte), the results had improved to better than 99.6% accuracy in distinguishing the two classes. Furthermore, the system can examine hundreds of phytoliths (enough to produce statistically significant results) from more species of corn or other grasses in one month than have been done by hand and eye in the last 20 years. The same system has recently been used for classification of squash seeds (Rovner, personal communication).

kNN and cluster analysis

Other methods are used to establish limits for classes in parameter space. The two most widely used, *k*-nearest neighbor (*k*NN) and cluster analysis, share the drawback that unlike the histogram and linear discriminant method described earlier, it is necessary to save the actual coordinates for each identified feature, which means that storage requirements grow continually if the system is to continue learning. The other difficulty with these methods is that the time required to make an identification rises with the number of stored values, even with efficient algorithms to sort or prune the data set and work with only a reasonable number of candidate points. On the other hand, these methods do not presuppose any particular shape for the class regions, such as the rectangular prism, ellipsoid, or polyhedral methods described previously. It is even possible to handle such situations as shown in **Figure 25**, in which one class is nonconvex, disjoint, or is largely or completely surrounded by another.

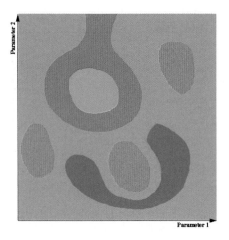

The *k*-nearest neighbor classification works by searching the database of previously identified features for those which are "most like" the current measurement, as shown in **Figure 26**. This amounts to finding the distance between the coordinates of the current feature's parameters, and those for other features. The distance is generally calculated in a simple Pythagorean sense (square root of the sum of squares of differences), but this overlooks the important fact that the different axes in parameter space have very different units and metrics. Usually the distance along each axis is simply expressed as a fraction of the total range of values for that parameter, but there is no real justification for such an assumption. It would be better to use some normalizing scale such as the standard deviation of values within each class, if this is available (the same logic with Mahalanobis distance as used above for the ellipsoid class limits).

In the simplest form of *k*-neighbor comparison, *k* is one, and the search is simply for the one single prior measurement that is most similar, and which is then assumed to identify the class of the new feature. For features near the boundary between classes, single-nearest-neighbor matching proves to be quite noisy and produces irregular boundaries that do not promote robust identification, as shown in **Figure 27**. Using the identification of the majority of five, nine, or even more nearest-neighbors produces a smoother boundary between classes, but is still highly sensitive to the relative size of the populations. If one population has many more members than the other, it effectively shrinks the class limits for the minor group by making it more likely that the majority of matches will be with members of the more numerous population.

The methods described so far presume that some training population in which the features belong to known classes can be used to construct the class limits. As noted before, this is known as "supervised

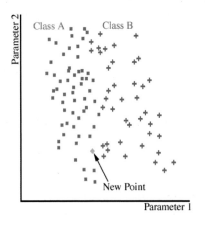

Figure 26. Three of the five nearest-neighbors to the new point lie in Class B, so it is assigned to that class.

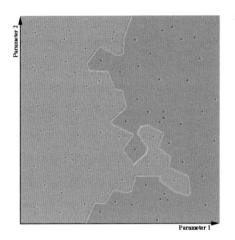

Figure 27. *The irregular boundary that forms between two classes (whose individual members have parameter values indicated by the colored points) using single-nearest-neighbor classification.*

learning" in which the operator identifies the actual class or population to which each feature belongs, and the software uses that information along with whatever measurement parameters are available to determine an identification strategy. There are some situations in which it is not known *a priori* what the classes are, or perhaps even how many of them are present. In these cases, it is still useful to plot each feature's measured parameters as values in a parameter space, and then look for clusters of points. Cluster analysis with non-supervised training is a rich topic that goes beyond the scope of this text (see, for example, Pentland, 1986; James, 1988; Bow, 1992; Fukunaga, 1990).

One typical way that cluster analysis proceeds uses the distance between points to identify the members of a cluster. For example, start with the two points closest together. Assume these represent a class, and add to the class other nearby points until the distance from the nearest point already assigned to the cluster exceeds some (arbitrary) limit, which may be calculated from the size of the growing class region. The method can obviously be generalized to use more than a single nearest-neighbor. Once a given class has stopped growing, begin again with the remaining points, and continue until all have been assigned. There are many refinements of this approach, which allow for assigned class regions to be merged or split.

A somewhat complementary method for finding clusters uses all of the points simultaneously. It starts by constructing a minimal spanning tree for all of the points present (an intensive amount of computation for large data sets). The links in this tree can be weighted either by their Euclidean or Mahalanobis length, or by the number of matches present in a table of *k*-nearest-neighbors for each point. In other words, if the same points are each listed in each other's nearest neighbor lists, they are probably in the same cluster. The spanning tree is then pruned by cutting the links with the greatest length or the smallest number of matches, to leave the identified clusters. **Figure 28** shows an example of a sparse cluster of points, the minimal spanning tree, and the clusters that result from pruning (after Bow, 1992).

Another, somewhat different approach to find clusters in data, particularly when there is only one significant measured variable, is the dendrogram. **Figure 29** shows an example. The features are ranked into order based on the value of the measured variable, such as formfactor. Then the features that have the smallest value differences are connected (numbers 7 and 21 in the example, followed by 4 and 23, 27 and 14, 13 and 16, etc.) by horizontal lines positioned according to the difference value. Groups of features are usually linked based on the smallest difference between any two members of the group, although it is also possible to use the difference between the mean or median values in each group. Eventually all of the features and groups are connected into a single tree.

If multiple measurement parameters (e.g., formfactor, diameter, and density) are used, the difference between features is calculated as the distance between the vector representation of the

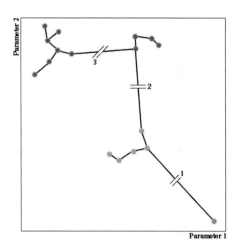

Figure 28. Parameter values plotted as points, and the minimal spanning tree connecting them. Cutting the branches with the greatest length separates the clusters (indicated by different colors).

multiple values in N-dimensional space. This typically presents a problem because the units of the various parameters are quite different, and the lengths of the various axes are not compatible so there is no natural way to scale them in proportion. This can sometimes be handled by normalizing each measured parameter based on (for example) the total range or standard deviation of the measured parameters, but such a method is inherently arbitrary. Without a full characterization of the statistical distributions of each parameter, it is not possible to calculate a true Mahalanobis distance for the parameter space.

Once the dendrogram has been constructed, it can be used to determine any number of clusters by selecting a different threshold value for the difference. For example, in **Figure 29** a value of 0.6 would yield two clusters while a value of 0.4 would yield four clusters and a value of 0.3 would yield 5 clusters. By definition, in the unsupervised clustering situation, we do not know *a priori* how many classes are present. Therefore, the decision requires human judgment.

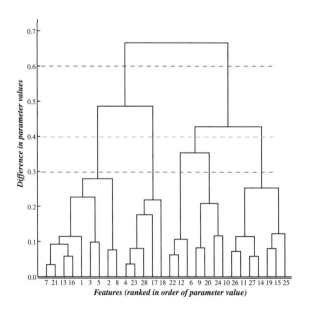

Figure 29. Example dendrogram as discussed in the text. The red, green, and blue lines indicate the effect of selecting different threshold values for the difference between feature measurements on the number of classes.

Expert systems

After clusters have been identified by one of these methods, the class limits must still be constructed by one of the methods shown earlier. This could be a geometric shape (rectangular prism, ellipsoid, polyhedron) or a *k*NN boundary. Now we will consider how to apply these class boundaries as a set of rules for the identification of subsequent features.

The simplest and most common method is the traditional expert system. A set of rules (such as the limits — either hard or fuzzy — for the class boundaries) is created which must be applied to each new set of feature measurements. Returning to the case of the letters A through E, **Figure 30** shows a very simple expert system with four rules, requiring measurement of only three parameters. In the most efficient implementation, only those parameters required would be measured, so for the letter B (which is identified by the number of holes in the shape) the roundness and aspect ratio parameters, which are not needed, would not be determined at all. When they are used, the cutoff values of the parameters for each letter type were determined experimentally, by measuring characters from a few different fonts. In situations such as this, it becomes important to design the system so that the least "expensive" parameters are determined first, to reduce the time needed for the overall identification. Counting holes requires less computation than measuring dimensions needed for the shape factors. Also notice that, unlike the template matching and cross correlation examples shown earlier, this method is insensitive to position, size or orientation of the letters, and tolerates several different fonts.

Simple classification systems such as this are sometimes called decision trees or production rules, consisting of an ordered set of IF/THEN relationships. Classic expert systems separate the data base (rules) from the inference engine used to find a solution (Black, 1986; Winstanley, 1987; Rolston, 1988; Slatter, 1987; Walters, 1988). One of the drawbacks to such systems is that the addition

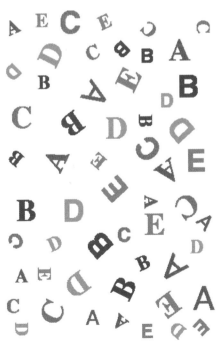

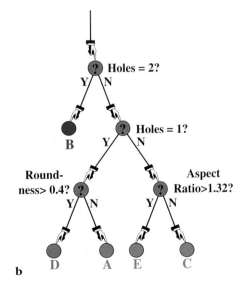

Figure 30. *Expert system to classify the letters A through E. The colors shown in*
(a) were assigned using the logic in
(b) Note that the shape factors used as parameters do not depend on size, orientation or position, and that several different fonts (with and without serifs) are present.

a

b

of another class (e.g., the letter F) does not simply graft on another step, but may completely reshuffle the order in which the rules should be applied, or even eliminate some rules altogether and replace them with others. The optimum decision tree is not necessarily the one with the fewest branches. "Knowledge shaping" procedures such as including the cost of obtaining each input value can greatly improve overall efficiency and determine an optimum search and solution tree (Cockett, 1987).

Most real expert systems have far more rules than this one and the order in which they are to be applied is not necessarily obvious. The complexity of decision paths increases rapidly with a large number of rules. General purpose expert systems try to find a path between the various input values and a conclusion in one of two ways. If, as shown in **Figure 31**, the number of observations is less than the number of possible conclusions, forward chaining that starts at the left and explores pathways through various rules toward a conclusion would be used. In other cases, backward chaining that works from conclusions back toward observations may be more efficient. In the very schematic diagram shown in the figure, there are 6 initial observations (measurements), 21 rules, and 12 possible conclusions; real systems are several orders of magnitude more complex. Some of the rules shown have more than two possible outcomes; in some systems, each possible outcome would represent a separate rule.

Normal forward searching for a successful path through this network would start at some point on the left, follow a path to a rule, and follow the outcome until a contradiction was met (a rule could not be satisfied). The system would then backtrack to the preceding node and try a different path, until a conclusion was reached. This approach does not test all possible paths from observations to conclusions. Heuristics to control the order in which possible paths are tested are very important. In cases of realistic complexity, it is not possible to test all consequences of applying one rule, and so simplifications such as depth-first or breadth-first strategies are employed. Pruning, or rejecting a path before working through it to exhaustion, is also used. (You may use as a rough analogy the search for a move in a chess program. Some initial moves are rejected immediately, while others are searched to various depths to evaluate the various responses possible and the outcomes). Reverse searching works in the same way, starting from possible conclusions and searching for paths that lead to observations. Some search "engines" combine both forward and reverse searching methods.

When fuzzy logic is used, the various rules contain probabilities. In that case, it is ideally necessary to construct a total probability by combining the values for nodes along each path, to select the most likely path and hence the most probable result. The heuristics that control search order are less important, but the total computation load can be much greater.

Figure 31. Schematic diagram for an expert system.

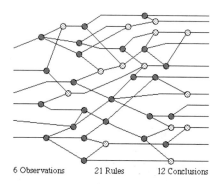

6 Observations   21 Rules   12 Conclusions

Neural nets

Searching the multiple pathways through an expert system, especially one utilizing fuzzy logic probabilities, is an inherently parallel problem. An attractive way to solve it uses neural networks, an implementation of a simplified and idealized model of the functioning of biological processes. Each element in a neural net is a threshold logic unit, illustrated in **Figure 32**. It is analogous to a simplified model of a functioning neuron, as shown in the classic McCulloch–Pitts model (McCulloch and Pitts, 1943; Rosenblatt, 1958; Lettvin et al., 1959; Minsky and Papert, 1969; Grossberg, 1988). Multiple inputs (which in the image analysis case could be either measured parameter values, or pixel intensities) are weighted and summed, and the total compared to a threshold value. If the threshold is exceeded, the neuron "fires." In a biological system, it sends a train of pulses as inputs to other neurons; in a neural network it transmits a calculated output value (a probability) to another threshold logic unit.

To understand the functioning of these simple units, it is worthwhile to consider a classical description of a theoretical construct called the "grandmother cell." Imagine a cell that has been trained to recognize your grandmother, and patiently examines every image that is transmitted from your eyes searching for clues. Earlier logic units, some of them in the eye and some in the visual cortex, find low level structures. So the presence of white hair, blue eyes, and the spacing of eyes, nose, mouth, cheekbones, etc., are all inputs to the grandmother cell. It has been shown that human vision is very efficient at locating facial features (even babies do it, immediately after birth), and that it is the ratios of spacings between these features that are important clues to recognition of individuals.

Other clues might include the presence of a familiar dress, jewelry, or glasses. Some of these are more important than others (have larger weighting), and some factors may simply be missing (e.g., if your view of the person prevents seeing the color of her eyes). There may also be some factors with large negative weights, such as the presence of a bushy red mustache or a height over

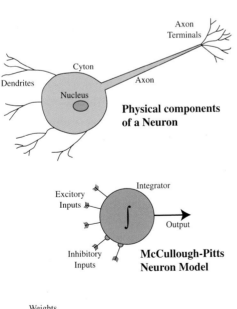

Figure 32. A threshold logic unit and an idealized neuron.

six feet tall. When all of the inputs are summed, if the total is large enough, the cell alerts your conscious brain that grandmother is present. Such a system accounts for the occurrence of false positives (thinking that you see someone familiar, who on close examination turns out not to be the expected person). The result will not always be correct (we may miss grandma in some situations, or mistake someone else for her occasionally), but it is very efficient and works quickly and well enough.

Connecting together a network of these simple devices (perceptrons) in multiple layers, with some low level decisions passing information to higher levels, produces a system capable of making decisions based on diverse types of inputs. The classic topology of a neural network is shown in **Figure 33**. Each artificial neuron calculates like the perceptron, producing an output that is a weighted combination (not necessarily linear) of its input values. These outputs are routed through at least one hidden layer before reaching the output layer. The output layer produces outputs that are discrete, selecting one (or at most a few) values. Training the neural net adjusts the weights in the neurons to produce the desired output patterns for the various training patterns (Hebbs, 1949). This is typically accomplished by training the system with examples. When a correct conclusion is reached, the weights of the inputs from the neurons that contributed to the decision are increased, and vice versa. This feedback system eventually results in pathways that correspond to descriptions of the objects being recognized. Various methods for adjusting the weights are in use, some working forward and some backwards through the network (Rumelhart et al., 1986).

In principle, the weights in the various units describe the shape of each class space in a high dimensional space (corresponding to the number of inputs). In practice, it is very difficult if not impossible to interpret the weights, particularly in the inner layers of the system. Dealing with overlapping classes (the possibility that the same set of inputs may lead to more than one output) is exactly analogous to the situation shown earlier in **Figure 11**. Many systems cannot explain the reasons for the answers they deliver; indeed, it is difficult to find just where the "knowledge" resides in the system (like our own brains, it seems to be distributed widely throughout the network). It is difficult to assign probabilities or confidence limits to the result, but neural net systems usually fail gracefully. Unlike classic expert systems, the solution time for a neural system decreases as more information is made available. Their principal shortcoming is the need for unusual computer architectures for efficient realization. Although the neural network is in theory a parallel device, many actual implementations use traditional serial computers to perform all of the calculations, simulating a parallel structure, and in this case the speed advantage is lost.

The weights in a neural network typically take a long time to stabilize, which is another way to say that it takes a lot of training to produce a network that gives correct answers most of the time. The same requirements for finding representative training populations exist as for the statistical classification methods discussed previously. The quality of the training is usually more important than how the solution is implemented. The only real difference between a neural network and one of the statistical methods shown above is the intricacy with which parameter space can be dissected

Figure 33. Schematic diagram of a minimal neural network with one hidden layer.

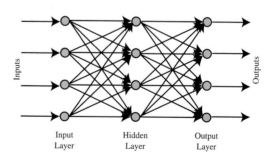

Input Layer   Hidden Layer   Output Layer

into the various class regions. Neural networks can fit very complex functions to describe surfaces separating regions, which may perform better in some cases than simple rectangular prisms, ellipsoids or polyhedra, without encountering the problems of storage, sensitivity to outliers, and slow speed inherent in kNN methods.

Syntactical models

Another approach to feature recognition is used, and it is quite different from the parameter space methods described earlier (Fu, 1974, 1982; Pavlidis, 1977; Tou and Gonzalez, 1981; Schalkoff, 1991). Syntactical models deal primarily with shape information, usually derived from the feature outline or skeleton. This is broken down into the important pieces, and their relative positions recorded. This recording can be likened to a set of characters that spell a word, and compared with other words on the basis of the number of missing, substituted, or rearranged characters.

To give an example, **Figure 34** shows the key elements of the letter A. The two branch points at the sides and the corner or apex at the top identify this letter visually, and no other letter in the alphabet has the same key points nor the same arrangement of them. The "springs" in the figure indicate that the key points can move around quite a bit without changing their usefulness for identification, as long as their relative positions remain in the same topological order. Extracting these key points and their arrangement provides a very robust identifier of the letter, which is quite insensitive to size and font. Some OCR (optical character recognition) programs that convert printed text to computer-readable files use similar methods.

Key points such as branches and ends can be obtained directly from the skeleton, as shown in Chapter 7. Corners can be isolated in several ways. **Figure 35** shows one, in which convolution with a simple 3×3 kernel can select a corner in any specified orientation. A more general corner-finding method traverses the skeleton or outline of the feature using chain code, introduced in Chapter 7. A sequence of links in the chain that gives a net 90-degree (or more) change in direction within a certain (arbitrary) distance along the chain is interpreted as a corner. Fitting functions — polynomials or splines — to the edge points can also be used to locate corners.

Figure 36 shows another example of letters A through E, in several fonts, with the key identifying points of each (ends, branches, and corners). There is actually more information than needed to uniquely identify each character; some of the points can be missing (e.g., due to extreme alterations in letter shape in handwritten characters) without compromising readability. Similar schemes are used in some of the efforts to develop computer programs that read handwriting. Syntactical characterization of the shape and density patterns in human chromosomes is routinely used in karyotyping.

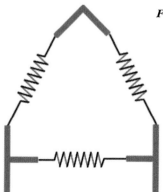

Figure 34. The important branch and corner points that identify the letter A. The springs that connect them indicate that shifting their positions, as long as their relative order remains the same, does not interfere with the identification.

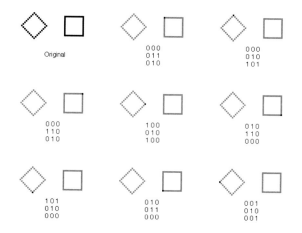

Figure 35. *Extracting corner points from a skeleton or outline by using a 3 × 3 convolution kernel. In general, any pattern can be found by applying a kernel that has the same shape as the desired pattern.*

Original

```
0 0 0
0 1 1
0 1 0
```

```
0 0 0
0 1 0
1 0 1
```

```
0 0 0
1 1 0
0 1 0
```

```
1 0 0
0 1 0
1 0 0
```

```
0 1 0
1 1 0
0 0 0
```

```
1 0 1
0 1 0
0 0 0
```

```
0 1 0
0 1 1
0 0 0
```

```
0 0 1
0 1 0
0 0 1
```

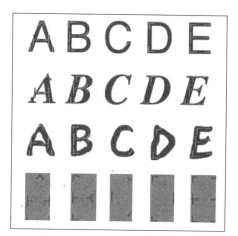

Figure 36. *The letters A through E with their key branches, corners, and end points.*

3D Image Acquisition

Volume imaging versus sections

Studying the three-dimensional (3D) structures of solid objects is often a goal of imaging. Many of the two-dimensional (2D) images used in the preceding chapters have been sections through three-dimensional structures. This is especially true in the various types of microscopy, where either polished flat planes or cut thin sections are needed in order to form the images in the first place. But the specimens thus sampled are three-dimensional, and the goal of the microscopist is to understand the three-dimensional structure.

There are quantitative tools of great power and utility that can interpret measurements on 2D images in ways that characterize 3D structures. As summarized in Chapter 8, these enable the measurement of volume fraction of phases, surface area of interfaces, mean thickness of membranes, and even the size distribution of spherical particles seen only in a random section. But there are many aspects of structure, both quantitative and qualitative, that are not accessible from 2D section images. Topological properties comprise a major category of such information, including such "simple" properties as the number of separate objects in a volume. Features visible in a single two-dimensional section do not reveal the actual three-dimensional structure present, as shown in **Figure 1**. In Chapter 8, a method was shown for unfolding the distribution of circles to determine the size distribution and total number of spheres in a sample, although this procedure requires making a critical assumption that the objects are all spheres. If the shape of features is unknown, can vary, or is a function of size, then this method fails.

Furthermore, as valuable as numerical measurement data may be, they cannot provide the typical viewer with a real sense of the structure. As pointed out in the first chapter, we are overwhelmingly visual creatures — we need to *see* the 3D structure. Furthermore, our world is 3D. We are accustomed to looking at external surfaces, or occasionally through transparent media, not at thin sections or polished cut surfaces. Try to imagine (again the need to resort to a word with its connotation of vision) standing by a busy street in which an imaginary plane exists transverse to traffic flow, and that you can see that plane but nothing else. What do cars and people look like as they pass through that plane?

If you have a well-developed geometric sense, or experience as a radiologist or draftsman, you may be able to accurately visualize the appearance of that plane as portions of torsos, engine

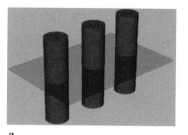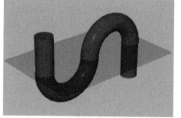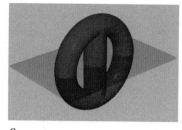

a   b   c

Figure 1. Examples of sections through three different structures that produce the same 2D sections:
(a) three discrete objects;
(b) one object with simple connectivity;
(c) one object with multiple connectivity.

blocks, even simple shapes such as tires, are cut by the plane. Most people will have difficulty imagining such collections of sections, and when asked to sketch the sections of even simple shapes will produce wildly inaccurate results.

If you doubt this, give yourself a simple test. Get some Cheerios®, or rotini noodles, or some other simple food object that has a well defined shape (**Figure 2**). Then mix up an opaque matrix (fudge is good) and stir in the objects. While it is hardening, try to draw what various representative random slices through the structure might look like. After it has hardened, cut slices through the sample and compare the actual results to your sketches. My experience with students is that they have a strong tendency to imagine sections through the object that are parallel to principal axes, and ones that pass through the geometrical center of the objects. For the Cheerios (little torii), few actual sections consist of two side-by-side circles or one annulus, and are not necessarily even convex (**Figure 3**). For the rotini, most people do not realize that sections through the curved surfaces actually produce straight lines.

As difficult as this particular visualization task may be, even fewer people can make the transition in the opposite direction: given a collection of section data, to reconstruct in the mind a correct representation of the 3D structure. This is true even of those who feel quite comfortable with the 2D images themselves. Within the world of the 2D images, recognition and understanding can be learned as a separate knowledge base that need not relate to the 3D world. Observing the

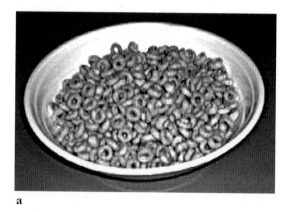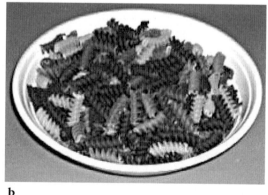

a   b

Figure 2. *Food objects (Cheerios® and rotini noodles) that are useful for experimenting with the relationship between 3D shapes and 2D section images. These are somewhat simpler and much more consistent than many natural structures we would like to understand.*

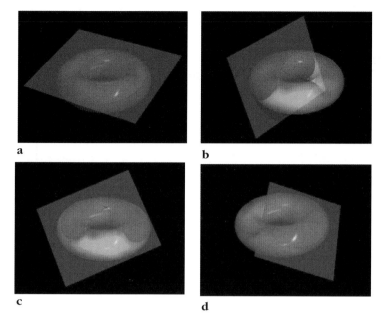

Figure 3. *A few sections through a torus, producing one or two intersections that may be either convex or concave.*

a

b

c

d

characteristic appearance of dendrites in polished metal samples, or that of mitochondria in thin electron microscope sections of cells, or internal organs in medical images (especially because these latter images are almost always oriented in transaxial, coronal, or sagittal views), does not necessarily mean that the complex 3D shapes of these objects become familiar. In fact, these examples are good illustrations of erroneous 3D interpretations that have persistently been made from 2D section images.

Because of this difficulty in using 2D images to study 3D structure, there is interest in 3D imaging. It may be performed directly, as discussed in this chapter, by actually collecting a 3D set of information all at once, or indirectly by gathering a sequence of 2D (slice) images and then combining them, as discussed in the next chapter. There are a variety of ways to acquire 2D images to assemble the data needed for 3D imaging, and also a great variety of ways to present the information to the user. Many of each are discussed in Chapter 12. The large number of approaches suggests that no one way is best, either for most viewers or for most applications.

Any method that reconstructs internal structural information within an object by mathematically reconstructing it from a series of projections is generally referred to as tomography. It may be used to obtain true 3D arrays of voxels (the 3D analog of the pixel in a 2D image), or to obtain a 2D image from a series of one-dimensional (1D) line projections. The latter method is used in most medical imaging, which is by far the most common application of CT (computed tomography) at the present time, although, the same basic techniques are used for 3D imaging and for other imaging signals.

Medical tomography primarily uses x-ray absorption, magnetic resonance imaging (MRI), positron-emission tomography (PET), and sound waves (ultrasound). Other fields of application and research use many different frequencies of electromagnetic radiation, from x- and gamma rays (nm wavelengths), through visible light and even microwave radiation (wavelengths from cm up). Besides photons, tomography is regularly performed using electrons and neutrons. In addition to absorption of the particles or radiation, tomography can be based on the scattering or emission of radiation as well. Tomography of mixing fluids can sometimes be performed by measuring the electrical resistance or impedance between multiple points around the containment vessel (Mann et al., 2001; York, 2001).

Sound waves produced by small intentional explosions or by "ground thumpers" are used to image underground strata for prospecting, while naturally occurring noise sources such as earthquakes are used to perform seismic tomography, imaging underground faults, rock density beneath volcanoes, and locating discontinuities between the mantle and core of the earth. Devices are also used for listening to moon- and mars-quakes, which will reveal their internal structure, and active studies of the seismic structure of the sun.

Basics of reconstruction

X-ray absorption tomography is one of the oldest, most widely used methods and will be used here to illustrate the various parameters, artefacts, and performance possibilities. Images produced by computerized axial tomography (CAT scans) and similar methods using magnetic resonance, sound waves, isotope emission, x-ray scattering or electron beams, deserve special attention. They are formed by computer processing of information from many individual pieces of projection information obtained nondestructively through the body of an object, which must be unfolded to see the internal structure. The mathematical description of the process presented here is that of x-ray absorption tomography, as it is used both in medical applications and in industrial testing (Herman, 1980; Kak and Slaney, 1988, 2001; Natterer, 2001; Natterer and Wubbeling, 2001). Similar sets of equations and methods of solution apply to the other signal modalities.

Absorption tomography is based on physical processes that reduce intensity as radiation or particles pass through the sample in straight lines. In some other kinds of tomography, the paths are not straight and the reconstruction takes place along curved lines (e.g., magnetic resonance imaging and x-ray scattering tomography), or even along many lines at once (seismic tomography). This makes the equations and graphics slightly more confusing, but does not affect the basic principles involved.

X-rays pass through material but are absorbed along the way according to the composition and density which they encounter. The intensity (number of photons per second) is reduced according to a linear attenuation coefficient μ, which for an interesting specimen is not uniform but has some spatial variation so that we can write $\mu(x,y,z)$, or for a 2D plane through the object, $\mu(x,y)$. The linear attenuation coefficient is the product of the density and the mass absorption coefficient, which depends on the local elemental composition. In medical tomography, the composition varies only slightly, and density variations are primarily responsible for producing images. For industrial applications, significant variations in composition are also usually present. The measured intensity along a straight line path through this distribution is given by

$$\int \mu(x,y)\,dS = \log_e \frac{I_o}{I_d} \qquad (1)$$

where I_o is the incident intensity (from an x-ray tube or radioisotope) that is known and generally held constant, and I_d is the detected intensity. This is called the ray integral equation and describes the result along one projection through the object.

If a series of parallel lines are measured, either one at a time by scanning the source and detector, or all at once using many detectors, a profile of intensity is obtained, which is called a view. As shown schematically in **Figure 4**, this function is usually plotted as the inverse of the intensity, or the summation of absorption along each of the lines. The function is written as $P(\phi,t)$ to indicate that it varies with position along the direction t as rays sample different portions of the object, and also with angle ϕ as the mechanism is rotated around the object to view it from different directions (or equivalently as the object is rotated).

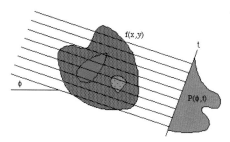

Figure 4. Illustration of a set of projections through an object at a viewing angle φ forming the function P.

Each of the views is a one-dimensional profile of measured attenuation as a function of position, corresponding to a particular angle. The collection of many such views can be presented as a 2D plot or image in which one axis is position *t* and the other is angle φ. This image is called a sinogram or the Radon transform of the 2D slice. **Figures 5** and **6** show a simple example. The construction of a planar figure as shown in **Figure 5a** is called a phantom, and is used to evaluate the important variables and different methods for reconstructing the object slice from the projection information. Such phantoms typically mimic the important structures of real interest, as an aid to evaluating reconstruction algorithms. Compare it to **Figure 5b** showing an actual MRI image of a brain tumor.

The individual projection profiles shown in **Figure 6** show some variation as the angle is changed, but this presentation is difficult to interpret. The sinogram in **Figure 6b** organizes the data so that it can be examined more readily. The name sinogram comes from the sinusoidal variation of position of projections through the various structures within the phantom as a function of rotation, which is evident in the example. The name Radon transform acknowledges the fact that the principles of this method of imaging were published in 1917 by Radon. However, the equations he presented did not provide a practical way to implement a reconstruction since they required a continuous array of projections, and it was not until Hounsfield and Cormack developed a practical reconstruction algorithm and hardware that CAT scans became a routine medical possibility. A. M. Cormack developed a mathematically manageable reconstruction method at Tufts University (Medford, MA) during 1963–1964, and G. N. Hounsfield designed a working instrument at EMI, Ltd. in England in 1972. They shared the Nobel prize in 1979.

The Fourier transform of the set of projection data in one view direction can be written as

$$S(\phi,\varpi)=\int P(\phi,t)\,e^{-j2\bar{s}\varpi t}dt \tag{2}$$

Figure 5. A phantom (test object with geometrical shapes of known density) and a real magnetic resonance image of a tumor (bright area) in a section through a head.

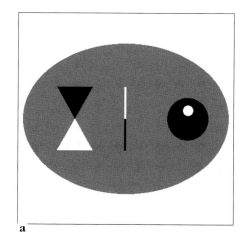

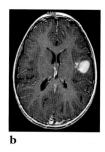

b

a

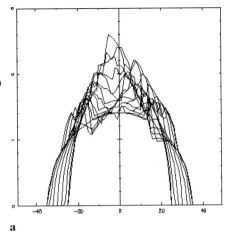
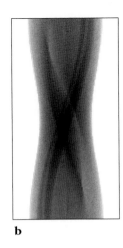

Figure 6. Sixteen attenuation profiles for the phantom in *Figure 5* *(a)* and the sinogram or Radon transform *(b)* produced by plotting 180 such profiles (each as one horizontal line).

a   b

Radon showed that this could also be written as

$$S(\phi,\varpi)=\iint f(x,y)e^{-j2\bar{s}\varpi(x\cos\phi+y\sin\phi)}dxdy \qquad (3)$$

which is simply the 2D Fourier transform $F(u,v)$ for the function $f(x,y)$ with the constraints that $u = \varpi \cos \phi$ and $v = \varpi \sin \phi$. This is consequently the equation of the line for the projection.

What this relationship means is that starting with the original image of the phantom, forming its two-dimensional Fourier transform as discussed in Chapter 5, and then looking at the information in that image along a radial direction from the origin normal to the direction ϕ would give the function S, which is just the 1D Fourier transform of the projection data in direction ϕ in real space. The way this can be used in practice is to measure the projections P in many directions, calculate the one-dimensional transforms S, plot the complex coefficients of S into a 2D transform image in the corresponding direction, and after enough directions have been measured, perform an inverse 2D Fourier transform to recover the spatial domain image for the slice. This permits a reconstruction of the slice image from the projection data, so that a non-destructive internal image can be obtained. It is the principle behind tomographic imaging.

Figure 7 shows an example. Eight views or sets of projections are taken at equal angle steps, the Fourier transform of each is calculated and plotted into a 2D complex image, which is then reconstructed. The image quality is only fair, because of the limited number of views. When 180 views at one-degree intervals are used, the result is quite good. The artefacts which are still present arise because of the gaps in the frequency space image. This missing information is especially evident at high frequencies (far from the origin) where the lines from the individual views become more widely spaced. All tomographic reconstruction procedures are sensitive to the number of views, as we will see.

By collecting enough views and performing this Fourier space reconstruction, it is possible to perform real tomographic imaging. In practice, few systems actually work this way. An exactly equivalent procedure that requires less computation is also available, known as filtered backprojection. This is the method used in most medical scanners and some industrial applications.

The principle behind backprojection is simple to demonstrate. The attenuation plotted in each projection in a view is due to the structure of the sample along the individual lines, or ray integrals. It is not possible to know from one projection just where along the line the attenuation occurs, but it is possible to evenly distribute the measured attenuation along the line. If this is done for only

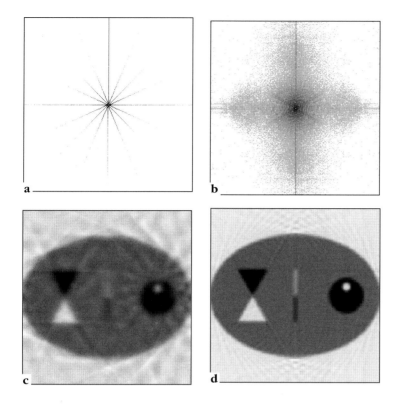

Figure 7. Reconstruction in frequency space. The (complex) 1D Fourier transforms of projection sets or views at different angles are plotted into a 2D frequency domain image, which is then reconstructed:
(a) *8 views in frequency space;*
(b) *180 views in frequency space;*
(c) *reconstruction from* ***a;***
(d) *reconstruction from* ***b***.

a single view, the result is not very interesting. If it is done along projections from several views, however, the superposition of the density or attenuation values should correspond to the features present in the structure.

Figure 8 illustrates this result for the same phantom. It is possible to see the dense (dark) cylinder with its hollow (light) core in the projections. Data from several views overlap to delineate the cylinder in the reconstructed image. There is a problem with this result, however. The attenuation or density of uniform regions in the original phantom is not constant, but increases toward the center of the section. Also, edges are blurred.

The cause of this problem can be described in several different but equivalent ways. The projections from all of the views contribute too much to the center of the image, where all projections overlap. The effect is the same as if the image was viewed through an out-of-focus optical system whose blur or point spread function is proportional to $1/r$, where r is the frequency, or the distance from the center of the frequency transform.

We saw in Chapter 5 how to remove a known blur from an image: apply an inverse function to the frequency space transform that attenuates low frequencies before retransforming. Based on the Fourier approach, and writing the reverse transformation in terms of polar coordinates, this gives

$$f(x,y) = \int\limits_{0^-}^{\bar{s}} \int S(\phi,\varpi)\,|\varpi|\,e^{j2\bar{s}\varpi t}\,d\varpi d\phi \tag{4}$$

or, in terms of x and y,

$$f(x,y) = \int\limits_{0}^{\pi} Q_\phi(x\cos\phi + y\sin\phi)\,d\phi \tag{5}$$

Figure 8. Back projection in the spatial domain. The attenuation values in each view are projected back through the object space along each projection line. Adding together the data from many view directions does show the major features, but the image is blurred:
(a) *1 view;*
(b) *6 views;*
(c) *30 views;*
(d) *180 views.*

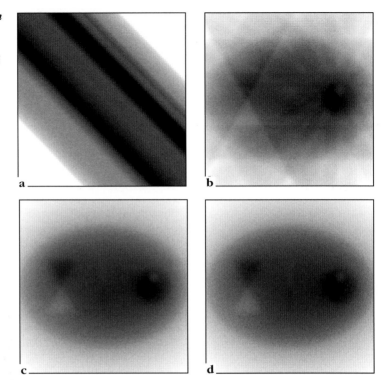

where

$$Q_\phi = \int\limits_{-}^{+} S(\phi,\varpi)|\varpi|e^{j2\bar{s}\varpi t}d\varpi \tag{6}$$

This is just the convolution of S, the Fourier transform of the projection, by $|\omega|$ the absolute value of frequency. In frequency space, this is an ideal inverse filter which is shaped as shown in **Figure 9**. But, as was pointed out in Chapter 5, convolutions can also be applied in the spatial domain. The inverse transform of this ideal filter is also shown in **Figure 9**. Note its similarity to the shape of a Laplacian or difference of Gaussians as discussed in Chapter 4.

As a 1D kernel or set of weights, this function can be multiplied by the projection P just as kernels were applied to 2D images in Chapters 3 and 4. The weights are multiplied by the values, and the sum is saved as one point in the filtered projection. This is repeated for each line in the projection set or view. **Figure 10** shows the result for the projection data, presented in the form of a sinogram. Edges (high frequencies) are strongly enhanced, and low-frequency information is suppressed.

The filtered data are then projected back, and the blurring is corrected as shown in **Figure 11**. Filtered backprojection using an ideal or inverse filter produces results identical to the inverse Fourier transform method described previously. The practical implementation of filtered back projection is easier because the projection data from each view can be filtered by convolution (a 1D operation) and the data spread back across the image as it is acquired, with no need to store the complex (i.e., real and imaginary values) frequency space image needed for the Fourier method, or retransforming it afterward.

Notice in **Figure 11** that the quality of the image, and the effect of number of views on the artefacts, is identical to that shown for the frequency space method in **Figure 7**. In the absence of noise in the data and other effects which will be discussed in the next section, these two methods are exactly equivalent.

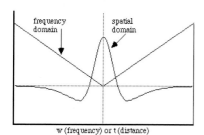

w (frequency) or t (distance)

Figure 9. *An ideal inverse filter, which selectively removes low frequencies, and its spatial domain equivalent kernel.*

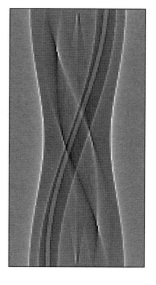

Figure 10. *The filtered projection data from* **Figure 6***, shown as a sinogram.*

Algebraic reconstruction methods

The problem of solving for the density (actually, for the linear attenuation coefficient) of each location in the image can also be viewed as a set of simultaneous equations. Each ray integral (or summation, in the finite case we are dealing with here) provides one equation. The sum of the attenuation coefficients for the pixels (or voxels) along the ray, each multiplied by a weighting factor that takes into account the actual path length of that ray through the pixel, is equal to the measured absorption. **Figure 12** illustrates the relationship between the pixels and the ray integral equations.

The number of unknowns in this set of equations is the number of pixels in the image of the slice through the specimen. The number of equations is the number of ray integrals, which is generally the number of detectors used along each projection profile times the number of view angles. This is a very large number of equations, but fortunately many of the weights are zero (most pixels are not involved in any one particular ray integral equation). Furthermore, the number of equations rarely equals the number of unknowns. But fortunately there are a number of practical and well tested computer methods for solving such sets of sparse equations when they are under- or overdetermined.

It is not our purpose here to compare the various solution methods. A suitable understanding of the method can be attained using the simplest of the methods, known as the algebraic reconstruction technique or ART (Gordon, 1974). In this approach, the equations are solved iteratively. The set of equations can be written as

$$A^{m \bullet n} x^n = b^m \tag{7}$$

Figure 11. Filtered back projection. The method is the same as in Figure 8, except that the values for each view have been filtered by convolution with the function in Figure 9:

(a) 1 view;
(b) 2 views;
(c) 4 views;
(d) 8 views;
(e) 16 views;
(f) 32 views;
(g) 180 views.

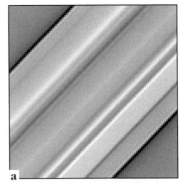

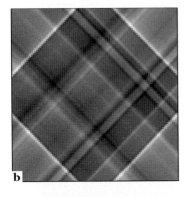
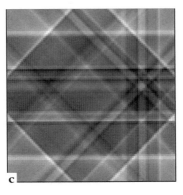
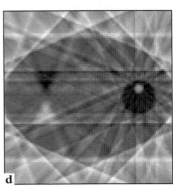

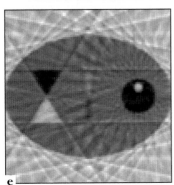
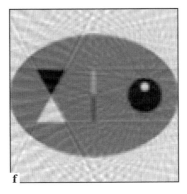
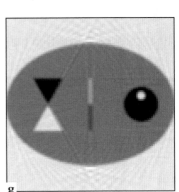

where n is the number of voxels, m is the number of projections, and **A** is the matrix of weights that correspond to the contribution of each voxel to each ray path. The voxel values are the **x** values and the projection measurements are the **b** values. The classic ART method calculates each iterative set of **x** values from the preceding ones as

$$\mathbf{x}^{k+1} = \mathbf{x}^k + A_i (b_i - A_i^\lambda \mathbf{x}^k) \| A_i \|^2 \tag{8}$$

The value of λ, the relaxation coefficient, generally lies between 0 and 2, and controls the speed of convergence. When λ is very small, this becomes equivalent to a conventional least squares solution. Practical considerations, including the order in which the various equations are applied, are dealt with in detail in the literature (Censor, 1983, 1984).

Figure 13 shows a simple example of this approach. The 16×16 array of voxels has been given density values from 0 to 20 as shown in **Figure 13b**, and three projection sets at view angles of

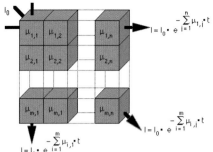

$$I = I_0 \cdot e^{-\sum_{i=1}^{n} \mu_{1,i} \cdot t}$$

$$I = I_0 \cdot e^{-\sum_{i=1}^{m} \mu_{i,i} \cdot t}$$

$$I = I_0 \cdot e^{-\sum_{i=1}^{m} \mu_{i,1} \cdot t}$$

Figure 12. *Schematic drawing of pixels (or voxels, because they have depth) in a plane section of the specimen, and the ray integral equations which sum up the attenuation.*

Figure 13. *Example of the application of an iterative solution. Three projection sets were calculated for an array of 25 detectors, with view directions of 0°, 90°, and 180° **(a)** The simulated specimen **(b)** contains a 16 × 16 array of voxels. The calculation results after **(c)** one, **(d)** five, and **(e)** 50 iterations are shown.*

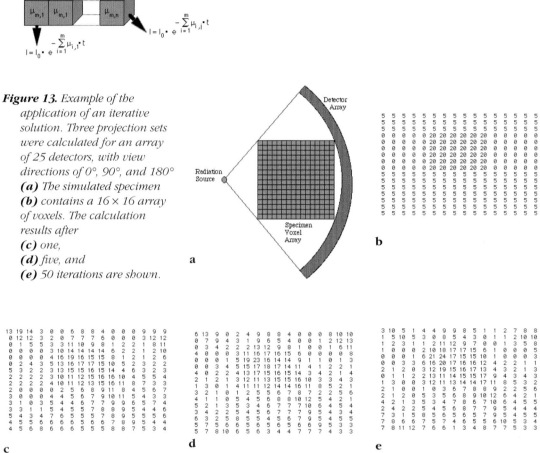

0°, 90°, and 180° calculated for the fan beam geometry shown in **Figure 13a**. For an array of 25 detectors, this gives a total of 75 equations in 256 unknowns. Starting with an initial guess of uniform voxels (with density 10), the results after one, five and fifty iterations are shown. The void areas and internal square appear rather quickly, and the definition of boundaries gradually improves. The errors, particularly in the corners of the image where fewer ray equations contain any information, and at the corners of the internal dense square, where the attenuation value changes abruptly, are evident. Still, considering the extent to which the system is underdetermined, the results are rather good.

Kacmarz' method for this solution is illustrated in **Figure 14**, for the very modest case of three equations and two unknowns, and λ = 1. Beginning at some initial guess, for instance that all of the pixels have the same attenuation value, one of the equations is applied. This is equivalent to moving perpendicular to the line representing the equation. This new point is then used as a starting point to apply the next equation, and so on. In the real case the equations do not all meet in a perfect point. Because of finite precision in the various measurements, counting statistics,

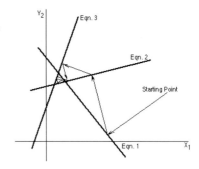

Figure 14. *Schematic diagram of Kacmarz' method for iteratively solving a set of equations, shown here for the case of two unknowns.*

machine variation, etc. there is no single point that represents a stable answer. Instead, the solution converges toward a region that is mostly within the region between the various lines, and then oscillates there. In a high-dimensionality space with some noisy equations, however, it is possible for the solution to leave this region and wander away after many iterations.

In real cases with many dimensions, the convergence may not be very fast. The greatest difficulty in using the iterative algebraic technique is deciding when to stop. Logically, we would like to continue until the answer is as good as it can get, but without knowing the "truth" this stopping point is not possible to judge exactly. Some methods examine the change in the calculated image after each iteration and attempt to judge from that when to stop (for instance, when the normalized total variation in pixel values falls below some arbitrary limit, or when it increases from the previous iteration). This method is prone to serious errors in a few cases, but is used nonetheless. It should be noted that the penalty for continuing the iteration is not simply the computational cost, but also the possibility that for some sets of data, the answer may start to diverge (leave the bounded region near the crossover point). This condition is, of course, highly undesirable.

Given the drawbacks to the algebraic approach, and the relative simplicity and straightforward approach of the filtered back projection method, why would we use this method? There are several potential advantages of algebraic methods such as ART. First, the filtered back projection method, and the Fourier transform method which it embodies, require that the number of views be rather large, and that they be equally spaced so that frequency space is well filled with data. Missing angles, or entire sets of angles which may be unattainable due to physical limitations, present problems for filtered back projection and introduce significant artefacts. ART methods can still produce an acceptable reconstruction. There may still be lack of detail in portions of the reconstructed image which are undersampled by the projections, but the artefacts do not spread throughout the entire image. In fact, acceptable reconstructions are often obtained with only a very few views (examples are shown in the following).

Another advantage to ART is the ability to apply constraints. For instance, it is possible in a filtered back projection or Fourier transform method to calculate negative values of density (attenuation) for some voxels, because of the finite measurement precision. Such values have no physical meaning. In the iterative algebraic method, any such values can be restricted to zero. In the schematic diagram of **Figure 14**, this amounts to restricting the solution to the quadrant of the graph with positive values.

In fact, any other prior knowledge can also be applied. If it is known that the only possible values of density and attenuation in the specimen correspond to specific materials, then the values can be easily constrained to correspond. Any geometric information, such as the outside dimensions of the object, can also be included (in this case, by forcing the voxels outside the object boundaries to zero).

It is even possible to set up a grid of voxels that are not all of the same size and spacing. This setup might allow, for instance, the use of a fine voxel spacing in the interior of an object where great detail is desired, but a much coarser grid outside (or vice versa). This would still allow the calculation of the contribution of the outside material to the ray integrals, but would reduce the number of unknowns to produce a better solution for any given number of views and projections. Sets of non-square pixels or non-cubic voxels can also be used when necessary to conform to specific object shapes and symmetries.

The flexibility of the algebraic method and its particular abilities to use *a priori* information often available in an industrial tomography setting compensates for its slowness and requirements for large amounts of computation. The calculation of voxel weights (the **A** matrix) can be tedious, especially for fan beam or other complex geometries, but no more so than backprojection in such cases, and it is a one-time calculation. The use of other solution methods than the simple iterative approach described here can provide improved stability and convergence.

Maximum entropy

There are other ways to solve these huge sets of sparse equations. One is the so-called maximum entropy approach. Maximum entropy was mentioned as an image processing tool to remove noise from a 2D image, in Chapter 3. Bayes' theorem is the cornerstone for the maximum entropy approach, given that we have relevant prior information which can be used as constraints. In the case where no prior information is available but noise is a dominant factor, Bayes' theorem leads to the classical or "least squares" approximation method. It is the use of prior information that permits a different approach.

The philosophical justification for the maximum entropy approach comes from Bayesian statistics and information theory. It has also been derived from Gibbs' concept of statistical thermodynamics (Jaynes, 1967). For the nonspecialist, it can be described as follows: find the result (distribution of brightnesses in pixels of image, distribution of density values in a voxel array, or practically anything else) that is feasible (consistent with the known constraints, such as the total number of photons, the non-negativity of brightness or density at any point, the physics involved in the detector or measurement process, etc.) and has the configuration of values which is most probable.

This probability is defined as being able to be formed in the most ways. For an image formed by photons, all photons are considered indistinguishable, and the order in which they arrive is unimportant, so the distribution of photons to the various pixels can be carried out in many ways. For some brightness patterns (images) the number of ways to form the pattern is much greater than others. We say that these images with greater multiplicity have a higher entropy. Nature can form them in more ways, so they are more likely. The entropy is defined as $S = - p_i \log p_i$, where p_i is the fraction of pixels with brightness value i.

The most likely image (from a simple statistical point of view) is for all of the pixels to get the same average number of photons, producing a uniform grey scene; however, this result may not be permitted by our constraints, one of which is the measured brightness pattern actually recorded. The difference between the calculated scene and the measured one can only be allowed to have a set upper limit, usually based on the estimated noise characteristics of the detector, the number of photons, etc. Finding the feasible scene which has the highest multiplicity is the maximum entropy method.

For instance, in solving for the tomographic reconstruction of an object from the set of ray integral equations obtained from various view angles, we have a large set of simultaneous equations in many unknowns. Instead of formally solving the set of simultaneous equations, for instance by a traditional Gauss–Jordan elimination scheme which would take far too many steps to be practical, the maximum entropy approach recasts the problem. Start with any initial guess (in most "well-behaved" cases, the quality of that guess matters little in the end result) and then iteratively, starting at that point, find another solution (within the class of feasible solutions as defined by the constraints) that has a higher entropy. Deciding which way to move in the space defined by the parameters (the values of all the voxels) is usually done with LaGrange multipliers by taking partial derivatives and trying always to move "uphill" where the objective function used to evaluate each set of values is the entropy.

It is usually found that the solution having the maximum feasible entropy (i.e., permitted by the constraints) is hard against the boundary formed by those constraints, and if they were relaxed the solution would move higher (towards a more uniform image). Knowing or assuming that the solution lies along the constraint boundaries allows use of more efficient schemes for finding the best solution. For the noise removal problem discussed in Chapter 3, the constraint is commonly the chi-squared value of the smoothed image as compared to the measured one. This is generally assumed to be due to classical noise, and so should have an upper limit and a known distribution.

For tomographic reconstruction, the constraints are based on satisfying the ray integral equations. These are not all consistent, so a weighting scheme must be imposed on the error; linear weighting is the simplest and most often used. It turns out that in most cases, the cluster of solutions with high entropies, all permitted by the constraints, are virtually indistinguishable. In other words, the maximum entropy method does lead to a useful and robust solution. While the solution is still iterative, the method is quite efficient as compared to other solution techniques.

Defects in reconstructed images

The reconstructed example shown above in **Figures 7** and **11** was calculated using projection data simulated by computation, with no noise or any other defects. In real tomography, a variety of defects may be present in the projection sets that propagate errors back into the reconstructed image. Using the same phantom, several of the more common ones can be demonstrated.

Ideally, a large number of view angles and enough detector positions along each projection set will be used to provide enough information for the reconstruction. In the event that fewer projections in a set or fewer views are used, the image has more reconstruction artefacts and poorer resolution, definition of boundaries, and precision and uniformity of voxel values. **Figure 15** shows the effect of fewer projections in each set but still uses 180 view angles. The reconstructed images are displayed with 100×100 pixels. This ideally requires a number of ray integrals in each projection set equal to at least $\sqrt{2}$ times the width, or 141 equations for each view. With fewer, the resolution of the reconstruction degrades.

If fewer view angles are used (but the angular spacing is still uniform), the artefacts in the reconstruction increase as was shown above in **Figure 11.** If the view angles are not uniformly spaced, the results are much worse as shown in **Figure 16**.

In real images, the number of x-ray photons detected at each point in the projection set is subject to fluctuations due to counting statistics. In many cases, both in medical and industrial tomography, the number of photons is limited. In medical applications, it is important to limit the total exposure to the subject. In industrial applications, the limitation is due to the finite source strength of either the x-ray tube or radioisotope source, and the need to acquire as many views as possible within a reasonable time. In either case, the variation in the number of detected x-rays varies in a Gaussian or normal distribution whose standard deviation is the square root of the number counted. Counting an average of 100 x-rays produces a variation whose standard deviation is 10% ($\sqrt{100}$ = 10), while an average of 10,000 x-rays is needed to reduce the variation to 1% ($\sqrt{10^4} = 10^2$).

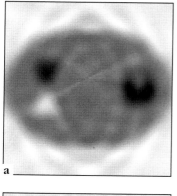

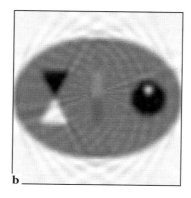

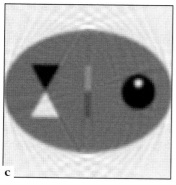

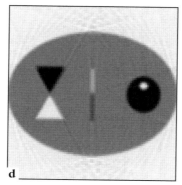

Figure 15. Effect of number of ray integrals in the projection set on reconstructed image quality. Each image is reconstructed with 100 × 100 pixels, and is calculated from 180 view angles. The images show the use of
(a) 25;
(b) 49;
(c) 75, and
(d) 99 ray projections, respectively.

Figure 16. Effect of using a set of view angles that do not uniformly fill the angular range:
(a) 150-degree coverage;
(b) 120-degree coverage;
(c) 90-degree coverage;
(d) a different 90-degree range.

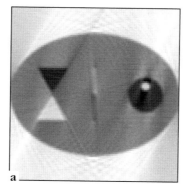

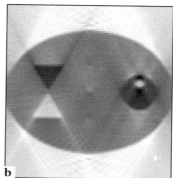

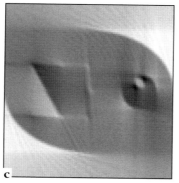

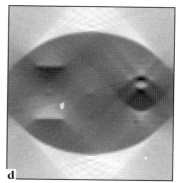

The process of reconstruction amplifies the effect of noise in the projections. This is the same effect of noise seen in Chapter 5 for removing blur by deconvolution, and arises from the same mathematical procedures. The filtering process suppresses the low frequencies and keeps the high frequencies, and the counting fluctuations vary randomly from point to point and so are represented in the highest frequency data. **Figure 17** shows the result. Adding a statistical or counting fluctuation of a few percent to the simulated projection data produces a much greater noise in the reconstructed image. Although the density differences in the three regions of the phantom vary by 100%, some of the regions disappear altogether when 10% or 20% noise is added to the projection data.

Suppression of the high-frequency noise in the projection data by the filtering process can reduce the effect of the noise somewhat, as shown in **Figure 18**. Notice that the noise variations in the reconstructed images are reduced, but that the high frequency data needed to produce sharp edges and reveal the smaller structures are gone as well.

Several different filter shapes are used for this purpose. **Figure 19** shows representative examples, in comparison to the shape of the ideal inverse filter that was discussed above. The plots are in terms of frequency. All of the filters reduce the low frequency values, which is required in order to prevent blurring, and all of the noise reduction filters also attenuate the high frequencies in order to suppress the noise.

Another important source of errors in the reconstruction of images is imprecise knowledge of the location of the center of rotation, or variation in that center due to imperfect mechanical mechanisms (Barnes et al., 1990). As shown in **Figure 20**, this variation also produces an effect in the reconstructed image which is magnified. The characteristic "U" shaped arcs result from an off-center rotation, because view angles in a range of 180° were used. If 360-degree rotation is used, a complete circular arc is present (**Figure 21**) that also distorts the reconstruction but is more difficult to recognize. Note that it is not common to collect data over a complete 360-degree set of

Figure 17. Effect of counting statistics on reconstruction. The images were reconstructed from simulated projection data to which Gaussian random fluctuations were added:
(a) 2%;
(b) 5%;
(c) 10%;
(d) 20%.

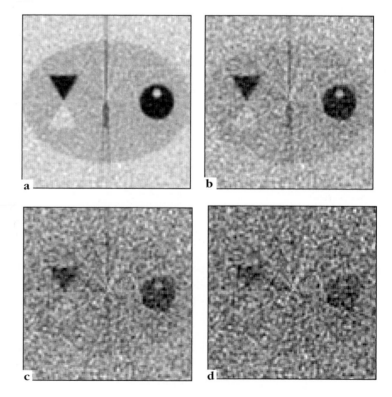

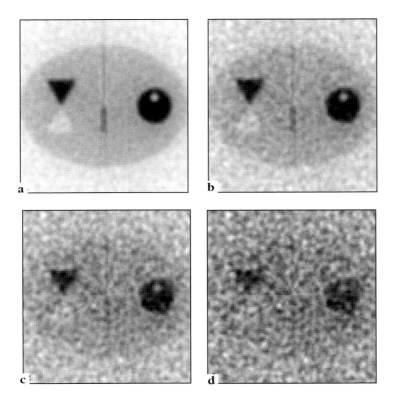

Figure 18. *Reconstructions from the same projection data with superimposed counting statistics variations as in **Figure 17**, but using a Hann filter instead of an ideal inverse filter to reduce the high-frequency noise.*

angles, because in the absence of off-center rotation or beam hardening (discussed below) the second half of the data would be redundant. The effect of a variable center is equal in magnitude with 360-degree rotation, but harder to recognize. In general, it is required that the location of the center of rotation and its constancy should be less than about one-tenth of the expected spatial resolution in the reconstructed images.

Similarly, the motion of the object should be restricted during the collection of the multiple views. In medical imaging, where the most common imaging geometry is to place the subject inside a circular track on which the source and/or detectors rotate, this means that the patient must not breathe during the scanning process. If the images are expected to show the heart, the entire collection of views must be obtained in a time much shorter than the single beat, or else some stroboscopic triggering scheme must be used to collect images at the same relative timing over many beats.

Figure 19. Filter profiles for noise reduction in filtered back projection:

Ideal inverse: Weight = $|f|$

Hann: Weight = $|f| \cdot \{0.5 + 0.5 \cos [(\pi/2) (f/fm)]\}$

Hamming: Weight = $|f| \cdot \{0.54 + 0.46 \cos (\pi f/fm)\}$

Butterworth (n = 3): Weight = $|f| \cdot 1/(1+(f/2fm)2n)$

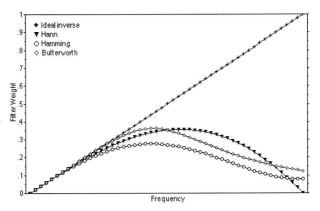

Figure 20. Effect of errors in the center of rotation on the reconstructed image. In each of these images, the center is consistent, but displaced from the location assumed in the rotation by a fraction of the image width:
(a) 0.5%;
(b) 1.0%,
(c) 2.5%;
(d) 5.0%

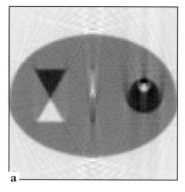

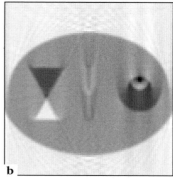

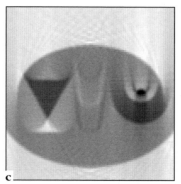

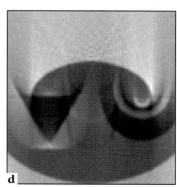

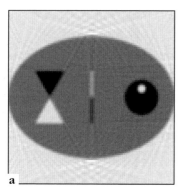

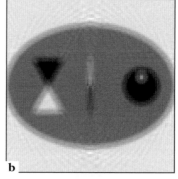

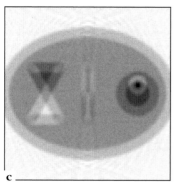

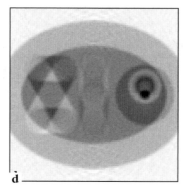

Figure 21. Repeating the reconstructions of Figure 20 using the same number of views (180) but spread over 360° instead of 180°, with the center of rotation displaced from the assumed location by a fraction of the image width:
(a) 0.5%;
(b) 1.0%;
(c) 2.5%;
(d) 5.0%

Beam hardening

Beam hardening is the name used to describe the effect in which the lower energy or "softer" x-rays from a polychromatic source such as a conventional x-ray tube are preferentially absorbed in a sample. The consequence is that the effective attenuation coefficient of a voxel is different depending on whether it is on the side of the specimen near the source or farther away. This variation along the path is indicated schematically in **Figure 22**. Beam hardening is not a major problem in medical tomography because the variation in composition of the various parts of the human body is only slight. Everything is mostly water with some addition of carbon, a trace of other elements, and for bones, some calcium. The density is variable, and is in fact what the reconstructed image shows, but the range of variation is small. This uniformity makes x-ray tubes an acceptable source, and simple back projection a suitable reconstruction method.

Industrial applications commonly encounter samples with a much greater variation in composition, ranging across the entire periodic table and with physical densities that vary from zero (voids) to more than ten times the density of biological tissue. This large range of variation makes beam hardening an important problem. One solution is to use a monochromatic source such as a radioisotope or a filtered x-ray tube. Another is to use two different energies (Schneberk et al., 1991) or a combination of absorption and x-ray scattering data (Prettyman et al., 1991) and to use the two projection sets to correct for the change in composition in the reconstruction process; however, this method increases the complexity significantly and requires an algebraic solution method rather than back projection or Fourier techniques.

Figure 23 shows a representative example of the beam hardening effect in the same phantom used previously. In this case, the sample composition is specified as void (the lightest region and the surroundings), titanium (the medium grey region of the elliptical object), and iron (the dark region). The total width is 1 cm, and the x-ray tube is assumed to be operating at 100 kV. This is in fact a very modest amount of beam hardening. A larger specimen, a lower tube voltage, higher atomic number elements, or a greater variation in atomic number of density, would produce a much greater effect.

Figure 24 shows reconstructions of the image using view angles which cover 180° and 360°, respectively. In most tomography, 180° is adequate since the projections are expected to be the same regardless of direction along a ray path. This assumption is not true in the case of beam hardening (as it was not for the case of off-center rotation), and so better results are obtained with a full 360° of data. Notice, however, that artefacts are still present. This is particularly true of the central feature, in which the narrow void is hardly visible. **Figure 25** shows the same phantom with no beam hardening, produced with a monochromatic x-ray source.

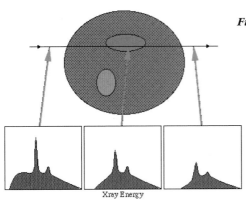

Figure 22. Schematic diagram of beam hardening. The energy spectrum of x-rays from an x-ray tube is shown at the beginning, middle, and end of the path through the specimen. As the lower energy x-rays are absorbed, the attenuation coefficient of the sample changes independent of any actual change in composition or density.

Figure 23. Example of beam hardening effect on the sinogram or Radon transform
(a) and the inverse filtered data
(b). Notice that the contrast of each feature changes according to where it lies within the rotated object.

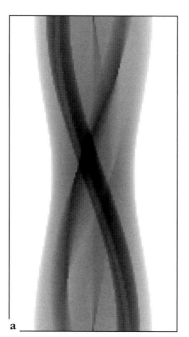

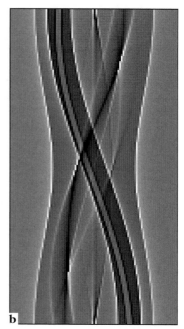

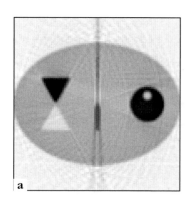

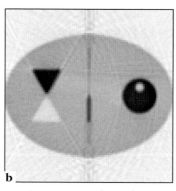

Figure 24. Reconstruction of the beam-hardened data from Figure 23:
(a) 180 views covering 180°;
(b) 180 views covering 360°.

When x-rays pass through material, the attenuation coefficient that reduces the transmitted intensity consists of two principal parts: the absorption of the x-rays by the excitation of a bound electron, and the scattering of the x-rays either coherently or incoherently into a different direction. In either case, the photons are lost from the direct ray path, and the measured intensity decreases. In the case of scattering, however, the x-rays may be redirected to another location in the detector array (see the discussion of the geometries of various generations of instrument designs, in the following paragraphs).

When this scattering takes place, the measured projection profiles contain additional background on which the attenuation data are superimposed. The presence of the background also produces artefacts in the reconstruction as shown in **Figure 26**. The effect is visually similar to that produced by beam hardening.

In addition, the uniform regions in the object are reconstructed with a variable density due to the background. **Figure 27** shows this reconstruction for a simple annular object (a crude model for a bone cross-section), and **Figure 28** shows plots across the center of the reconstructions. The deviation from a uniform density in the reconstruction is called cupping. Note that this example uses

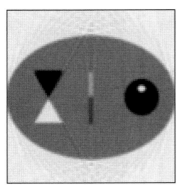

Figure 25. Reconstruction of the same phantom as Figure 23 but using a monochromatic 50 kV x-ray source. Notice particularly the void in the center of the object, which is not visible in Figure 24.

Figure 26. Reconstruction of the phantom in Figure 25 when the measured projection sets include scattered background radiation of
(a) 5;
(b) 10;
(c) 20; and
(d) 40% of the average intensity. The effect on the image is similar to beam hardening. Small features are obscured by artefacts, and the overall contrast changes.

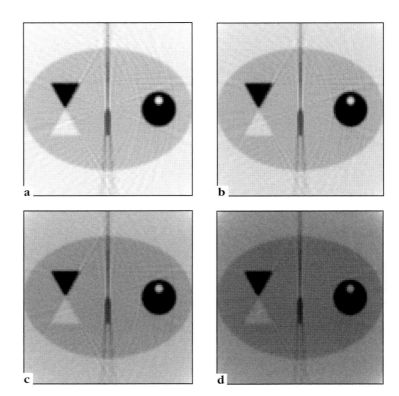

materials similar to those in the human body. Medical tomography is not usually required to produce a quantitatively accurate measure of density; however, it is used to show the location of internal structures and boundaries (this may not be true in all cases; for example radiography and computed tomography are used to measure bone density loss due to osteoporosis). Industrial tomography is often called upon to measure densities accurately so as to quantify gradients in parts due to processing, and this source of error is therefore of concern.

Although medical applications rarely need to measure densities exactly, they do require the ability to show small variations in density. A test phantom often used to demonstrate and evaluate performance in this category is the Shepp and Logan (1974) head phantom. Composed of ellipses with densities close to 1.0, it mimics in simplified form the human head, surrounded by a much denser skull, and containing regions very slightly lower or higher in density that model the brain structure and the presence of tumors. The ability to image these areas is critical to the detection of anomalies in real head scans.

Figure 27. *Reconstruction of a simple annulus with outer composition of calcium carbonate (an approximation to bone) and an inner composition of water (an approximation to tissue):* **(a)** *no scattered background;* **(b)** *10% scattered background in projection data.*

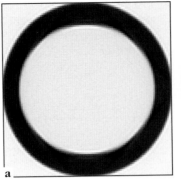 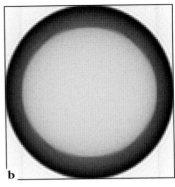

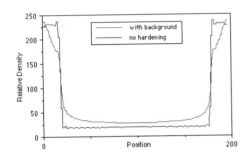

Figure 28. *Line profiles of the density in the images in* **Figure 27.**

Figure 29. *Shepp and Logan phantom, intended to represent the difficulty of visualizing a tumor inside the human head. The regions of varying density inside the "brain" range of relative densities of 1.0 to 1.04, while the "skull" has a density of 2.0. They are not visible in the reconstructed image* **(a)** *unless some contrast expansion is applied. Here, histogram equalization is used* **(b)** *to spread the grey scale nonlinearly to show the various ellipses and their overlaps (and also to increase the visibility of artefacts in the reconstruction). The brightness histograms* **(c, d)** *show the effect of the equalization.*

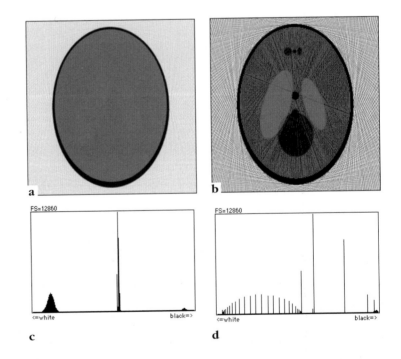

Figure 29 shows a reconstruction of this phantom. Using the full dynamic range of the display (values from 0 to 255) linearly to represent the image does not reveal the internal detail within the phantom. Applying histogram equalization (as discussed in Chapter 4) expands the contrast in the center of the histogram so that the different regions become visible. The figure shows the cumulative histograms of display brightness for the original and histogram-equalized images. In the former, the steps show the principal density values; after equalization the values approximate a straight line, and the steps show the distinction between similar regions. A profile plot across the center of the structure shows the different regions with quite uniform density values (**Figure 30**).

As noted previously, tomography can be performed using modalities other than x-ray absorption. One is emission tomography, in which a radioactive isotope is placed inside the object and then reveals its location by emitting gamma ray photons. Collimated detectors around the object can specify the lines along which the source of the photons lie, producing data functionally equivalent to the attenuation profiles of the conventional case.

Figure 31 shows an example of emission tomography using real data, in which another artefact is evident. The bright areas in the reconstruction are cavities within a machined part that contain a radioactive isotope. The sinogram shows the detected emission profiles as a function of view angle. Notice that the width of the regions varies with angle. This variation is due to the finite width of the collimators on the detectors, which cover a wider dimension on the far side of the object as indicated schematically in **Figure 32**. This effect is also present in x-ray absorption tomography, due to the finite size of apertures on the source and the detectors. If the angle of the collimators is known, this effect can be included in the reconstruction, either by progressively spreading the data as the filtered profile is spread back across the voxel array, or by adjusting the voxel weights in the algebraic reconstruction technique.

Figure 30. Brightness profiles across the images in Figure 29, showing the uniformity and sharpness of transitions for the regions, and the effect of histogram equalization.

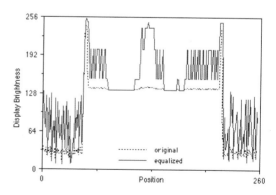

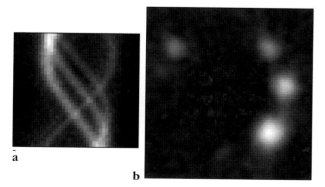

*Figure 31. Emission tomography. The sample is a block of aluminum containing several cylindrical cavities containing radioactive cobalt. The detector collects a series of intensity profiles as a function of rotation, shown in the form of a sinogram (**a**). Note that the width of the trace for each cylinder varies as the sample is rotated, due to the finite angle of the entrance collimator to the detector. The reconstruction of the cross-section is shown in (**b**).*

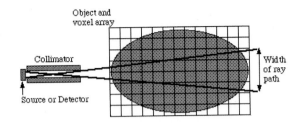

Figure 32. *Schematic diagram showing the effect of a finite collimator angle on the dimensions and voxels covered in different parts of the object.*

Imaging geometries

First-generation tomographic systems collected projection sets at a variety of view angles by moving a source and detector just as shown above in **Figure 3**. **Figure 33** shows the procedure used to collect a complete set of projection data. This is called a pencil-beam or parallel-beam geometry, in which each ray integral is parallel and the projection set can be directly backprojected. It is not very efficient, since only a small solid angle of the generated x-rays can be used, and only a single detector is in use, but is still used in a few industrial imaging situations where time of data acquisition is not a major concern.

Second-generation instruments added a set of detectors so that a fan beam of x-rays could be detected and attenuation measured along several lines at the same time, as shown in **Figure 34**. This procedure requires fewer view angles to collect the same amount of data, but the attenuation measurements from each detector are actually for different angles and there is some re-ordering of the data needed before it can be used.

The so-called fan-beam geometry is appealing in its efficiency, and the next logical step, in so-called third-generation instruments used for medical imaging, was to use a larger array of detectors (and to arrange them on an arc so that each covered the same solid angle and had normal x-ray incidence) and a single x-ray tube. The detectors and tube rotate together about the object as the x-ray tube is pulsed to produce the series of views (**Figure 35**). In fourth-generation systems, a complete ring of detectors is installed and only the source rotates (**Figure 36**). Notice that the x-rays are

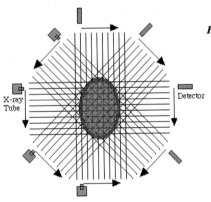

Figure 33. *First-generation geometry. The detector and source move together to collect each projection set, and rotate to many view angles to collect all of the required data.*

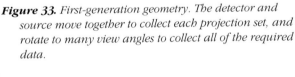

Figure 34. *Second-generation geometry. The detector array simultaneously measures attenuations in a fan beam, requiring fewer view angles than first generation systems to collect the data.*

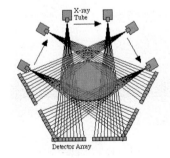

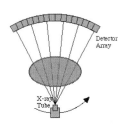

Figure 35. Third-generation geometry. The x-ray tube and detector array rotate together around the object being imaged, as the tube is rapidly pulsed to produce each view.

no longer normally incident on the detectors in this case. There is a fifth-generation design in which even less hardware motion is required: the x-rays are generated by magnetically deflecting an electron beam against a fixed target ring, rotating the source of x-rays to produce the same effective geometry as in fourth-generation systems, but with even shorter exposure times.

These latter types of geometry are less used in industrial tomography, since they are primarily intended for imaging speed, to minimize exposure and acquire all of the projections before anything can move in the person being imaged. First- or second-generation (pencil or fan beam) methods in which a series of discrete views are collected provide greater flexibility in dealing with industrial problems. All of the methods are equivalent, however, if the various ray integrals using individual detectors in the fan-beam geometry are sorted out according to angle, and either backprojected, used in a Fourier transform method, or used to calculate an algebraic reconstruction with appropriate weights.

Some imaging technologies use different geometries and reconstructions. For instance, ultrasound images, most familiarly used for examining a fetus in utero, are obtained as fan-beam sections, but can be reconstructed to show surfaces (**Figure 37**). Positron-emission tomography (PET), single-photon

Figure 36. Fourth-generation geometry. The detector array forms a complete ring and is fixed. The x-ray tube rotates around the object and is pulsed. Data from the detectors is sorted out to produce the projection sets.

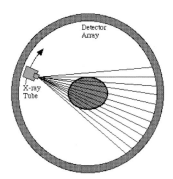

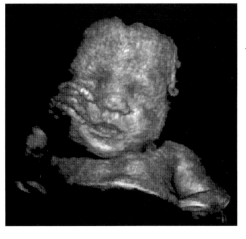

Figure 37. Surface reconstruction from ultrasound scans (image courtesy William Beaumont Hospital).

emission spectroscopy (SPECT), and magnetic resonance imaging (MRI) are similar in geometry to CT scans, but record different information about internal structure.

PET and SPECT localize specific atomic isotopes by their decay. In PET, the positron produced by the atomic nucleus gives rise to a pair of 511 keV photons that travel in exactly opposite directions. Detecting them with a ring of detectors locates the original isotope tag somewhere on the line between the two points, which becomes the line integral used in the reconstruction. SPECT detects gamma rays from isotope decay with collimated detectors. An array of detectors collects information from a parallel set of projections, and is scanned across and around the subject to collect multiple projections.

When protons are placed in a magnetic field, they oscillate (resonate — thus "magnetic resonance imaging" or MRI) at a frequency that depends on the field strength, and absorb energy at the oscillation frequency. This energy is reradiated as the protons return to their ground state. The reradiation involves processes (relaxation of the magnetization components parallel and perpendicular to the field) with different time constants T1 and T2. MRI signal strength depends on the proton concentration (essentially the water concentration in the tissue for medical imaging) but the contrast depends on T1 and T2, which are strongly influenced by the fluid viscosity or tissue rigidity. Weighting the combination of the two signals provides control over the observed image.

PET and MRI data can be very complementary to the density information from x-ray tomography, and in many cases scans using the different modalities are combined by overlaying the section images in registration (**Figure 38**).

Three-dimensional tomography

Although the most common application of tomography is still to form images of planar sections through objects without physical sectioning, the method can be directly extended to generate complete three-dimensional images. Chapter 10 shows several examples of 3D displays of volume data. Most of these, including many of the tomographic images, are actually serial section images.

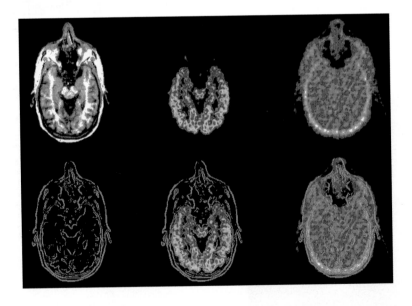

Figure 38. _Co-registration of PET and MRI scans (images courtesy K. A. Paller, Northwestern University)._

Whether formed by physical sectioning, optical sectioning (for instance, using the confocal light microscope), or conventional tomographic reconstruction, these methods are not true 3D data sets.

The distinction is that the pixels in each image plane are square, but as they are extended into the third dimension as voxels, they do not necessarily become cubes. The distance between the planes, or the depth resolution, is not inherently the same as the pixel size or resolution within the plane. In fact, few of these methods have depth resolution that is even close to the lateral resolution. Some techniques such as physical or optical sectioning have much poorer depth resolution. Others such as the secondary ion mass spectrometer have depth resolution that is far better than the lateral resolution of images. This has profound effects for 3D image presentation, for image processing, and especially for three-dimensional structural measurement.

True 3D imaging is possible with tomographic reconstruction. The object is represented by a three-dimensional array of cubic voxels, and the individual projection sets become two-dimensional arrays (projection images). Each projection is from a point, and is referred to as a cone-beam geometry (by analogy to the fan-beam method used for single slice projections). The set of view directions must include orientations that move out of the plane and into three dimensions, described by two polar angles. This does not necessarily require rotating the object with two different polar angles, since using a cone-beam imaging geometry provides different angles for the projection lines, just as a fan beam geometry does in two dimensions. The best reconstructions, however, are obtained with a series of view angles that cover the 3D orientations as uniformly as possible.

Several geometries are possible. One of the simplest is to rotate the sample about a single axis as shown in **Figure 39**. This method offers the advantage of precise rotation, since as seen before, the quality of the reconstruction depends on the consistency of the center of rotation. On the other hand, artefacts in the reconstructed voxels can be significant, especially in the direction parallel to the axis and near the north and south poles of the sample. The single-axis rotation method is most often used with x-ray, neutron, or gamma ray tomography because the samples may be rather large and are relatively equiaxed so that the distance that the radiation must pass through the sample is the same in each direction. Improved resolution in the axial direction can be obtained using a helical scan (Wang et al., 1991) in which the specimen rotates while moving in the axial direction (**Figure 40**). This has become the preferred geometry, particularly for small industrial objects.

For electron tomography, most samples are thin sections, and few transmission electron microscope stages permit complete movement of the sample about its axis. For a sample that is essentially

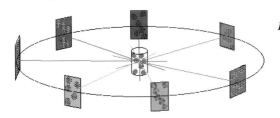

Figure 39. Geometry for volume imaging using radial projections obtained by rotating the sample about a single axis.

Figure 40. In helical scanning, the specimen is raised as it rotates so that multiple views measure absorption along different angles through the voxels.

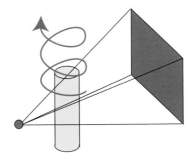

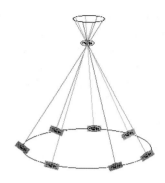

Figure 41. *Tilting the sample in a conical pattern produces a series of projections used for reconstruction in transmission electron microscopy. The spacing along the cone trace is generally not uniform.*

slab-like, the geometry that is usually adopted is a series of tilt angles that project along the limbs of a cone, as shown in **Figure 41**. Collecting these projections by controlling the tilt and rotation of the sample in its holder with enough precision to allow good reconstructions is very difficult. Some TEM samples consist of many repeating structures (macromolecules, virus particles, etc.), and a single orientation of the sample can collect enough different views to be used for reconstruction. Because of the use of many different individual objects with various orientations, this method is called random-conical, as compared with the use of equal angular increments. The very small aperture angle of the beam in the TEM produces essentially parallel rather than cone-beam projections, which does simplify the reconstruction and makes backprojection straightforward, but the use of a limited set of views arranged in a cone produces artefacts because little information is available in the axial direction (sometimes referred to as the missing cone of information). Frank (1992) presents a thorough review of the current state of the art in electron microscope tomography.

From a theoretical viewpoint, the best reconstruction for any given number of projections is obtained when they are uniformly distributed in 3D space (**Figure 42**). Constructing a mechanism to achieve accurate rotations about two precisely centered axes is difficult and this technique not widely used.

The reconstruction can be performed with any of the methods used in two dimensions. For Fourier inversion, the frequency space is also a 3D array, and the 2D images produced by each projection are transformed and the complex values plotted on planes in the array. As for the 2D case, filling the space as completely and uniformly as possible is desirable. The Fourier inversion is performed in three dimensions, but this is a direct extension of methods in lower dimensions and in fact the inversion can be performed in one dimension at a time (successively along rows in the u, v, and w directions).

Backprojection can also be used for 3D reconstruction, and as in the 2D case is simply an implementation of the Fourier transform mathematics. The filtering of the 2D images must be performed

Figure 42. *Optimum 3D reconstruction is possible when a series of 3D projections is used, by rotating the sample about two axes.*

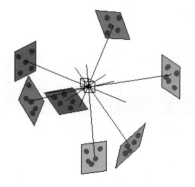

with a 2D convolution, which can be carried out either by kernel operation in the spatial domain or by multiplication in the Fourier domain. The principal difficulty with the backprojection method is that calculation of the matrix of weights can be quite tricky for cone-beam geometry, especially when combined with helical scanning. These values represent the attenuation path length along each of the ray integrals through each of the voxels. The use of backprojection requires a large number of views to avoid artefacts and is most commonly used with single-axis rotation or with helical scans about a single rotational axis, with either cone-beam or parallel-beam projections (Feldkamp et al., 1984; Smith, 1990; Shih et al., 2001). It is difficult to apply to a full 3D set of cone beams because they are spaced at relatively large angles.

Algebraic reconstruction technology (ART) methods are also applicable to voxel arrays. The difficulty in obtaining a uniform set of view angles, which is particularly the case for electron microscopy, can make ART methods more attractive than the inverse Fourier approach. In fact, when using an iterative technique such as ART, the best results are often obtained with a surprisingly small number of views. **Figures 43** and **44** show an example. The specimen (about 2 cm on a side) consists of three different metal cylinders in a plastic block. Chromium, manganese and iron are consecutive elements in the periodic table, with similar densities. Tomographic reconstruction from only 12 views with 3D rotations, using a low power industrial x-ray source, shows the inserts quite well (Ham, 1993).

Of course, more views should produce a better reconstruction. But in most tomography situations, the total dose is a fixed constraint. In some cases, this can be because of concerns about radiation

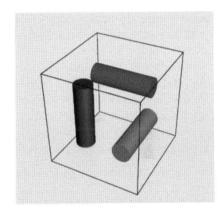

Figure 43. Geometry of a test sample. Three cylindrical inserts of different metals (Cr, Mn, and Fe) are placed in a plastic block (2 cm on a side).

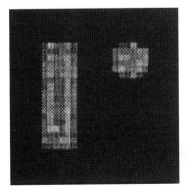 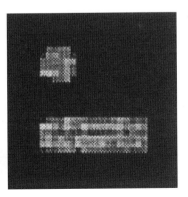 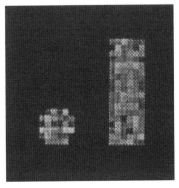

Figure 44. Tomographic reconstruction of three planes in the xy, yz, and zx orientations passing through the metal inserts in the plastic block shown in Figure 43, reconstructed using just 12 cone beam projections with rotations in 3D.

damage to the sample. Dosage to the sample is a concern for medical x-ray tomography, of course; but it also creates problems for electron tomography. The amount of energy deposited in each cubic nanometer of the sample from a focused electron beam is great enough to cook biological tissue, disrupt molecules, and change the structure we want to image.

Even for industrial tomography, the total flux of radiation that can be generated and the time spent acquiring the images usually is limited. A necessary trade-off must be made between the number of projections and the time spent acquiring each one. More time on each projection improves the statistical quality of the view image, so acquiring more projections makes each one noisier, and vice versa. In some experiments with a limited total photon budget, the best quality reconstructions with full 3D rotation were obtained with only 12 projections (Ham, 1993). This small number of views requires an iterative method rather than backprojection.

The limited number of photons becomes particularly critical when low-intensity sources are used. Synchrotrons are excellent sources of x-rays with high brightness and the ability to select a specific monochromatic energy, but are not usually conveniently available for tomographic work. Radioactive sources of gamma rays present handling difficulties and have low intensities as well. X-ray tubes are a convenient source for tomography, with adjustable voltage and a variety of target materials that emit different x-ray spectra. Such a source is not monochromatic, which may cause significant beam hardening effects for many specimens, as discussed previously.

Absorption filters can be used to select just a single band of energies from a polychromatic source. For each view angle, two projection images are collected using filters whose absorption edge energies are different. The ratio of the two images yields the attenuation information for the elements whose absorption edges lie between the two filter energies, as indicated in **Figure 45**. A series of such image pairs can provide separate information on the spatial distribution of many elements. **Figure 46** shows an example in which the use of filters has selected two of the three metal inserts in the sample. The use of the filters reduces the already low intensity from the x-ray tube, and the use of the ratio of the two images presents a further limitation on the statistical quality of the projections. It is therefore important to use a small number of views to obtain the best possible projection images. In this example, 12 projections with full 3D rotation of axes were obtained. **Figure 47** shows the artefacts present in the reconstruction when the same number of views is obtained with single-axis rotation.

The electron microscope produces images in which contrast is due to attenuation, and a series of views at different angles can be reconstructed to show 3D structure. The use of an arbitrary series of angles is quite difficult to achieve for materials specimens because of diffraction of the electrons from planes of atoms in the crystal structure. This source of contrast is not easily modeled by the usual attenuation calculation since one voxel may have quite different values in different directions. For noncrystalline materials such as biological specimens, however, the reconstruction is straightforward (Engel & Massalski, 1984; Hegerl, 1989).

Figure 45. *Diagram of the use of balanced absorption edge filters to isolate a single energy band. The plots show the absorption coefficient as a function of energy for two different filters containing the elements chromium and nickel. Elements in the sample with absorption edges between these two energies, such as manganese, iron, and cobalt, will be imaged in the ratio of the two intensities.*

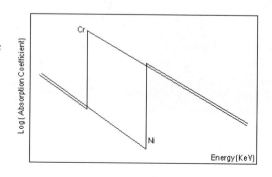

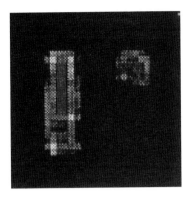 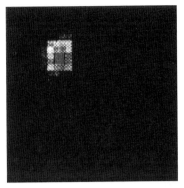 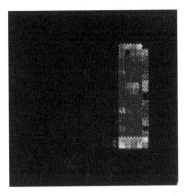

*Figure 46. Reconstruction of the same three planes as shown in **Figure 44**, but using images obtained as a difference between two projections through different filters (Cr and Fe metal foils), which form a bandpass filter to select a narrow band of x-ray energies. Note that one of the inserts (Cr) is missing but the Mn and Fe inserts are visible. Reconstructed using 12 cone beam projections with rotations in 3D.*

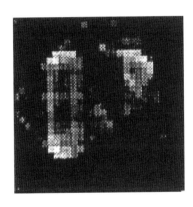

*Figure 47. Reconstruction of the same plane as shown in **Figure 46**, reconstructed in the same way using two filters, but using 12 radial projections (rotating the sample about one axis only). Note the artefacts between and within the inserts.*

Even more efficient than collecting a series of different views using multiple orientations of a single specimen is using images of many different but identical specimens that happen to have different orientations, as mentioned above. **Figure 48** shows an example. The two-dimensional image is an electron micrograph of a single virus particle. The specimen is an adenovirus that causes respiratory ailments.

The low dose of electrons required to prevent damage to the specimen makes the image very noisy. In a typical specimen, however, many such particles are present, each in a different, essentially random orientation. Collecting the various images, indexing the orientation of each image by referring to the location of the triangular facets on the virus surface, and performing a reconstruction produces a 3D reconstruction of the particle in which each voxel value is the electron density. Modeling the surface of the outer protein coat of the virus produces the surface-rendered image shown in **Figure 49** (Stewart and Burnett, 1991).

At a very different scale, tomography has also been performed on the earth itself using seismography. Seismic waves are created by earthquakes or large explosions such as nuclear weapons tests. Such large-magnitude events generate two types of waves that propagate through the earth to receivers (seismographs) at many different locations. P-waves (pressure waves) are compressional pulses which can penetrate through every part of the earth's interior, while S-waves (shear waves) are transverse deformations that cannot propagate through the liquid core. In fact, the presence of a liquid core was deduced in 1906 by the British seismologist, R. D. Oldham, from the shadow cast by the core in seismic S-wave patterns.

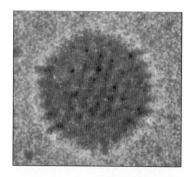

Figure 48. Transmission electron microscope image of single adenovirus particle.

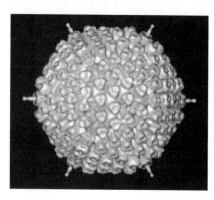

Figure 49. Reconstruction of the adenovirus particle from many transmission images.

The paths of seismic waves are not straight (**Figure 50**), but bend because of the variations in temperature, pressure and composition within the earth which affect the speed of transmission just as the index of refraction of glass affects light and causes it to bend in a lens system. Also similar to the behavior of light, the seismic waves may reflect at interfaces where the speed of propagation varies abruptly. This happens at the core-mantle boundary and the surface of the inner core. The propagation velocities of the P- and S-waves are different, and respond differently to composition.

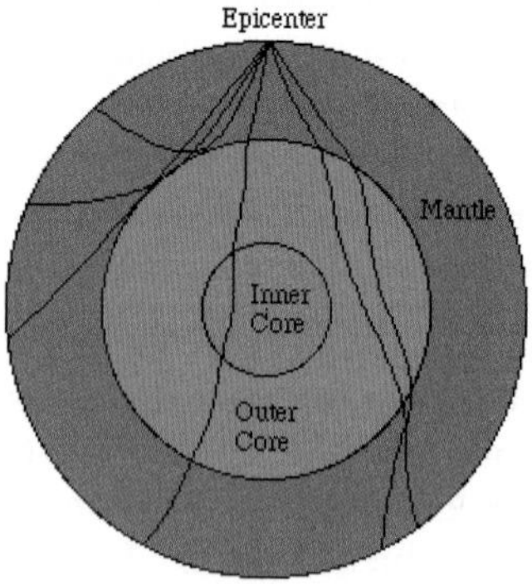

Figure 50. Diagram of paths taken by pressure and shear waves from earthquakes, which reveal information the density along the paths through the core and mantle, and the location of discontinuities.

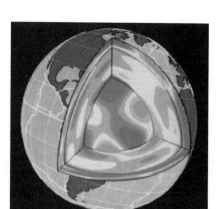

Figure 51. Computed tomogram of the mantle, showing rock densities (light shades are hot, light rocks which are rising, and conversely).

Collecting many seismograms from different events creates a set of ray paths that do not uniformly cover the earth, but rather depend on the chance and highly nonuniform distribution of earthquakes and the distribution of seismographs. Nevertheless, analysis of the travel times of waves that have taken different paths through the earth permits forming a tomographic reconstruction. The density of the material (shown by shading in **Figure 51**) indicates the temperature and the direction of motion (cool, dense material is sinking through the mantle toward the core, while hot, light material is rising). Convection in the mantle is the driving force behind volcanism and continental drift.

Also of great utility are waves that have reflected (one or more times) from the various surfaces. For instance, the difference in travel times of S-waves that arrive directly vs. those which have reflected from the core-mantle boundary permit mapping the elevation of that boundary with a resolution better than 1 kilometer, and reveal that the boundary is not a smooth spherical surface. Because the relatively viscous mantle is floating on a low velocity liquid core, and it is the relatively fast motion of the latter that produces the earth's magnetic field, the study of this interface is important in understanding the earth's dynamics.

Global tomographic reconstruction is generally insensitive to the small details of structure such as faults, but another ongoing program to perform high-resolution tomography under the state of California (where many faults exist, which are of more than casual interest to the surface-dwelling humans) employs an array of high sensitivity seismographs, and uses the very frequent minor earthquakes there to map out the faults through the reflections that they produce.

High resolution tomography

Medical tomography has a typical resolution of about 1 mm, which is adequate for its purpose, and radiologists generally feel comfortable with a series of planar section images in standardized orientations in which they have been trained to recognize normal and abnormal features; but there is considerable interest in applying true 3D tomographic imaging to study the microstructure of various materials including metals, ceramics, composites and polymers, as well as larger industrial components. Some of the structural features cannot be determined from conventional 2D microscopy of cross section surfaces. This includes determining the number of particles of arbitrary or variable shape in a volume, and the topology of networks or pore structures, which control the permeability of materials to fluids.

This information can only be determined by having the full 3D data set, with adequate resolution, and ideally with cubic voxels. Resolution of the order of 1 µm has been demonstrated using a synchrotron as a very bright point source of x-rays. Resolution of about 10 µm is possible using more readily available sources such as microfocus x-ray tubes. Filtering such sources to produce element-specific imaging is also possible, as illustrated.

Cone-beam geometry is well suited to this type of microstructural imaging because it provides magnification of the structure (Johnson et al., 1986; Russ, 1988; Kinney et al., 1989, 1990; Deckman, 1989). **Figure 52** shows this schematically. The magnification is strictly geometric because x-rays

Figure 52. Diagram of a cone-beam imaging system. The projection image magnification is the ratio of b:a. The attainable resolution is limited by the spot size of the x-ray source.

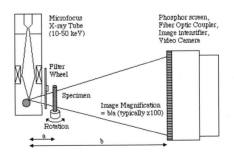

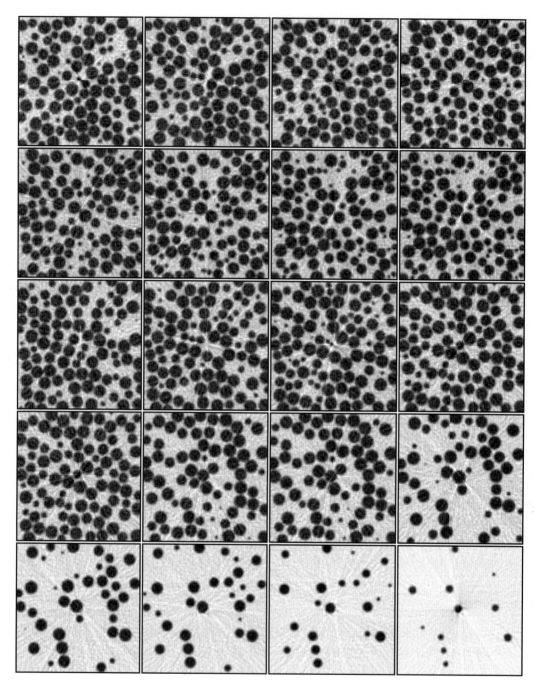

Figure 53. *Twenty individual planes of reconstructed voxels showing a sintered alumina ceramic consisting of 100-μm diameter spheres.*

are not refracted by lenses, but can amount to as much as 100:1. The projected images can be collected using conventional video technology, after conversion to visible light by a phosphor or channel plate and suitable intensification. The intensity of conventional small-spot, x-ray sources is very low, so the use of high-brightness sources, such as those available at a synchrotron, is particularly desirable for high-resolution imaging, as is image averaging, which may be done by using the same cooled charge coupled device (CCD) cameras used for astronomical imaging.

As discussed in Chapter 10, 3D imaging requires many voxels, and the reconstruction process is very computer intensive. The time required to perform the reconstruction is, however, still shorter than that required to collect the various projection images. These images are generally photon-limited, with considerable noise affecting the reconstruction as indicated above. In order to collect reasonable-quality projections from a finite intensity source, the number of view angles is limited. Ideally the views should be arranged to cover the polar angles optimally in 3D space. This arrangement of course places demands on the quality of the mechanism used to perform the rotations and tilts, because the center of rotation must be constant and located within a few micrometers to preserve the image quality as discussed above. Helical scanning is usually easier to accomplish, and more commonly used.

The presentation of 3D information requires extensive use of computer graphics methods as shown in Chapter 10. **Figure 53** shows a simple series of planes of voxels from a 3D tomographic reconstruction of a porous alumina ceramic. The individual particles are approximately 100 µm diameter spheres that fill about 60% of the volume of the sample. The voxels are 10 µm cubes. **Figure 54** shows one of the projection sets through this specimen, a two-dimensional image in which the spherical particles overlap along the lines of sight and are partially transparent. A three-dimensional presentation of this data is shown in **Figure 55**.

Since the first edition of this book (1990) showed these examples from our own experimental setup, several commercial implementations of such instruments have become available (Wang and Vannier, 2001). Figure 56 shows images of bone that have approximately 10 µm resolution, reconstructing up to 1000 slices of 1000 × 1000 voxels in a 1 mm^3 specimen. Reconstructions that in 1990 required a Cray supercomputer are now being performed on a standard desktop machine.

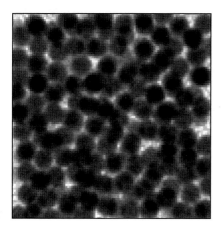

Figure 54. A single 2D projection set through the structure shown in *Figure 53*.

Figure 55. Three-dimensional presentation of the data from *Figure 53*.

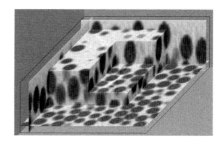

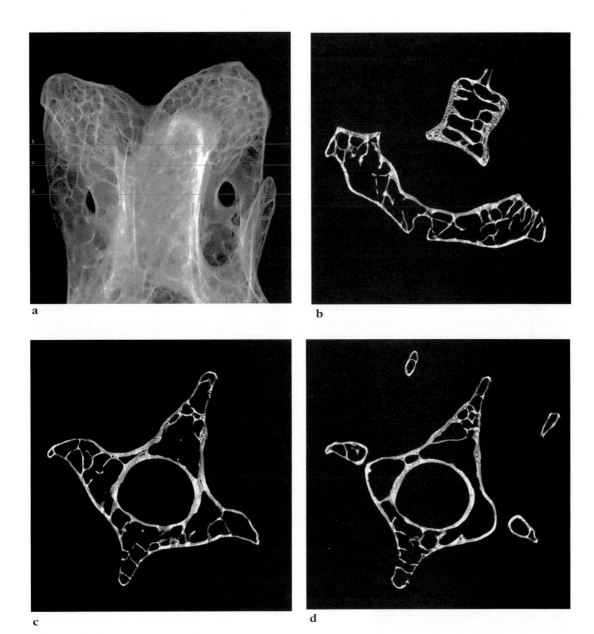

Figure 56. Microtomography of bone:
(a) one projected view image;
(b–d) reconstructed transverse slices at the positions marked in image **a** (images courtesy Skyscan, Aartselaar, Belgium).

3D Image Visualization

12

Sources of 3D data

True three-dimensional (3D) imaging is becoming more accessible with the continued development of instrumentation. Just as the pixel is the unit of brightness measurement for a two-dimensional (2D) image, the voxel (volume element, the 3D analog of the pixel or picture element) is the unit for 3D imaging; and just as processing and analysis is much simpler if the pixels are square, so the use of cubic voxels is preferred for three dimensions, although it is not as often achieved.

Several basic approaches are used for volume imaging. In Chapter 11, 3D imaging by tomographic reconstruction was described. This is perhaps the premier method for measuring the density and in some cases the composition of solid specimens. It can produce a set of cubic voxels, although that is not the only or even the most common way that tomography is presently used. Most medical and industrial applications produce one or a series of 2D section planes, which are spaced farther apart than the lateral resolution within the plane (Baba et al., 1984, 1988; Briarty and Jenkins, 1984; Johnson and Capowski, 1985; Kriete, 1992).

Tomography can be performed using a variety of different signals, including seismic waves, ultrasound, magnetic resonance, conventional x-rays, gamma rays, neutron beams, and electron microscopy, as well as other even less familiar methods. The resolution may vary from kilometers (seismic tomography), to centimeters (most conventional medical scans), millimeters (typical industrial applications), micrometers (microfocus x-ray or synchrotron sources), and even nanometers (electron microscope reconstructions of viruses and atomic lattices). The same basic presentation tools are available regardless of the imaging modality or the dimensional scale.

The most important variable in tomographic imaging, as for all of the other 3D methods discussed here, is whether the data set is planes of pixels, or an array of true voxels. As discussed in Chapter 11, it is possible to set up an array of cubic voxels, collect projection data from a series of views in three dimensions, and solve (either algebraically or by backprojection) for the density of each voxel. The most common way to perform tomography however, is to define one plane at a time as an array of square pixels, collect a series of linear views, solve for the 2D array of densities in that plane, and then proceed to the next plane. When used in this way, tomography shares many similarities (and problems) with other essentially 2D imaging methods that we will collectively define as serial imaging or serial section techniques.

A radiologist viewing an array of such images is expected to combine them in his or her mind to "see" the 3D structures present. (This process is aided enormously by the fact that the radiologist already knows what the structure is, and is generally looking for things that differ from the familiar, particularly in a few characteristic ways that identify disease or injury.) Only a few current-generation systems use the techniques discussed in this chapter to present 3D views directly. In industrial tomography, the greater diversity of structure (and correspondingly lesser ability to predict what is expected), and the greater amount of time available for study and interpretation, has encouraged the use of computer graphics. But such displays are still the exception rather than the rule, and an array of 2D planar images is more commonly used for volume imaging. This chapter emphasizes methods that use a series of parallel, uniformly spaced 2D images, but present them in combination to show 3D structure.

These images are obtained by dissecting the sample into a series of planar sections, which are then piled up as a stack of voxels. Sometimes the sectioning is physical. Blocks of embedded biological materials, textiles, and even some metals, can be sliced with a microtome, and each slice imaged (just as individual slices are normally viewed). Collecting and aligning the images produces a 3D data set in which the voxels are typically very elongated in the "Z" direction because the slices are much thicker or more widely spaced than the lateral resolution within each slice.

At the other extreme, the secondary ion mass spectrometer uses an incident ion beam to remove one layer of atoms at a time from the sample surface. These pass through a mass spectrometer to select atoms from a single element, which is then imaged on a fluorescent screen. Collecting a series of images from many elements can produce a complete 3D map of the sample. One difference from the imaging of slices is that there is no alignment problem, because the sample block is held in place as the surface layers are removed. On the other hand, the erosion rate through different structures can vary so that the surface does not remain planar, and this roughening or differential erosion is very difficult to account for. In this type of instrument, the voxel height can be very small (essentially atomic dimensions) while the lateral dimension is many times larger.

Serial sections

Most physical sectioning approaches are similar to one or the other of these examples. They are known collectively as serial section methods. The name serial section comes from the use of light microscopy imaging of biological tissue, in which blocks of tissue embedded in resin are cut using a microtome into a series of individual slices. Collecting these slices (or at least some of them) for viewing in the microscope enables researchers to assemble a set of photographs which can then be used to reconstruct the 3D structure.

This technique illustrates most of the problems that may be encountered with any 3D imaging method based on a series of individual slices. First, the individual images must be aligned. The microtomed slices are collected on slides and viewed in arbitrary orientations. So, even if the same structures can be located in the different sections (not always an easy task, given that some variation in structure with depth must be present or there would be no incentive to do this kind of work), the pictures do not line up.

Using the details of structure visible in each section provides only a coarse guide to alignment. The automatic methods generally seek to minimize the mismatch between sections either by aligning the centroids of features in the planes so that the sum of squares of distances is minimized, or by overlaying binary images from the two sections and shifting or rotating to minimize the area resulting from combining them with an Ex-OR (exclusive OR) operation, discussed in Chapter 7.

This procedure is illustrated in **Figure 1**. When grey-scale values are present in the image, cross-correlation can be used as discussed in Chapter 5. Unfortunately, neither of these methods is easy to implement in the general case when sections may be shifted in X and Y and also rotated. Solving for the "best alignment" is difficult and must usually proceed iteratively and slowly.

Furthermore, there is no reason to expect the minimum point reached by these algorithms to really represent the true alignment. As shown in **Figures 2** and **3**, shifting or rotating each image to visually align the structures in one section with the next can completely alter the reconstructed 3D structure. It is generally assumed that given enough detail present in the images, some kind of average alignment will avoid these major errors; however, it is far from certain that a best visual alignment is the correct one nor that automated methods, which overlap sequential images, produce the proper alignment.

One approach that improves on the use of internal image detail for alignment is to incorporate fiducial marks in the block before sectioning. These could take the form of holes drilled by a laser, threads or fibers placed in the resin before it hardens, or grooves machined down the edges of the block, for example. With several such marks that can reasonably be expected to maintain their shape from section to section and continue in some known direction through the stack of images, much better alignment is possible. Placing and finding fiducial marks in the close vicinity of the structures of interest is often difficult. In practice, if the sections are not contiguous there may still be difficulties, and alignment errors may propagate through the stack of images.

Most fiducial marks are large enough to cover several pixels in each image. As discussed in Chapter 8, this size allows locating the centroid to a fraction of one pixel accuracy, although not all systems take advantage of this capability. Once the alignment points are identified (either from fiducial marks or internal image detail), the rotation and translation of one image to line up with the next is performed as discussed in Chapter 3. Resampling of the pixel array and interpolation to prevent aliasing produces a new image. This process takes some computational time, but this is a minor problem in comparison to the difficulty of obtaining the images in the first place.

Unfortunately, for classic serial sectioning the result of this rotation and translation is not a true representation of the original 3D structure. The act of sectioning using a microtome generally produces

Figure 1. *Alignment of serial sections by "best fit" of features seeks to minimize mismatched area, measured by ExOR function, as a function of translation and rotation.*

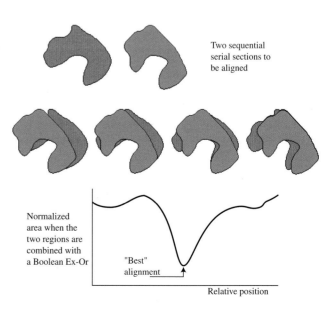

Two sequential serial sections to be aligned

Normalized area when the two regions are combined with a Boolean Ex-Or

"Best" alignment

Relative position

Figure 2. Alignment of serial sections with translation. Sections through an inclined circular cylinder may be misconstrued as a vertical elliptical cylinder.

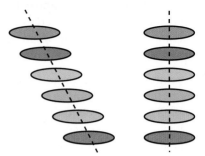

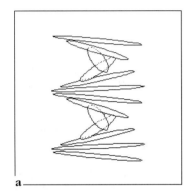
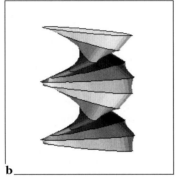
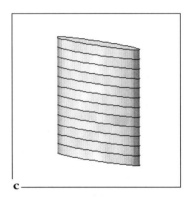

a   b   c

Figure 3. Alignment of serial sections with rotation:
   (a) actual outlines in 3D serial section stack;
   (b) surface modeling applied to outlines, showing twisted structure;
   (c) erroneous result without twist when outlines are aligned to each other.

some distortion in the block. This 5–20% compression in one direction is usually assumed to be nearly the same for all sections (since they are cut in the same direction, and generally have only small differences in structure that would alter their mechanical properties). If the fiducial marks have known absolute coordinates, then stretching of the images to correct for the distortion is possible. It is usually assumed that the entire section is compressed uniformly, although for some samples this may not be true.

Otherwise, it may be possible to use internal information to estimate the distortion. For example, if there is no reason to expect cells or cell nuclei to be elongated in any preferred direction in the tissue, then measurement of the dimensions of many cells or nuclei may be used to determine an average amount of compression. Obviously, this approach includes some assumptions and can only be used in particular circumstances.

Another difficulty with serial sections is calibration of dimension in the depth direction. The thickness of the individual sections is only known approximately (for example, by judging the color of the light produced by interference from the top and bottom surfaces, or based on the mechanical feed rate of the microtome). It may vary from section to section, and even from place to place within the section, depending on the local hardness of the material being cut. Constructing an accurate depth scale is quite difficult, and dimensions in the depth direction will be much less accurate than those measured within one section plane.

If only some sections are used, such as every second or fifth (in order to reduce the amount of work required to image them and then align the images), then this error becomes much worse.

It also becomes difficult to follow structures from one image to the next with confidence. Before computer reconstruction methods became common, however, this kind of skipping was often necessary simply to reduce the amount of data that the human observer had to juggle and interpret.

Using only a fraction of the sections is particularly common when ultra-thin sections are cut for viewing in an electron microscope instead of the light microscope. As the sections become thinner, they increase in number and are more prone to distortion. Some may be lost (for instance due to folding) or intentionally skipped. Portions of each section are obscured by the support grid, which also prevents some from being used. At higher magnification, the fiducial marks become larger, less precisely defined, and above all more widely spaced so that they may not be in close proximity to the structure of interest.

Figure 4 shows a portion of a series of transmission electron microscope (TEM) images of tissue in which the 3D configuration of the membranes (dark, stained lines) is of interest. The details of the edges of cells and organelles have been used to approximately align pairs of sections through the stack, but different details must be used for different pairs as there is no continuity of detail through the entire stack. The membranes can be isolated in these images by thresholding (**Figure 5**), but the sections are too far apart to link the lines together to reconstruct the 3D shape of the surface. This problem is common with conventional serial section images.

Metallographic imaging typically uses reflected rather than transmitted light. As discussed in the next section, serial sectioning in this context is accomplished by removing layers of materials sequentially by physical polishing. The need to locate the same sample position after polishing, and to monitor the depth of polishing, can be met by placing hardness indentations on the sample, or by laser ablation of pits. These serve as fiduciary marks for alignment, and the change in size of the mark reveals the depth. In archaeological excavation the fiduciary marks may be a network of strings and a transit, and the removal tool may be a shovel. In some mining and quarrying examples it may be a bulldozer, but the principles remain the same regardless of scale.

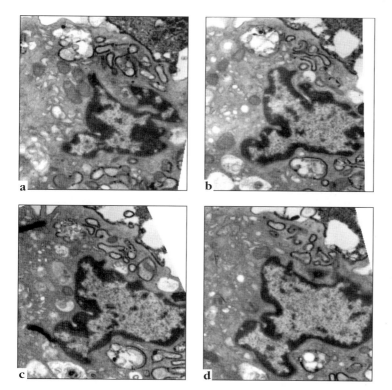

Figure 4. Four serial section images from a stack (courtesy Dr. C. D. Bucana, University of Texas M. D. Anderson Cancer Center, Houston, TX), which have already been rotated for alignment. The membranes at the upper left corner of the images are thresholded and displayed for the entire stack of images in *Figure 5.*

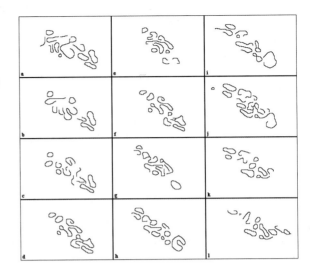

Figure 5. Membranes from the sequential images illustrated in Figure 4, showing the changes from section to section. Because of the separation distance between the planes, these variations are too great to model the shape of the surfaces in 3D.

In most of these surface imaging methods, the sequential 2D images represent the sample along planes that are separated in the z direction. The intervening material that has been removed must be inferred or interpolated from the planes. In the cases, the voxel value is not really an average over its extent, as most pixel values are. Nor is the voxel truly a discrete point value in space, because it does represent an average in the section plane. Interpolation between sections that are too far apart (in terms of the scale of the structure) can lead to some serious errors and misinterpretation.

For the serial sectioning method in which slices are viewed in transmission the voxel value is a volume average, which is easier to interpret. In most cases, the voxel value is a measure of density of the material. Depending on what the radiation is (visible light, x-rays, electrons, neutrons, sound, and so forth), the value may represent the local concentration of some element or compound. In some cases, emitted radiation from voxels also gives concentration information (examples include fluorescence light microscopy and positron-emission tomography).

Optical sectioning

Physical sectioning on any scale is a difficult technique that destroys the sample. Controlling and measuring the section thickness and aligning the sections or at least locating the same position on the sample can become a major source of error. In some cases, it is possible to image sections through a sample without performing physical sectioning. The confocal scanning light microscope (CSLM) offers one way to accomplish this. Depth information can also be obtained in some cases by interpreting the phase shift introduced by objects viewed in light microscopy, as well as by neutron or x-ray transmission imaging (Barty et al., 2000).

The normal operation of the transmission light microscope does not lend itself to optical sectioning. The depth of field of high numerical aperture optics is small (just a few times the lateral resolution), so that only a small "slice" of the image will be sharply focused; however, light from locations above and below the plane of focus is also transmitted to the image, out of focus, and this both blurs the image and includes information from an extended distance in the z direction. In some cases, deconvolution of the point spread function can be accomplished (as discussed in Chapter 5), but in many cases this is of limited value since the blurring varies from one location to another. An example shown in the section on "stereo viewing," (**Figure 36**) under the topic of stereo imaging shows that it is possible to process the images to remove some of the artefacts that result from the passage of light through the sample above and below the plane of focus.

The confocal microscope eliminates this extraneous light, and so produces useful optical section images without the need for processing. This is possible because the sample is imaged one point at a time (thus, the presence of "scanning" in the name). The principle was introduced in Chapter 4 (Image Enhancement), in conjunction with some of the ways that images of light reflected from surfaces can be processed. The principle of the confocal microscope is that light from a point source (often a laser) is focused on a single point in the specimen and collected by an identical set of optics, reaching a pinhole detector. Any portion of the specimen away from the focal point, and particularly out of the focal plane, cannot return light to the pinhole light to interfere with the formation of the image. Scanning the beam with respect to the specimen (by moving the light source, the specimen, or using scanning elements in the optical path) builds up a complete image of the focal plane.

If the numerical aperture of the lenses is high, the depth of field of this microscope is very small, although still several times the lateral resolution within individual image planes. Much more important, the portion of the specimen that is away from the focal plane contributes very little to the image. This makes it possible to image a plane within a bulk specimen, even one that would ordinarily be considered translucent because of light scattering. This method of isolating a single plane within a bulk sample, called optical sectioning, works because the confocal light microscope has a very shallow depth of field and a high rejection of stray light. Translating the specimen in the z direction and collecting a series of images makes it possible to build up a three-dimensional data set for viewing.

Several imaging modalities are possible with the confocal light microscope. The most common are reflected light, in which the light reflected from the sample returns through the same objective lens as used to focus the incident light and is then diverted by a mirror to a detector, and fluorescence in which light is emitted from points within the specimen and is recorded using the same geometry. It is also possible, however, to use the microscope to view transmitted light images using the geometry shown in **Figure 6**. This permits acquiring transmitted light images for focal plane sectioning of bulk translucent or transparent materials. **Figure 7** shows an example of a transmitted light focal plane section.

Both transmitted and reflected-light images of focal plane sections can be used in 3D imaging for different types of specimens. The characteristic of reflected-light confocal images is that the intensity of light reflected to the detector drops off very rapidly as points are shifted above or below the focal plane. Therefore, for structures in a transparent medium, only the surfaces will reflect light.

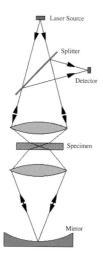

Laser Source

Splitter

Detector

Specimen

Mirror

Figure 6. *Transmission confocal scanning light microscopy (CSLM) can be performed by passing the light through the specimen twice. Light is not imaged from points away from the in-focus point, which gives good lateral and excellent depth resolution compared to a conventional light microscope. (The more common reflected light confocal microscope omits the optics beneath the specimen.)*

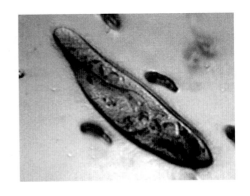

Figure 7. *CSLM image showing a $\frac{1}{30}$ second image of a paramecium swimming in a droplet of water, as it passed through the focal plane of the microscope.*

For any single image plane, only the portion of the field of view where some structure passes through the plane will appear bright, and the rest of the image will be dark. This characteristic permits some rather straightforward reconstruction algorithms.

A widely used imaging method for the confocal microscope is emission or fluorescence, in which the wavelength of the incident light is able to cause excitation of a dye or other fluorescing probe introduced to the specimen. The lower-energy (longer wavelength) light emitted by this probe is separated from the incident light, for instance by a dichroic mirror, and used to form an image in which the location of the probe or dye appears bright. Building up a series of images in depth allows the structure labeled by the probe to be reconstructed.

The transmitted-light mode, while it is the most straightforward in terms of optical sectioning, is little used as yet. This situation is partly due to the difficulties in constructing the microscope with matched optics above and below the specimen, as compared with the reflection and emission modes in which the optics are only above it; however, the use of a lens and mirror beneath the specimen to return the light to the same detector as present in the more standard microscope design can produce most of the same imaging advantages (the only loss is that in passing through the specimen twice, some intensity is lost).

The principal advantages of optical sectioning are avoiding physical distortion of the specimen due to cutting, and having alignment of images from the various imaging planes. The depth resolution, although inferior to the lateral resolution in each plane by about a factor of two to three times, is still useful for many applications. This difference in resolution, however, does raise some difficulties for 3D image processing, even if the distance between planes is made smaller than the resolution so that the stored voxels are cubic (which is by no means common).

By measuring or modeling the 3D shape of the microscope's point spread function, it is possible by deconvolution to improve the resolution of the confocal light microscope. The method is identical to that shown in Chapter 5 for 2D images.

Sequential removal

Many materials are opaque and therefore cannot be imaged by any transmission method, preventing any type of optical sectioning. Indeed, metals, composites, and ceramics are usually examined in the reflected light microscope, although it is still possible to collect a series of depth images for 3D reconstruction by sequential polishing of such materials, as mentioned earlier.

The means of removal of material from the surface depends strongly on the hardness of the material. For some soft metals, polymers, and textiles, the microtome can be used just as for a block of biological material, except that instead of examining the slice of material removed, the surface left behind is imaged. This approach avoids most problems of alignment and distortion, especially if the cutting can be done *in situ* without removing the specimen from the viewing position in the microscope. It is still difficult to determine precisely the thickness of material removed in each cut and to assure its uniformity, but it is generally estimated from the mechanical settings on the device (ignoring any permanent or temporary distortion in the material).

For harder materials, the grinding or polishing operations used to produce conventional sections for 2D images can be used. Such operations generally require removing and replacing the specimen, so again fiducial marks are needed to locate the same region. Probably the most common approach to this marking is the use of hardness indentations. Several pyramid-shaped impressions are made in the surface of the specimen so that after additional abrasion or polishing, the deepest parts of the indentations are still visible. These can be accurately aligned with the marks in the original image. In addition, the reduction in size of the impression, with a shape that is known, gives a measure of the depth of polish and hence of the spacing between the two images. With several such indentations, the overall uniformity of polish can also be judged, although local variations due to the hardness of particular phases may be present.

For still harder materials or ones in which conventional polishing might cause surface damage, other methods may be used. Electrolytic or chemical etching is generally difficult to control and little used. Ion beam erosion is slow, but is already in use in many laboratories for the cutting and thinning of transmission electron microscope specimens, and may be utilized for this purpose. Controlling the erosion to obtain uniformity and avoid surface roughening presents challenges for many specimens.

In situ ion beam erosion is used in the scanning electron microscope and scanning Auger microscope, for instance to allow the removal of surface contamination. Focused ion beams (FIB) are also used to cut slices in the **z** direction to examine microstructures. This capability can be used to produce a series of images in depth in these microscopes, which generally have resolution far better than the light microscope. The time involved in performing the erosion or slicing may be quite long (and thus costly), however, and the uniformity of eroding through complex structures (the most interesting kind for imaging) may be poor.

One kind of microscope performs this type of erosion automatically as part of its imaging process. The ion microscope or secondary ion mass spectrometer (SIMS) uses a beam of heavy ions to erode a layer of atoms from the specimen surface. The secondary ions are then separated according to element in a mass spectrometer and recorded, for example using a channel plate multiplier and more-or-less conventional video or digital camera, to form an image of one plane in the specimen for one element at a time. The depth of erosion is usually calibrated for these instruments by measuring the signal profile of a known standard, such as may be produced by the same methods used to produce modern microelectronics.

The rate of surface removal is highly controllable (if somewhat slow) and capable of essentially atomic resolution in depth. The lateral resolution, by contrast, is of about the same level as in the conventional light microscope, so in this case instead of having voxels which are high in resolution in the plane but poorer in the depth direction, the situation is reversed. The non-cubic voxels create problems for processing and measurement.

Furthermore, the erosion rate for ion beam bombardment in the ion microscope or SIMS may vary from place to place in the specimen as a function of composition, structure, or even crystallographic orientation. This variation does not necessarily show up in the reconstruction, since each set of data is assumed to represent a plane, but can cause significant distortion in the final interpretation. In principle, stretching of the data in 3D can be performed just as images can be corrected for deformation in 2D, although without fiducial marks or accurate quantitative data on local erosion rates, it is hard to accomplish this with real data.

The ability to image many different elements with the SIMS creates a rich data set for 3D display. A color 2D image has three channels (whether it is saved as RGB or HSI, as discussed in Chapter 1), and satellite 2D images typically have as many as seven bands including infrared. The SIMS may have practically any number. The ability of the instrument to detect trace levels (typically ppm or better) of every element or even isotope in the periodic table, plus molecular fragments, means that even for relatively simple specimens the multiband data present a challenge to store, display and interpret.

Another type of microscope that removes layers of atoms as it images them is the atom probe ion microscope. In this instrument, a strong electrical field between a sharply curved sample tip and a display screen causes atoms to be desorbed from the surface and accelerated toward the screen where they are imaged. The screen may include an electron channel plate to amplify the signal so that individual atoms can be seen, or may be used as a time-of-flight mass spectrometer with pulsed application of the high voltage so that the different atom species can be distinguished. With any of the instrument variations, the result is a highly magnified image of atoms from the sample, showing atom arrangements in 3D as layer after layer is removed.

Examples of images from all these types of instruments were shown in Chapter 1.

Stereo measurement

There remains another way to see 3D structures. It is the same way that humans see depth in some real-world situations — having two eyes that face forward so that their fields-of-view overlap permits us to use stereoscopic vision to judge the relative distance to objects. In humans, this is done point by point, by moving our eyes in their sockets to bring each subject to the fovea, the portion of the retina with the densest packing of cones. The muscles in turn tell the brain what motion was needed to achieve convergence, and so we know whether one object is closer or farther than another.

Further into this section, we will see stereo vision used as a means to transmit 3D data to the human viewer. It would be wrong to think that all human depth perception relies on stereoscopy. In fact, much of our judgment about the 3D world around us comes from other cues such as shading, relative size, precedence, atmospheric effects (e.g., fog or haze), and motion flow (nearer objects move more in our visual field when we move our head) that work just fine with one eye and are used in some computer-based measurement methods (Roberts, 1965; Horn, 1970, 1975; Woodham, 1978; Carlsen, 1985; Pentland, 1986). For the moment, however, let us see how stereoscopy can be used to determine depth information to put information into a 3D computer database.

The light microscope has a rather shallow depth of field, which is made even less in the confocal scanning light microscope discussed previously. Consequently, looking at a specimen with deep relief is not very satisfactory except at relatively low magnifications; however, the electron microscope has lenses with very small aperture angles, and thus has very great depth of field. Stereoscopy is most commonly used with the scanning electron microscope (SEM) to produce in-focus images of rough surfaces. Tilting the specimen, or electromagnetically deflecting the scanning beam, can produce a pair of images from different points of view that form a stereo pair. Looking at one picture with each eye fools the brain into seeing the original rough surface.

Measuring the relief of surfaces from such images is the same in principle and in practice as using stereo pair images taken from aircraft or satellites to measure the elevation of topographic features on the earth or another planet. The richer detail in the satellite photos makes it easier to find matching points practically anywhere in the images, but by the same token requires more matching points to define the surface than the simpler geometry of typical specimens observed in the SEM. The mathematical relationship between the measured parallax (the apparent displacement of points in the left and right eye image) and the relative elevation of the two points on the surface was presented in Chapter 1.

Automatic matching of points from stereo pairs is a difficult task for computer-based image analysis (Marr and Poggio, 1976; Medioni and Nevatia, 1985; Kayaalp and Jain, 1987). It is usually performed by using the pattern of brightness values in one image, for instance the left one, as a template to perform a cross-correlation search for the most nearly identical pattern in the right image. The area of search is restricted by the possible displacement, which depends on the angle between the two views and the maximum roughness of the surface, to a horizontal band in the second image. Some points will not be matched by this process because they may not be visible in both images (or are lost off the edges of one or the other image). Other points will match poorly because the local pattern of brightness values in the pixels includes some noise, and several parts of the image may have similar noise levels.

Matching many points produces a new image in which each pixel can be given a value based on the parallax, and hence represents the elevation of the surface. This range image will contain many false matches, but operations such as a median filter usually do a good job of removing the outlier points to produce an overall range image of the surface. In the example of **Figure 8**, cross-correlation matching of every point in the left-eye view with points in the right produces a disparity map (the horizontal distance between the location of the matched points) that contains false matches, which are filled in by a median filter as shown. The resulting elevation data can be used for measurement of points or line profiles, or used to reconstruct surface images, as illustrated. This use of surface range data is discussed further in Chapter 13.

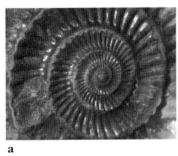

Figure 8. Elevation measurement using stereo pair images:
(a, b) left and right eye views of a microfossil;
(c) raw cross-correlation disparity values;
(d) median filter applied to c;
(e) surface height values measured from a mean plane, displayed as grey-scale values;
(f) rendered perspective-corrected surface model using the values in e;
(g) the same surface reconstruction using elevation values from e with surface brightness values from a.

a

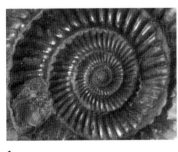

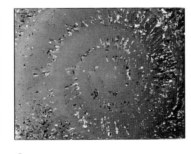

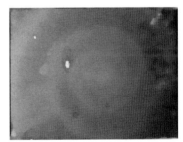

b

c

d

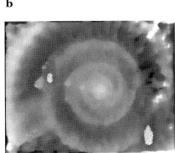

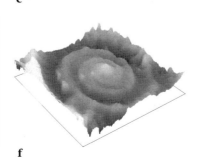

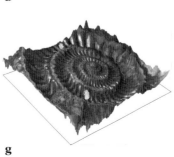

f

g

e

A second approach to matching stereo pairs is based on the realization that many of the points in each image will not match well because they are just part of the overall surface or structure and not the "interesting" points where surfaces meet or other discontinuities are present. This approach is presumably related to human vision, which usually spends most of its time concentrating on only the few points in each scene where discontinuities are found. Locating these interesting points based on some local property such as the variance, entropy, or result of a high-pass filter, produces a comparatively short list of points to be matched between the two images (Moravec, 1977; Quam and Hannah, 1974). A typical case may have only thousands of points, instead of the million or so pixels in the original images.

Somewhat better results are obtained by fitting a cubic polynomial to the pixel brightness values in each neighborhood. Then, if the polynomial is written as

$$f(i, j) = c_1 + c_2 x + c_3 y + c_4 x^2 + c_5 xy + c_6 y^2 +$$

$$+ c_7 x^3 + c_8 x^2 y + c_9 xy^2 + c_{10} y^3 \tag{1}$$

the Zuniga–Haralick operator (Zuniga and Haralick, 1983; Haralick and Shapiro, 1992) used to detect corner points is

$$\frac{-2 \cdot (c_2^2 c_6 - c_2 c_3 c_5 - c_3^2 c_4)}{(c_2^2 + c_3^2)^{3/2}} \tag{2}$$

The points on the resulting short list are then matched in the same way as above, by correlation of their neighborhood brightness patterns. Additionally, for most surfaces the order of points is preserved. This, and the limits on possible parallax for a given pair of images, reduces the typical candidate list for matching to ten or less, and produces a list of surface points and their elevations. It is then assumed that the surface between these points is well behaved and can be treated as consisting of planar facets or simple spline patches, which are constructed by linking the points in a Delaunay tesselation. If the facets are small enough, it is possible to generate a contour map of the surface as shown in **Figure 9** by interpolating straight line segments between points along the edges of each planar facet. A complete display of elevation, called a range image, can be produced by interpolation as shown in **Figure 10**.

The TEM also has a very large depth of field. In most cases, the specimens observed in the TEM are very thin (in order to permit electron penetration), and the optical depth of field is unimportant. With recent generations of high-voltage microscopes, however, comparatively thick samples (of the order of micrometers) may be imaged. This thickness is enough to contain a considerable amount of 3D structure at the resolution of the TEM (of the order of a few nanometers). Thus, using the same approach of tilting the specimen to acquire stereo pair images, it is possible to obtain information about the depth of points and the 3D structure.

Figure 9. Drawing contour lines (iso elevation lines) on the triangular facets joining an arbitrary arrangement of points with elevations that have been determined by stereoscopy.

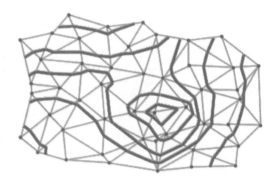

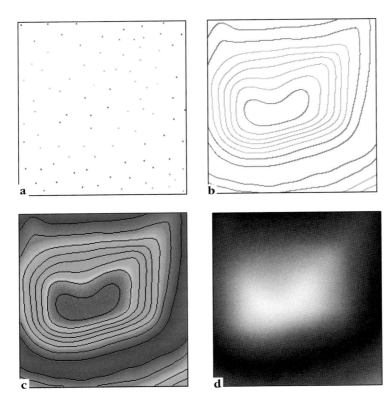

Figure 10. Interpolation of a range image:
(a) *isolated, randomly arranged points with measured elevation (color coded);*
(b) *contour lines drawn through the tesselation;*
(c) *smooth interpolation between contour lines;*
(d) *the constructed range image (grey scale).*

Presenting the images to a human viewer's eyes so that two pictures acquired at different times can be fused in the mind and examined in depth is not difficult. It has been accomplished for years photographically, and is now often done with modest tradeoff in lateral resolution using a computer to record and display the images. The methods discussed in the following paragraphs, which use stereo pair displays to communicate 3D information from generated images are equally applicable here.

It is far more difficult, however, to have the computer determine the depth of features in the structure and construct a 3D database of points and their relationship to each other. Part of the problem is that so much background detail is available from the (mostly) transparent medium surrounding the features of interest that it may dominate the local pixel brightnesses and make matching impossible. Another part of the problem is that it is no longer possible to assume that points maintain their order from left to right. In a 3D structure, points may change their order as they pass in front or in back of each other.

The consequence of these limitations has been that only in a very few, highly idealized cases has automatic fusion of stereo pair images from the TEM been attempted successfully. Simplification of the problem using very high contrast markers, such as small gold particles bound to selected surfaces using antibodies, or some other highly selective stain, helps. In this case, only the markers are considered. Only a few dozen of these exist, and similar to the interesting points mentioned previously for mapping surfaces, they are easily detected (being usually far darker than anything else in the image) and only a few could possibly match.

Even with these markers, a human may still be needed to identify the matches. Given the matching points in the two images, the computer can construct a series of lines that describe the surface which the markers define, but this surface may be only a small part of the total structure. **Figure 11** shows an example of this method in which human matching was performed. Similar methods can be applied to stained networks (Huang et al., 1994), or the distribution of precipitate particles in materials, for example.

Figure 11. *Example of decorating a surface with metal particles (Golgi stain) shown in transmission electron micrographs (Peachey and Heath; 1989) with elevations that are measured stereoscopically to form a network describing the surface (**b**).*

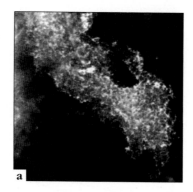
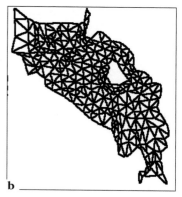

In most matching procedures, the points in left and right images are defined in terms of pixel addresses. The error in the vertical dimension determined by stereoscopy is typically an order-of-magnitude greater than the precision of measurement of the parallax, because the vertical height is proportional to the lateral parallax times the cosecant of the small angle between the views. Improving the measurement of parallax between features to subpixel accuracy is therefore of considerable interest. Such improvement is possible in some cases, particularly when information from many pixels can be combined. As described in Chapter 9, the centroids of features or the location of lines can be specified to an accuracy of one-tenth of a pixel or better.

3D data sets

In the case of matching of points between two stereo pair images, the database is a list of a few hundred or perhaps thousands of coordinates that usually define either a surface or perhaps nodes in a network structure. If these points are to be used for measurement, the coordinates and perhaps some information on which points are connected to which points are all that is required. If image reconstruction is intended, it will be necessary to interpolate additional points between them to complete a display. This is somewhat parallel to the use of boundary representation in two dimensions. It may offer a very compact record of the essential (or at least of the selected) information in the image, but it requires expansion to be visually useful to the human observer.

The most common way to store 3D data sets is as a series of 2D images. Each single image, which we have previously described as an array of pixels, is now seen to have depth. This depth is present either because the plane is truly an average over some depth of the sample (as in looking through a thin section in the light microscope) or based on the spacing between that plane and the next (as for instance a series of polished planes observed by reflected light). Because of the depth associated with the planes, we refer to the individual elements as voxels (volume elements) rather than pixels (pixel elements).

For viewing, processing and measurement, the voxels will ideally be regular and uniformly spaced. This goal is often accomplished with a cubic array of voxels, which is easiest to address in computer memory and corresponds to the way that some image acquisition devices function (e.g., the confocal scanning light microscope). Other arrangements of voxels in space offer some advantages. In a simple cubic arrangement, the neighboring voxels are at different distances from the central voxel, depending on whether they share a face, edge or corner. Deciding whether voxels touch and are part of the same feature requires a decision to include 6-, 18- or 26-neighbor connectedness, even more complicated than the 4- or 8-connectedness of square pixels in a 2D image, discussed in Chapter 6.

More symmetrical arrangements are possible. The arrangements of atoms in metal crystals typically occupy sites in one of three lattice configurations: body-centered cubic (BCC), face-centered cubic (FCC), or hexagonal close packed (HCP). The first of these surrounds each atom (or voxel) with eight touching neighbors at the same distance, and the other two have 12 equidistant neighbors.

The advantage of these voxel-stacking arrangements is that processing of images can treat each of the neighbors identically, and that measurements are less biased as a function of direction. A more symmetrical neighborhood with neighbors at uniform distances also simplifies processing, including the application of filters and morphological operations. Of course, in order to fill space, the shapes of the voxels in these cases are not simple. Storing and addressing the voxel array is difficult, as is acquiring images or displaying them. Usually the acquired image must be re-sampled by interpolation to obtain voxels in one of these patterns, and a reverse interpolation is needed for display. For most purposes, these disadvantages outweigh the theoretical advantages, just as the use of a hexagonal pixel array is rarely used for two-dimensional images. Cubic arrays are the most common 3D arrangement of voxels.

If the voxels are not cubic because the spacing between planes is different from the resolution within each plane, it may be possible to adjust things so that they are. In the discussion that follows, we will assume that the depth spacing is greater than the spacing within the plane, but an analogous situation could be described for the reverse case. This adjustment could be done by interpolating additional planes of voxels between those that have been measured. Unfortunately, doing this will not help much with image processing operations, since the assumption is that all of the neighbors are equal in importance, and with interpolation they become redundant.

The alternative approach is to reduce the resolution within the plane by sampling every nth pixel, or perhaps by averaging pixels together in blocks, so that a new image is formed with cubic voxels. This resolution reduction also reduces the amount of storage that will be required, since many fewer voxels remain. Although it seems unnatural to give up resolution, in a few cases where cubic voxels are required for analysis this is done.

A variety of different formats are available for storing 3D data sets, either as a stack of individual images or effectively as an array of voxel values with x, y, z indices. Such arrays become very large, very fast. A 512×512 or 640×480 pixel 2D image, which represents a very common image size for digitizing video images, occupies 250 or 300K bytes of storage, using one byte per pixel (256 grey values). This is easily handled in the memory of a desktop computer, or recorded on a floppy disk. Even with modern digital cameras, a typical 1024×1024 color image occupies only a few M bytes. A $512 \times 512 \times 512$ 3D image would occupy 128 megabytes of memory, about the upper limit for practical processing on a desktop machine. Larger files present difficulties just in storing or transmitting from place to place, let alone processing. Most of the data sets in this chapter are much smaller, for instance $256 \times 256 \times 50$ (3.2 megabytes). The same operations shown here can be used for larger data sets, given time, computer power (speed and memory), or both.

Compression can reduce the size of the storage requirements. The individual 2D images can be compressed either using run-length encoding (especially useful for binary images), or by the JPEG (Joint Photographers Expert Group) compression algorithms based on a discrete cosine transform, discussed in Chapter 2. There is not yet a standardized algorithm extending to 3D images, but there are emerging standards for time sequences of images. One, the MPEG (Moving Pictures Expert Group) approach, is based on the fact that in a time series of images, most of the pixels do not change much in successive frames. Similar assumptions have been used to transmit video conferences over telephone lines; only the changing pixels must be transmitted for each frame.

This high correlation from frame to frame is also usually true for a series of planes in 3D, and may lead to standardized algorithms for compacting such images. They will still require unpacking for display, processing and measurement, however, and the significant artefacts introduced by these lossy compression methods (discussed in Chapter 2) argues against their use. For 3D image stacks compressed using MPEG methods, the artefacts in the z-direction (interpreted as time) are even worse than those in each individual x-y plane.

It is instructive to compare this situation to that of computer-aided design (CAD). For manmade objects with comparatively simple geometric surfaces, only a tiny number of point coordinates are required to define the entire 3D structure. This kind of boundary representation is very compact, but it often takes some time (or specialized display hardware) to render a drawing with realistic surfaces from such a data set. For a voxel image, the storage requirements are great but information is immediately available without computation for each location, and the various display images shown in this chapter can usually be produced very quickly (sometimes even at interactive speeds) by modest computers.

For instance, given a series of surfaces defined by boundary representation or a few coordinates, the generation of a display may proceed by first constructing all of the points for one plane, calculating the local angles of the plane with respect to the viewer and light source, using those to determine a brightness value, and plotting that value on the screen. At the same time, another image memory is used to store the actual depth (z-value) of the surface at that point. After one plane is complete, the next one is similarly drawn except that the depth value is compared point by point to the values in the z-buffer to determine whether the plane is in front of or behind the previous values. Of course, each point is only drawn if it lies in front. This procedure permits multiple intersecting planes to be drawn on the screen correctly. (For more information on graphic presentation of 3D CAD data, see Foley and Van Dam, 1984; or Hearn and Baker, 1986.)

Additional logic is needed to clip the edges of the planes to the stored boundaries, to change the reflectivity rules used to calculate brightness depending on the surface characteristics, and so forth. Standard texts on computer graphics describe algorithms for accomplishing these tasks and devote considerable space to the relative efficiency of various methods because the time involved can be significant. By comparison, looking up the value in a large array, or even running through a column in the array to add densities or find the maximum value, is very fast. This is particularly true if the array can be held in memory rather than requiring disk access.

The difficulties of aligning sequential slices to produce a 3D data set were discussed above. In many cases, there may be several 3D data sets obtained by different imaging techniques (e.g., magnetic resonance imaging (MRI), x-ray, and PET images of the head) which must be aligned to each other. They also commonly have different resolutions and voxel sizes, so that interpolation is needed to adjust them to match one another. The situation is a direct analog to the 2D problems encountered in geographical information systems (GIS) in which surface maps, images in different wavelengths from different satellites, aerial photographs and other information must be aligned and combined.

The general problem is usually described as one of registering the multiple data sets. The two principal techniques, which are complementary, are to use cross-correlation methods on the entire pixel or voxel array as discussed in Chapter 5, or to isolate specific features in the multiple images and use them as fiducial marks to perform warping (Brown, 1992; Besl, 1992; van den Elsen et al., 1993, 1994, 1995; Reddy and Chatterji, 1996; Frederik et al., 1997; West et al., 1997).

Slicing the data set

Most 3D image data sets are actually stored as a series of 2D images, so it is very easy to access any of the individual image planes, usually called slices. Playing the series of slices back in order to create an animation or "movie" is perhaps the most common tool available to let the user view the data. It is often quite effective in letting the viewer perform the 3D integration, and as it recapitulates the way the images may have been acquired (but with a much compressed time base), most viewers can understand images presented in this way. A simple user interface need only allow the viewer to vary the speed of the animation, change direction or stop at a chosen slice, for example. The same software now widely available to play back movies on the computer screen can be used for this purpose.

One problem with presenting the original images as slices of the data is that the orientation of some features in the 3D structure may not show up very well in the slices. It is useful to be able to change the orientation of the slices to look at any plane through the data, either in still or animated playback. This change in orientation is quite easy to do as long as the orientation of the slices is parallel to the x-, y-, or z-axes in the data set. If the depth direction is understood as the z-axis, then the x- and y-axes are the horizontal and vertical edges of the individual images. If the data are stored as discrete voxels, then accessing the data to form an image on planes parallel to these directions is just a matter of calculating the addresses of voxels using offsets to the start of each row and column in the array. This addressing can be done at real-time speeds if the data are held in memory, but is somewhat slower if the data are stored on a disk drive because the voxels that are adjacent along scan lines in the original slice images are stored contiguously on disk and can be read as a group in a single pass. When a different orientation is required the voxels must be located at widely separated places in the file, however and it takes time to move the head and wait for the disk to rotate.

Displaying an image in planes parallel to the x-, y-, and z-axes was introduced in Chapter 11. **Figure 12** shows another example of orthogonal slices. The images are MRIs of a human head. The views are generally described as transaxial (perpendicular to the subject's spine), sagittal (parallel

*Figure 12. A few slices from a complete set of MRI head scan data. Images **a** through **c** show transaxial sections (3 from a set of 46), images **d** and **e** are coronal sections (2 from a set of 42), and **f** is a sagittal section (1 from a set of 30).*

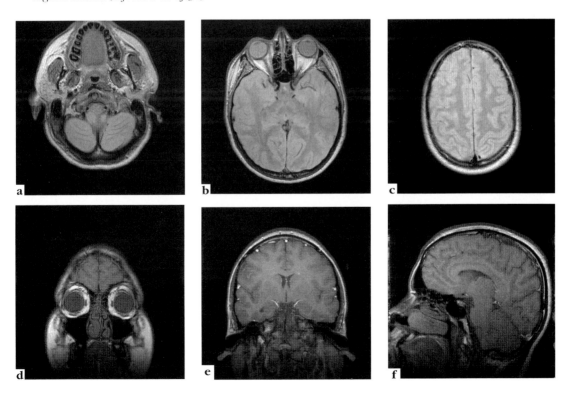

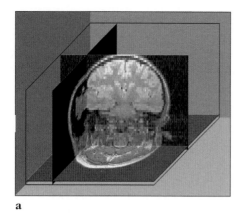
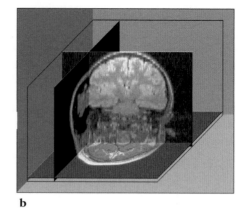

a b

Figure 13. Comparison of two vertical slices through the 3D MRI data set from Figure 12:
 (a) *slices extended vertically;*
 (b) *linear interpolation between slices.*

to the spine and to the major axis of symmetry), and coronal (parallel to the spine and perpendicular to the "straight ahead" line of sight). Several individual sections are shown representing each orientation.

It is actually not too common to perform this kind of resectioning with MRI data (or most other kinds of medical images) because the spacing of the planes is usually greater than the resolution in the plane, and the result is a visible loss of resolution in one direction in the resectioned slices due to interpolation in the z direction. The alternative to interpolation is to extend the voxels in space; in most cases, this is even more distracting to the eye, as shown in **Figure 13**. Interpolation between planes of pixels can be done linearly, or using higher-order fits to more than two planes, or more than just the two pixels immediately above and below. But while interpolation produces a visually acceptable image, it can ignore real structure or create apparent structure. **Figure 14** shows an example of interpolation, which creates an impression of structure that is not actually present (and hides the real structure).

When data can be obtained with cubic voxels this interpolation is not a problem. In several of the figures later in this chapter, much greater loss of resolution in the z direction will be evident when plane images are reconstructed by sampling and interpolation of the original data. In the case of **Figure 12**, the MRI images were actually obtained with uniform resolution in each of the three directions.

Combining several views at once using orthogonal planes adds to the feeling of three-dimensionality of the data. **Figure 15** shows several examples of this using the same MRI head data based

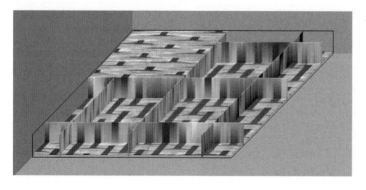

Figure 14. *Interpolation in a 3D array. In this example, only two images of the top and bottom of a woven fabric are used. The points between the two surfaces are linearly interpolated and bear no relationship to the actual 3D structure of the textile.*

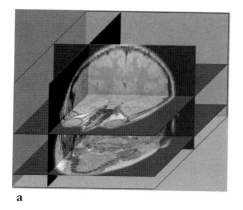 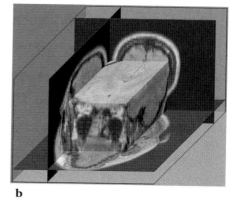

a   b

*Figure 15. Several views of the MRI head data from **Figure 12** along section planes normal to the axes of the voxel array. The voxels were taken from the trans-axial slices, and so the resolution is poorer in the direction normal to the planes than in the planes.*

on plane images obtained in the transaxial direction. The poorer resolution in the z direction is evident, but still the overall impression of 3D structure is quite good. These views can also be animated, by moving one (or several) of the planes through the data set while keeping the other orthogonal planes fixed to act as a visual reference.

Unfortunately, there is no good way to demonstrate this time-based animation in a print medium. Once upon a time, children's cartoon books used a "flip" mode with animation printed on a series of pages that the viewer could literally flip or riffle through at a fast enough rate to cause flicker-fusion in the eye and see motion. That form of animation takes a lot of pages and is really only good for very simple images such as cartoons. It is unlikely to appeal to the publishers of books and technical journals. All that can really be done here is to show a few of the still images from such a sequence and appeal to the reader's imagination to supply a necessarily weak impression of the effect of a live animation. Many online Web sites can show such animations as Quicktime® movies.

Figure 16 shows a series of images that can be used to show "moving pictures" of this kind. They are actually a portion of the series of images which Eadweard Muybridge recorded of a running horse by setting up a row of cameras that were tripped in order as the moving horse broke threads attached to the shutter releases. His purpose was to show that the horse's feet were not always in contact with the ground (in order to win a wager for Leland Stanford, Jr.). The individual still pictures show that. Once it was realized that such images could be viewed in sequence to recreate the impression of smooth motion, our modern motion picture industry (and ultimately television) became possible.

It is difficult to show motion using printed images in books. There is current interest in the use of videotape or compact disk for the distribution of technical papers, which will perhaps offer a medium that can use time as a third axis to substitute for a spatial axis and show 3D structure through motion. The possibilities will be mentioned again in connection with rotation and other time-based display methods.

Motion, or a sequence of images, is used to show multidimensional data in many cases. "Flipping" through a series of planes provides a crude method of showing data sets that occupy three spatial dimensions. Another effective animation shows a view of an entire 3D data set while varying the opacity of the voxels. Even for a data set that occupies two spatial dimensions, transitions between many kinds of information may be used effectively. **Figure 17** shows this multiplicity with weather data, showing temperature, wind velocity and other parameters displayed onto a map of the U.S. In general, displays that utilize a 2D map as an organizing basis for multidimensional data

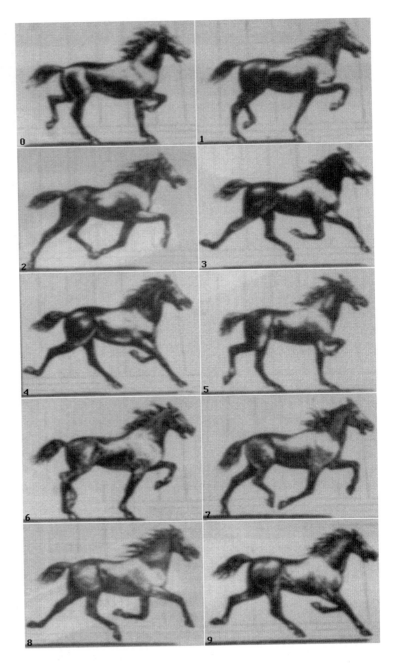

Figure 16. A few of the series of historic photographs taken by Eadweard Muybridge to show the motion of a running horse. Viewed rapidly in succession, these create the illusion of continuous motion.

such as road networks, geological formations, and so on, called GIS, have many types of data and can only display a small fraction of it at any one time.

Of course, time itself is also a valid third dimension and the acquisition of a series of images in rapid succession to study changes in structure or composition with time can employ many of the same analytical and visualization tools as images covering three space dimensions. **Figure 18** shows a series of images recorded at video rate (30 frames per second) from a confocal light microscope. Such data sets can be assembled into a cube in which the z direction is time, and changes studied by sectioning this volume in planes along the z direction, or viewed volumetrically, or as a time sequence.

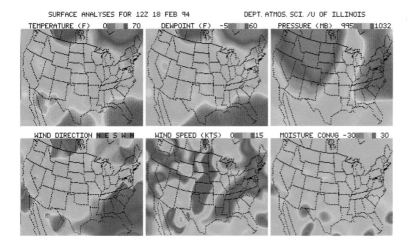

SURFACE ANALYSES FOR 12Z 18 FEB 94   DEPT. ATMOS. SCI. /U OF ILLINOIS

Figure 17. Weather data for the U.S. is a richly multidimensional data set tied to a geographic base.

Figure 18. A series of images of adult rat atrial myocytes loaded with the calcium indicator fluo-3. The images were recorded at video rate (30 frames per second) from a confocal light microscope (images courtesy of Dr. William T. Mason and Dr. John Hoyland, Department of Neurobiology, Babraham Institute, Cambridge, U.K.).

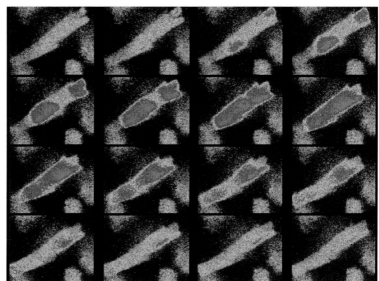

Arbitrary section planes

Restricting the section planes to those perpendicular to the x-, y-, or z-axes is obviously limiting for the viewer. It is done for convenience in accessing the voxels in storage and creating the display. If some arbitrary planar orientation is selected, the voxels must be found that lie closest to the plane. As for the case of image warping, stretching and rotating discussed in Chapter 3, these voxels will not generally lie exactly in the plane, nor will they have a regular grid-like spacing that lends itself to forming an image. **Figure 19** shows an example of a plane section through an array of cubic voxels, in which portions of various size and shape are revealed. These variations complicate displaying the voxel contents on the plane.

The available solutions are either to use the voxels that are closest to the section plane, plot them where they land, and spread them out to fill any gaps that develop, or to establish a grid of points in the section plane and then interpolate values from the nearest voxels, which may be up to eight in number. As for the case of rotation and stretching, these two solutions have different shortcomings. Using the nearest voxel preserves brightness values (or whatever the voxel value represents) but may distort boundaries and produce stair-stepping or aliasing. Interpolation makes the boundaries appear straight and smooth, but also smooths the brightness values by averaging so that

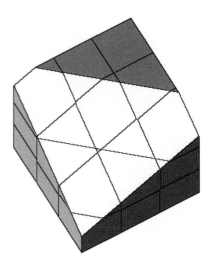

steps are blurred. It is also slower, because more voxels must be located in the array and the interpolation performed.

Producing an animation by continuously moving a section plane at an arbitrary orientation requires a significant amount of computation, even if it is simple calculation of addresses and linear interpolation of values. Instead of doing this calculation in real time, many systems instead create new images of each of the plane positions, store them, and then create the animation by playing them back. This procedure is fine for demonstrating something that the user has already found, but because of the time delay is not a particularly good tool for exploring the 3D data set to discover the unexpected.

The ultimate use of planar resectioning would be to change the location and orientation of the section plane dynamically in real time, allowing instant response to the scene. Chapter 1 pointed out that humans study things by turning them over, either in the hand or in the mind. This kind of "turning-over" is a natural way to study objects, but requires a fairly large computer memory (to hold all of the voxel data), a fairly speedy processor and display, and a user interface that provides the required number of degrees of freedom. Modern desktop computers are approaching this level of performance; **Figure 20** shows a typical display.

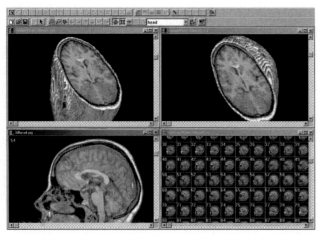

Figure 20. *Presentation of serial sections, 3D reconstruction, and arbitrary plane slice on a desktop computer (courtesy Able Software).*

Positioning an arbitrary plane can be done in two different ways, which, of course, produce the same results but feel quite different to the user. One is to move the plane with respect to a fixed 3D voxel array. This can be done, for example, by dragging the corners of the plane along the x-, y-, z-axes, or by positioning a center point and then tilting the plane around two axes through that point. A different method is to keep the section plane fixed perpendicular to the direction of view while allowing the data set to be rotated in space. Combined with the ability to shift the section plane toward or away from the viewer (or equivalently to shift the data set), this method allows exactly the same information to be obtained.

The principal difference between these approaches is that in the latter case the image is seen without perspective or foreshortening, so that size comparisons or measurements can be made. Obtaining such data may be important in some applications. On the other hand, keeping the data set fixed and moving the section plane seems to aid the user in maintaining orientation within the structure. There are as many different modes of human interaction with 3D data sets as there are programs, and as yet no general consensus on which are most useful has emerged.

Figure 21 shows the voxels revealed by an arbitrary section plane through the 3D data set from the MRI image series. The appearance of the voxels as a series of steps is rather distracting, so it is more common to show the value of the nearest voxels to the plane, or to interpolate among the voxels to obtain brightness values for each point on the plane as shown in **Figure 22**.

Also useful is the ability to make some of the pixels in section planes transparent, allowing the viewing of other planes behind the first, and making the 3D structure of the data more apparent. **Figure 23** shows an example of this for the spherical particle data shown in Chapter 11. The series of parallel slices are not contiguous planes of voxels, and the separation of the planes has been increased by a factor of two in the z direction. The voxels whose density falls below a threshold that roughly corresponds to that of the particles have been made transparent. This allows seeing voxels which are part of particles in other section planes behind the first.

Figure 24 shows a similar treatment for the MRI data set of the human head. The threshold for choosing which voxels to make transparent is more arbitrary than for the spheres, because void and low-density regions exist inside as well as outside the head. However, the overall impression of 3D structure is clearly enhanced by this treatment.

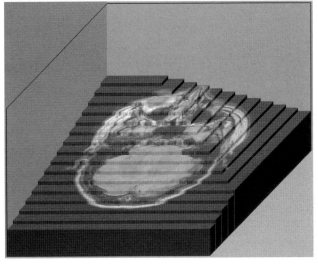

Figure 21. Sampling voxels along inclined planes in a 3D array. Showing the entire voxel is visually distracting and does not produce a smooth image

Figure 22. *Smooth interpolation of image pixels on arbitrary planes positioned in a voxel array.*

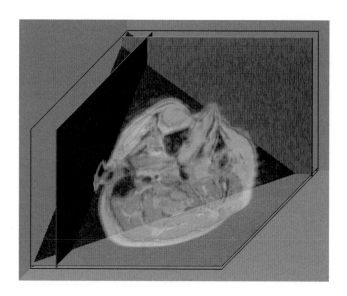

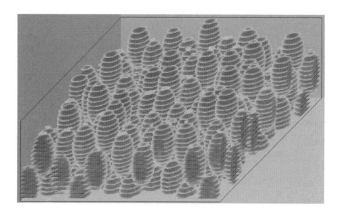

Figure 23. *"Exploded" view of voxel layers in the tomographic reconstruction of spherical particles (**Figures 54–55, Chapter 11**). The low-density region surrounding the particles is shown as transparent.*

Figure 24. *View of several orthogonal slices of the MRI head data with transparency for the low-density regions in the planes.*

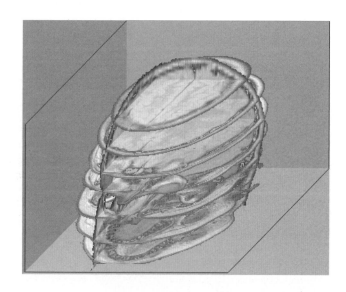

The use of color

Assignment of pseudo-colors to grey-scale 2D images was discussed in earlier chapters. It sometimes permits distinguishing subtle variations that are imperceptible in brightness in the original; but, as noted before, it more often breaks up the overall continuity and gestalt of the image so that the image is more difficult to interpret. Of course, the same display tricks can be used with 3D sets of images, with the same consequences.

A subtle use of color or shading is to apply slightly different shading to different planar orientations shown in **Figures 15** and **22** to increase the impression of three-dimensionality. In this example, a grey-scale difference between the x, y, and z orientations is evident. Light tints of red, green and blue can be used for this as well.

It is more useful to employ different color scales to distinguish different structures, as was also demonstrated for 2D images. It requires separate processing or measurement operations to distinguish the different structures. When applied to 3D data sets, the colored scales assist in seeing the continuity from one image to another, while providing ranges of brightness values for each object.

One of the most common ways that multiple colors can be used to advantage in 3D image data is to code multiband data such as the elemental concentrations measured from the secondary ion mass spectrometer. This use of pseudo-color is analogous to similar coding in 2D images, very frequently used for x-ray maps from the SEM and (of course) for remotely sensed satellite images, in which the colors may either be "true" or used to represent colors beyond the range of human vision, particularly infrared. Of course, the other tools for working with multiband images in 2D, such as calculating ratios, can also be applied in 3D.

Figure 25 shows example images for the SIMS depth imaging of elements implanted in a silicon wafer. Comparing the spatial location of the different elements is made easier by superimposing the separate images and using colors to distinguish the elements. This is done by assigning red, green and blue to each of three elements and then combining the image planes, with the result shown in **Figure 26**.

Volumetric display

Sectioning the data set, even if some regions are made transparent, obscures much of the voxel array. Only the selected planes are seen and much of the information in the data set is not used. It has been pointed out before that the topological properties of 3D structures are not revealed on

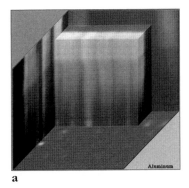 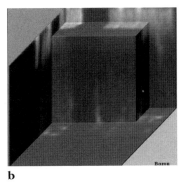 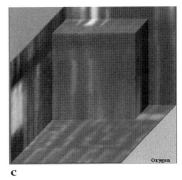

a   b   c

Figure 25. Views of plane sections for the elements aluminum, boron, and oxygen in a silicon wafer, imaged by secondary ion mass spectrometry. Figure 26 shows a color image of all three elements on another orthogonal set of planes.

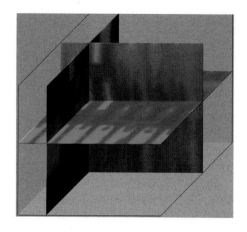

Figure 26. Color coding of elemental intensity from SIMS images in Figure 25. The multiband 3D data set is sectioned on x, y, and z planes, and the 256-level (8-bit) brightness scale for the elements Aluminum, Boron, and Oxygen are assigned to red, green, and blue, respectively.

section planes. The volumetric display method shows all of the 3D voxel information. For simple structures displaying everything can be an advantage, while for very complex ones the overlapping features and boundaries can become confusing.

A volumetric display is produced by ray tracing. In the simplest model used, a uniform, extended light source is placed behind the voxel array. For each parallel straight line ray from the light source to a point on the display screen, the density value of each voxel that lies along the path is used to calculate a reduction in the light intensity following the usual absorption rule:

$$\frac{I}{I_0} = e^{-\sum \rho}$$

(3)

Performing this calculation for rays reaching each point on the display generates an image. The total contrast range may be adjusted to the range of the display by introducing an arbitrary scaling constant. This scaling can be important because the calculated intensities may be quite small for large voxel arrays.

Notice that this model assumes that the voxel values actually correspond to density, or to some other property that may be adequately modeled by the absorption of light. The images shown in **Figures 54** and **56a** in **Chapter 11** correspond closely to this model, since they show the projected view through a specimen using x-rays, although the geometry is cone beam rather than parallel projection. In fact, x-ray tomographic reconstruction, discussed in the preceding chapter, proceeds from such views to a calculation of the voxel array. Having the array of voxel values then permits generating many kinds of displays to examine the data. It seems counter-productive to calculate the projection view again, and indeed in such a view as shown in those figures, the ability to distinguish the individual features and see their relationship is poor.

One of the advantages of this mode is that the direction of view can be changed rather easily. For each, it is necessary to calculate the addresses of voxels that lie along each ray. When the view direction is not parallel to one of the axes, this addressing can be done efficiently using sine/cosine values or a generalization of the Bresenham line drawing algorithm. Also in this case, an improved display quality is obtained by calculating the length of the line segment along each ray through each pixel. The absorption rule then becomes

$$\frac{I}{I_0} = e^{-\sum \rho t}$$

(4)

This method is far short of a complete ray tracing, although it is sometimes described as one. In a true ray-traced image, refraction and reflection of the light is included along with the absorption.

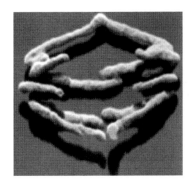

Figure 27. Reconstruction of chromosomes in a dividing cell from CSLM 3D data. The chromosomes are opaque and the matrix around them transparent, and shadows have been ray cast on the rear plane to enhance the 3D appearance.

Figure 27 shows an example in which the inclusion of shadows greatly increases the 3D impression. More complex shading, in which features cast shadows on themselves and each other, requires calculations that are generally too time-consuming for routine use in this application. With the simple absorption-only method, it is possible to achieve display speeds capable of rotating the array (changing the view direction) interactively with desktop computers.

Of course, it is always possible to generate and save a series of projection images that can then be played back as an animation or movie. These are primarily useful for communicating some information already known to another viewer, however, while interactive displays may assist in discovering the structural relationships in the first place.

These types of volumetric displays are often isometric rather than perspective-corrected. In other words, the dimension of a voxel or feature does not change with distance. This is equivalent to looking at the scene through a long focal length lens, and given the inherent strangeness of data in most 3D image sets does not generally cause significant additional discomfort to viewers. True perspective correction requires that x,y dimensions on the screen be adjusted for depth. Particularly for rotated views, perspective adds a significant amount of computation.

Figure 28 shows such a view through a joint in the leg of a head louse. The original series of images were obtained with a transmission confocal light microscope, with nearly cubic voxels (the spacing between sequential focal planes was 0.2 μm in depth). The individual muscle fibers are visible but overlapped. Shifting the stack to approximate rotation as described below gives the viewer the ability to distinguish the various muscle groups. Again, a time sequence (hard to show in print media) is used as a third dimension to display 3D data as the planes are shifted, and since no complex arithmetic is needed to run this sequence it is practical to create such animations in a small computer.

A much more limited approach to volumetric presentation is to show one portion of the image as a surface rendered model, as discussed below, but to show the surrounding tissue as a transparent

Figure 28. Volumetric projection image through a stack of 60 CSLM images of a joint in the leg of a head louse. Each plane is displaced by one voxel dimension to produce a view at 45°.

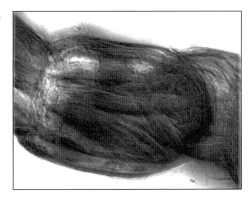

Figure 29. *Viewing the surface reconstruction from serial sections through a knee joint with the surrounding tissue shown as a transparent volume with no internal detail.*

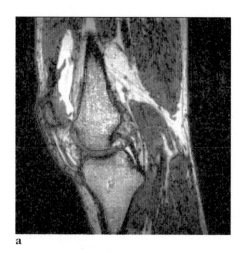

a

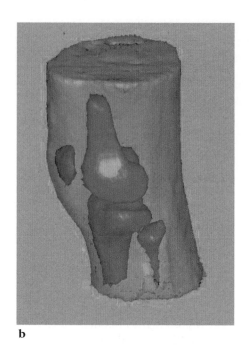

b

volume. Usually no detail is preserved in this volume, and it is present only to provide a point of reference for the structure of interest, as shown in **Figure 29**.

Very rapid generation of projection images is possible if the addressing can be simplified and the variation in distance through different voxels can be ignored. **Figure 30** shows an approximation that facilitates these changes. Each plane of voxels is shifted laterally by a small amount, which may be an integer number of voxel spaces making the address calculation particularly simple, but in any case requires no more than simple 2D interpolation. The planes remain normal to the view direction, so that all distances through pixels are the same. This kind of shifting can give the impression of rotation for small angles. Beyond about 30°, the distortion of the 3D structure due to stretching may become visually objectionable; however, this method provides a fast way to cause some relative displacement of features as a function of depth to better understand the structure.

Stereo viewing

In many of the images in this chapter, two adjacent images in a rotation or pseudo-rotation sequence can be viewed as a stereo pair. For some readers looking at them will require an inexpensive viewer which allows one to focus on the separate images while keeping the eyes looking straight ahead (which the brain expects to correspond to objects at a great distance). Other readers may have mastered the trick of fusing such printed stereo views without assistance. Some,

Figure 30. *Schematic diagram of shifting image planes laterally to create illusion of rotation, or to produce stereo-pair images for viewing.*

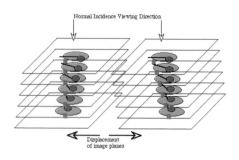

unfortunately, will not be able to see them at all. A significant portion of the population seems not to actually use stereo vision, due for instance to uncorrected amblyopia ("lazy eye") in childhood.

Stereo views are so useful to a reasonable fraction of people that it may be useful to display them directly on the viewing screen. Of course, with a large screen, it is possible to draw the two views side by side. **Figures 31** and **32** show examples of stereo pair presentation of 3D images using both the volumetric display method discussed above and the surface-rendered method discussed below, for the same specimen (derived from confocal light microscope images of a sea urchin embryo). **Figure 33** shows another stereo pair presentation of skeletonized data obtained from neurons imaged in the confocal light microscope.

A more direct stereo display method uses color planes in the display for the left- and right-eye views. For instance, **Figure 34** shows a stereo pair of blood vessels in the skin of a hamster, imaged live using a confocal light microscope in fluorescence mode. The 3D reconstruction method used pseudo-rotation by shifting of the focal section planes with the emission rules discussed

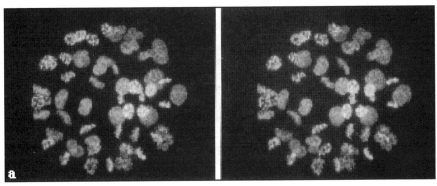

Figure 31. *Stereo pair presentation of Feulgen-stained DNA in a sea urchin embryo. The cells form a hollow sphere, evident in the stereo images, with some cells in the act of cell division. This image shows a volumetric image that is "ray cast" or "ray traced," using an emission model, with different offsets for the individual optical sections to produce a stereo effect. See also **Figure 32** for a surface image of the same data (From Summers, R.G. et al. (1991).* J. Electron Microscope Tech. *18:24–30. With permission.)*

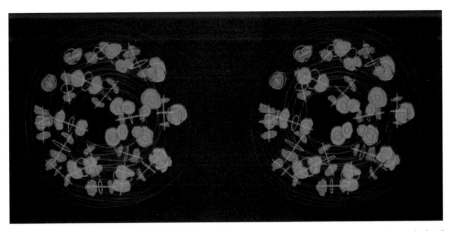

Figure 32. *Stereo view of the data set from **Figure 31**, but surface is rendered and color coded. The surface image shows contours within each section which render the surfaces of the chromosomal masses but obscure any internal detail or structures to the rear. Contour lines for the embryo are also shown.*

Figure 33. Stereo images of skeletonized
lines (manually entered from serial
section data) from two neurons in
hippocampus of 10-day old rat, showing
branching and 3-D relationships (From
Turner, J.N. et al. (1991). J. Electron
Microscope Tech. 8:11–23. With
permission.)

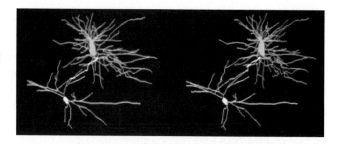

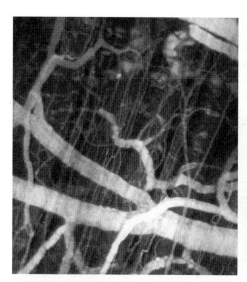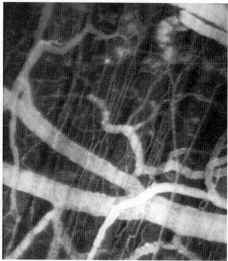

Figure 34. Stereo view of multiple focal plane images from a confocal light microscope showing light
emitted from fluorescent dye injected into the vasculature of a hamster and viewed live in the skin. This
image is also shown in **Figure 35** (images courtesy Chris Russ, University of Texas, Austin TX).

below. Combining these images using red and green to display two views of the same 3D data set is shown in **Figure 35**. The images are overlapped, and the viewer (equipped with glasses having appropriate red and cyan filters) can easily look at the combined images. Of course, this method cannot be used for color images, as discussed in the following paragraphs.

These stereo views were constructed from multiple sections by projecting or ray tracing through a stack of images as shown in **Figure 30**. The individual sections were obtained by confocal microscopy, which, due to its very shallow depth of field, can be used to obtain a continuous set of voxel planes. Other techniques that produce continuous arrays of thin sections can also be used, of course; but it is even possible to perform this type of reconstruction using a conventional optical microscope, despite the blurring of the images due to the large depth of field and the effect of light passing through the specimen above and below the image planes.

Removing artefacts such as blur from images by processing in frequency space was discussed in Chapter 5. For three dimensions the procedure is identical except that the point spread function and the Fourier transform are three dimensional. **Figure 36** shows an example of using Wiener inverse filtering to accomplish this deblurring in the creation of a stereo pair. The images were reconstructed from 90 optical sections spaced through a 50-μm thick section, which is much closer than the depth of field of the optics. The use of the inverse filter removes most of the artefacts from the images and produces a clear stereo pair image (Lin et al., 1994). Another approach to the same kind of sharpening is to apply an iterative procedure that uses neighboring images to estimate the

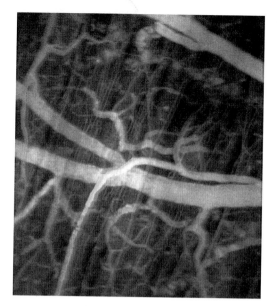

Figure 35. Stereo pair of the same image pair shown in *Figure 34*, using red and cyan for the different eye views. This allows viewing the image with normal eye vergence, using glasses (red lens on left eye, green or blue on right).

Figure 36. Sharpening of focal sections by Wiener filtering. The stereo-pair images are produced by ray tracing two projections at angles of about ±2.4° through 90 serial optical sections in a 50 µm thick section. **The sample is Spirogyra.**
(a) original images;
(b) Wiener inverse filtered (From Lin, W. et al. (1994). J. Comput. Assisted Microsc. 6(3):113–128. With permission.)

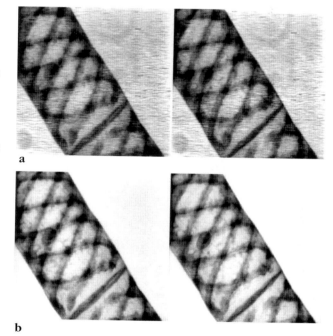

a

b

artefacts in each plane. This Van Cittert filter requires using neighbor planes on each side out to about twice the dimension of the point spread function, which in this case is the depth of optical focus (Jain, 1989).

For projection of stereo pair images, it is possible to use two slide projectors equipped with polarizing filters that orient the light polarization at right angles (usually 45° to the right and left of vertical). Viewers wearing polarized glasses can then see the stereo effect, and color can still be used. This display method requires special specular projection screens that reflect the light without losing the polarization, and works best for viewers in line with the center of the screen. However, it has become a rather popular method of displaying 3D data. Of course, it is not as practical for interactive exploration of a data set since photographic slides must be made first. Polarization can also be used with live computer displays, as discussed in the next paragraph.

The difference in viewing angle for the two images can be adjusted somewhat arbitrarily to control the visual impression of depth. The angle can be made to correspond to the typical vergence angle of human vision for normal viewing. Using a typical interocular distance of 7.5 cm, and a viewing distance of 1 meter, the actual vergence angle is 4.3°. For closer viewing, larger angles are appropriate. The judgment of depth thus depends on our brain's interpretation of the viewing distance, which is based on the focus distance to the image in combination with the vergence angle of the eyes in their sockets. If the angle is varied, the impression of depth can be adjusted to expand or compress the z dimension, as shown in **Figure 37**.

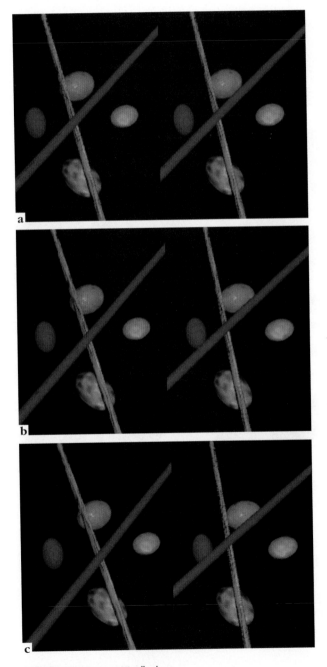

Figure 37. Stereo pair images of a generated structure with varying angles to control the apparent depth of the structure in the z direction: **(a)** ±1°; **(b)** ±3°; **(c)** ±5°. Visual fusion of the images become increasingly difficult with the larger angles.

Special display hardware

Other specialized display hardware for 3D image analysis may be useful in some cases. Holography offers the promise of realistic 3D display that can be viewed from different directions (Blackie et al., 1987). Attempts to generate such displays by calculating the holograms have been experimentally successful, although they are still too slow for interactive use (and far from the "stand alone" 3D presentation of Princess Leia in *Star Wars*). At present, the best holograms are displayed using coherent light from a laser and high resolution film. In order to produce live displays from a computer, multiple screens such as the LCDs used for conference room projection can be used in place of the film; however, the resolution and control of the light modulation (relative intensity) is not really adequate.

Another custom approach is called a varifocal mirror (Fuchs et al., 1982). Each plane of voxels in the 3D array is drawn one at a time on the display CRT. The screen is not viewed directly by the user, but is reflected from a mirror. The mirror is mounted on a speaker voice coil so that it can be moved. As each different plane of voxels is drawn, the mirror is displaced slightly as shown schematically in **Figure 38**. This movement changes the distance from the viewer's eye to the screen, and gives the impression of depth. In order to achieve high drawing speeds (so that the entire set of planes can be redrawn at least 30 times per second), this technique is usually restricted to simple outline drawings rather than the entire voxel data set. The successive outlines are perceived as surfaces in three dimensions.

The mirror technique also suffers from a slowdown if the planes are not normal to the x-, y-, and z-axes so that trigonometric calculations are required to access the data. The alternative approach is to continue to draw outlines in the major orthogonal planes, but to move the mirror during the drawing of each outline to correspond to the tilting of the plane. This requires a much higher and more complex frequency response from the mechanical devices used to control the mirror.

Another, more recent development for real-time viewing of 3D computer graphics displays uses stereo images. The computer calculates two display images for slightly different orientations of the data set or viewing positions. These are displayed alternately using high-speed display hardware which typically shows 120 images per second. Special hardware is then used to allow each eye to see only the correct images, at a rate of 60 times per second, fast enough to eliminate flicker (the minimum rate for flicker fusion above which we see continuous images rather than discrete ones is usually at least 16 frames per second; commercial moving pictures typically use 24 frames, and television uses 25 for European and 30 in U.S. systems).

The visual switching may be done by installing a liquid crystal device on the display monitor that can rapidly switch the polarization direction of the transmitted light, so that viewers can watch through glasses containing polarizing film. A second approach is to wear special glasses containing active liquid crystal devices that can rapidly turn clear or opaque. Synchronizing pulses from the computer cause the glasses to switch as the images are displayed, so that each eye sees the proper view.

Figure 38. *Diagram of the operation of a varifocal mirror to show depth in images. The speaker voice coil rapidly varies the position of the mirror, which changes the distance from the viewer's eye to the cathode ray tube display as it draws information from different depths in the data set.*

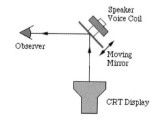

Such devices have been used primarily for graphics design, in which substantial computer resources are used to model 3D objects, generate rendered surface views, and allow the user to freely rotate and zoom. With the number of disciplines interested in using 3D computer graphics, it seems assured that new hardware (and the required corresponding software) will continue to evolve for this purpose. The economic breakthrough that would impact scientific uses will probably come when game console manufacturers decide to deliver 3D displays.

These various display tools can be adapted to the display of 3D image data and used at scales ranging from nanometers (electron and ion microscopy) to kilometers (seismic exploration). It is possible to imagine using other senses than visual to deal with multiband data (e.g., sound which changes pitch and volume to reveal density and composition as you move a cursor over the display of a voxel array), but as emphasized in Chapter 1, we are overwhelmingly visual creatures who expect to get information through images. Existing technologies such as force-feedback gloves that would allow the user to "reach into" structures and feel or manipulate them, and virtual reality "caves" using lightweight headsets with stereo displays that sense the user's head position and generate appropriate images that allow one to wander through the microstructure, are still much too costly for routine use. Because vision is our primary sense, however, it appears likely that most methods will be primarily visual, and the researcher who is color-blind or cannot see stereo will remain disadvantaged.

Also, no consensus has been reached on the best input and control devices for complex computer graphics displays. Rotating or shifting the viewpoint in response to horizontal or vertical motion of the now ubiquitous mouse gives a rather crude control. For moving points, lines, and planes in 3D, some more flexible device will be required. Simply locating a specific voxel location in the array can be done in several different ways. One is to use an x,y input device (mouse, trackball, etc.) for two axes and periodically shift to a different control, which may be a scroll bar on the screen, to adjust the distance along the third axis. Another is to move two cursors, one on an x-y projection and one on an x-z projection, for example. Such approaches usually feel rather clumsy because of the need to move back and forth between two areas of the screen and two modalities of interaction. Appropriate color-coding of the cursor to report depth can help.

Three-axis joysticks and sonic digitizers that allow the user to point in space (multiple sensors triangulate the position) exist but are hardly standard. The dataglove, an instrumented glove or framework that fits on the hand and reports all motion of joints to the computer, has been used to move molecules around each other to study enzyme action. Supplemented by force feedback, this method gives the researcher rich information about the ways that molecules can best fit together.

At the other extreme, it is important to remember the history of 3D visualization (Cookson, 1994), which began with physical models constructed of wood, plastic or plaster. Building such a model from a series of section planes was very difficult and time-consuming, and still could not reveal all of the internal detail. Computer modeling has progressed from simple outlines to hidden line removal, surface construction, shading and rendering, and full volumetric or ray-traced methods.

Ray tracing

The example of volumetric display shown above performed a simplified ray tracing to sum the density values of voxels and calculate a brightness based on light being absorbed as it propagated from back to front through the 3D data set. Although this model does correspond to some imaging situations, such as the transmission light or electron microscope and tomography, different rules are appropriate in many other situations.

In the process of traversing a voxel array, following a particular line of sight that will end in one pixel of a ray-traced image, the variables that are available include:

1. The brightness and perhaps color of the original light source placed behind the array, and whether it is an extended source (producing parallel rays of light) or a point source (producing a cone beam of light). This illumination source will control the contribution that transmission makes to the final image.
2. The location of the first and last voxels with a density above some arbitrary threshold taken to represent transparency. These voxels will define surfaces that can be rendered using reflected light. Additional rules for surface reflectivity, the location, brightness, and color of the light sources, and so forth, must be added.
3. The location of the maximum or minimum values or large gradients, which may define the location of some internal surface for rendering.
4. The rule for combining voxel values along a path. This may be multiplication of fractional values, which models simple absorption according to Beer's law for photons provided that the voxel values are linear absorption values. In some cases density is proportional to attenuation, so this rule can produce interpretable images. There are other convolution rules available as well, including linear summation and retention of maximum or minimum values. Although these may also correspond to some physical situations, their greatest value is that they produce images which can delineate internal structure.
5. The relationship between the voxel values and the intensity (and perhaps color) of light originating in each voxel, which represents fluorescence or other emission processes.

The combining rules mentioned briefly in part 4 of the above list correspond to the various image processing tools described in Chapters 3 and 4 for combining pixels from two or more images. They include arithmetic (multiplication, addition), rank ordering (minimum or maximum value), and Boolean logic. It is also possible to include lateral scattering so that point sources of light spread or blur as they pass through the voxel array, or even to combine several modes. This approach to realism through computation is rarely justified because the measured voxel values are not generally physically related to light transmission or scattering.

A software package for 3D visualization may make any or all of these parameters accessible to the user, along with others. For example, control of the surface reflectivity and roughness, and the location of the incident light source(s), affects the appearance of rendered surfaces. In performing a convolution of transmitted light along ray paths from a light source behind the voxel array, the relationship between the voxel values and the absorption of the light is another parameter that offers control. By varying the relationship between voxel value and opacity (linear attenuation coefficient), or selectively introducing color, it is possible to make some structures appear or to remove them, allowing others to be seen.

Figure 39 shows an example of this presentation. The data set is the same as used above; the voxel values come from the MRI measurement technique and approximately correspond to the amount of water present. Not enough information is given to fully describe the structures actually present in a human head, so there is no "correct" relationship between voxel value and light absorption for the volumetric rendering. Using different, arbitrary curves, it is possible to selectively view the outer skin, bone structure, or brain.

Using color permits even more distinctions to be made. **Figure 40** shows images of a hog heart reconstructed using different relationships for opacity vs. voxel value that emphasize the heart muscle or the blood vessels. In this example, each voxel is assumed both to absorb the light from the source placed behind the voxel array and to contribute its own light along the ray in proportion to its value and with color taken from an arbitrary table. The result allows structures with different measured values to appear in different colors.

Of course, with only a single value for each voxel it is not possible to model absorption and emission separately. By performing dual-energy tomography in which the average atomic number and

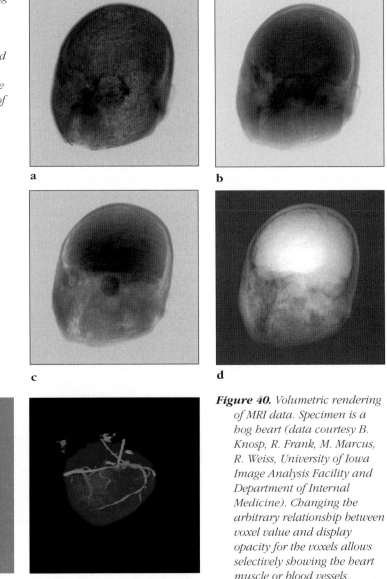

Figure 39. *Volumetric imaging of the MRI head data from* **Figure 12**. *Varying the relationship between voxel values and the opacity used to absorb light transmitted along each ray through the structure allows selection of which structures are revealed.*

a

b

c

d

Figure 40. *Volumetric rendering of MRI data. Specimen is a hog heart (data courtesy B. Knosp, R. Frank, M. Marcus, R. Weiss, University of Iowa Image Analysis Facility and Department of Internal Medicine). Changing the arbitrary relationship between voxel value and display opacity for the voxels allows selectively showing the heart muscle or blood vessels.*

average density are both determined, or multi-energy tomography in which the concentration of various elements in each voxel is measured, or by using the T1,T2 relaxation time signals from MRI, such techniques become possible. They represent straightforward implementation of several of the multiband and color imaging methods discussed in earlier chapters, but are not yet common as neither the imaging instrumentation nor the computer routines are yet widely available. It is consequently usually necessary to adopt some arbitrary relationship between the single measured set of voxel values and the displayed rendering that corresponds to the major voxel property measured by the original imaging process.

For example, in fluorescence light microscopy, or x-ray images from the SEM, or ion microscopy, the voxel value is a measure of emitted brightness that is generally proportional to elemental concentration. These 3D data sets can also be shown volumetrically by a simplified ray tracing.

Instead of absorbing light from an external light source, the rule is to sum the voxel values as brightnesses along each path.

Figure 34 showed an application using the fluorescence confocal light microscope. A dye was injected into the blood vessel of a hamster, which was excited by the incident light from the microscope. The emitted light was collected to form a series of 2D images at different focal depths, and these were then arranged in a stack to produce a 3D data set. In this case the spacing between the planes is much greater than the resolution within each image plane. Sliding the image stack laterally as discussed above produces an approximation of rotation and impression of depth. The brightness values for each voxel are then summed along vertical columns to produce each image.

This emission model is very easy to calculate but does not take into account any possible absorption of the emitted light intensity by other voxels along the ray path. Generally, simple 3D data sets have only one piece of data per voxel and there is no separate information on density and emission brightness, so no such correction is even possible. Sometimes a simple reduction in intensity in proportion to the total number of voxels traversed (known as a "distance fade") may be used to approximate this absorption effect. Usually, it is assumed that the emission intensity is sufficiently high and the structure sufficiently transparent that no such correction is needed, or that it would not change the interpretation of the structure, which is in any case qualitative rather than quantitative.

When multiband data are available, as for instance in the SIMS data set used in **Figures 25** and **26**, emission rules can be used with the assignment of different colors (at least up to three) to different signals. **Figures 41** and **42** show a volumetric view of these data using emission rules, presented as a stereo pair. The monochrome figure shows a single element (boron) while in the color image, multiple elements are combined. The use of color in the images forces the use of two

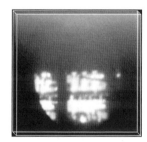
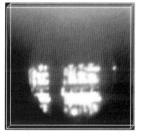

Figure 41: Stereo-pair display of emission rule volumetric images of Boron concentration in a silicon wafer, imaged by a secondary ion mass spectrometer.

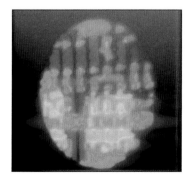
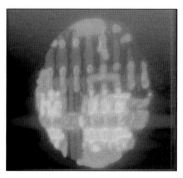

Figure 42. Stereo pair of volumetric images from the SIMS data set. Colors assigned to the different elements are Red = Aluminum, Green = Boron, and Blue = Oxygen, with 256 brightness levels of each. The use of color for elemental information precludes color coding of views for stereo viewing. The density of information in this display is so great that fusing the images to see the depth is quite difficult.

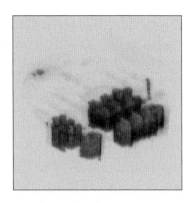

Figure 43. Surface rendered display of the same data as in Figure 42. The internal surface of the boron-rich region is determined by arbitrary thresholding, and then rendered using an arbitrarily placed light source.

side-by-side images for viewing, and the density of information in the images that results from overlaying the 8-bit (256 grey-level) values from each element at every point makes it quite difficult to fuse these images for satisfactory stereo viewing.

Using the same data set, it is possible to use the location of the frontmost voxel along each line of sight whose value is above an arbitrary threshold to define the location of an internal boundary. If this resulting surface is then rendered as a solid surface with incident reflected light, another representation of the data is obtained as shown in **Figure 43**.

An internal surface can be displayed in several different ways. **Figure 44** shows several views of the spiral cochlear structure from the ear of a bat (Keating, 1993). Slices through the 3D voxel array do not show that the structure is connected. Thresholding to show all of the voxels within the structure reveals the topology of the spiral. A series of section images can be shown as either wire frame outlines, or with the surface rendered. The outlines are more convenient for rotating to view the structure from different directions.

When color coding of structures, volumetric rending, and selective transparency are combined with the display of internal surfaces (with shading as discussed in the next section), the results can be quite striking. **Figure 45** shows an example, the brain of a fruit fly (*Drosophila melanogaster*), using data recorded with a confocal laser scanning microscope. The 3D reconstruction shows surfaces rendered as partially transparent in a transparent medium, to reveal the surfaces of other structures behind them. Although effective at communicating specific information to the viewer, these displays require prior decisions and selection and are not so useful for exploring unknown data sets, as noted previously.

Reflection

Another important imaging modality is reflection. The conventional CSLM, seismic reflection mapping, acoustic microscopy, ultrasound imaging, and so forth, acquire a 3D image set whose voxel values record the reflection of the signal from internal locations. **Figure 46** shows the use of ultrasound to show the surface of a fetus in utero. In most of these technologies, a voxel array is generated and used to locate boundaries where strong reflections occur, within a matrix that may be otherwise opaque. In the CSLM, the matrix is transparent (either air or liquid) and the strongest reflection at each *x,y* point is where the specimen surface is in focus. This means that recording a set of images as a 3D data array makes it possible to locate the surface in three dimensions. Most systems use the processing methods discussed in Chapter 4 to find the brightest value at each pixel, and thus construct the surface range image.

Figure 44. Cochlear structure from the ear of a bat (Keating, 1993):
  (a) arbitrary planar slices through the voxel array;
  (b) array of parallel slices through the array;
  (c) surface revealed by thresholding the voxels;
  (d) outlines delineating the structure in all voxel planes;
  (e) surface reconstructed from the outlines in *d*;
  (f) the same structure as shown in *e*, rotated to a different point of view.

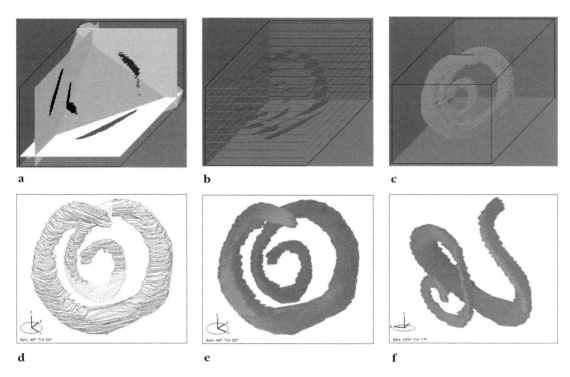

a b c

d e f

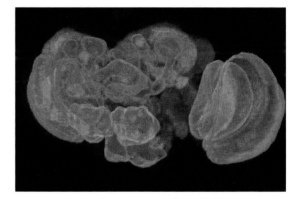

Figure 45. *Reconstruction of a fruit fly brain with transparent surfaces. Data courtesy of K. Rein (Department of Genetics, University Wuerzburg), visualization by M. Zoeckler (ZIB) using the Amira software (www.amiravis.com).*

One way to generate such a display is to go down columns of the data array (just as in volumetric ray tracing), looking for the maximum voxel value, or the first value to exceed some threshold. Keeping only that value produces an image of the entire surface in focus, as was shown in Chapter 4. The same methods for rotating or shifting the data array to alter the viewing direction can be used; therefore, it is also possible to find the maxima or surface points along any viewing direction and display the surface as an animation sequence or to construct a stereo pair. In principle, fitting a curve based on the known depth-of-field characteristics of the optics to the brightness values along a vertical column of voxels can locate the surface with sub-voxel accuracy. **Figure 47**

Figure 46. The face of a 26-week-old fetus, imaged by ultrasound.

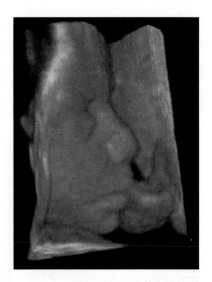

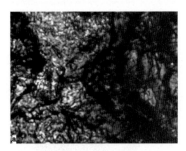

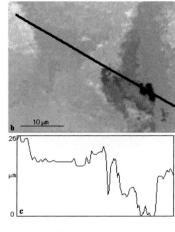

Figure 47. Depth measurement using the confocal scanning light microscope:
(a) extended focus image of an alumina fracture surface obtained by keeping the brightest value from many focal planes at each pixel location;
(b) range image obtained by assigning a grey scale value to each pixel according to the focal plane image in which the brightest (in focus) reflectance is measured;
(c) elevation profile along the traverse line shown in figure b.

shows the alumina fracture (from **Chapter 4, Figure 80**) both as an extended-focus image and as a range image (in which pixel brightness is proportional to elevation). Several presentation modes for range images are available to assist in visualizing the 3D shape of the surface. One, shown in the figure, is simply to plot the brightness profile along any line across the image, which gives the elevation profile directly.

Figure 48 shows several of the presentation modes for range images (Chapter 13 goes into more detail). The specimen is a microelectronics chip imaged by reflection CSLM, so both an extended-focus image and a range image can be obtained from the series of focal plane sections. From the range image data, plotting contour maps, grid or mesh plots, or rendered displays is a straightforward exercise in computer graphics.

One of the classic ways to show surface elevation is a contour map (**Figure 49**), in which isoelevation lines are drawn, usually at uniform increments of altitude. These lines are of course

***Figure 48. Presentation modes for surface information from the CSLM (specimen is a
microelectronics chip):***

(a) *the in-focus image of the surface reflectance obtained by keeping the brightest value at each pixel
address from all of the multiple focal plane images;*
(b) *the elevation or range image produced by grey-scale encoding the depth at which the brightest pixel
was measured for each pixel address;*
(c) *contour map of the surface elevation with color coding for the height values;*
(d) *perspective-corrected rendering of the surface with grid lines and pseudo-color;*
(e) *the same image as **d** with realistic shading;*
(f) *the rendering from **e** from two points of view, combined as a stereo pair.*

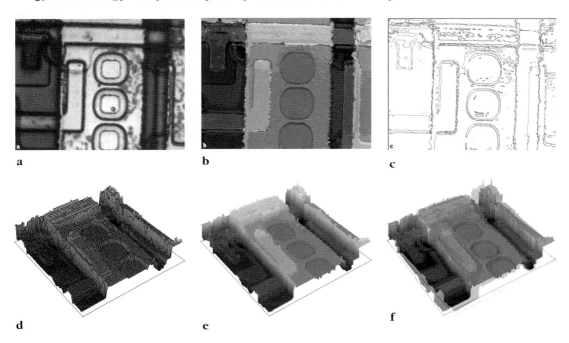

a   b   c

d   e   f

Figure 49. *Fragment of a
conventional topographic
map (Phantom Ranch in the
Grand Canyon) showing
isoelevation contour lines.*

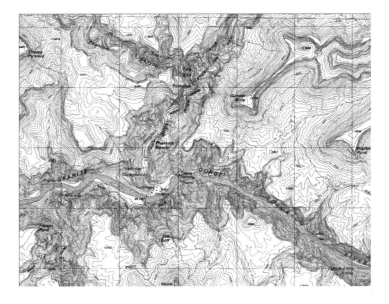

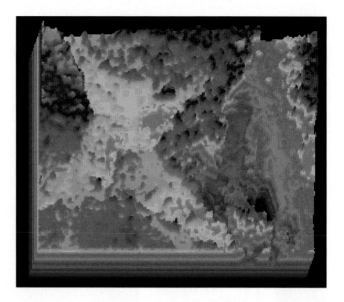

Figure 50. *Isometric view of elevation data for the alumina fracture surface shown in* **Figure 47**. *A rapidly varying color palette is used to reveal small changes.*

continuous and closed. This is the way topographic maps are drawn, and the same methods are useful at any scale. The contour map reduces the pixel data from the original range image to boundary representation, so the method for forming the boundaries is the same as discussed in Chapter 5 for segmentation. The lines may be labeled or color-coded to assist in distinguishing elevations.

A shortcut way to draw contour lines on a range image is to present the data as a shaded isometric view, as in **Figure 50**, which shows the elevation data for the alumina fracture surface of **Figure 47**. In this image, a 3D representation (without perspective) is used to draw a vertical line for each pixel in the range image to a height proportional to the value. The image is also shaded so that each point has its grey-scale value. Replacing the grey-scale values with a pseudo-color table allows communication of the elevations in a particularly easy-to-interpret way, and in fact many topographic maps use similar methods to show elevations.

Constructing a contour map can be either simple or complex. The simplest method merely locates those pixels that have neighbors that are above and below the threshold level. As shown in **Figure 51**, however, this produces a very coarse approximation. Interpolating between pixel addresses produces a much better map, as shown in the figure.

Figure 52 shows an example that looks broadly similar to **Figure 51**, but represents data at a very different scale. This is a three-dimensional view of Ishtar Terra on Venus. The data come from the spacecraft Magellan's side-looking mapping radar. This synthetic-aperture radar bounces 12.5-cm-wavelength radar waves off the surface, using the echo time delay for range, and the Doppler shift to collect signals from points ahead of and behind the direct line of sight. The 2D images obtained by processing the signals are similar in appearance to aerial photographs.

Rendering of a surface defined by a range image produces a realistic image of surface appearance, as compared to grid or isometric contour map displays that are more abstract and more difficult for visual interpretation, as shown in **Figure 53**; however, the quantitative interpretation of the surface data is more readily accessible in the range image. Also, it is difficult to select realistic surface colors and textures to be applied. It is possible to apply brightness values to an isometric display of range data that come from another image of the same area, such as the original reflectivity or texture information. When multiband images are recorded, this combination is particularly effective.

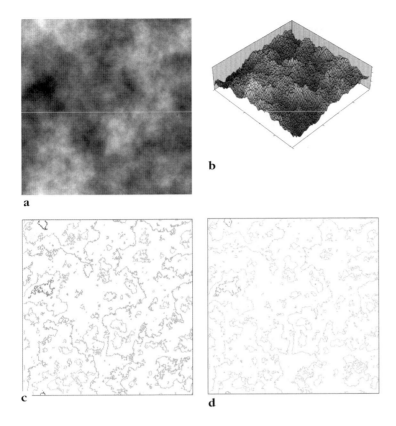

a

b

c

d

Figure 51. Surface of a metal fracture:
(a) range image (grey scale proportional to elevation);
(b) shaded grid;
(c) contour map produced by selecting pixels with neighbors above and below each of five thresholds;
(d) contour map produced by linear interpolation.

Figure 52. Reconstructed surface image of Ishtar Terra on Venus, looking northeast across Lakshmi Panum toward Maxwell Montes with an exaggerated vertical scale (From Saunders, S. (1991). Eng. Sci. Spring 1991:15–27. With permission.)

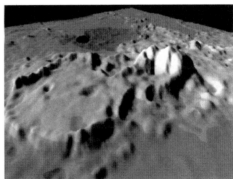

The surfaces discussed in the preceding section are in fact external physical surfaces of the specimen. Internal surfaces may be defined as boundaries between distinct regions, or in more subtle ways. For instance, **Figure 54** shows the data from the SIMS example used above, in which the depth of the voxel having the maximum concentration of silicon at any location is shown. This surface isolation provides a visualization of the shape of the implanted region. The image is shown as a shaded isometric display, as discussed previously.

Surfaces

Surfaces to be examined may be either physical surfaces revealed directly by reflection of light, electrons or sound waves, or surfaces internal to the sample and revealed only indirectly after the entire 3D data set has been acquired. The use of computer graphics to display them is closely related to other graphics display modes used in CAD, for example; however, the typical CAD object

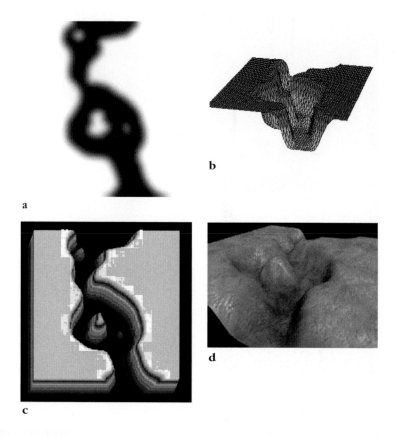

**Figure 53. Display modes
for surface
information:**
(**a**) *range image;*
(**b**) *grid mesh;*
(**c**) *isometric view;*
(**d**) *rendered terrain.*

a

b

c

d

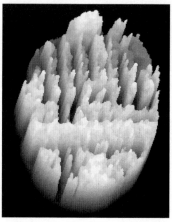

Figure 54. *Isometric display of elevation data within a volume. The height of the surface having the maximum concentration on Si in the SIMS voxel array.*

has only a few numbers to describe it, such as the coordinates of vertices. Generating the interpolated surfaces and calculating the local orientation and hence the brightness of the image at many points requires a significant amount of computing.

In contrast, the image data discussed here is typically a complete 3D data set, or at least a complete 2D range image derived from the 3D set. Consequently, there is elevation data at every pixel location in the display image, which allows for an extremely rapid image generation. Rendering the surface images shown here took only a few seconds on a desktop computer. Doing the same for a typical CAD object would take longer.

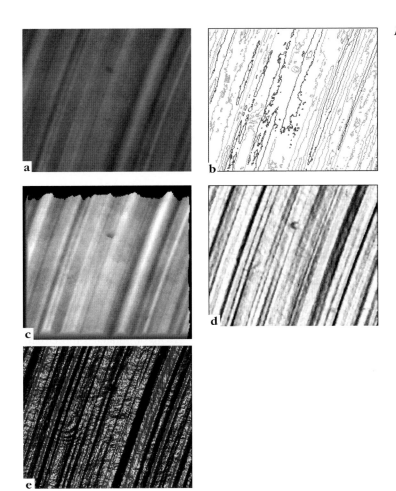

Figure 55. Presentation modes for the surface elevation data from an optical interferometer (specimen is the machined surface of nickel):

(a) original image, in which the grey-scale brightness encodes height;

(b) a contour map with grey-scale shading to indicate the height of lines;

(c) isometric view with superimposed grey scale values from image *a*;

(d) the surface data rendered as it would appear with a diffuse material;

(e) the surface data rendered as it would appear with a specular material.

Some instruments produce range images directly. Large-scale examples include radar mapping, elevation measurement from stereo pair calculations, and sonar depth ranging. At a finer scale, a standard tool for measuring precision machined surfaces is interferometry, which produces images as shown in **Figure 55**. The brightness is a direct measure of elevation, and the image can be comprehended more easily with appropriate rendering. Notice that the lens artefact (the faint ring structure at the left side of the image) is not true elevation data and when presented as such looks quite strange.

Displays of surface images (more formally of range images, because real surfaces may be complex and multivalued, but range images are well behaved and single valued) can use any of the techniques described above. These include wire mesh or line profile displays, contour maps, and shaded isometric displays, all described in more detail in Chapter 13. These all involve a certain level of abstraction.

A simple set of line profiles gives an impression of surface elevation and requires no computation, although the need to space the lines apart loses some detail. Consequently, it is sometimes used as a direct display mode on instruments such as the SEM or scanning tunneling microscopy (STM). Unfortunately, the signal that is displayed in this way may not actually be the elevation, and in this case the pseudo-topographic display can be quite misleading. Adding grid or mesh lines in both directions requires additional computation, but also increases the effective spacing and decreases the lateral resolution of the display.

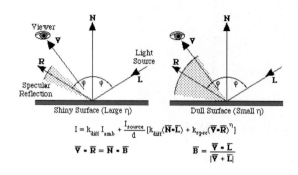

Figure 56. *Lambertian rules for light scattering from surfaces with different specularity. The vectors are N (surface normal), L (light source), R (reflection), and V (viewing direction). the k factors are the diffuse and specular reflection coefficients. The I values are the intensities of the principal and ambient light sources, and h is a constant describing the breadth of the specular reflection, which depends on the fine-scale surface roughness.*

Generating an image of a surface that approximates the appearance of a real, physical surface is known generically as rendering and requires more computational effort. The physical rules that govern the way real surfaces look are simple and are summarized in **Figure 56**. The important variables are the intensity and location of the light source and the location of the viewer. Both are usually given in terms of the angles between the normal vector of the surface and the vectors to the source and viewer. The absolute reflectivity of the surface (or albedo) must be known; if this varies with wavelength we say that the surface is colored because some colors will be reflected more than others.

Finally, the local roughness of the surface controls the degree of variation in the angle of reflection. A very narrow angle for this spread corresponds to a smooth surface that reflects specularly. A broader angle corresponds to a more diffuse reflection. One of the very common tricks in graphic arts, which can be seen any evening in television advertising, is the addition of bright specular reflections to objects to make them appear metallic and hopefully more interesting.

For a typical surface defined by a few points, as in CAD drawings, the surface is broken into facets, often triangular, and the orientation of each facet is calculated with respect to the viewer and light source. The reflected light intensity is then calculated, and the result plotted on the display screen or other output device to build the image. This would seem to be a rather fast process with only a small number of facets, but the problem is that such images do not look natural. The large, flat facets and the abrupt angles between them do not correspond to the continuous surfaces we encounter in most real objects.

Shading the brightness values between facets (Gouraud shading) can eliminate these abrupt edges and improve the appearance of the image, but requires much interpolation. Better smoothing can be achieved (particularly when there are specular reflections present) by interpolating the angles between the centers of the facets rather than simply the mean brightness values. The interpolated angles are used to generate local brightness values, which vary nonlinearly with angle and hence position. This Phong shading is even more computer-intensive.

For continuous pixel images, each set of three pixels can be considered to define a triangular facet as shown schematically in **Figure 57**. The difference in value (elevation) of the neighboring pixels gives the angles of the local surface normal directly. A precalculated lookup table (LUT) of the image brightness values for a given light source location and surface characteristics completes the solution with minimum calculations. This is done at the pixel or voxel level in the display; therefore, no interpolation of shading is needed.

When the surface rendering is accomplished in this way using section planes that are relatively widely spaced, it often produces artefacts in the reconstruction that appear to be grooves parallel to the section direction (**Figure 58**). The use of relatively large voxels can produce rendered

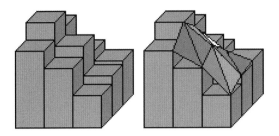

Figure 57. Diagram showing the construction of a triangular tesselation on a surface formed by discrete height values for an array of pixels.

Figure 58. Rendered surface of a fractured pelvis created from sequential tomographic section images. Note the appearance of grooves and other surface artefacts due to the section plane spacing.

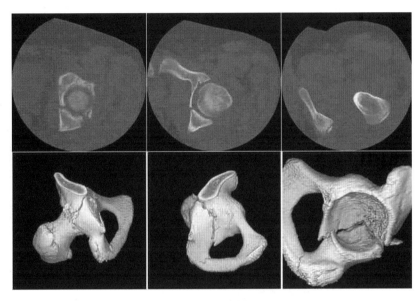

results that have an artificial blocky appearance (**Figure 59**). Applying image processing operations beforehand to range image data is often used to improve the resulting surface image. Smoothing with kernels that calculate a weighted average can produce Phong shading. Applying a median filter removes noise that would show up as local spikes or holes in the surface. The names of filters such as the rolling ball operator discussed in Chapter 3 come directly from their use on range images. This particular operator tests the difference between the minimum value in two neighborhood regions of different sizes and eliminates points that are too low. The analogy is that depressions which a ball of defined radius cannot touch as it rolls across the surface are filled in.

Rendering a surface (calculating its brightness according to its orientation relative to the viewer and light source) using the lookup table approach is fast, provided that the appropriate tables for different light source locations and surface characteristics have been calculated beforehand.

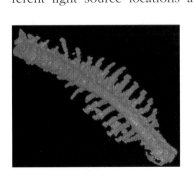

Figure 59. Rendered surface of a spine in which the coarse voxel size produces a blocky appearance.

The tables are not large and can be stored for a reasonable number of cases. The tables permit a nearly real-time animation of a rendered surface with a moving light source, which is another way to use the dimension of time to reveal 3D spatial information. Changing the surface characteristics, from diffuse to specular or from white reflection to colored, can be used to show multiband data.

Surface rendering of structures isolated within a voxel array can be enhanced by adding stereo views (**Figure 60**) and shadows (**Figure 61**). Rendered surface images have the appearance of real, physical objects and so communicate easily to the viewer, although, they obscure much of the information present in the original 3D image data set from which they have been extracted. More complex displays, which require real ray tracing, can make surfaces that are partially reflecting and partially transmitting so that the surface can be combined with volumetric information in the display. This presentation has somewhat the appearance of embedding the solid surface in a partially transparent medium, similar to fruit in Jello. Such displays can be dramatic in appearance and useful for communicating complex 3D information, but are too slow to generate and have too many variable parameters to be used for most explorations of complex data sets interactively.

Figure 60. CT slices of arteries in a human heart, combined and surface rendered, shown as stereo pair (courtesy of General Electric Co.).

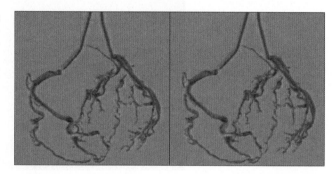

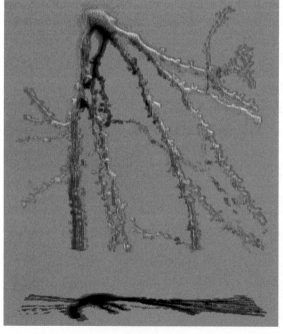

Figure 61. Stereo view of rendered dendrites, with shadows.

Multiply connected surfaces

Rendering techniques are most needed for complex, multiply connected surfaces, since the topology of such surfaces cannot be studied in 2D images. Rendering these more complex surfaces is also possible but takes a little longer. **Figure 62** shows a series of 2D planes in a 3D data set from an ion microscope. The sample, a two-phase metal alloy, shows many regions in each image. It is only in the full 3D data set that the connection between all of the regions is evident. In fact, each of the two phase regions in this specimen is a single, continuous network intimately intertwined with the other. This cannot be seen even by using resectioning in various directions (**Figure 63**).

Volumetric displays of this data set can show some of the intricacy, especially when the live animation can be viewed as the rotation is carried out. **Figure 64** shows a few orientations of the data set using ray tracing to produce a volumetric display; viewed rapidly in sequence, these produce the visual effect of rotation. The complexity of this structure and the precedence in which features lie in front and in back of others, however, limits the usefulness of this approach. Isolating the boundary between the two phases allows a rendered surface to be constructed as shown in **Figure 65**. With the faceting shown, this display can be drawn quickly enough (a few seconds on a desktop computer) to be useful as an analysis tool. A complete smoothed rendering (**Figure 66**) takes longer (several minutes on the same computer) or requires access to graphics workstations.

Figure 62. Sequential images from an ion microscope, showing two phase structure in an Fe-45% Cr alloy aged 192 hours at 540°C (courtesy M. K. Miller, Oak Ridge National Laboratories, Oak Ridge, TN).

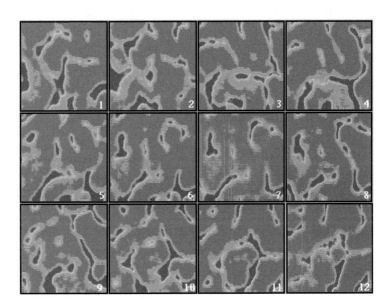

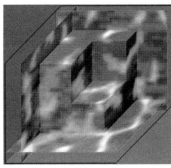

a

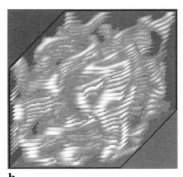

b

Figure 63. Section views of the 3D voxel array formed from the images in Figure 62: (a) stored brightness values along several arbitrary orthogonal planes; (b) stored values on a series of parallel planes with dark voxels made transparent.

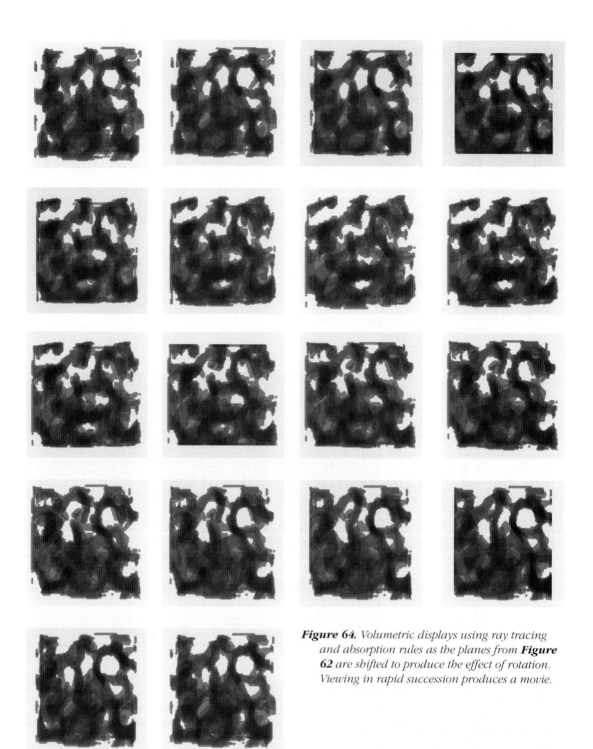

Figure 64. *Volumetric displays using ray tracing and absorption rules as the planes from **Figure 62** are shifted to produce the effect of rotation. Viewing in rapid succession produces a movie.*

The rendering of the surface follows the determination of the various surface facets. The simplest kind of facet is a triangle. In the example shown in **Figure 65**, a series of narrow rectangles or trapezoids are used to connect together points along each section outline. For features in which the sections are similar in shape and size, this faceting is fairly straightforward. When the shapes change considerably from section to section, the resulting facets offer a less realistic view of the surface shape.

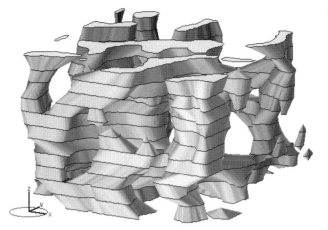

Figure 65. Simple rendering of the boundary surface between the two phases in the specimen from *Figure 62*, by interpolating planar facets between the planes.

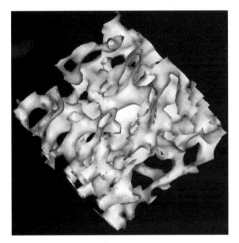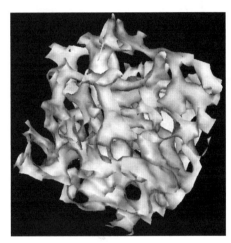

Figure 66. Two high-resolution rendered views of the boundary surface between the two phases in the specimen from *Figure 62*.

The greatest difficulty is dealing with splits and merges in the structure. This means that the number of outlines in one section is greater than in the next, and so the surface must somehow divide. **Figure 67** shows two ways to do this. In one, the junction actually lies in one of the planes. It may either be located manually or by various algorithms, such as dividing the feature normal to its moment axis at a point which gives area ratios equal to those of the two features in the next section. The rendered result is fairly easy to draw because no surface facets intersect.

The second method constructs surface facets from sets of points along the feature boundaries from the single feature in one section to both of the features in the next section plane. This technique moves the junction into the space between planes, and produces a fairly realistic picture, but requires more calculation. The intersecting planes must be drawn with a z-buffer, a computer graphics technique that records the depth (in the viewing direction) of each image point, and only draws points on one surface where they lie in front of the other.

The major drawback to this kind of surface rendering from serial section outlines is that the surfaces hide what is behind them, and even with rotation it may not be possible to see all parts of a complex structure. Combining surface rendering with transparency (so that selective features are shown as opaque and others as partially transparent, letting other structures behind become

Figure 67. Two ways to render the surface on serial section outlines where splits or merges occur: (**a**) *dividing one plane into arbitrary regions which correspond to each branch;* (**b**) *continuous surfaces from each branch to the entire next outline, with intersection between the planes.*

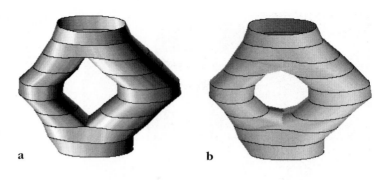

a b

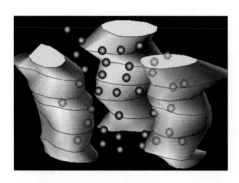

Figure 68. Combining surface rendering with partial transparency to show structures otherwise hidden by surfaces in front. The spheres which lie behind the frontmost surfaces are dimmed or shown in a different color. Notice that this is only partial transparency in that the front vertical column is completely opaque to the rear one, and the spheres are dimmed uniformly without regard to the actual amount of material in front of them.

visible) offers a partial solution. **Figure 68** shows an example in which one kind of feature (the spheres) has been given the property to show with a reduced brightness through any superimposed surface. This allows the spheres to be seen where they lie behind the columns. The dimming is not realistic (since the density of the columns is not known), however, and other structures behind the columns are completely hidden.

In the example shown previously in **Figure 65**, the boundary was determined by thresholding in each of the 2D image planes, since the plane spacing was not the same as the in-plane resolution. A certain amount of interpolation between the planes is required, which makes the curvature and roughness of surfaces different in the depth or z direction. For data sets with true cubic voxels, as for example the tomographic reconstructions shown in **Figure 23** and examples in Chapter 11, the resolution is the same in all directions, and greater fidelity can be achieved in the surface rendering. **Figure 69** shows the surface rendered image from that data set.

Multiple colors are needed to distinguish the many features present (about 200 roughly spherical particles) in this structure. This use of pseudo-color is particularly important to identify the

Figure 69. Rendered surface image of spherical particles from tomographic reconstruction (see **Chapter 11, Figure 51**) *created by interpolating surface tiles between the slices shown in* **Figure 23**, *and assigning arbitrary colors to each feature.*

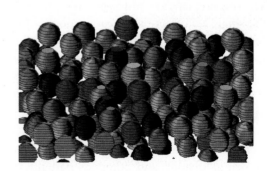

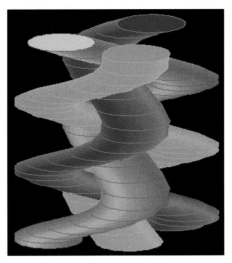

continuity of multiply connected surfaces. **Figure 70** shows another example in which the structural organization of the braid is much easier to see when each fiber is assigned a unique color palette.

The braided fibers in **Figure 70** emphasize that serial section reconstruction for 3D displays is certainly not restricted to microscopy and medical applications. The study of woven textiles and fibers used in composite materials uses the same methods (Gowayed et al., 1991). **Figure 71** uses color coding to identify the muscles and bones in a common everyday example of serial sectioning. The images were acquired by visiting the local supermarket and photographing each roast sliced from a side of beef. After aligning the images and thresholding them to delineate the various structures, the stack of slices can be rendered to reveal the 3D structure of the muscles and bones. Remember, though, that the volume, surface area and length of these structures can be determine much more efficiently by using stereological procedures to draw grids and count hits on the individual slices as discussed in Chapter 8.

Image processing in 3D

The emphasis so far has been on the display of 3D image data, with little mention of processing. Most of the same processing tools that were described in the preceding chapters for 2D images can

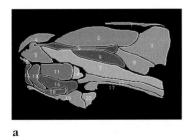

a

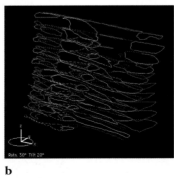

b

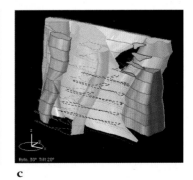

c

Figure 71. Serial sections through a side of beef:
   (a) one section with features numbered;
   (b) stack of slices;
   (c) rendered result, showing selected muscles with solid surfaces and several bones with dashed outlines.

be applied more or less directly to 3D images for the same purposes (Nikolaidis and Pitas, 2001). Arithmetic operations such as ratios in multiband data are used, for instance, in exactly the same way. Each voxel value is divided by the value of the voxel at the same location in the second image. This kind of operation does not depend on the images having cubic voxels.

Many processing operations that use neighborhoods (e.g., for kernel multiplication, template matching, rank operations, etc.), however, do expect cubic voxel arrays. In a few instances, a kernel may be adapted to non-cubic voxels by adjusting the weight values so that the different distance to the neighbors in the z direction is taken into account. This adjustment only works when the difference in z distance is small as compared to the x,y directions, for instance a factor of 2 or 3 as may be achieved in the confocal light microscope. It will not work well if the image planes are separated by ten (or more) times the magnitude of the in-plane resolution. And any departure from cubic voxel shape causes serious problems for ranking or template-matching operations.

In these cases, it is more common to perform the processing on the individual planes and then form a new 3D image set from the results. **Figure 72** shows a series of pseudo-rotation views of the MRI head images used above. Each slice image has been processed using a Frei and Chen operator to extract edges. These edges show the internal structure as well as the surface wrinkles in the brain. Furthermore, image processing was used to form a mask to delineate the brain (defined

Figure 72. Several views of the brain from the MRI data set. The skull has been eliminated, individual image planes have been processed with an edge operator, and the resulting values have been used with emission rules to create a volumetric display. Lateral shifting of the planes produces pseudo-rotation. Each pair of images can be viewed in stereo, or the entire sequence used as an animation. Structures are visible from the folds in the top of the brain to the spinal column at the bottom.

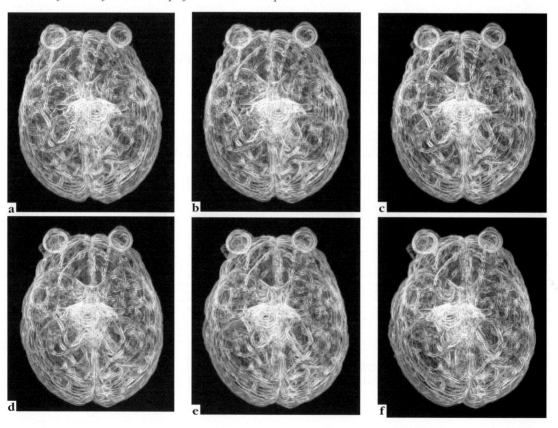

as the central bright feature in each slice) and isolate it from other portions of the image. The result is a series of slice images that show only the brain, processed to show the internal edges.

Another display trick has been used here. It is not clear just what volumetric display mode is appropriate for such processed images. Instead of the conventional absorption mode, in which transmitted light is passed through the data array, these images use the emission mode, in which each voxel emits light in proportion to its value. That value is the edgeness of the voxel as defined by the Frei and Chen operator. In other words, we see the edges glowing in space. In a live animation, or for those readers who can use pairs of the images to view the 3D data set stereoscopically, this image creates a fairly strong impression of the 3D structure of the brain. The same type of display of lines in space can be used to display contours within a 3D data set.

This illustration may serve as an indication of the flexibility with which display rules for 3D images can be bent. Nontraditional display modes, particularly for processed images, are often quite effective for showing structural relationships. There are no guidelines here, except for the need to simplify the image by eliminating extraneous detail to reveal the structure that is important. An experimental approach is encouraged.

The use of 2D processing of image planes in a 3D data set should be used with some care. It is only justified if the planes have no preferred orientation and are random with respect to the structure, or conversely if the planes have a very definite but known orientation that matches that of the structure. The latter situation applies to some situations involving coatings. When possible, 3D processing is preferred, even though it imposes a rather significant computing load. The size of neighborhoods increases as the cube of dimension. A kernel of modest size, say 7×7, may be fast enough for practical use in 2D, requiring 49 multiplications and additions for every pixel. In 3D, the same $7 \times 7 \times 7$ kernel requires 343 multiplications and additions per voxel, and of course the number of total voxels has also increased dramatically so that processing takes much more time.

For complex neighborhood operations such as gradient or edge finding in which more than one kernel is used, the problem is increased further because the number of kernels must increase to deal with the higher dimensionality of the data. For instance, the 3D version of the Sobel gradient operator would use the square root of the sum of squares of derivatives in three directions. And since it takes two angles to define a direction in three dimensions, an image of gradient orientation would require two arrays, and it is not clear how it would be used.

The Frei and Chen operator (Frei and Chen, 1977), a very useful edge detector in 2D images introduced in Chapter 4, can be extended to three dimensions by adding to the size and number of the basis functions. For instance, the first basis function (which measures the gradient in one direction and corresponds to the presence of a boundary) becomes

$$
\begin{array}{ccccccccc}
-\sqrt{3}/3 & -\sqrt{2}/2 & -\sqrt{3}/3 & & & & & & \\
-\sqrt{2}/2 & -1 & -\sqrt{2}/2 & 0 & 0 & 0 & & & \\
-\sqrt{3}/3 & -\sqrt{2}/2 & -\sqrt{3}/3 & 0 & 0 & 0 & +\sqrt{3}/3 & +\sqrt{2}/3 & +\sqrt{3}/3 \\
& & & 0 & 0 & 0 & +\sqrt{2}/2 & +1 & +\sqrt{2}/2 \\
& & & & & & +\sqrt{3}/3 & +\sqrt{2}/2 & +\sqrt{3}/3
\end{array}
$$

It should be noted that in three dimensions, it is possible to construct a set of basis functions to search for lines as well as surfaces. It remains to find good ways to display the boundaries which these operators find.

Three-dimensional processing can be used in many ways to enhance the visibility of structures. In **Figure 42**, the boron concentration was shown volumetrically using emission rules, although, the overlap between front and rear portions of the structure makes it difficult to see all of the details.

The surface rendering in **Figure 43** is even worse in this regard. **Figure 73** shows the same structures after 3D processing. Each voxel in the new image has a value that is proportional to the variance of voxels in a 3 × 3 × 3 neighborhood in the original image set. These values are displayed volumetrically as a transmission image. In other words, the absorption of light coming through the 3D array is a measure of the presence of edges; uniform regions appear transparent. The visibility of internal surfaces in this "cellophane" display is much better than in the original, and the surfaces do not obscure information behind them, as they would with rendering.

The time requirements for neighborhood operations are even worse for ranking operations. The time required to rank a list of values in order increases not in proportion to the number of entries, as in the kernel multiplication case, but as $N \bullet \log(N)$. This assumes a maximally efficient sorting algorithm and means that ranking operations in really large neighborhoods take quite a long time.

For template-matching operations such as those used in implementing erosion, dilation, skeletonization, and so forth, the situation is worse still. The very efficient methods possible in 2D by using a lookup or fate table based on the pattern of neighbors will no longer work. In 2D, there are eight neighbors so a table with $2^8=256$ entries can cover all possibilities. In 3D, there are 26 adjacent neighbors and $2^{26} = 67$ million patterns. Consequently, either fewer neighboring voxels can be considered in determining the result (e.g., just the six face-touching neighbors), or a different algorithm must be used.

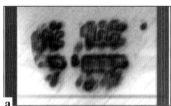

Figure 73. Volumetric display of Boron concentration from SIMS image data set. The series of images shows pseudo-rotation by shifting of planes, using the local 3D variance in pixel values to locate edges. The magnitude of the variance is used as an effective density value to absorb light along rays through the voxel array.

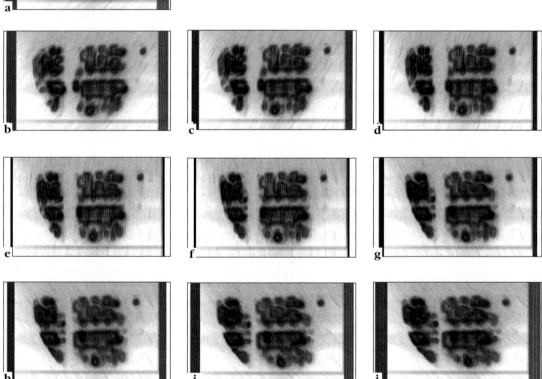

All of the morphological operations (erosion, dilation, etc.) have direct generalizations in three dimensions (Gratin and Meyer, 1992). Normally, for practical reasons, cubic voxels are used. This means that consideration must be given to the difference between face-, edge- and corner-touching neighbors. In principle, the more symmetrical arrangements of voxels mentioned previously would allow simpler erosion/dilation rules and more uniform processing, but these are rarely used. Just as in two dimensions it is necessary to distinguish between 4-connectedness (touching pixels share an edge) and 8-connectedness (touching pixels share a corner), in three dimensions 6-, 18-, and 26-connectedness possibilities exist for voxels (sharing a face, edge, or corner, respectively). For practical reasons, many methods use 6-connectedness as the simplest definition.

This has particular impact on thresholding and feature enumeration. In many 3D data arrays, thresholding based on voxel value is a simple and effective method. But in complex structures methods based on region growing are widely used, in which the user identifies a seed pixel and then all connected voxels having values within some tolerance band are selected. Another approach to segmentation of features uses a 3D extension ("balloons") of the active contours ("snakes") used in two dimensions (Kaes et al., 1987; Cohen, 1991).

The 3D analog of a Euclidean distance map can be constructed by a direct extension of the 2D method, and has the same advantages both for improving isotropy and for distance measurement from surfaces or boundaries (Borgefors, 1996). Watershed segmentation in three dimensions, however, has only rarely proved satisfactory.

Skeletonization in 3D analogous to that in 2D would remove voxels from a binary image if they touched a background or "OFF" voxel, unless the touching "ON" voxels did not all touch each other (Borgefors et al., 1999; Halford and Preston, 1984; Lobregt et al., 1980). If touching is considered to include the corner-to-corner diagonal neighbors as well as edge-to-edge touching and face-to-face touching, then a minimum skeleton can be constructed; however, if a table for the 26 possible touching neighbors cannot be used, then it is necessary to actually count the touching voxels for each neighbor, which is much slower.

It should be noted that skeletonization in 3D is entirely different from performing a series of skeletonizations in the 2D image planes and combining or connecting them. In 3D, the skeleton becomes a series of linear links and branches that correctly depict the topology of the structure. If the operation is performed in 2D image planes, the skeletons in each plane form a series of sheetlike surfaces that twist through the 3D object and have a different topological relationship to the structure. The skeleton of linear links and branches in 3D has been formed by connecting the ultimate eroded points (UEPs) in each section. A different skeleton can be constructed by joining the branch points in the 2D sections.

Measurements on 3D images

As discussed in Chapters 8 and 9, it is clear that one of the reasons to collect and process images is to obtain quantitative data from them. This is true for 3D imaging as well as 2D, and consequently some additional comments about the kinds of measurements that can be performed, their practicality and the accuracy of the results appear appropriate.

Measurements are broadly classified into two categories: feature-specific and global or scene-based. The best known global measurement is the volume fraction of a selected phase or region. Assuming that the phase can be selected by thresholding (perhaps with processing as discussed in Chapter 3), then the volume fraction could be estimated simply by counting the voxels in the phase and dividing by the total number of voxels in the array or in some other separately defined reference volume. The result is independent of whether the voxels are cubic. In fact, the same result can be obtained by counting pixels on image planes and does not depend in any way on the arrangement of the planes into a 3D array.

A second global parameter is the surface area per unit volume of a selected boundary. There are stereological rules for determining this value from measurements on 2D images, as presented in Chapter 8. One method counts the number of crossings that random lines (for a random structure, the scan lines can be used) make with the boundary. Another method measures the length of the boundary in the 2D image. Each of these values can be used to calculate the 3D surface area.

It might seem that directly measuring the area in the 3D data set would be a superior method that does not require so many assumptions. In practice, it is not clear that this is so. First, the resolution of the boundary, particularly if it is irregular and rough, depends critically on the size of pixels or voxels. The practical limitation on the number of voxels that can be dealt with in 3D arrays may force the individual voxels to be larger than desired. It was pointed out before that a 1024 × 1024 image in 2D requires 1 megabyte of storage, while the same storage space can hold only a 128 × 128 × 64 3D array.

The use of smaller pixels to better define the boundary is not the only advantage of performing measurements in 2D. The summation of boundary area in a 3D array must add up the areas of triangles defined by each set of three voxels along the boundary. A table can be constructed giving the area of the triangle in terms of the position differences of the voxels, but the summation process must be assured of finding all of the parts of the boundary. No unique path can be followed along a convoluted or multiply-connected surface that guarantees finding all of the parts.

For other global properties, such as the length of linear features or the curvature of boundaries, similar considerations apply. The power of unbiased 2D stereological tools for measuring global metric parameters is such that the efficiency and precision of measurement makes them preferred in most cases.

Feature-specific measurements include measures of size, shape, position, and density. Examples of size measures are volume, surface area, length (maximum dimension), and so forth. In three dimensions, these parameters can be determined by direct counting. The same difficulties for following a boundary in 3D mentioned previously still apply. But in 2D images the measurements of features must be converted to 3D sizes using relationships from geometric probability. These calculations are based on shape assumptions and are mathematically ill-conditioned. This means that a small error in measurements or assumptions is magnified in the calculated size distribution.

Simple shapes, such as spheres, produce good results. **Figure 74** shows the result for the tomographic image of spherical particles shown in **Figure 65**. The measurement on 2D plane slices gives circle areas that must be unfolded to get a distribution of spheres as discussed in Chapter 8. The result shows some small errors in the distribution, including negative counts for some sizes that are physically impossible, but the total number and mean size are in good agreement with the results from direct 3D measurement and require much less effort.

When feature shapes are more complicated or variable, 2D methods simply do not work. If information on the distribution of shapes and sizes is needed, then measurement in 3D, even with the problem of limited resolution, is the only available technique.

Position of features in 3D is not difficult to determine. Counting pixels and summing moments in three directions provides the location of the centroid and the orientation of the moment axes. Likewise, feature density can be calculated by straightforward summation. These properties can be determined accurately even if the voxels are not cubic and are affected only slightly by a reduction in voxel resolution.

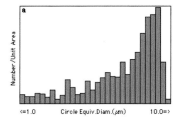 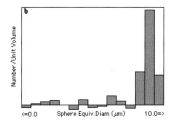 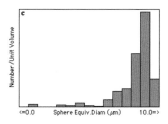

a   b   c

Figure 74. Comparison of 2D and 3D measurement of size of spherical particles in structure shown in Figure 69:
(a) size distribution of circles in 2D plane sections;
(b) estimated size distribution of spheres by unfolding the circle data in figure a (note negative values);
(c) directly measured size distribution of spheres from 3D voxel array.

Shape is a difficult concept even in two dimensions. The most common shape parameters are formally dimensionless ratios of size, such as (volume) $^{1/3}$/(surface area) $^{1/2}$ or length/breadth (length is easy to define as the longest dimension, but just as for the 2D case, the proper definition and measurement procedure for breadth is not so obvious). The selection of a parameter which has meaning in any particular situation is very ad hoc, either based on the researcher's intuition or on trial-and-error and statistical regression. In 3D, the values may be less precise because of the poorer voxel resolution, but the accuracy may be better because the size parameters used are less biased. It may also be important to the user's intuition to consider 3D shape factors, which are less unfamiliar than 2D ones.

The other approaches to shape in 2D are harmonic analysis (which unrolls the feature boundary and performs a Fourier analysis on the resulting plot), and fractal dimension determination; both were discussed in Chapter 9. These parameters can be determined rather efficiently in two dimensions, but only with great difficulty in three dimensions. The 2D results are related stereologically to 3D structure, so it is preferable to perform these measurements on the individual 2D image planes.

Closely related to shape is the idea of topology. This is a non-metric description of the basic geometrical properties of the object or structure. Topological properties include the numbers of loops, nodes and branches (Aigeltinger et al., 1972). The connectivity per unit volume of a network structure is a topological property that is directly related to such physical properties as permeability. It is not possible to determine topological properties of 3D structures from single 2D images (although minimal 3D probes such as the disector can provide unbiased estimates). These can be measured directly on the 3D data set, perhaps after skeletonization to simplify the structure (Russ and Russ, 1989). Another example, a reconstruction showing the topology of an overhand knot, was shown in Chapter 8.

Conclusion

There is little doubt that 3D imaging will continue to increase in capability and popularity. It offers direct visualization and measurement of complex structures and 3D relationships, which cannot be as satisfactorily studied using 2D imaging. Most of the kinds of imaging modalities that produce 3D images, especially tomographic reconstruction and optical sectioning, are well understood, although the hardware will benefit from further development (as will the computers and software). Current display methods are barely adequate to the task of communicating the richness of 3D image data sets to the user. New display algorithms and interface control devices will surely emerge, driven not only by the field of image processing but also by other related fields such as visualization of supercomputer data and interactive computer games. The continued increase in computer power and memory is certain. Watching and using these developments offers an exciting prospect for the future.

13

Imaging Surfaces

In many different disciplines, surfaces are more important than bulk structures. Mechanical interaction between parts involves friction and wear between surfaces, many chemical interactions take place on surfaces (including catalysis) and most modern electronic devices consist of thin layers of materials laid down in intricate patterns on the surface of substrates. The appearance of objects is dominated by their surface characteristics, textures, and coatings. In all these cases and many more, scientists and engineers need to characterize surfaces and the ways in which fabrication and use modify them. Imaging plays important roles in obtaining the information as well as presenting it for human visualization and analysis.

Producing surfaces

Surfaces are produced in a wide variety of processes, some tightly controlled and some quite chaotic. One of the oldest techniques by which mankind has produced intentional surfaces is by removal of material, for instance creating a statue or a stone tool by removing chips from a larger block of stone. Modern fabrication of parts typically involves machining, grinding, and polishing to remove material and to create a surface with specific macroscopic dimensions and also microscopic roughness.

Machining is a process in which a cutting tool removes chips from the material as it is moved relative to the workpiece. The shape of the tool's cutting tip or edge, its speed and the depth of cut, control the dynamics of chip formation which can be either ductile (long, continuous chips) or brittle (short, broken ones). The surface typically displays long grooves in one direction whose shape is determined in large part by the shape of the tool. Grinding is a process in which many small cutting points, typically facets of hard particles cemented together into a wheel, simultaneously remove material from a surface. Polishing results when many loose hard particles slide and roll between two surfaces, removing material as the surfaces move relative to one another. Impact erosion (such as sandblasting) uses particles to produce small craters on the surface. Each of these processes involve both plastic deformation and fracture, and have many variables such as applied forces, the presence of liquids, etc., which dramatically modify the appearance and performance of the resulting surface (as well as the tools or particles doing the work). A wide variety of other methods are used, ranging from fracture to electrical spark discharges, plastic deformation of surfaces by rolling, forging or extrusion, chemical etching, and so on, which modern technology employs to produce surfaces of parts by the removal or rearrangement of material. **Figure 1** shows a few different surfaces.

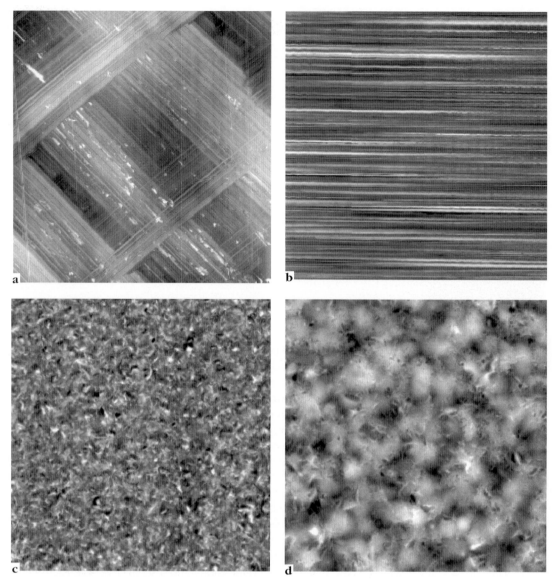

Figure 1. Range images of metal surfaces (each shows 1 square millimeter with grey scale proportional to elevation):
(a) machined (flycut) surface of aluminum;
(b) ground surface of stainless steel;
(c) vapor-polished surface of aluminum;
(d) shot-blasted surface of brass. Images courtesy Rank Taylor Hobson Ltd., obtained with a scanning probe instrument with 5 μm radius diamond stylus.

Other methods can build up surfaces by deposition. Again, this may be physical or chemical. Liquids solidify to leave solid coatings, sometimes accompanied by polymerization or formation of crystalline structures. Liquids may solidify in a mold which controls some of the surface morphology, while in some cases other forces such as viscosity and surface tension are more important than the actual mold surface. Freezing of liquids or gases onto a substrate may produce either very smooth or extremely rough surfaces depending on how the particles and molecules can move on the surface (**Figure 2**). Electroplating typically produces quite smooth surfaces by deposition of

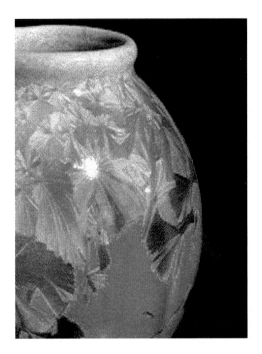

Figure 2. *Photograph of a glaze covering a ceramic pot. The glaze flows down the surface in a molten state and solidifies to an amorphous glass under the forces of surface tension. Subsequently, the atoms rearrange themselves to form crystals which nucleate and grow in the glaze, producing visually interesting patterns and also modifying the surface geometry.*

atoms from chemical solution, while ballistic deposition and aggregation of particles may generate ones with porous fractal surfaces. Some deposited layers are then subjected to selective removal, either by chemical or physical processes. This is the process by which complex multilayer electronic chips and a coming proliferation of micromechanical devices are fabricated.

Another concern about surfaces is their cleanliness. The presence of particulates, either lying loosely on the surface or attached by electrostatic or chemical forces, can disrupt the deposition of the carefully controlled layers used in microelectronics, so elaborate clean rooms and handling methods are required. Surface defects such as pits and scratches are also of concern. Chemical modification of surfaces is called contamination, oxidation, or corrosion depending on the circumstances. This is strongly controlled by the environment. Sometimes such processes may be carried out intentionally to protect the original surface from other environmental effects (for instance, aluminum is anodized to produce a thin oxide layer that provides a chemically inert, mechanically hard surface resistant to further contamination in use). Electrical and optical properties of surfaces can be modified greatly by extremely thin contamination layers.

In all these cases, there is a great need to characterize the surfaces so that the topography of the surface, and perhaps other properties such as chemical composition or electrical parameters, can be determined. Some of the surface characterization data are obtained directly by imaging methods. Even when the data are obtained in other ways, visualizing the surfaces is an imaging technique, relying on the human interpretation of the images to detect important information about the surfaces. Measurement follows to reduce the image data to a few selected numbers that can be used for process control, and to correlate the structure of the surfaces with their fabrication history on the one hand and with their performance and behavior on the other.

Devices that image surfaces by physical contact

Most of the measurement methods used to characterize surfaces are based on either some kind of microscope that provides magnified images of the surface, or scattering of radiation or particles from the surface. The methods may provide measurement of either composition or geometry, including the thickness of thin layers. Many different kinds of microscopes (and some tools that may not be conventionally thought of or named as microscopes) are used to study surfaces (Castle and Zhdan, 1997; Van Helleputte et al., 1995; Russell and Batchelor, 2001). Many of these require no surface preparation, or at most minimal cleaning; a few such as the scanning electron microscope (SEM) may require applying conductive coatings to electrical insulators. The common methods use visible light, electrons, ions, physical contact, electron tunneling, sound waves, and other signals to produce images that sometimes can be directly related to the surface geometry and in other cases are primarily influenced by the surface slope, composition, coating thickness, or microstructure. The most immediately useful imaging methods are those where the output consists of "range" values in which the elevation of the surface is directly represented in the values often shown as either profile traces or grey scale images. Although most of the examples shown here will be ones in which the grey scale directly encodes elevation, it should be understood that a similar display of chemical information or elemental concentration can be dealt with using the identical measurement and visualization tools.

One method that covers some of the newest devices, such as the atomic force microscope (AFM), and quite old and well-established methods used in industrial manufacturing, such as profilometers, is the use of a mechanical stylus that is dragged across the surface. Motion of the stylus is amplified to record the elevation of the surface point by point. If a full raster scan is used, this produces an array of elevation data that can be displayed as an image, as shown by the examples in **Figure 1**. If the mass of the moving parts of the stylus assembly is kept as low as possible, forces of a few milligrams can keep the stylus in contact with the surface (at least for surfaces that have slopes up to about 45°) at quite high scanning rates. The images in **Figure 1** were obtained in about 50 seconds each, as an array of 500×500 points covering a 1-mm square area.

Stylus instruments used in industry typically use diamond-tipped styli with a tip radius of about 1μ, which defines the lateral resolution that the instruments can provide. Vertical motion may be sensed using inductive, capacitance or interference gauges, which are capable of sub-nanometer sensitivity. With suitable calibration, which is typically provided by scanning over known artefacts, these methods are routinely used to quantitatively measure surface elevations in many industrial settings to measure surface finish, the thickness of layers, etc. These instruments have primarily been used with metal and ceramic parts, but are also capable of measuring a wide variety of softer and more fragile materials as shown in **Figure 3**.

The AFM also uses a stylus but a much smaller one (Quate, 1994; Binnig et al., 1986; Wickramasinghe, 1991). The scanning tunneling microscope (STM) stimulated a range of new microscopies which use essentially the same scanning and similar feedback principles to obtain nanometer resolution images. The AFM was introduced in 1986 as a new instrument for examining the surface of insulating crystals, and it was clear from the beginning that it would be capable of resolving single atoms, although unambiguous evidence for atomic resolution did not appear until 1993. The AFM has evolved into a flexible instrument that provides new insights in the fields of surface science, electrochemistry, biology and physics, and new adaptations of the technology continue.

By etching silicon or silicon nitride to a sharp point, or by depositing carbon in such a way that it grows into a long thin spike, a stylus can be fabricated with a tip radius of a few nanometers (**Figure 4**). This allows much greater lateral resolution than profilometer styli. But such tips are extremely fragile and easily deformed, so a variety of techniques have been devised to utilize them to probe a surface. Typically, the tip is used as a reference point and the surface is translated in the z (elevation) direction to contact it. The tip is attached to or a part of a cantilever arm whose deflection is monitored by deflection of a light beam on the rear face or sometimes by interference measurement, and vertical sensitivity below one nanometer is easily obtained. Either the sample or the stylus can be translated in an X, Y raster pattern to cover the entire surface to create a complete image. The translation is typically accomplished with piezoelectric devices, which limits the total range of motion.

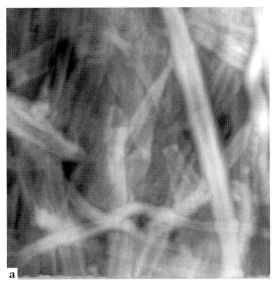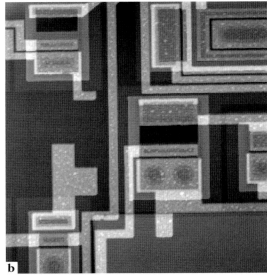

a b

Figure 3. Range images obtained with a scanned stylus instrument: (a) *paper;* **(b)** *microelectronic chip.*

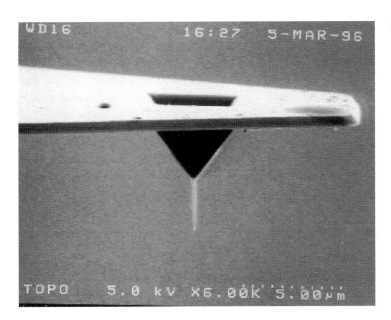

Figure 4. *Scanning electron microscope image of an ultrafine tip used for high-resolution atomic force microscopy (image courtesy Topometrix Corp.).*

The traditional and still most common mode of operation places the tip in sliding contact with the surface. In order to reduce the lateral and shear forces on the stylus and the surface, the stylus may be rapidly raised and lowered ("tapping mode"), or the lateral forces may be measured by the twisting of the stylus to determine the elastic modulus of the surface material, or the friction between the stylus and surface. Additional modes can be used in which physical contact is not actually required. For example, the stylus can track the surface without touching it with somewhat lower resolution by using attractive Van der Waals forces. In addition, some systems use strategies such as heating the tip and measuring the heat loss when it is close to the surface, vibrating it and measuring a change in characteristic frequency when it is close to the surface, or using it as a guide for light photons that interact with the surface and detect its presence without contact. The electric or magnetic force gradient and distribution above the sample surface can be measured using amplitude, phase or frequency shifts, while scanning capacitance microscopy measures carrier (dopant) concentration profiles on semiconductor surfaces. The original operational mode, which won a Nobel prize for its development, was scanning tunneling microscopy (STM), which measures the surface electronic states in semiconducting materials. The variety of operational modes of the scanned probe microscope seems nearly unlimited as manufacturers and users experiment with them, but many of these techniques are applicable only to a particular set of materials and surface types. The same technology has been used to modify surfaces, either by pushing individual atoms around or by writing patterns into masks used for lithographic manufacture of microelectronic and micromechanical devices.

One of the problems faced by AFMs is the difficulty in making quantitative dimensional measurements. Most designs use open-loop piezoelectric ceramic devices for scanning, which suffer from hysteresis and non-linearity. Software correction, no matter how elegant, can only go so far in correcting the resulting image distortions and measurement errors due to its inability to adapt to the topography of each individual sample. This particularly affects the use of the AFM in the metrology-intensive semiconductor industry. A few recent designs use a much more expensive approach which employs a separate measurement device in each axis to provide a closed-loop measurement of the piezo scanner's movement. Using either interference or capacitance gauges, these permit accurate measurements to be made on small structures such as microelectronic and micromechanical devices, magnetic storage devices, and structures such as the compact disk stamper shown in **Figure 5**.

The AFM is limited in the area that it can scan and the speed with which it can do so, and in the relief of the specimen which can be present without interfering with the cantilever arm. Special designs which attempt to alleviate one or more of these limitations are required for specific applications, as is true for all surface measurement approaches. But it is useful to have an overview of the general range of capabilities of the different techniques. **Figure 6** shows of graph (a Stedman diagram named after Margaret Stedman of the British National Physical Laboratories) that plots the range of lateral and vertical distances which can be accommodated by various surface measurement techniques. Notice that the minimum vertical dimensions detected by several methods is about the same, but the AFM has much better lateral resolution and the stylus instruments have a much larger range. Some of the other techniques plotted on the diagram will be discussed later in this chapter, but none of them offers a perfect combination of range and resolution in both vertical and lateral directions along with quantitative accuracy and an ability to deal with most kinds of surfaces.

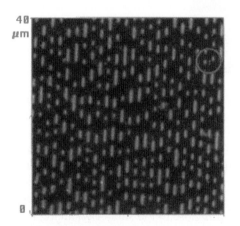
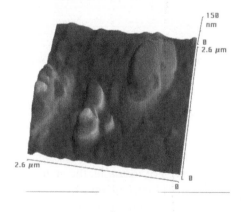

Figure 5. *AFM image of a defect on a CD stamper (image courtesy Topometrix Corp.). The presentation modes are discussed in the text.*

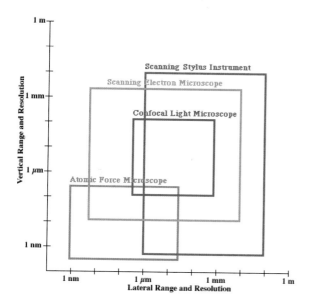

Figure 6. *Comparison of the typical range and resolution of several surface imaging technologies.*

Noncontacting measurements

Stylus instruments are limited in speed by the need to move a probe with finite mass across the specimen one line at a time. They also touch the surface which raises concerns about specimen damage. Indeed, AFMs have been used to create surface topography as well as to image it, and industrial stylus instruments are often accused of leaving surface markings where they have been used on soft metal surfaces. For some surfaces, the best solution is to make a replica that can be scanned. Plastic replicas can preserve fine detail as shown in **Figure 7**, and remove concern about damage to the original specimen.

It would appear that using light as a probe would make it possible to overcome concerns about speed or damage. Unfortunately, it also raises others. The principle drawback is that the light does not interact with the same surface that the tip feels, so that the measured elevation does not agree with that from the stylus methods (which are accepted according to various international standards for surface measurement). In many materials the light waves penetrate to a small distance

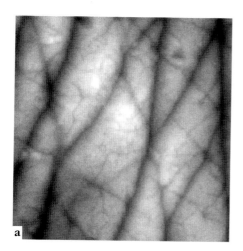

a

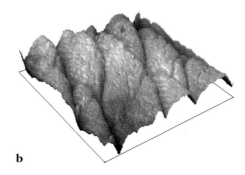

b

Figure 7. Scanned stylus image of a plastic replica of human skin:
(a) *grey-scale representation of the elevation data;*
(b) *photorealistic visualization of the surface.*

beneath the surface as they are reflected, and this surface impedance depends upon the dielectric properties of the material (which may be modified near the surface by contamination or oxidation layers). Very fine scale structure can also produce speckle and interference effects that alter the returned light in ways that mimic quite different surface structures and give incorrect results. Also, the presence of contaminant or oxidation films or local surface tilt angles of more than a few degrees can reduce the amount of light scattered back to the detector so that some points on the surface are not measured at all.

Light can be used to probe surfaces in a wide variety of ways. One choice is to use a beam of light focused to a point that is then scanned over the sample in the same way that a stylus would be, while other instruments image light from the entire area of interest at once. Point probes may use confocal optics to detect the distance to the specimen (also called focus detection), which also requires vertical scanning of either the sample or the optics. This can be done for each point, which is slow because of the need to move a finite mass, or the scan can be performed over the entire area for each Z setting as in most confocal light microscopes. In this method, the light intensity at each location is stored for each Z setting and then the peak intensity value (which may be interpolated between settings) is used to determine the surface elevation at that location. It is also possible to construct an optical point probe that uses a lens with large chromatic aberrations, and to detect the wavelength of light that is most strongly reflected. Because the lens brings each wavelength to focus at a different working distance, this provides a measure of the surface elevation. Other optical techniques such as triangulation are very sensitive to the local surface slope and have relatively poor lateral resolution.

The method which provides the greatest resolution over the greatest range is interference, and this can be done with either a point probe or for the entire surface, and with either monochromatic (usually laser) light or with white light. The classic Michelson–Morley interferometer uses mirrors to send light along two pathways, and then recombines them to produce interference patterns that show fringes corresponding to differences in dimensions that can be much smaller than the wavelength of the light. When one leg of the interferometer reflects light from the sample surface, these fringes can be used to directly measure surface elevations. The lateral resolution is only as good as the light microscope used to collect the reflected light, or about 1 µm, but the depth resolution can be 1 nm or better. For samples that do not reflect light well or that have steep cliffs or deep pits, however, there may not be enough light reflected, or the spacing of the fringes may be too close together, to provide results.

When monochromatic light is used it is possible to interpolate the elevation of a point to about 1 nm, about 1/1000th the wavelength of light; however, the fringes must be far enough apart (the surface elevation must vary gradually) that it is possible to keep track of the changes in elevation because the interference pattern repeats with every multiple of the light wavelength. Many modern systems use more than one wavelength of light or white light instead. This produces constructive interference only at one focal depth, where the path lengths are equal and all of the wavelengths are in phase. When a surface is being imaged, this means that only points along one iso-elevation contour are bright. Varying the distance between the specimen and the optics allows scanning in Z to determine the elevation of points over the entire image. This takes longer than a simple monochromatic interference pattern and is limited in precision of elevation values to the performance of the scanning hardware but can handle surfaces with much more relief and steeper slopes.

Indirect interference techniques such as projection of grids to produce moiré patterns, also produce two-dimensional arrays of elevation data. Imagine light streaming through venetian blinds onto the floor of a room. If the floor is flat, the strips of light will be straight when viewed from above. If there are irregularities, they show up directly as deviations in the lines of light and shadow. When it is scaled down to the dimensions of interest on surfaces or, at least, to distances of a few micrometers, which is the resolution of the light optics used to view the stripes, this same structured light method is easily used to measure surface geometry. Image processing can be used to detect the edges of the shadows, interpolating along each scan line to accuracies much better than the pixel spacing. Depending on the geometry this can produce vertical measurement accuracy similar to the lateral resolution of the optics (typically about 1 μm), but, of course, for only a few locations across the sample surface unless the line pattern is scanned. Toolmakers' microscopes and quality control examination of planed surfaces of lumber (among other applications) use the same basic method.

In a modern modification of the technique, mirrors or prisms are used to deflect a beam of laser light in patterns across the work piece to produce the same type of image. This has the advantage of being able to measure in various orientations and directions. Closely related to the idea of structured light is shadowing of surfaces with evaporated or deposited metal or carbon coatings, followed by measurement of the shadows cast by features and irregularities on the surface. If the image of the grid pattern in the incident light passes through another similar grid, it produces a moiré pattern, with dark lines that can be used to reveal the shape of the object. This technique is particularly useful for revealing local strains and deviations of surfaces from ideal geometric forms. Because it is fast and noncontacting, this method is often used in medical applications, ranging from orthopedic work on curvature of the spine to measuring the curvature of the lens of the eye before and after corrective surgery.

Microscopy of surfaces

Most forms of microscopy produce images in which intensity is related to the reflection of light (or some other signal) from the surface. This is only indirectly related to the surface geometry, and includes other information such as composition. Despite the difficulties in interpretation, this is still the most widespread procedure for surface examination.

The standard light microscope at moderately high magnification has a comparatively shallow depth of field. This creates many problems for examining surfaces. If the surface is not extremely flat and perpendicular to the optical axis (for example, a metallographically polished specimen), it cannot all be focused at the same time. Only low-magnification light microscopes can be used to examine rough surfaces (e.g., for fractography), and do not give much information about surface geometry. The pattern of light scattered by rough surfaces under diffuse lighting can be used to determine the roughness. It has been shown (Russ, 1994; Pentland, 1984) that a surface with fractal geometry will scatter diffuse light to produce a fractal pattern, and that there is a relationship between the fractal dimension of the surface and that of the light. This has also been reported for scanning electron microscope images of such surfaces. But measuring the overall roughness dimension of the surface is not the same thing as determining the actual coordinates of points on the surface.

On the other hand, the depth of field of the conventional light microscope is too great to measure the important dimensions in the vertical direction on rough surfaces. Paradoxically, the confocal light microscope has a much shallower depth of field (and more importantly rejects stray light from locations away from the plane and point of focus), which allows it to produce true range images from irregular surfaces. In the confocal microscope, the image is built up one point at a time (usually in a raster pattern). Each image corresponds only to points at a particular focal depth, but repeating this operation at many focal depths produces both an extended focus image in which the entire surface is imaged, and a range image in which the elevation at each point is recorded. The resolution in both vertical and lateral directions is much worse than the scanned probe microscopes, but quite useful for many surface measurement applications including metrology of some microelectronic devices.

Because of its very large depth of field, coupled with excellent resolution (typically <10 nm, much better than the light microscope) the SEM is often a tool of choice for the examination of rough surfaces. Furthermore, the appearance of the secondary electron image that is most often recorded from this instrument looks reasonably "familiar" to most observers, who therefore believe they can interpret the image to obtain geometric information. Unfortunately, this is not at all simple. **Figure 8** shows an SEM image of a surface, sintered tungsten carbide particles. This is a relatively simple surface composed of uniform composition particles with relatively flat facets. But there is no unique or simple relationship between elevation or slope and the local pixel brightness. For relatively smooth surfaces, "shape from shading" methods can convert changes in intensity to changes in slope and thus extract the geometry. The influence of fine-scale roughness, edges, surface contamination, or compositional variation prevents this from being a general purpose approach. Backscattered electron imaging is less sensitive to many of these effects and is used for some metrology applications, but only gives "real" geometric dimensions when comparison to standards is available or extensive modeling of the interactions between electron and sample is performed.

The great frustration in using the SEM to examine surfaces is that while the images look quite natural to human viewers, and seem to represent surface elevation in a familiar way, determining actual dimension values from them is nearly impossible except in very constrained cases. Metrology of integrated circuits is used to determine lateral dimensions, but even in these cases the definition of just what the relationship is between the physical contour of an edge and the voltage profile of the signal is far from certain (and highly dependent upon the voltage used, the material being imaged, the detector type and location, etc.). Metrology is used for quality control in which consistency rather than absolute accuracy is important, and there is no attempt to extract measurements in the Z direction from such images (indeed, even the visibility of points near the bottoms of grooves or contact holes is a problem).

Stereometric imaging in which two (or more) different views of the surface are combined to measure elevation is the same in principle as the generation of topographic contour maps from aerial photographs (Wong, 1980; Wang, 1990). This is not an easy technique to automate (Wrobel, 1991; Heipke, 1992; Barnard and Thompson, 1980; Zhou and Dorrer, 1994; Abbasi-Dezfouli and Freeman, 1994) however, and even with careful control of imaging conditions and measurement of

Figure 8. *SEM image of the surface of sintered tungsten carbide.*

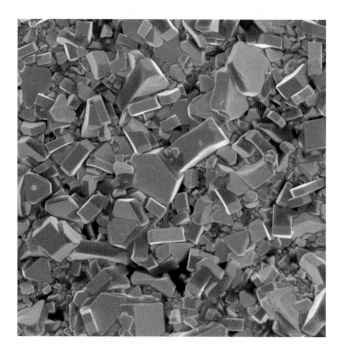

angles, the vertical resolution is typically much worse than the lateral resolution of the individual images. This is because the tilt angle δ between the two views must usually be small (7–10° is typical) to prevent points being hidden in one of the two views, and the angle enters the calculation as $1/\sin(\delta)$. The precision of lateral dimensions is magnified by any uncertainty in angle and limits the precision of the final result.

Measurement of the elevation difference between individual points is usually quite straightforward using a human to locate the same points in the two images. Then the parallax or offset of the points gives the elevation by straightforward trigonometry; however, to generate an elevation map for an entire surface requires matching a great many points, and requires automation to be practical. The two methods used for this are area-based or feature-based. Area-based matching uses cross correlation (either in the spatial domain or the frequency domain) to find the location of an area in the second image that most closely matches each area in the first. Changes in the visibility or contrast of the area between the two images, the presence of specular reflections, or repetitive structures that produce multiple matches, produce problems for this approach.

Figure 9 shows a typical result (from Chapter 12) in which two stereo images have been matched by cross correlation, testing each point in the left-eye view with possible points in the right-eye view to find the best match. The horizontal displacement (disparity or parallax) where the match was found measures the elevation of the point. Mismatched or unmatched points are typically present, and are filled in using a median filter. The calculated elevation values can then be used for measurement or visualization.

Feature matching detects locations in each image which have some characteristic such as a maximum local value of variance. These points are then matched against the similar list of points in the other image. This is generally more successful, but may match only a few thousand locations in the two images out of perhaps a million pixels, so that the intervening locations can only be interpolated. In all cases, constraints such as preserving the order of points from left to right and knowing the direction of tilt so that searching for matches need only occur in a small fraction of the total image area are important aids to the practical implementation of the methods.

Because of its great depth of field, the scanning electron microscope is very often used to obtain stereo pair images of surfaces. The SEM is also used to generate x-ray maps of surface composition, discussed separately in the next section. Instead of using electrons, light, or other radiation to form an image of the surface, quite a lot of information is available from the scattering or diffraction patterns that are produced. X-ray patterns contain data about the structure of either crystalline

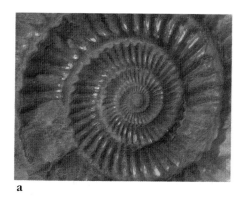 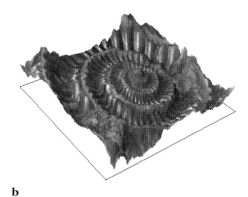

a   b

Figure 9. Surface reconstruction from stereo pair images:
    (a) left and right views of a microfossil superimposed as a color composite for viewing;
    (b) rendered surface reconstruction.

or amorphous layers. Electron scattering patterns contain information on the crystallographic arrangement and also on local strains in the material (which shows up as the displacement or broadening of lines in the pattern). Scattered patterns of electromagnetic radiation are in effect the Fourier transform of the elevation profiles of the surface and their measurement is therefore a direct method to study the surface elevation in a way that separates the information on the form or figure (the intended large scale geometry of the part), the waviness (medium scale departures from the figure), and the texture or roughness (the fine scale details on the surface). In many cases, the scattering of reflected light may also be directly related to the intended use of the surface, for instance if it is a high-precision mirror. Images such as diffraction patterns can be processed and measured using many of the same techniques as more conventional images, but are not discussed here in detail.

Surface composition imaging

The variety of techniques for probing surfaces is astoundingly broad. Some of the more common ones are the SEM using an x-ray detector, the ion microscope or microprobe using secondary ion mass spectrometry (SIMS), and Fourier transform infrared (FTIR) spectroscopy. There are many other tools used as well, particularly for measuring the thickness and composition of coatings. These include the backscattering of particles, which samples the composition and density of the sample at depths up to several micrometers beneath the surface. Also of rather specialized interest is acoustic microscopy, which is sensitive to debonding between the coating layer and substrate. Gigahertz acoustic waves have a wavelength similar to visible light, and can be used to image surface and near-surface structures that are difficult to detect with other signals. Surface waves are strongly reflected by cracks (even closed ones that cannot be seen otherwise) and bulk waves are similarly reflected by the surfaces of pores (although these subsurface waves only propagate at lower frequencies, with correspondingly poorer resolution). The speed of sound in the material can also be measured to determine the modulus of elasticity and other physical properties. Ellipsometry takes advantage of the fact that for many types of thin layer coatings, the plane of polarized light is rotated as it passes through the coating. Measurement of that rotation can provide highly precise coating thickness measurements, and when different wavelengths of light are used (or a spectrometer is used to scan an entire range of wavelengths) can also reveal details about the internal structure of the coating. This method is primarily used to measure relatively large spots, however, and not to produce images of the surface. Similarly, another spot-analysis analytical technique uses a laser-beam directed at a selected point on the surface with a light microscope to vaporize material from a pit (typically several μm across and deep) blasted from the surface so that the atomic and molecular fragments can be weighed in a mass spectrometer.

Several different types of ion microscopes are used. Many can produce elemental composition maps of the surface, or a series of such images at various depths in the material. An incident beam of ions knocks the uppermost layer of atoms loose from the specimen, either one point at a time (the ion microprobe) or over the entire surface at once. These atoms are ionized and are then accelerated into a mass spectrometer which separates them according to their mass/charge ratio, identifying specific elements and isotopes. A detector or detector array then produces an image. This typically represents the spatial distribution of one selected element at a time across the imaged area, with a lateral resolution of about 1 μm (depending on the diameter of the incident beam in the case of the ion microprobe and the resolution of the ion optics in the case of the ion microscope) but with a depth resolution of one atomic layer. Rapid switching from one element to another as layers are removed produces complete data sets of the structure of the material.

Compositional mapping of surfaces is particularly important for examination of deposited coatings and the identification of contamination. The most common approach to this mapping uses a raster-scanned electron beam to generate characteristic x-rays from the atoms present, which are then detected. The unique energy or wavelength of the x-rays identify the elements, and calculations based on the physics of x-ray generation can be used to determine their amounts. The lateral and depth resolution is limited to the order of 1 µm by the range of the electrons. Several different types of x-ray spectrometers are used; the diffractive or wavelength-dispersive type measures x-rays from one element at a time but with good trace element sensitivity while the more common type energy-dispersive type can measure all of the elements present at the same time, but with poorer detectability. These typically produce "dot map" images for several elements at once (**Figure 10**), which only approximately delineate the regions containing the elements and must be processed and combined as discussed in the following section. Other signals, such as Auger electrons, come from a smaller region near the point of entry of the focused electron beam and have better spatial and depth resolution, but because the signal to noise level is poor are not so good at detecting minor and trace elements.

Figure 10. X-ray maps from a mineral (mica) showing the location of several elements (as labeled on each image). Each dot corresponds to the location of the beam when one x-ray with the proper energy was detected, but some of these x-rays are the Bremsstrahlung background and are not characteristic x-rays of the element selected. This produces a finite background level in parts of the image where the specimen may not contain the element. Only in high-concentration areas are the boundaries of phase regions well delineated (images courtesy Pia Wahlberg, Danish Technological Institute).

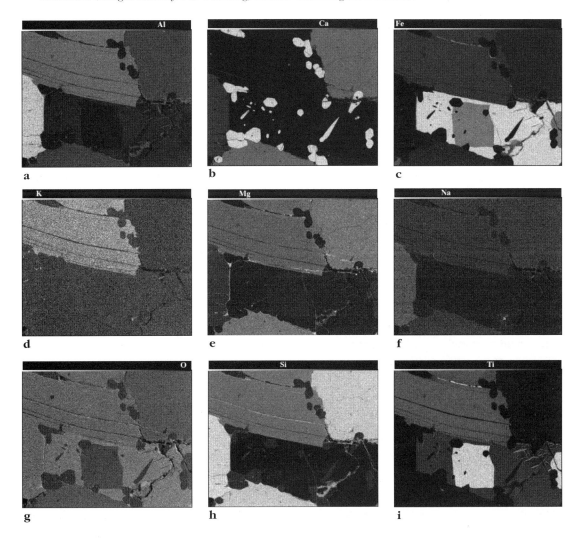

Molecular identification of coatings and contamination can be made using infrared spectroscopy, in which various vibratory modes of the molecules are excited to produce characteristic spectral peaks. This method is most suitable to the analysis of organic materials and coatings, such as plastics. The spatial resolution of this approach is limited to several micrometers by the light optics used.

Processing of range images

Elevation data from surfaces produced by the various methods discussed above are typically recorded as 8- or 16-bit grey-scale images. Each pixel has a value that represents the physical elevation or composition of the corresponding surface location. Because most of the techniques described look vertically down upon the surface, the data are single valued and represent only the uppermost point for surfaces whose irregularity is so great that undercuts and bridges can occur. The SEM is an exception to this, as shown in **Figure 11**, which shows a complex polymer surface with undercuts and bridges which a range image cannot reveal. Integer data stored for each pixel in a range image can be converted to an elevation value in appropriate units (nm, μm, etc.) using scale data that are usually stored in the file header. Unfortunately, no standard format is used for this data. Not only does each manufacturer have its own format (which is not always generally readable or well documented), but some have more than one format that corresponds to different instruments.

Reading in these different file formats and storing the data in some standardized format such as TIFF files may require custom programming. Some image processing and display programs do have the ability to read arrays of data (i.e., images) in a wide variety of data formats provided that the user can specify (or deduce) the necessary format information. This typically includes at least the length of the header and perhaps where specific scaling or other information is stored within in, the dimensions of the array and whether the data are stored in rows or columns, and the data format (byte, integer, long integer, real, etc., and whether the byte order is Intel or Motorola — low word first or high word first).

Once the data are available, the kinds of processing that are required for surface images depend strongly on what kind of instrument was used. Some examples will serve to illustrate the possibilities:

Interference microscopes often have drop-out pixels where the local slope of the surface was too great (more than a few degrees from normal) to return enough light to the optics to permit

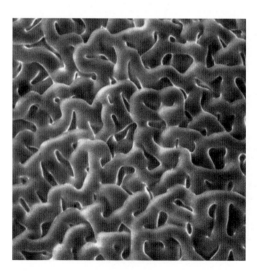

Figure 11. *Scanning electron microscope of the complex surface of a polymer, with undercuts and bridges.*

measurement. These points can be detected by filling the array beforehand with an illegal or impossible value that is replaced by real measurement data. Any pixel that retains the original value is a drop out point and must be filled in, and the most common way to do this is with a median or smoothing filter. A simple median would suffice for single points, but in many cases regions several pixels across or arranged as a line corresponding to some step or ridge on the surface may be dropped out. In this case a modification of the median approach is necessary. For example, for each dropout pixel, build an array of the neighborhood pixels that are not dropouts. If this is not an empty list, rank them into order and find the median, and place it into the missing location. After this has been done for all of the dropout pixels in the image, see if any remain. If so, repeat the process until every point has been filled in. This will fill in even large areas from their periphery and is sometimes preferable to linear or spline interpolation between pixels around the drop out, which produces blurred and smoothed edges.

A slight improvement in the basic iterated median can be achieved by using a weighted median in which pixels contribute to the decision on the value to be entered into the central pixel in proportion to how far away they are. For a 3×3 neighborhood, the corner pixels are $\sqrt{2}$ farther away than the ones that share an edge. Placing each corner pixel value into the list of values to be sorted twice and placing the edge pixel values into the list three times gives a ratio of 1.5 which is close to 1.414... and produces the desired weighted median when the list is sorted. For a 5-pixel-wide circular neighborhood (**Figure 12**) the pixel distances are 1, $\sqrt{2}$, 2, and $\sqrt{5}$. Weights of 3 for the edge neighbors, 2 for the corner neighbors, and 1 each for the more distant pixels approximate the relative contribution of the neighbors according to their distance. Note that this weighting increases the length of the list of values that must be sorted, which slows the operation significantly and is why larger integer weights which would more closely match the inverse distances are not used. For a single dropout pixel with all 20 neighbors in a 5-pixel-wide circle contributing, the sorting list grows from 20 values to 32, approximately doubling the sorting time. If the list of values is even in length rather than odd, the average of the two central values in the sorted list may be used.

Reducing or removing noise in range images uses the same methods as other images: either a median filter or some type of averaging filter such as the Gaussian. For surface images, however, they are best not applied in the same type of round neighborhood as shown in Chapter 3. Instead, the neighborhood is restricted to pixels that lie on the same portion of the surface, excluding points at a different elevation or on a surface with a different slope. This is an example of an adaptive neighborhood filter, similar to the procedures used to smooth geographic data (also a range map) called kriging. In the example shown (**Figure 13**), the neighborhood restriction provides superior noise reduction while preserving fine lines and corners.

Stylus instruments, whether macroscopic ones with diamond tips several micrometers in diameter or atomic force microscopes using Buckytubes to probe much smaller lateral dimensions, share some of the same image analysis problems and require anisotropic filtering. The scan rate along each line (the X-direction) is typically determined by the dynamics of the stylus itself — the mass of the moving tip and the applied force — which determines the maximum speed at which the tip

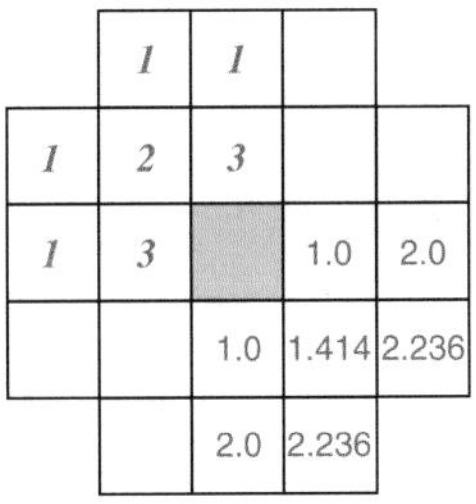

Figure 12. *Weighted median filter duplicates pixel values 2 or 3 times for the closest pixels (red) approximately in inverse proportion to their distance from the center, as shown in blue.*

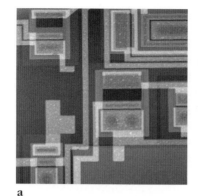
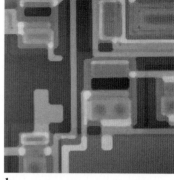

Figure 13. Noise reduction using a restricted neighborhood:
(a) *original image showing noise;*
(b) *conventional median filter (7-pixel diameter) applied;*
(c) *mean filter in a 9-pixel diameter and a threshold to exclude values more than 40 grey levels different from the local surface;*
(d) *median filter with the same neighborhood as **c**.*

a   b

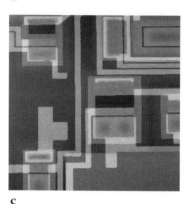
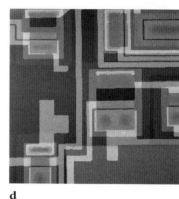

c   d

can move across the surface while remaining in contact with it. Too high a force will result in damage to the surface or the tip, but too low a restoring force will allow the tip to skip over holes or fly from rising slopes. Depending on whether the stylus moves some sensing element (an interferometer, capacitance or inductance gauge for example, or perhaps just a beam of light) or the surface is moved to null the position of the stylus (the typical AFM mode of operation) and the signal to the piezoelectric drivers is recorded, the output signal for the surface elevation is usually an electrical voltage. This must be amplified and then digitized, and in the process suitable filtering can be applied with a time constant appropriate for the scanning speed. This reduces the noise along each scan line, and eliminates the need for subsequent digital filtering to be required to reduce noise. Filtering may be used as discussed in the following paragraphs to separate the low-frequency signals related to surface form and waviness from the high-frequency roughness value, but that is part of the process of measurement rather than image enhancement.

The situation is quite different in the Y-direction (from one line to the next). A significant amount of time passes between sequential lines in the raster scan, allowing for changes in the mechanical and electronic components. Most systems scan in one direction only (to minimize hysteresis problems) and have a retrace scan during which the stylus is raised and not in contact with the sample. Repositioning the stylus to the exact same value is very difficult when the resolution of these methods in the vertical direction is of the order of 1 nm, The result is that subsequent scan lines tend to be offset from each other. Because the eye is sensitive to abrupt changes in brightness that extend over large distances, this produces images in which a visible horizontal stripe pattern may be seen. Some AFM manufacturers attempt to alleviate this problem by adjusting each line so that the average value is the same as that of the preceding line. This is rarely a good idea — it means for example that if there is a rising peak somewhere in the image area, the background around the peak will be depressed as the peak rises, producing false data and even an incorrect visual impression of the surface, as shown in **Figure 14**.

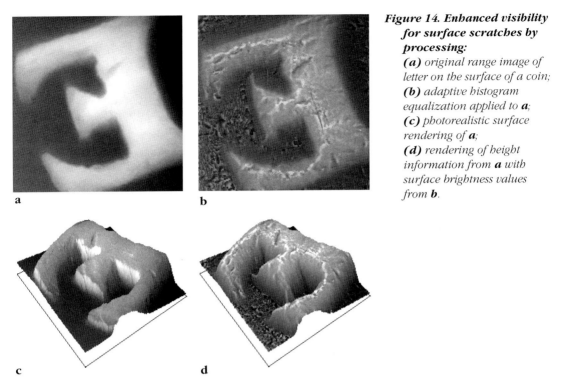

Figure 14. Enhanced visibility for surface scratches by processing:
(a) *original range image of letter on the surface of a coin;*
(b) *adaptive histogram equalization applied to **a**;*
(c) *photorealistic surface rendering of **a**;*
(d) *rendering of height information from **a** with surface brightness values from **b**.*

A better solution can be used instead of mean or average value for this line-to-line adjustment, although it requires more computation. The ideal solution would be to align the mode values of sequential lines of data. Under the assumption that the surface consists primarily of a background level with some roughness superimposed on it, plus major features of interest that rise or fall with respect to that plane, the mode is by definition the most probable surface elevation value. For a relatively small collection of data points (most area scans have only a few hundred data points along each line), the mode is not robustly determined. But for any distribution the median is closer to the mode than is the mean. Just as the median value is preferred over the mean for filtering noise from an array of pixels, so the median offers a workable solution for adjusting the scan lines in a raster scan stylus image. **Figure 15** shows this method applied to a typical image of a rough surface.

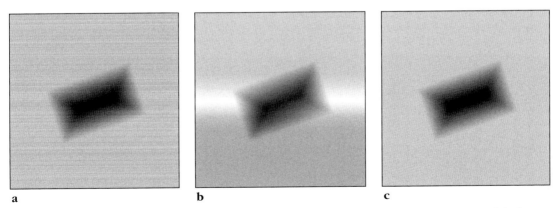

Figure 15. AFM scan of an etch pit in silicon, showing the line offsets in the raw image (a), *the darkening artefact resulting from correction by adjusting the mean value of each line **(b)**, and the improved result using the median value **(c)**.*

Another artefact in AFM images that is best avoided by proper attention to the hardware but which seems in principle to be correctable to some extent in software, is the deconvolution of tip shape from the images. As shown in Chapter 5, if the point spread function of an image can be measured, dividing the Fourier transform of the image by the transform of the point spread function can remove much of the smearing or loss of resolution, so that the inverse transform yields an improved image. Real AFM tips are far from perfect, exhibiting various departures from a ideal symmetrical point. Scanning the tip over a known artefact such as a circular disk (Jarausch et al, 1996; Keller, 1991; Keller and Franke, 1993; Markiewicz and Goh, 1994, 1995; Villarrubia, 1994, 1996, 1997) allows calculation of the tip shape, and permits this deconvolution. In practice, the tips have a short life and no two are identical, so that frequent recalibration is required; however, tip deconvolution is only important at the highest magnification and finest resolution levels.

Processing of composition maps

Most surface composition maps that are obtained by ion mass spectroscopy, x-ray energy spectroscopy, or other methods, suffer from low signal levels. As discussed in Chapter 3, this can in principle be rectified by collecting more data, but this is generally not desirable on economic grounds and sometimes is impossible because the analysis alters or consumes the surface. Thus, noise reduction methods, such as weighted smoothing or median filtering, are often applicable. **Figure 16** shows the Potassium x-ray map from **Figure 10** processed with a Gaussian smoothing operator, a conventional median and a hybrid median. The latter gives the best preservation of edges, corners and fine lines.

When multiple images are obtained of the same area showing the spatial distribution of different elements or other chemical data, it is very important to find ways to display them in combinations that will communicate the information to the observer, and to find ways to delineate and distinguish the various phases that are present. Combining multiple images as color planes offers one approach to this, as shown Chapter 1 and repeated in **Figure 17**; however, because of the way that the display hardware (and human vision) works, this allows only three planes (R, G, and B) to be assigned and there may be many more individual images available than that. The situation is analogous to the situation for remote sensing images; the Landsat thematic mapper records seven wavelength bands from the visible into the infrared, and other satellites capture even more. There is no straightforward way to "see" all this information at one time; the choice of which planes to show and in which colors can be quite subjective and can reveal (or conceal) quite different aspects of the information.

If the individual elemental maps can be thresholded to correspond to the intensity levels from individual phases, then Boolean combinations of the planes using "AND" and "NOT" permits forming binary images of each phase, which can then be measured. This process corresponds to setting up threshold ranges in an N-dimensional intensity space corresponding to the number of elements present, in which the ranges are rectangular prisms in shape. This is often adequate to distinguish

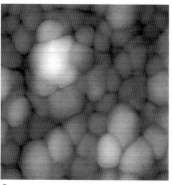

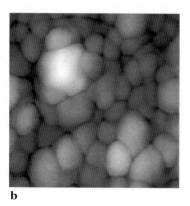

Figure 16. AFM scan of a chemically deposited surface before and after the correction of line offsets.

a   b

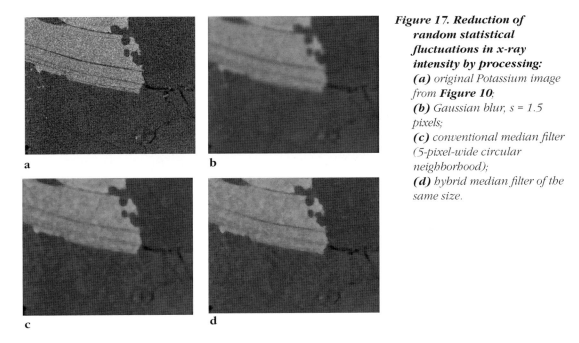

Figure 17. Reduction of random statistical fluctuations in x-ray intensity by processing: (a) original Potassium image from **Figure 10**; *(b)* Gaussian blur, s = 1.5 pixels; *(c)* conventional median filter (5-pixel-wide circular neighborhood); *(d)* hybrid median filter of the same size.

the phases present in real materials, but a more free-from shape that corresponded to the natural variations in intensity for each phase would be preferred.

Some statistical techniques plot the intensity of each pixel in each of the image planes as a vector or point in n-space (nine dimensions for the example shown here) and then search for clusters in that space. Once clusters are identified and the boundaries around them defined, the various phases present can be identified (MacQueen, 1968; Anderberg, 1973; Hartigan, 1975). This is a direct extension of methods discussed in Chapter 10. The pixels whose values lie within each cluster are then classified as belonging to the corresponding phase, and a new image can be generated with unique colors for each class so that the phases are delineated (Bright et al., 1988; Mott, 1995; DeMandolx and Davoust, 1997). **Figure 18** shows the results of an unsupervised cluster analysis technique using principal components analysis applied to the raw data from **Figure 10**; seven phases are identified and arbitrarily color coded.

When there is *a priori* information about the composition of the various phases expected to be present, this method works quite well. Cluster detection without such information, however, suffers from several problems. First, the statistical techniques will always be better able (in a statistical sense) to segment the space by defining more clusters, so unless the number of phase clusters is known the results are suspect. Second, clusters for minor phases representing only a few percent by volume of the structure will be represented by only a few percent of the points. Although these phases may be very important (e.g., for the properties of materials and the economics of mineral ores) they will be poorly defined in the n-space plot and very hard to detect. They are likely to be overlooked amid the background of points from pixels that straddle boundaries between major phases. Principal components methods, for example, are more likely to segment single phase regions based on minor gradients in composition or statistical variations in intensity, instead of identifing the presence of important minor phase regions.

Data presentation and visualization

Many types of surface measurement instruments produce data arrays with very large range to resolution ratios. In other words the number of bits that encode the elevation or other surface

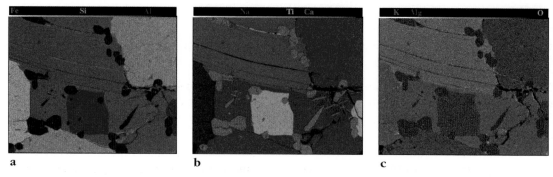

a   b   c

*Figure 18. Color combinations from the nine elemental x-ray maps in **Figure 10**. Each of the three planes (RGB) can be assigned to any of the nine planes, so this one data set can be displayed in more than 500 different ways.*

characterization data are very large. Most image processing and display programs cope adequately with 256 grey levels, but even this exceeds the ability of human vision to distinguish them on a computer screen. Resolution of 1 nm over a range of 1 mm, which is quite possible with a high-precision stylus or interferometric instrument, produces a million levels (20 bits). This far exceeds the capabilities of displays or of perception. Consequently, the display routines must either select one part of the entire range to display, or compress the data to show the entire range. Processing can help, for instance by dealing with local slopes or derivatives rather than absolute values, but this also requires some user experience to interpret.

The very large dynamic range of the data from surface measuring tools can only be displayed on the computer screen at the cost of making small but measurably different value appear with indistinguishably small differences in brightness. One particularly effective way of assisting in the visualization of such small changes, often associated with dirt or defects, is the adaptive neighborhood histogram equalization introduced in Chapter 4. **Figure 19** shows an example, a range image of the raised surface of a letter on a coin. Scratches on both the lower coin face and the raised letter can barely be detected in the original, but become visually quite evident after applying the equalization procedure, which makes small differences larger while suppressing large ones. Other processing techniques, discussed in preceding chapters, can also of course be employed on range images, but should be done so always recognizing that the actual numeric elevation values are altered and can no longer be used for measurement purposes.

Range images, in which the grey scale value at each pixel represents the elevation (or some other surface parameter) at that point, contain all of the raw information in the data array. Even if the range can be accommodated by the display (for instance by dividing down the resolution with

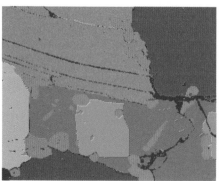

*Figure 19. Color-coding of the seven major phases in the mica sample from **Figure 10**, as identified by an unsupervised cluster analysis method.*

which the data were acquired, using a local equalization technique, or creative use of false colors), the resulting image is an unfamiliar one to human observers, and requires experience to interpret. Using false colors to increase the ability to visually discriminate small changes makes the resulting images even more unfamiliar.

Contour maps draw isoelevation lines, which are exactly the same as topographic maps of the earth's surface. These are familiar to many people and can be more easily be interpreted because they make it easy to follow the contour lines to identify the shape of protrusions and valleys, and to identify points at the same elevation. Of course, they also eliminate a great deal of information (the elevation data for all of the other pixels on the surface), but this is part of the simplification that makes interpretation easier. **Figure 20** shows the elevation of a familiar coin displayed as a grey-scale range image, one that has been color-coded, and one reduced to a small number of contour lines (which have also been color coded to make it easier to distinguish their elevation values).

Contour maps are less successful at communicating visual information when the lateral scale of detail is finer, or when the surface if very anisotropic, as shown in **Figure 21**. In these cases the individual lines are close together and hard to distinguish, and the lines do not tie together different areas of the surface very well. Whenever contour lines become close together because of the presence of fine detail or steep slopes, it is necessary to reduce the number of contour lines to help clarify the map.

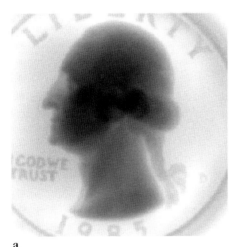

a

Figure 20. Range image of a coin (from a scanning stylus instrument, data courtesy of Paul Scott, Rank Taylor Hobson Ltd.), displayed as
(a) *a grey-scale range image;*
(b) *a color-coded range image;*
(c) *a color-coded contour map with ten isoelevation lines.*

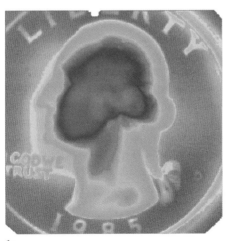

b

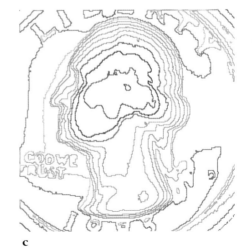

c

Figure 21. *Range images and contour maps (with five isoelevation lines) for an injection molded polymer surface (**a,b**) and a ground metal surface (**c,d**).*

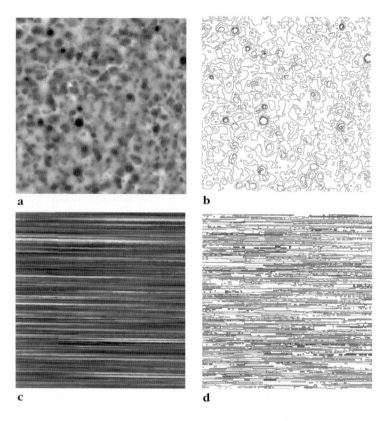

a   b

c   d

The visual impression of surface relief can be improved by processing. A directional derivative creates an "embossed" appearance with light and dark contrast along edges and gradients. As discussed in Chapter 5, a convolution kernel of weights of the form

$$
\begin{array}{ccc}
+1 & +1 & 0 \\
+1 & 0 & -1 \\
0 & -1 & -1
\end{array}
$$

produces the effect of lighting the surface from the upper left corner and produces the effect of shadows which the eye interprets as relief. The direction should always be from the top; if bright edges appear on the bottoms of edges the human vision system (which is accustomed to lighting from above) inverts the interpretation of the data and perceives hills as pits and vice versa.

The derivative image shows fine detail but hides the overall elevation changes in the data. This can be alleviated by combining the greyscale range image with the derivative. This may be done by adding the two (simply change the central value in the kernel from 0 to 1), but results that correspond more closely to the way vision perceives texture on surfaces can be obtained by multiplying the two images together. This is shown in **Figure 22**. A particularly attractive version of this display can be constructed by using the information from a color coded range image as well. In **Figure 22d** a hue, saturation, intensity (HSI) model was used with the elevation assigned to the hue for each pixel and the derivative assigned to the intensity (saturation is set to 50%). The shadows create an impression of relief while the color informs the eye about overall elevation values.

These results compare quite favorably to the results of a true rendering of the surface using each triangle of neighboring pixels as a facet and calculating the reflection of light from a light source in a fixed position as shown in **Figure 23**. In this type of calculation the surface can be given various reflectivity characteristics, either more diffuse or more specular. In the examples shown a full

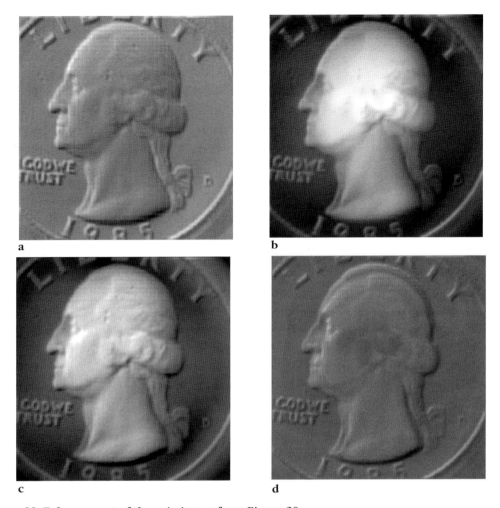

Figure 22. Enhancement of the coin image from Figure 20:
(*a*) *directional derivative;*
(*b*) *the derivative added to the original grey values;*
(*c*) *the derivative multiplied by the original elevation values;*
(*d*) *color image with the elevation in the hue plane and the derivative in the intensity image.*

ray-tracing and Phong shading was used. The latter method varies the shade across each facet according to the angle variation between neighboring facets, and produces a very smooth and realistic rendered surface as used in computer-aided design (CAD) workstations. The rendered image can also be color-coded, by using the grey-scale rendering of reflectivity as the intensity channel and the elevation as the hue channel as discussed above. Examples of this are shown in **Figure 24**.

Altering the displayed lighting and shading of surfaces can be an extremely powerful visualization tool for surface examination, taking advantage of the abilities to interpret surface images that humans have evolved in response to real-world experiences. Specular enhancement of surface appearance has been demonstrated by (Malzbender et al., 2001). They use multiple light sources (40 in the examples shown) to illuminate a specimen, which enables the local surface orientation at each location to be determined by shape-from-shading, also called photometric stereo. This data set is then represented mathematically as a polynomial map of orientation and texture, so that the appearance can be computed with altered surface reflectivity characteristics and any selected

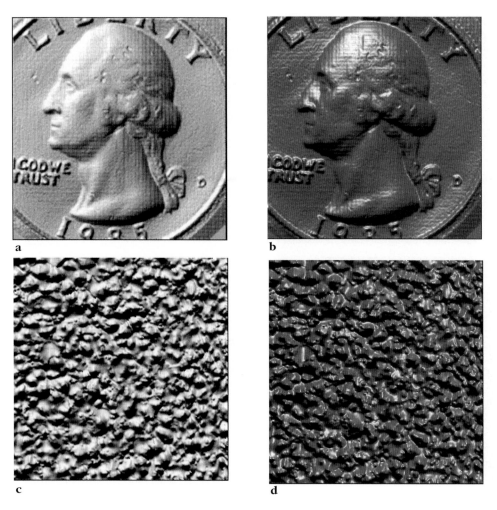

a   b

c   d

*Figure 23. Rendered surfaces of the coin (from **Figure 20**) and the polymer (from **Figure 21**), treating the surface as though it were a diffuse scatterer (plaster of Paris) or a specular one (shiny plastic or metal). The grid pattern visible in the coin image is an artefact of the scanner used to obtain the images, which becomes more visually evident in this display mode.*

illumination direction. **Figure 25** shows the enhanced appearance of a Cuneiform tablet with synthetic specular shading computed from the estimated surface orientation.

With this data set, it is also possible to interactively alter the illumination direction by moving the mouse over the image. **Figure 26** shows four images from this procedure, in which fine details on the surface can be studied as the lighting is altered. For instance, one interesting note is the fingerprint left in the wet clay by the scribe who prepared this tablet 4000 years ago in Sumeria, which can be discerned as a series of ridges near the upper left corner of the tablet. Such fine details are generally not observable without this enhancement technique.

Rendering and visualization

The views shown previously all look onto the surface from directly above. This normal view shows all of the data, but is not the most familiar to a human observer. The use of computer graphics to

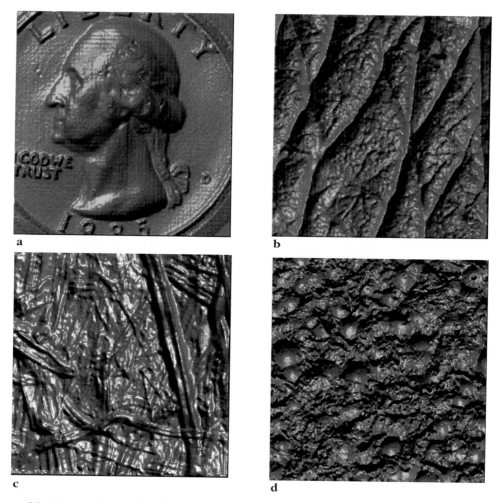

Figure 24. Color coded rendered surfaces using a hue/intensity combination:
   *(a) coin (from **Figure 20**);*
   *(b) skin (from **Figure 7**);*
   *(c) paper (from **Figure 3**);*
   *(d) shotblasted metal (from **Figure 1d**).*

render the surface from an oblique point of view (which many programs allow to be selected or even interactively rotated) produces an image that makes it easier to visualize the surface morphology, and perhaps to detect the features of interest. The oldest and simplest approach to this is to plot elevation profiles along some of the horizontal rows of pixels, displacing each line vertically and laterally to create the effect of a surface, and skipping some rows so that the lines are adequately spaced apart. **Figure 27** shows two examples of this. In the first, the coin image from **Figure 20**, the lines are well spaced and the surface slopes gradual enough that there are only a few places where lines are hidden (and erased). The result is a fairly easy surface to interpret. In the second example, the polymer image from **Figure 21**, the presentation is harder to interpret because so many lines cross each other and the overall morphology is obscured. Also in these displays the width of each line profile is the same, so that there is no perspective applied to the view. In this type of isometric presentation the human familiarity with the rules of perspective causes this constant width of the data to be misinterpreted as giving the array a wider apparent dimension at the back than at the front.

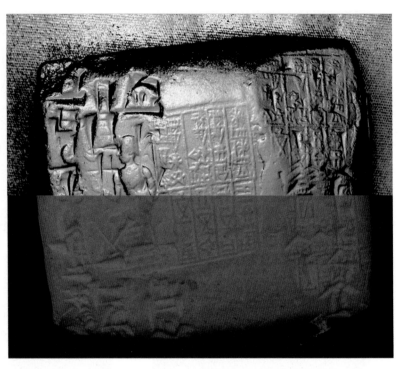

Figure 25. Specular enhancement of the image of a cuneiform tablet by computing the rendered reflection from the surface based on orientation data calculated by shape-from-shading using multiple images with different light source locations (image courtesy Tom Malzbender, Hewlett Packard Labs, Palo Alto, CA). Bottom half of the image shows the original surface appearance.

With the continued advance in computer graphics capabilities, in the form of more processing power and displays with more grey levels and colors, much more realistic presentations can be generated. Adding perspective also makes the data seem more realistic, and adding cross lines that connect together points on success line profiles breaks the surface up into an array of square or rectangular tiles that improve the interpretability of the surface morphology by showing slopes in the second direction. Increasing the line density provides more information, but still must omit many lines and rows of pixels in order to avoid overwhelming the eye with too many disappearing lines. Coloring in the tiles according to the elevation of the points provides additional cues to depth. The results (shown in **Figure 28**) represented the state of the art for desktop computers only a few years ago, but this is now easily performed on the typical desktop machine.

The most visually realistic presentation uses actual surface rendering to control the brightness of each facet on the surface. Instead of square tiles that must be bent to fit the four corner points (which in general will not lie in a plane), triangular tiles are simpler to deal with. Three corner points define the triangle and the orientation of the facet with respect to the line of sight and a light source location permits calculation of the intensity to be assigned to the facet. This can be done with complete photorealism given the time and computing power, but there will in general be a very large number of facets to render and faster methods are sought. We can perform this operation by shading each facet according to the product of its absolute height and its derivative to produce a very quick and visually realistic rendering.

Figure 29 illustrates this method. In **Figure 29a**, the edges of the individual triangular facets are drawn in for clarity. But with this method it is practical to create a facet for every pixel and its immediate neighbors, so the full resolution of the data set can be displayed. The result is shown in **Figure 29b**. In computer graphics (as used in CAD programs for example) it is common to apply shading to facets so that they blend in with their neighbors (Gourard or Phong shading) and to not reveal lines where they meet. But while that method is important for the small number of large facets encountered in CAD renderings, it is unnecessary for the tiny facets that correspond to each pixel, because the facets may cover only 1 or 2 pixels on the display. This also speeds up the process.

It is useful to compare this method against the slightly simpler display procedure of using the elevation to shade the facets, or using false colors to indicate elevation, as shown in **Figure 30**. These methods produce much less realistic results for visualization, and require a more educated eye on the part of the user. It is important to understand that human vision is an important tool for examining surface images, since the presence of defects or other features of interest is usually far more readily discerned by an experienced observer than is possible with computer pattern recognition programs.

It is also possible to introduce color to these displays using the same procedure as shown in **Figure 24**, applying the elevation as a color in the hue channel and the slope or Phong-rendered values in the intensity channel, while drawing each facet in its appropriate place on the screen to generate a perspective-corrected visual representation of the surface geometry. This is far more visually interpretable than simply applying false color, as shown in **Figure 31**. Generating such displays requires only seconds on a typical modern desktop computer.

Using this type of presentation communicates a much more effective representation of the surface geometry to most users, even ones with some experience, than does the simple grey-scale range image. **Figure 32** shows this mode of presentation for the same surface images presented in **Figure 1**. Even though the range images contain all of the data, and the perspective-corrected visualizations actually obscure some of it, comparison suggests that the latter are more realistic in appearance and hence more useful for visual recognition of characteristics or defects.

Modern computer graphics is also capable of rapidly redrawing surface views from different viewpoints. This can be used in several ways. Generating two realistic renderings of a surface from slightly different points of view allows using human stereo vision to interpret the depth of a surface. Creating a series of such images from different viewpoints can be used to display a "movie" showing a fly-over across the surface, and with enough computer horsepower this can be done in real time as an operator manipulates a joystick to interactively control the flight path. Combining this with the stereo display (**Figure 33**) creates a virtual reality world in which the surface can be viewed in detail.

Analysis of surface data

There is no doubt that human visual examination of well-presented visualizations of the surface geometrical and compositional information offers a powerful tool for recognizing defects and other specific characteristics of the surface. For many purposes, numerical measures of the surface are needed, which can be used for control purposes and to correlate the surface geometry or compositional variations with the creation and processing history of the surface, and with its performance behavior. For these purposes, analytical methods relying on computer processing of the data are needed, and it is far from clear just what should be measured to provide effective parameters for any given requirement.

The traditional measures of surfaces include the thickness of coatings, and the geometric features of the surface geometry. Most of these values, although quite precise, are highly dependent on other factors such as the material composition (and spatial variations of composition), the particular measurement procedure used, and the size of the measured area. Most thickness measuring procedures and some elevation measuring instruments naturally average over a lateral distance that is at least several micrometers and often much more. This is much larger than the vertical resolution most techniques are capable of, and may hide important details of the coating. Sampling strategies must be employed to determine spatial uniformity.

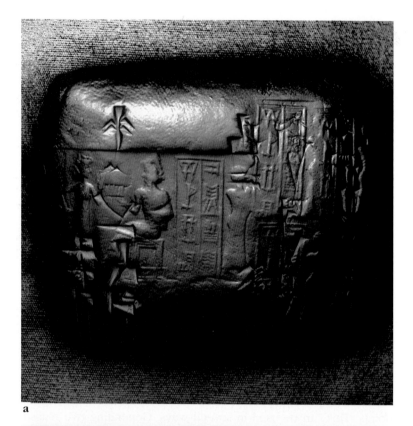

a

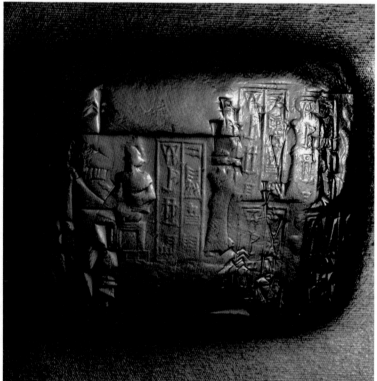

b

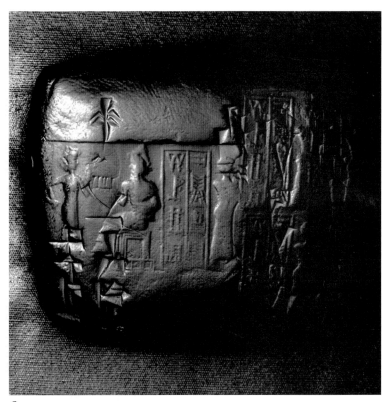

c

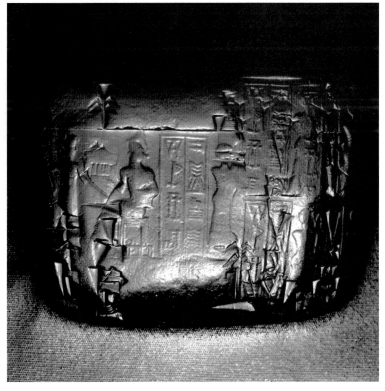

d

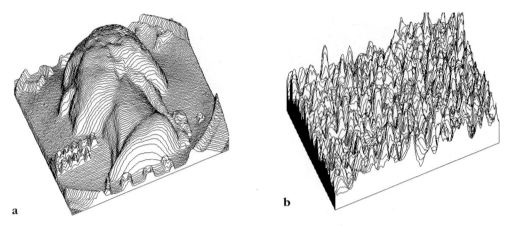

Figure 27. *Isometric line profile displays of the coin image from* **Figure 20** *and the polymer image from* **Figure 21.**

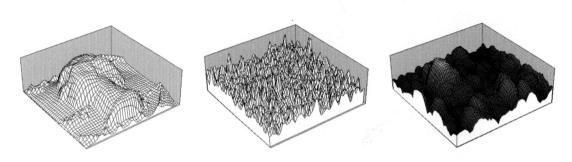

Figure 28. *Grid or mesh displays of the coin (***Figure 20***), polymer (***Figure 21***) and deposited surface (***Figure 16***).*

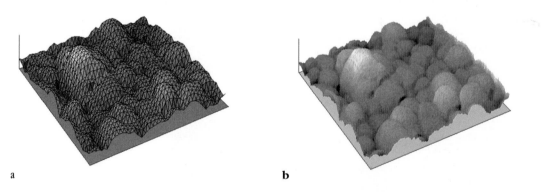

a   b

Figure 29. Deposited surface rendered with triangular facets where brightness is the product of the elevation and slope:
 (a) *large facets that are 6 pixels wide;*
 (b) *facets connecting each pixel and its immediate neighbors.*

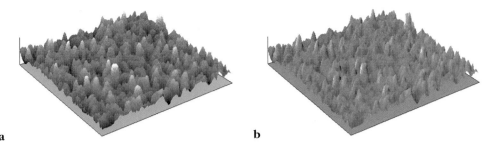

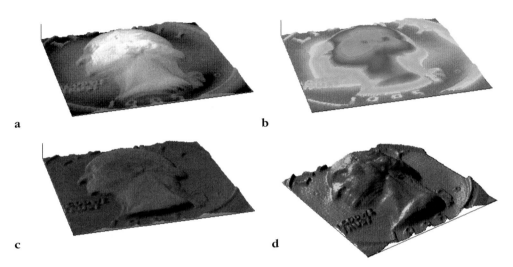

Figure 30. Data from the polymer surface:
   (*a*) *elevation value used to shade the facets;*
   (*b*) *product of elevation and slope.*

Figure 31. Presentation of elevation data
   from the coin image:
   (*a*) *each facet shaded according to the product of elevation and slope;*
   (*b*) *each facet assigned a color representing elevation;*
   (*c*) *Using the hue to represent elevation and the intensity to represent slope;*
   (*d*) *using hue for elevation and the Phong-rendered surface values for intensity.*

Dimensional measurement of surfaces is one application where coordinate measuring machines, stylus instruments and optical interference techniques are all used. In many cases very exact dimensions are specified in the design of the part, and so the measurement does not require an area scan or an image, but simply the proper alignment of the measuring tool with the component. However, as dimensions become small, as in the case of microelectronic devices, it may be necessary to acquire an image to locate the point where measurement is to be performed. **Figure 34** shows an elevation profile taken from one scan line of an AFM, from which highly precise measurements can be taken on the width and height of the steps present.

Because the AFM is a relatively slow device which has difficulty handling large parts, and because there is always concern about surface damage when a physical contact is made, many of the metrology measurements on these devices are presently made by SEM. (The light microscope was used with earlier generations of devices, but the dimensions are now too small for the wavelength of light to resolve them.) **Figure 35** shows an SEM image of two lines of photoresist on a silicon wafer. Unfortunately, the SEM image is only indirectly related to the surface geometry.

Figure 32. The surface data from the four surfaces in *Figure 1* and the two surfaces in *Figure 3* rendered to show perspective-corrected visualizations with facets shaded according to the product of slope and elevation. The graphics have been expanded in the vertical (Z) direction to increase the perception of roughness and relief in the data.

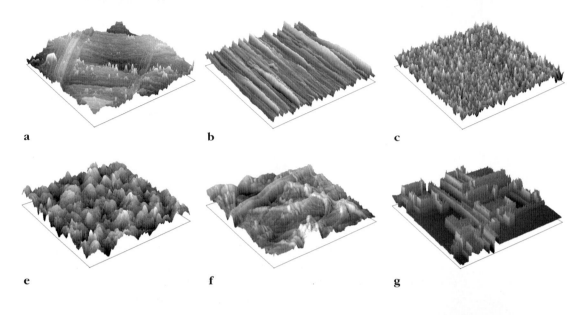

a   b   c

e   f   g

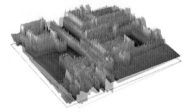

Figure 33. The surface rendering of *Figure 32f* performed from two slightly different viewpoints, which are combined to form a stereo pair.

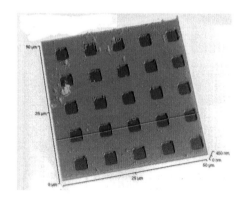

Figure 34. AFM image of a lithographic test pattern used to select the location for a single line scan used for dimensional measurement. When used for this purpose, the AFM requires quantitative position sensing such as an interferometer, instead of relying on measuring the signals sent to the piezoelectric positioners.

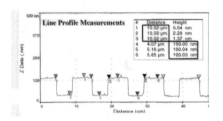

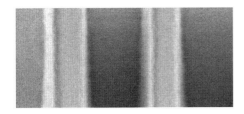

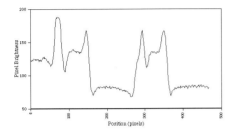

Figure 35. *Portion of an SEM image of two parallel lines of photoresist on a silicon wafer and the signal profile across them. The relationship between the physical profile and the signal depends upon the slope and roughness of the sides of the lines, the composition of the material, the electron accelerating voltage used, and the electron detector used.*

Consequently the signal profile along a scan line (actually averaged over multiple scan lines to improve the signal to noise ratio) is difficult to interpret to determine the line width. The pitch or spacing of the lines can be determined with fair accuracy under the assumption that the lines have the same shape, and thus generate the same signal profile. Consequently selecting any reproducible characteristic of the signal — the peak, or the maximum slope, etc., can be used to measure the distance between the lines. In order to measure the peak width accurately, however, there must be some absolute determination of where the edge lies (and even what that means given the slightly irregular shape of typical lines).

Computer modeling of the process of generating the SEM image signal can be carried out for various specimen geometries (and as a function of composition, electron beam voltage, and detector characteristics and placement). This is a time consuming process but still easier than fabricating physical standards for comparison. Even so, little accurate metrology is done in reality. Most manufacturers that use SEM images for metrology select some arbitrary feature of the signal that can be easily and reproducibly measured, such as the point of maximum slope or halfway between the darkest and lightest signal levels, and use that to monitor changes in dimension but without trying to determine the actual dimension. This is the classic difference between accuracy and precision, and works adequately for production control but is not adequate to support the development of new geometries and devices.

Profile measurements

Unlike the SEM, most instruments considered here do produce actual physical elevation profiles. Surface measurements have historically been assessed from these elevation profiles rather than using full two-dimensional images (because the instrumentation is simpler and the time required is much less, and hence because familiarity with the methods became established). By applying filters to the data (either digitally or in the amplifier electronics), different ranges of frequencies in the profiles can be separated which are traditionally described as the figure or form, waviness, and texture or roughness (**Figure 36**). Form is the overall gross geometrical shape, which is generally specified in engineering drawings, controlled by set dimensions, and described by conventional Euclidean geometry. The medium frequencies are called waviness and the high frequencies the texture or roughness. In machining processes, waviness is assumed to result from vibrations or deflections in the machine, while roughness results from more local interactions between the tool and the local microstructure in the material. These divisions are somewhat arbitrary and may differ

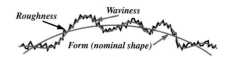

according to the size of the part. The cutoff frequencies used to define the filters are typically set to wavelengths from about 0.25 mm up to several mm to separate waviness from roughness. International standards specify these as part of the measurement procedure for many mechanical engineering applications.

Filtering to separate roughness from waviness and form data was originally done using analog RC filters in the electronics. In modern systems digital processing is used, with a least-squares line or arc fitted to remove the form and spatial Gaussian filter to separate the waviness and roughness. This generalizes directly to area scans which can also be filtered with an equivalent Gaussian filter, or the Fourier transform of the image can be filtered to select the desired range of frequencies. The form data are most often separated by least squares fitting of a plane, or some other Euclidean shape such as a cylinder or sphere that corresponds to the known intended form, or a generalized polynomial. **Figure 37** shows a simple example of form removal, in which roughness on a

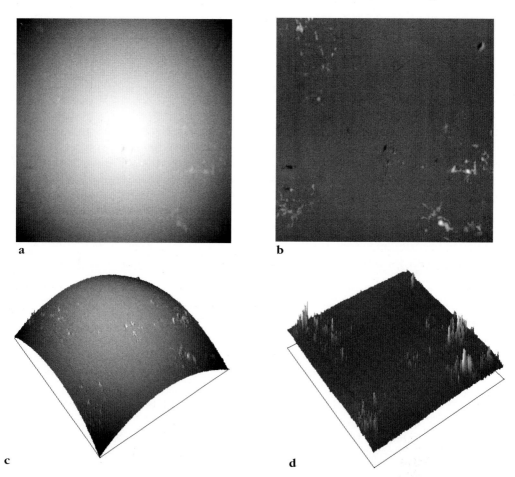

Figure 37. *Range images and surface visualizations of a ball bearing surface showing the overall form (a,c) and the results of flattening the data by subtracting the spherical shape (b,d). Grey-scale and vertical expansion of the data is possible after form removal.*

ball bearing (spherical) surface is made more evident visually and also becomes easier to measure after the general curvature is subtracted. Deviations are then measured from the nominal form of the ball.

The roughness of surfaces is typically determined from the roughness profile after the low(er)-frequency components have been removed. A wide variety of measurement parameters are used, some of them codified in various International Standards Organization (ISO) or other international standards, and some of them corresponding to specific industries or equipment manufacturers (Rosen and Crafoord, 1997). A complete review of instrumentation and methods is in Whitehouse (1994), and up-to-date reviews of analysis procedures are covered in Thomas (1999) and Mainsah et al. (2001). The most widely used procedures perform statistical analysis on the elevation data without regard to its spatial arrangement. Examples include the maximum peak-to-valley range of elevations along the profile, the average absolute value of the deviation from the mean (Ra), or the statistical standard deviation of the elevation data (Rq). Another measure of the magnitude of the roughness is the difference in elevation between the five highest peaks and five lowest valleys (Rz), but this requires defining a peak or a valley. This problem becomes more difficult when applied to area scans or images.

Information on the spatial distribution of the elevation data includes parameters such as the number of peaks along the profile and the correlation length. The latter may be defined as the average distance between successive peaks, or between points at some specific elevation such as the mean elevation line left by removing the form and waviness. A more general definition of the correlation length comes from a plots as shown in **Figure 38**; this is just the magnitude of the autocorrelation function which can be determined from the Fourier transform of the profile. The autocorrelation function (ACF) is also of interest because, for surfaces produced by a large number of independent events (shot blasting, grinding, ballistic deposition, etc.), it has the same shape as the ACF of the "average event" that produced the surface.

Functional parameters are also used, which are presumed to correspond to particular usage of the surfaces. The "Abbott curve" is simply the cumulative histogram of the elevation data (**Figure 39**); it gives the area of contact which would be obtained by removal of a portion of the surface, either by in-service wear or by an additional fabrication step such as plateau honing of automotive cylinder liners.

Another approach called "motif," originally introduced in the French automobile industry and now used throughout Europe (Dietzsch et al., 1997), simplifies the profile to just the peaks which would contact another surface based on the height of the peaks relative to the intervening valleys and the width of the valleys. **Figure 40** shows the principle. Peaks are characterized by their depth (the height above the valley) and their separation distance. Peak and valley patterns are then combined according to their separation distance and depth to eliminate the small peaks on the sides of larger ones, until a minimum is reached which contains just the most important peaks.

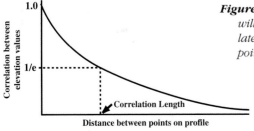

Figure 38. The correlation plot shows the probability that points will have the same elevation value as a function of their lateral separation. The correlation length is defined as the point at which this plot drops to 1/e or 36.79%

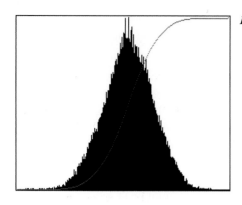

Figure 39. The histogram (black) of the shotblasted surface range image (*Figure 1d*) and the same data shown as a cumulative histogram (red). This plots the fraction of points on the surface whose elevation is less than the value on the horizontal axes, and is called the Abbott–Firestone curve.

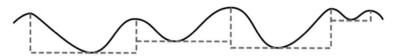

Figure 40. The basics of Motif combination — each peak and valley motif is measured by the depth (height of the smaller peak above the valley) and width. Motifs which have peaks smaller than the neighbor on either side, a width less than an arbitrary cutoff, and a depth less than 60% of the largest depth in the profile are combined with their neighbors to reduce the number of motifs present.

All these methods have serious limitations. They are highly dependent on the length of the profile scanned and the lateral resolution of the data points. They involve some very arbitrary definitions of what constitutes a peak or valley, ignore the fact that the profile path will not cross the highest or lowest points of most surface peaks and valleys, and do not correlate very well with the real subjects of interest, which are the processes by which surfaces are produced and their behavior for whatever service they are used. They are primarily suitable for specific quality control applications in which the real meaning of the parameters is hidden but consistency of measurement results can be used to keep a working process in control. Furthermore, they are very difficult to generalize to surface images produced by area scans of elevation.

All profile methods suffer from the fact that most real surfaces are not isotropic but have some directionality that results either from the way the surface was generated, the characteristics of the material itself, or the use it has been subjected to. This so-called "lay" of the surface can be simple (e.g. the ground surface in **Figure 1** is highly directional) or very complex and subtle. Measuring a profile perpendicular to the principal lay direction is the recommended approach, but for complicated surfaces this misses much of the actual character of the surface.

Because the history of profile measurements had generated (or accumulated) a rash of parameters, an effort is being made to rationalize the measurement of area scans. Supported by the ISO committee and spearheaded by researchers at the University of Birmingham (Stout et al., 1993), a set of statistical, spatial and functional parameters have been proposed which will probably evolve to form the basis of future international standards. These still contain some of the same limitations as the profile measures, such as the need to define what constitutes a peak and a strong dependence upon the size of the scan area and the lateral resolution of the points. Also, they do not include some of the potentially important methods such as topographic analysis, envelope or motif analysis, and fractal geometry. Because they represent an important starting point for surface description, some consideration of them is appropriate.

The Birmingham measurement suite

Four classes of measurement parameters are proposed, ones that deal with the elevation values without regard to their location (called amplitude parameters), ones that deal with lateral distances on the surface (called spatial parameters), ones that combine these together (called hybrid parameters), and ones that are believed to have some direct correlation with surface history and properties (called functional parameters). Within each group only a very few parameters, ones which have the most direct relationship to the more widely accepted profile measurement parameters, are selected. The symbols proposed for these parameters us the same nomenclature as those for profiles except that S (surface) is substituted for the R used in profile standards.

The amplitude parameters are simple extensions to area scans of the statistical measures that are used with profile plots. For instance, Sa is the analog to Ra, the arithmetic mean deviation. For an area scan it is the arithmetic mean of the absolute values of the elevation values from the mean plane (fit as discussed previously). Sa is preserved only because Ra is widely used, and that is so in turn because it was comparatively easy in the pre-computer days to design instruments to measure it. The root-mean-square deviation of the elevation points is a more robust measure, which is simply the standard deviation of the distribution of the elevation values, Sq. The variance (the square of the standard deviation) is the second moment of the distribution. The third and fourth moments are the skew and kurtosis, respectively, and these are also used as amplitude measurement parameters, called Ssk and Sku, respectively. For simple distributions which are not bimodal, these three parameters offer a reasonably compact statistical description of the surface heights.

The histogram of the surface elevation data (examples are shown in **Figure 41**) shows the overall range of surface elevation. The skew in the distribution distinguishes such cases as the narrow and deep grooves that may be important for distributing lubricant on plateau-honed cylinder liners in automobile engines (**Figure 41c**). In this case most of the surface has a very narrow range of elevations but the grooves, which cover only a small fraction of the area, reach down to much

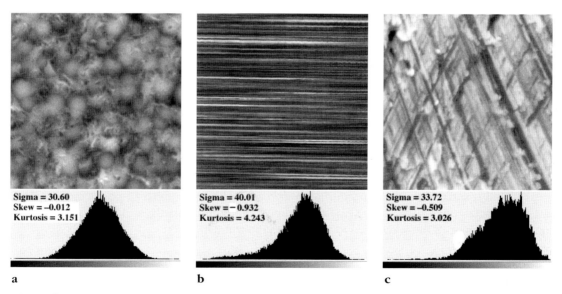

a   b   c

Figure 41. Histograms of elevation values for a few metal surfaces:
(a) shotblasted brass, which has a symmetrical distribution;
(b) ground stainless steel, which has a slight negative skew due to the presence of a few deep but separated parallel grooves;
(c) a plateau-honed cylinder liner with a negative skew resulting from the deep intersecting grooves which distribute lubricant.

Figure 42. The 20 highest peaks (red) and lowest valleys (green) on the shotblasted (a), ground *(b), and plateau-honed (c)* surfaces shown in *Figure 41.*

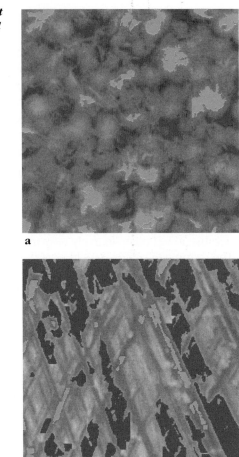

a

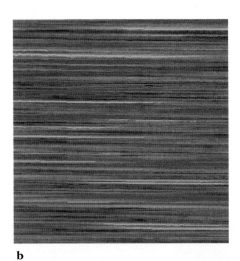

b

c

lower depths. A skew in the opposite direction would correspond to a surface with just a few high peaks or ridges rising up from a relatively smooth surface. But the histogram by itself contains no information on the spatial arrangement of the pits and valleys or the peaks and ridges. The same histogram would result from a surface with all of the high points collected together in one continuous ridge or distributed as thousands of tiny separate peaks. The properties of these two extreme surfaces would be quite different.

Just as for profiles, these statistical measures of amplitude are sensitive to the size of the sampled area. For most surfaces the standard deviation increases with the number of points measured, in fact for a fractal rough surface the slope of a curve plotting the variance as a function of size on log-log axes is one of the ways used to measure the fractal dimension.

For profiles, the parameter Rz is the difference in elevation between the average of the five highest peaks and five lowest valleys. For an area scan of a surface this is generalized to Sz, the difference between the ten highest peaks and ten lowest valleys. This is not purely an amplitude parameter, however, because it depends critically on the definitions of a peak and a valley. They cannot be simply the highest and lowest points on the surface (or pixels in the surface image), because these could be (and often will be) adjacent to each other and would all represent a single peak and valley. For a profile, the presence of a low point separating two high points might be taken to indicate separate peaks. This is a flawed definition because infinitesimal irregularities should not be considered significant, and so some criterion for the depth of the valley between the peaks is required; but, on an area scan of a surface, even more is needed because the peak (or valley) covers an area and two or more local peaks may connect along intricate paths (a ridge) to be considered part of the same peak (and vice versa for valleys). In tracing this connectivity, it matters whether pixels are considered to touch all eight of their immediate neighbors or only the four that share edges with them.

There is much more information in the identification of peaks and valleys than just the Sz parameter that is the elevation difference between the average of the ten highest and ten lowest. Different surfaces give rise to very different shapes for peaks and valleys, and their sizes and shapes, orientation and spacing may all contain important characterization information. In **Figure 42** several examples are shown in which peaks are defined as eight-connected (pixels touch eight neighbors), and are required to be distinct down to 80% of the height of the peak. Valleys are defined in the same way. In this example the 20 highest peaks and lowest valleys are found. The method is similar to the "flood fill" algorithm used in image processing, starting with the highest local maximum (and proceeding down) and including all touching pixels that extend down to the 80% limit, while checking to see if the peak merges into an existing labeled peak. Notice that for the shot-blasted surface the valleys are relative smooth in outline while the peaks are very irregular. Also, for the ground surface the peaks (ridges) tend to be broader than the valleys (crevices), and for the honed surface the peaks are very large while the valleys are much smaller. All of these differences are consistent with our understanding of how such surfaces are produced, and they may give important insights into other surfaces and their functional performance.

Another parameter involving the peaks present in the surface is the number of them per unit area, called Sds. Again, this depends upon the definition of a peak as discussed above. It is likely that secondary information about the peaks will also be important in a variety of applications. For instance, the uniformity of spacing of the peaks may play a role in cases where the surfaces are involved in electrical or thermal contact, friction and wear, or to judge the visual and aesthetic appearance. As discussed under image measurement, the mean nearest neighbor distance can be used to determine the tendency toward uniform spacing or clustering by comparing the value to the mean distance that a Poisson random distribution of the same number of points per unit area would have. **Figure 43** shows the surface of an injection molded polymer in which the peaks are relative evenly spaced (a complex function of the surface finish of the die, the temperature, pressure and viscosity of the polymer, and its molecular weight). This uniformity coupled with a spacing between peaks that is close to the spatial resolution limit of human vision produces an aesthetically pleasing appearance for the product.

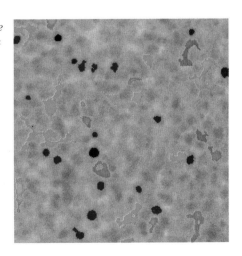

Figure 43. The highest 20 peaks and lowest 20 valleys in a one square millimeter area of the molded polymer surface from ***Figure 21***. *The peaks are color coded from purple to red according to height and the valleys from green to cyan. Notice that one valley completely surrounds a small peak, and that the peaks are much more regular in shape than the valleys.*

Note in the figure that the valleys have a very different shape and distribution than do the peaks. In some other applications the same information about the density and uniformity of pits rather than peaks would be of interest. An example is the surfaces of plates used to retain ink for printing applications.

Surfaces with anisotropy or lay can be characterized by spatial parameters derived from the autocorrelation function. As discussed in the chapter on Fourier space processing, the autocorrelation function (ACF) is obtained by squaring the magnitude of the complex variables in the Fourier transform while setting the phase to zero, which removes all spatial location information. The inverse transform produces the two-dimensional spatial image of the ACF. The parameters defined from this function are the texture aspect ratio *Str*, the texture direction *Std*, and the autocorrelation length *Sal*. Understanding these may be helped by examining the ACF images in **Figure 38.** The autocorrelation length is defined in the Birmingham report as the shortest distance in which the magnitude of the ACF drops to 20%. For the examples shown, this is the minimum radius of the contour line drawn at the 20% intensity level. The texture aspect ratio is the ratio of the minimum radius to the maximum radius, and the texture direction is the orientation of the maximum radius.

For the examples in **Figure 44**, the ACF of the polymer surface (**Figure 21**) is quite isotropic (indicating that the surface is also isotropic), so the aspect ratio is unity and there is no pronounced direction. The ground surface (**Figure 1b**) on the other hand as a strong preferred orientation

Figure 44. **Autocorrelation function calculated for: (a)** *the polymer surface from* **Figure 21;** *(c) the ground surface from* **Figure 1b;** *(e) the flycut surface from* **Figure 1a,** *with superimposed contour lines* **(b, d, f)** *indicating the shape of the function and the distance at which it drops to 20%.*

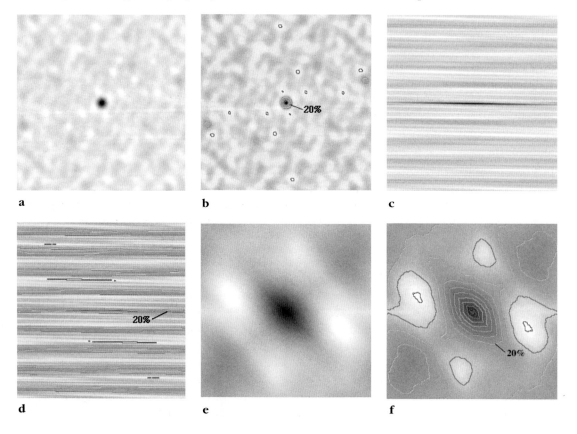

which is evident in the ACF and can be measured there. For the flycut surface (**Figure 1a**) the texture is more complicated, as is indeed evident in the original image which shows two predominant machining directions. The *Str, Std,* and *Sal* values as defined can of course be measured from the ACF but it is not clear that they contain all of the information about the surface lay that would be desired for characterization.

The hybrid properties involve both the elevation and lateral data (as indeed do many of the preceding parameters). *SΔq* is the root-mean-square slope of the surface, which can be calculated from the same triangular tiling procedure used to generate the visualizations shown earlier. Formally it is defined as the square root of the mean value of the sum of squares of the derivatives of the image in the vertical and horizontal directions, which can be determined simply as the local difference of elevation values between adjacent pixels. The mean summit curvature Ssc is similarly related to the second derivatives of elevation, but calculated only for those pixels located at peaks. This depends, of course, on first arriving at a meaningful and accepted definition of which peaks are to be included. The third hybrid property is the ratio of the actual surface area to the projected area *Sdr*. This can be obtained by summing up the areas of the triangles making up the visualization.

None of these hybrid properties is very difficult to compute, but they all depend critically on the sampling interval or spacing of the pixels. Changing lateral resolution will alter the parameter values dramatically so that they are not really functions of the surface but of the measurement technique, and can be used only for comparisons in the most limited way. This is also the case for many of the profile-based measurements, but one of the goals in moving to area-based measurements was to overcome some of the limitations of the older methods. In fact, many engineering surfaces have been shown to have a fractal geometry whose actual surface area is undefined (it increases without limit as the lateral resolution of the measurements improves).

It is a more subtle point, but measurements like these also depend upon whether the elevation data at each pixel are samples of the surface or averages over the pixel area. The mathematics apply for the case of sampling, where the elevation at each pixel is measured at a precise mathematical point and whatever happens between that pixel and the next is not taken into account. In fact, many measurement methods such as conventional stylus instruments and optical interferometers perform some averaging of measurement over the entire area of the pixel, which may either report the maximum value in that area or a weighted average of the elevation values. The mathematics appropriate to these cases has not been worked out and would affect not just the hybrid parameters but all of the parameters described here.

Functional parameters are intended to relate surface geometric data to specific aspects of surface performance, and these are generally related to mechanical engineering applications since the greatest use of surface metrology has thus far been in that field. One typical examples is the surface bearing area ratio Stp, which is the fraction of the image area that would be in contact with a flat plane parallel to the base if a given height of all peaks was removed by wear (**Figure 45**). This value, of course, can be read directly from the histogram of the elevation data in the image.

Similarly, the amount of volume removed in the process (the material volume ratio *Smr*) can be calculated by integrating the histogram, or using the cumulative histogram. The void volume ratio *Svr* is the volume of empty space within the surface of the specimen, which may be available for retaining or distributing a lubricant. It is measured by integrating the spaces at each elevation level, but this can also be done efficiently using the cumulative histogram. **Figure 46** shows the same data from **Figure 45** but as a surface visualization that reveals the nature of the contact surface and the void volume after some of the peaks have been removed by wear (but assuming that there is no deformation of the remaining surface nor filling in of pits with debris).

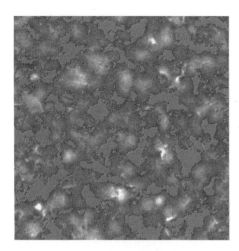

Figure 45. Thresholding the range image (in this example, the shotblasted surface from Figure 1d) at any particular elevation (in this example 31% below the maximum value) shows the surface area that would be in contact with a plane after a corresponding amount of wear (in the absence of any elastic or plastic deformation).

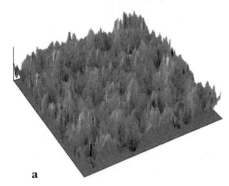

a

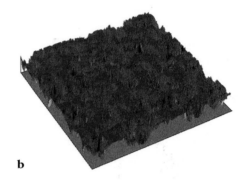

b

Figure 46. Visualization of the data from Figure 45:
(**a**) *the original shotblasted surface;*
(**b**) *the same surface truncated 31% below the top of the highest peak, showing the contact areas and the void volume.*

More information is really needed about the contact areas than these parameters provide. The size of the individual contacts is important for heating and deformation, and the void volume may either be completely connected, or consist of isolated pockets, or be a mixture of the two, with very different consequences for lubrication. There are other functional parameters proposed to deal with these and other aspects of surface performance, but these become very specific to each application and will require considerable research to properly define. Many of them are handicapped to a significant degree because the surface elevation data in a range image are single valued. The elevation recorded at each pixel is the maximum height at that point, as detected by a stylus or optical reflection, etc. Undercuts, caves, or pores within the surface that do not show up in the range image may become important if wear removes some of the surface overburden.

Image processing and analysis using the tools already developed in preceding chapters can be used to obtain many of the parameters of interest for surfaces from range images. For example, min and max ranking operators (grey-scale erosion and dilation) can be used to modify the image to form the envelope of the surface which a contact of known form would feel, basically a two-dimensional form of the motif logic mentioned above for profiles. Cross correlation with the image of a defect (crack, dust particle, etc.) can be used to locate such defects. Measurement of features obtained by thresholding can provide data on the contact areas and their distribution after wear has modified a surface. Skeletonization of the pore volume can be used to determine its connectivity as a pathway to distribute lubricants. Using these tools is straightforward once the significant parameters have been determined so that their relationships to surface behavior and history can be assessed.

New approaches — topographic analysis and fractal dimensions

The limitations and inadequacies of the traditional methods of analysis discussed above prevent them from fully describing real surfaces. They are primarily being used for process control applications in mechanical engineering, where comparison of measurements with prior history provides an indication of change, so long as the measurement technique and instrumentation remains unchanged. Newer methods have become available, but their full meaning and interpretation still remain to be explored. It is hoped that these new approaches that may provide more insight into the description and makeup of surfaces.

Human vision uses global topographic information to organize information on surfaces (Scott, 1995). The arrangement of hills and dales, ridges, courses and saddle points, contains quite a bit of information for describing a surface. A landscape or surface can be divided into regions consisting of hills (points from which all uphill paths lead to one particular peak) and dales (points from which all downhill paths lead to a pit). Boundaries between hills are courses and boundaries between dales are ridge lines (**Figure 47**).

A Pfalz graph (Pfalz, 1976) or change tree (**Figure 48**) connecting the peaks and dales through the respective saddle points where ridge and course lines meet summarizes the topological structure. The change tree can represent directly the height difference and lateral distance between features, which makes decisions straightforward about eliminating features that have either small vertical or lateral extent. This is a direct extension to surfaces of the motif combination used for profiles. Scott (1997) has proposed methods for dealing with the finite extent of real images and the corrections necessary for dealing with the intersection of ridges and courses with the edges of the image area. It is not yet clear just how this information will be used for surface measurement, but parameters such as the volume of connected valleys, the spatial distribution of valleys and peaks across the surface, and orientation of watercourses and ridges seem likely to be important for surface characterization.

At quite a different extreme of local roughness, many surfaces (but emphatically not all) are characterized by a self-similarity (more exactly, a self-affinity) that can be described by a fractal dimension. There are several ways to measure this (which do not exactly agree numerically) plus the need to provide an additional parameter that describes the magnitude of the roughness, and perhaps others to describe the directionality of the surface. The appeal of the fractal dimension is that it is not dependent on the measurement scale, and that it summarizes much of the "roughness" of surfaces in a way that seems to correspond to both the way nature works and the way humans perceive roughness. Given a series of surfaces, the "rougher" the surface as it appears to human

Figure 47. *A contour map representing a surface, with the peaks (red), valleys (green) and saddle points (purple) marked.*

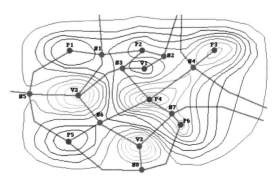

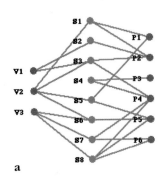
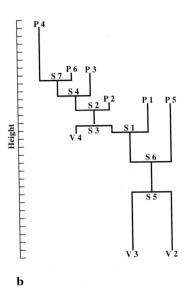

Figure 48. The Pfalz graph (a) showing which peaks, saddle points, and valleys are connected in Figure 47, and the change tree (b) that can be drawn to show the height difference and lateral distance between them.

a

b

interpretation (for a variety of basic reasons), the higher the fractal dimension. At the same time it must be noted that the recognition of fractal geometry (even the name) is comparatively new, and there is a "bandwagon" tendency that probably causes it to be applied where it should not be, or with more enthusiasm than critical thinking.

The fractal dimension of a surface is a real number greater than 2 (the topological dimension of the surface) and less than 3 (the topological dimension of the space in which the surface exists). A perfectly smooth surface (dimension 2.0) corresponds to Euclidean geometry, and a plot of the actual area of the measured area as a function of measurement resolution would not change. But for real surfaces an increase in the magnification or resolution with which it is examined will reveal more nooks and crannies and the surface area will increase. For a surprising variety of natural and man-made surfaces, a plot of the area as a function of resolution is linear on a log-log graph, and the slope of this curve gives the dimension D as shown in **Figure 49**.

This description comes directly from the earlier recognition that boundary lines around islands had a length that depended upon the measurement scale. A so-called Richardson plot of the length of the west coast of Britain (Mandelbrot, 1967) as a function of the length of the measurement tool showed this log-log relationship and was one of the triggering ideas that led Mandelbrot to study the mathematics of self-similar structures (ones that appear equally irregular at all scales) and to coin the name fractal for the field. Many other subsequent publications have shown that an extremely broad variety of surfaces also exhibit this kind of geometry, investigated a number of ways to measure the dimension, and begun to study the relationships between the dimension and the history and performance characteristics of surfaces.

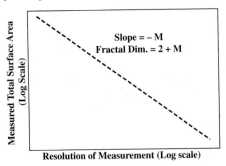

Figure 49. Schematic diagram of fractal dimension measurement. As the measurement resolution becomes smaller, the total measured area increases.

Measuring the surface area over a range of resolutions is in fact a rather difficult thing to do (one way is by adsorbing molecules of different sizes), and for basic reasons is not actually appropriate for many surfaces because they are not ideally self-similar. For most surfaces, the lateral directions and the normal direction are distinct in dimension and physical properties, which means that the scaling or self-similarity that exists in one direction may not be the same as the others. At a sufficiently large scale most surfaces approach an ideal Euclidean flat surface. For anisotropic surfaces this situation is more severe and even lateral directions are different. This means that the surfaces are mathematically self-affine rather than self-similar. The fact that elevation measurements are single valued and cannot reveal undercuts means that the measured data would be self-affine even for a truly self-similar surface (for instance one produced by diffusion-limited aggregation of particles on a substrate). For self-affine surfaces and data sets there are still a variety of correct and practical measurement techniques. A few of the more practical ones will be summarized here (and a more complete discussion is available in Russ, 1994).

In most cases, the most robust measure of the fractal dimension is the same procedure that can characterize surfaces that are not ideally fractal, nor perfectly isotropic (Russ, 2001). The Fourier power spectrum can also be used to characterize the instrumental response function, to distinguish it from the surface information. Instead of the usual display mode for the power spectrum, a plot of log (magnitude) vs. log (frequency) reveals a fractal surface as a straight line plot whose slope gives the dimension. The principal drawbacks to using the power spectrum plot to measure the dimension are that it tends to overestimate the numerical value of the dimension for relatively smooth surfaces (dimensions between 2.0 and about 2.3), and that the numerical precision of the measured value is lower than some of the other methods can provide for images of a given size. **Figure 50** shows an example of the power spectrum plot for a fractal surface, whose slope gives the fractal dimension.

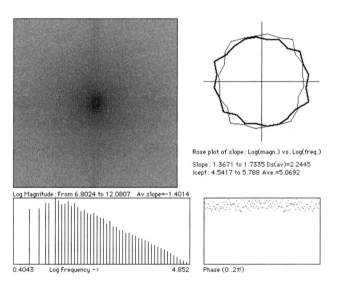

Figure 50. The Fourier transform power spectrum (upper left) of the shotblasted metal image (Figure 1d), with its subsequent analysis. The plot of log magnitude vs. log frequency (lower left) averaged over all directions shows a linear relationship which confirms the fractal behavior, and whose slope gives the dimension (2.24). A rose plot of the slope of as a function of orientation (upper left, bold line) shows that the surface is isotropic and has the same dimension in all directions. The thin line on the same plot shows the intercept of the plot as a function of direction, which is a measure of the amplitude of the roughness and also shows isotropy for this surface. Finally, a plot of the distribution of phases of the terms in the Fourier transform shows them to be uniformly random, which is required for a fractal.

Generating the two-dimensional Fourier transform of the surface range image reveals any fractal anisotropy (which can be either weak anisotropy in which the dimension is the same in all directions but the magnitude is not, or strong anisotropy in which the dimension also varies). Plotting the slope and intercept of the plot of log (magnitude) vs. log (frequency) as a function of orientation provides a quantitative tool to describe the fractal anisotropy. **Figure 51** shows an example. The separation of the low frequency data that describes the figure and high frequencies that often reveal instrument limitations from the intermediate frequencies can be used to isolate the surface fractal dimension.

By itself, the fractal dimension is only a partial description of surface roughness even for ideally fractal surfaces. Stretching the surface vertically to increase the magnitude of the roughness does not change the slope of the power spectrum or the fractal dimension. An additional measure, which has units of length, is needed to characterize the magnitude. The intercept of the plot of the power spectrum has units of length and can be used for this purpose. So can the topothesy, which is defined as the horizontal distance over which the mean angular change in slope is one radian.

A variety of other measurement approaches can be properly used with self-affine fractal surfaces. Two widely used techniques that deal with the range image of the area directly are the covering blanket and the variogram. Both work correctly for isotropic surfaces but do not reveal anisotropy and can produce nonsense values in those cases rather than an average. The latter is simply a plot of the variance in elevation values as a function of the size of the measured region. Values from small areas placed systematically or randomly over the surface are averaged, and a single mean value obtained. This process is repeated at many different sizes and a plot (**Figure 52**) made that gives the dimension.

The covering blanket or Minkowski method measures the difference (summed over the entire image) between an upper and lower envelope fitted to the surface as a function of the size of the neighborhood used. The minimum and maximum brightness rank operators discussed under image processing are applied with different diameter neighborhoods, and the total difference between them added up. This is analogous to the Minkowski dimension for a profile that was described in Chapter 7, obtained by using the Euclidean distance map to measure the area as a function of distance from the boundary line. The covering blanket method produces a plot as shown in **Figure 53** that gives a dimension. Notice that these three methods give only approximate

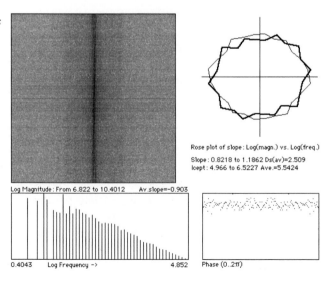

Figure 51. The same data presentation as in Figure 50, but for the anisotropic ground surface shown in Figure 1b. Both the slope and intercept of the power spectrum plot are different in the vertical and horizontal directions. The surface is an anisotropic fractal.

Rose plot of slope : Log(magn.) vs. Log(freq.)
Slope : 0.8218 to 1.1862 Ds(av)=2.509
Icept : 4.966 to 6.5227 Ave.=5.5424

Log Magnitude : From 6.822 to 10.4012   Av .slope=-0.903

0.4043   Log Frequency ->   4.852   Phase (0..2π)

Figure 52. *Plot of mean variance vs. neighborhood size to determine the fractal dimension of the shotblasted surface (same image as Figure 50).*

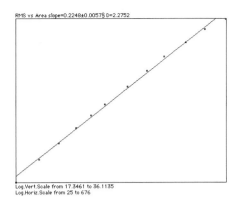

Figure 53. *Plot of the Minkowski cover volume as a function of neighborhood size to determine the fractal dimension (same image as Figures 50 and 52).*

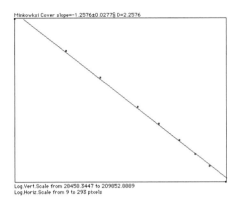

agreement as to the numerical value of the dimension. Part of this is just finite measurement precision, but part of the difference arises from the fact that all of these techniques measure something that is slightly different. These are limits to the actual dimension and in general will not agree, so when comparisons are being made between surfaces it is important to always use one technique for all of the measurements.

It is often attractive to perform measurements in a lower dimension, since a smaller number of data points are involved. Historically, much of the work with fractal measurement has been done with boundary lines, whose dimension lies between 1.0 (the Euclidean or topological dimension of a line) and 1.999 (a line whose irregularity is so great that it wanders across an entire plane). There is a way to do this with fractal surfaces, by intersecting the surface with a plane and then measuring the dimension of the line that is the intersection. It is vitally important however than this plane be parallel to the nominal surface orientation rather than a vertical cut. The vertical cut would produce the same profile as that obtained with a profilometer, but because the surface is self-affine and not self-similar the proper measurement of this profile is complicated and the common techniques such as the Richardson plot mentioned above do not apply. Also, of course, the profile will be oriented in a particular direction and cannot be used with anisotropic surfaces.

The horizontal cut is called a slit-island method, and it corresponds exactly to the case with which Richardson was dealing. The horizontal plane corresponds to sea level and the outlines are the coastlines of the islands produced by the hills that rise above the sea. A plot of the length of these coastlines as a function of measurement scale produces a dimension that is exactly one less than the surface dimension (the difference between the topological dimensions of a surface and a line). It is not usually convenient to measure the length of a coastline using a computer in the way Richardson did, by setting a pair of dividers to a particular scale length and "striding" around the

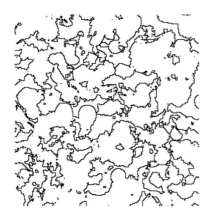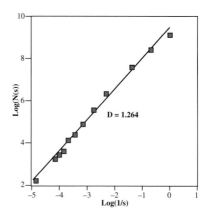

*Figure 54. Contour lines produced by thresholding the image from **Figure 1d** at 50% of its elevation range and the plot from a box-counting measurement.*

coastline so that the boundary length was the divider setting times the number of strides; but a variety of other methods are readily implemented in a computer.

The analog to the Minkowski blanket for the surface is a Minkowski sausage produced by thickening the boundary line by various amounts and plotting the area covered vs. the width of the stripe or sausage. The Euclidean distance map discussed in Chapter 7 on binary image processing accomplishes this procedure very efficiently and without the directional variation that results from conventional pixel-based dilation. Another method is box-counting (**Figure 54**) in which a grid is placed on the image and the number of squares through which the boundary line passes is counted as a function of the size of the grids. While these methods are quite fast, they are only applicable to isotropic surfaces.

It is beyond the scope of this text to discuss the relationships that have been found between fractal dimensions and various aspects of the history and properties of surfaces. In brief, most processes of surface formation that involve brittle fracture or deposit large amounts of energy in small regions tend to produce fractal surfaces, and the numerical value of the dimension is often a signature of the process that was involved (Russ, 1997). Likewise, many surface contact applications (electrical, thermal, etc.) depend upon the relationship between contact area and pressure and fractal geometry is pertinent to this case. Under some circumstances friction and wear may also be related to the surface dimension. Fractal description of surfaces is a new, and somewhat "trendy" approach to surface characterization. Although it clearly offers powerful methods that apply to some surfaces, for others such as ductile deformation it is inappropriate.

References

M. Abbasi-Dezfouli, T. G. Freeman (1994). Patch matching in stereo-images based on shape, *ISPRS Int. Arch. of Photogramm. and Remote Sensing* 30(3/1):1–8.

M. R. Anderberg (1973). *Cluster Analysis for Applications.* Academic Press, New York.

Agfa Compugraphic Division (1992). *Digital Color Prepress* (vols. 1 & 2). Agfa Corp., Wilmington, MA.

E. H. Aigeltinger, K. R. Craig, R. T. DeHoff (1972). Experimental determination of the topological properties of three-dimensional microstructures. *J. Microsc.* 95:69–81.

G. R. Arce, J. L. Paredes, J. Mullan (2000). Nonlinear filtering for image analysis and enhancement, in *Handbook of Image and Video Processing* (A. Bovic, Ed.). Academic Press, San Diego.

J. Astola, P. Haavisto, Y. Neuvo (1990). Vector median filters. *Proc. IEEE* 78:678–689.

N. Baba, M. Naka, Y. Muranaka, et al. (1984). Computer-aided stereographic representation of an object reconstructed from micrographs of serial thin sections. *Micron and Microsc. Acta* 15:221–226.

N. Baba, M. Baba, M. Imamura, et al. (1989). Serial section reconstruction using a computer graphics system: application to intracellular structures in yeast cells and to the periodontal structure of dogs' teeth. *J. Electron Microsc. Tech.* 11:16–26.

A. J. Baddeley, H. J. G. Gundersen, L. M. Cruz–Orive (1986). Estimation of surface area from vertical sections. *J. Microsc.* 142:259–276.

A. J. Baddeley, C. V. Howard, A. Boyde, et al. (1987). Three-dimensional analysis of the spatial distribution of particles using the tandem-scanning reflected light microscope. *Acta Stereol.* 6 (Suppl. II) 87–100.

R. Balasubramanian, C. A. Bouman, J. P. Allebach (1994). Sequential scalar quantization of color images. *J. Electron. Imaging* 3(1):45–59.

D. Ballard (1981). Generalizing the Hough transform to detect arbitrary shapes. *Pattern Recognition* 13(2):111–122.

D. H. Ballard, C. M. Brown (1982). *Computer Vision.* Prentice Hall, Englewood Cliffs, NJ.

D. H. Ballard, C. M. Brown, J. A. Feldman (1984). An approach to knowledge-directed image analysis, in *Computer Vision Systems* (A. R. Hanson, E. M. Riseman, Eds.) Academic Press, New York, NY, 271–282.

S. T. Barnard, W. B. Thompson (1980). Disparity Analysis of Images. *IEEE Trans. on Patt. Anal. Mach. Intell.* (PAMI) 2(4):333–340.

F. L. Barnes, S. G. Azavedo, H. E. Martz, G. P. Roberson, D. J. Schneberk, M. F. Skeate (1990). *Geometric Effects in Tomographic Reconstruction.* Lawrence Livermore National Laboratory Rept UCRL–ID–105130.

H. G. Barth, S-T. Sun (1985) Particle Size Analysis. *Anal. Chem.* 57:151.

A. Barty, K. A. Nugent, A. Roberts, et al. (2000). Quantitative Phase Tomography. *Optics Communications* 175:329–336.

J. K. Beddow, G. C. Philip, A. F. Vetter (1977). On relating some particle profiles characteristics to the profile Fourier coefficients. *Powder Technol.* 18:15–19.

G. Bertrand, J-C. Everat, M. Couprie (1997). Image segmentation through operators based on topology. *J. Electron. Imaging* 6(4):395–405.

V. Berzins (1984) Accuracy of Laplacian edge detectors. *Comput. Vis. Graph. Image Proc.* 27:1955–2010.

P. J. Besl, N. D. McKay (1992). A method for registration of 3-D shapes. *IEEE Trans. Patt. Anal. Mach. Intell.* 14(2): 239–256.

S. Beucher, C. Lantejoul (1979). Use of Watersheds in Contour Detection. *Proc. Intl. Workshop Image Process,* CCETT, Rennes, France.

G. B. Binnig, C. F. Quate, C. Gerber (1986). Atomic Force Microscope. *Phys. Rev. Lettr.* 52:930.

J. L. Bird, D. T. Eppler, D. M. Checkley, Jr. (1986). Comparisons of herring otoliths using Fourier series shape analysis. *Can. J. Fish. Aquat. Sci.* 43:1228–1234.

W. J. Black (1986). *Intelligent Knowledge-Based Systems: An Introduction.* Van Nostrand Reinhold, London.

R. A. S. Blackie, R. Bagby, L. Wright, J. Drinkwater, S. Hart (1987). Reconstruction of three-dimensional images of microscopic objects using holography. *Proc. R. Microsc. Soc.* 22:98.

F. Boddeke (1998). *Quantitative Fluorescence Microscopy. ASCI Dissertation Series.* Delft Univ. Press, Delft, Netherlands.

F. R. Boddeke, L. J. van Vliet, H. Netten, I. T. Young (1994). Autofocusing in microscopy based on the OTF and sampling. *Bioimaging* 2:193–203.

G. Borgefors (1996). On digital distance transforms in three dimensions. *Comp. Vision Image Understanding* 64(3):368–376.

G. Borgefors, I. Nystron, G. Sanniti di Baja (1999). Computing skeletons in three dimensions. *Patt. Recognition* 32(7):1225–1236.

S-T. Bow (1992). *Pattern Recognition and Image Preprocessing.* Marcel Dekker, New York.

A. Boyde (1973). Quantitative photogrammetric analysis and quantitative stereoscopic analysis of SEM images. *J. Microsc.* 98:452.

S. Bradbury, B. Bracegirdle (1998). *Introduction to Light Microscopy.* Bios Scientific Publishers, Oxford, U.K.

B. Bracegirdle, S. Bradbury (1995). *Modern Photomicrography.* Bios Scientific Publishers, Oxford UK.

R. N. Bracewell (1984). The fast Hartley transform. *Proc. IEEE* 72:8.

R. N. Bracewell (1986). *The Hartley Transform.* Oxford Univ. Press, Oxford, U.K.

R. N. Bracewell (June 1989). The Fourier Transform. *Scientific American,*

G. Braudaway (1987). A procedure for optimum choice of a small number of colors from a large color palette for color imaging. *Proc. Electronic Imaging 1987,* San Francisco, CA.

L. G. Briarty, P. H. Jenkins (1984). GRIDSS: an integrated suite of microcomputer programs for three-dimensional graphical reconstruction from serial sections. *J. Microsc.* 134:121–124.

D. S. Bright, D. E. Newbury, R. B. Marinenko (1988). Concentration-concentration histograms: scatter diagrams applied to quantitative compositional maps, in *Microbeam Analysis 1988* (D. E. Newbury Ed.). San Francisco Press, 18–24.

P. Brodatz (1966). *Textures: A Photographic Album for Artists and Designers*, Dover, New York.

L. G. Brown (1992). A survey of image registration techniques. *ACM Computing Surveys* 24(4):325–376.

R. K. Bryan, J. Skilling (1980). Deconvolution by maximum entropy, as illustrated by application to the jet of M87. *Mon. Not. R. Ast. Soc.* 191: 69–79.

V. Buzuloiu, M. Ciuc, R. M . Rangayyan, et al. (2001). Adaptive–neighborhood histogram equalization of color images. *J. Electron. Imaging* 10(2):445–459.

I. J. Canny (1986). A computational approach to edge detection. *IEEE Trans. Patt. Anal. Mach. Intell.* (PAMI) 8(6):679–698.

C. Carlsen (1985). Reconstruction of true surface topographies in scanning electron microscopes using backscattered electrons. *Scanning* 7:169–177.

W. A. Carrington (1990). Image restoration in 3D microscopy with limited data, in *Bioimaging and Two Dimensional Spectroscopy, Proc. SPIE,* Vol. 1205 (L. C. Smith, Ed.), 72–83.

E. Castle, P. A. Zhdan (1997). Characterization of surface topography by SEM and SFM: Problems and solutions. *J. Phys. D. App. Phys.* 30:722.

K. R. Castleman (1979). *Digital Image Processing* Prentice Hall, Englewood Cliffs, NJ.

R. L. T. Cederberg (1979). Chain-link coding and segmentation for raster scan devices. *Comput. Graph. Image Process* 10:224–234.

P. Chieco, A. Jonker, C. Melchiorri, et al. (1994). A user's guide for avoiding errors in absorbance image cytometry. Histochemical J. 26:1–19.

C. K. Chui (1992). *An Introduction to Wavelets.* Academic Press, London.

J. R. B. Cockett (1987). Decision expression optimization. *Fundamenta Informaticae X* 93–114.

L. Cohen (1991). On active contour models and balloons. *Comp. Vision, Graph. Image Process.* 53(2):211–218.

M. L. Comer, E. J. Delp (1999). Morphological operations for color image processing, *J. Electron. Imaging* 8:279–289.

J. Condeco, L. H. Christensen, S. F. Jorgensen, J. C. Russ, B-G. Rosen (2000). A comparative study of image stitching algorithms for surface topography measurements. *X. Intl Colloq. on Surfaces,* Germany.

J. Cookson (1994). Three-dimensional reconstruction in microscopy. *Proc. R. Microscopical Soc.* 29(1):3–10.

J. W. Cooley, J. W. Tukey (1965). An algorithm for the machine calculation of complex Fourier series. *Mathematics of Computation.*

A. M. Cormack (1963). Representation of a function by its line integrals with some radiological applications. *J. Appl. Phys.* 34:2722–2727.

A. M. Cormack (1964). Representation of a function by its line integrals with some radiological applications II. *J. Appl. Phys.* 35:2908–2913.

T. N. Cornsweet (1970). *Visual Perception,* Academic Press, New York.

L. F. Costa, R. M. Cesar (2001). *Shape Analysis and Classification.* CRC Press, Boca Raton, FL.

M. Coster, J.-L. Chermant (1985). *Précis D'Analse D'Images Éditions du Centre National de la Recherche Scientifique,* Paris.

L-M. Cruz-Orive (1976). Particle size-shape distributions: the general spheroid problem. *J. Microsc.* 107:235; 112:153.

L-M. Cruz-Orive (1983). Distribution-free estimation of sphere size distributions from slabs showing overprojections and truncation, with a review of previous methods. *J. Microsc.* 131:265.

P. E. Danielsson (1980). Euclidean distance mapping. *Comput. Graph. Image Process* 14:227–248.

I. Daubechies (1992). Ten Lectures on Wavelets. *CBMS-NSF Regional Conf. Series Applied Math*, Philadelphia, PA.

I. Daubechies (1996). Where do wavelets come from? — A personal point of view. *Proc. IEEE* 84(4):510–513.

D. G. Daut, D. Zhao, J. Wu (1993). Double predictor differential pulse coded modulation algorithm for image data compression. *Optical Engineering* 32(7):1514–1523.

J. Davidson (1991). Thinning and skeletonization: a tutorial and overview, in *Digital Image Processing: Fundamentals and Applications* (E. Dougherty, Ed.). Marcel Dekker, New York.

E. R. Davies (1988). On the noise suppression and image enhancement characteristics of the median, truncated median and mode filters, *Patt. Recog. Lett.* 7:87–97.

H. W. Deckman, K. L. D'Amico, J. H. Dunsmuir, B. P. Flannery, S. M. Gruner (1989). *Microtomography Detector Design Advances in X-ray Anal.* 32:641.

R. T. Dehoff, F. N. Rhines (1968). *Quantitative Microscopy,* McGraw-Hill, New York.

D. DeMandolx, J. Davoust (1997). Multicolor analysis and local image correlation in confocal microscopy. *J. Microsc.* 185:21–36.

M. De Marsicoi, L. Cinque, S. Levialdi (1997). Indexing pictorial documents by their content: a survey of current techniques. *Image Vision Computing* 15:119–141.

P. A. Devijver, J. Kittler (1980). *Pattern Recognition: A Statistical Approach.* Prentice Hall, Englewood Cliffs, NJ.

G. Diaz, A. Zuccarelli, I. Pelligra, et al. (1989). Elliptic Fourier analysis of cell and nuclear shapes. *Comput. Biomed. Res.* 22: 405–414. .

G. Diaz, D. Quacci, C. Dell'Orbo (1990). Recognition of cell surface modulation by elliptic Fourier analysis. *Comput. Meth. Prog. Biomedicine* 31:57–62.

M. Dietzsch, K. Papenfuss, T. Hartmann (1997). The MOTIF method (ISO 12085) — a suitable description for functional manufactural and metrological requirements, in *7th Intl Conf. on Metrology and Properties of Engineering Surfaces* (B. G. Rosen, R. J. Crafoord, Eds.). Chalmers Univ., Göteborg, Sweden, 231–238.

E. R. Dougherty, J. Astola (1994). *An Introduction to Nonlinear Image Processing.* SPIE, Bellingham, WA.

E. R. Dougherty, J. Astola (1999). *Nonlinear Filters for Image Processing.* SPIE, Bellingham, WA.

N. Draper, H. Smith (1981). *Applied Regression Analysis* (2nd edition). John Wiley & Sons, New York.

R. O. Duda, P. E. Hart (1972). Use of the Hough transform to detect lines and curves in pictures. *Commun. ACM* 15(1):11–15.

R. O. Duda, P. E. Hart (1973). *Pattern Classification and Scene Analysis.* John Wiley & Sons, New York, NY.

T. R. Edwards (1982). Two-dimensional convolute integers for analytical instrumentation. *Anal. Chem.* 54:1519–1524.

R. Ehrlich, B. Weinberg (1970). An exact method for characterization of grain shape. *J. Sediment. Petrol.* 40:205–212.

R. Ehrlich, S. K. Kennedy, S. J. Crabtree, R. L. Cannon (1984). Petrographic image analysis: 1. analysis of reservoir pore complexes. *J. Sediment Petrol.* 54:1365–1378.

A. Engel, A. Massalski (1984). 3D reconstruction from electron micrographs: its potential and practical limitations. *Ultramicroscopy* 13:71–84.

Y. Fahmy, J. C. Russ, C. Koch (1991). Application of fractal geometry measurements to the evaluation of fracture toughness of brittle intermetallics. *J. Mater. Res.* 6(9):1856–1861.

C. Faloutsos, W. Equitz, M. Flickner, et al. (1994). Efficient and effective querying by image content. *J. Intelligent Inf. Sys.* 3:231–262.

J. Feder (1988). *Fractals*. Plenum Press, New York NY.

L. A. Feldkamp, L. C. Davis, J. W. Kress (1984). Practical cone beam agorithm. *J. Opt. Soc. Am.* 1(6):612.

S. F. Ferson, F. J. Rohlf, R.K. Koehn (1985). Measuring shape variation of two-dimensional outlines. *Systematic Zoology* 34:59–68.

L. F. Firestone, K. Cook, et al. (1991). Comparison of autofocus methods for automated microscopy. *Cytometry* 12:195–206.

Y. Fisher, E.W. Jacobs, R. D. Boss (1992). Fractal image compression using iterated transforms, in *Image and Text Compression*. J. A. Storer, Ed. Kluwer Academic Publishers, Boston, MA, 35–61.

M. Flickner, H. Sawhney, W. Niblack, et al. (1995). Query by image and video content: the QBIC system, *IEEE Comput.* 28(9):23–32.

A. G. Flook (1978). Use of dilation logic on the Quantimet to achieve fractal dimension characterization of texture and structured profiles. *Powder Techn.* 21:295–298.

A. G. Flook (1982). Fourier analysis of particle shape, in *Particle Size Anal.* 1981-2 (N. G. Stanley-Wood, T. Allen, Eds.). Wiley Heyden, London.

J. D. Foley, A. Van Dam (1984). *Fundamentals of Interactive Computer Graphics* Addison Wesley, Reading, MA.

J. Frank, Ed. (1992). *Electron Tomography*. Plenum Press, NY.

R. J. Frank, T. J. Grabowski, H. Damasio (1995). Voxelwise percentage tissue segmentation of human brain magnetic resonance images, in *Abstracts, 25th Annual Meeting, Soc. for Neuroscience,* Washington, 694. Cited in M. Sonka, V. Hlavac, R. Boyle (1999). *Image Processing, Analysis and Machine Vision*. Brooks Cole, Pacific Grove, CA, 132.

M. Frederik, A. Collignon, D. Vandermeulen, et al. (1997). Multi-modality image registration by maximization of mutual Information, *IEEE Trans. Med. Imaging,* 16(2):187–198.

H. Freeman (1961). On the encoding of arbitrary geometric configurations. *IEEE Trans.* EC-10:260–268.

H. Freeman (1974). Computer processing of line–drawing images. *Comput. Surveys* 6:57-97

H. Freeman, L. S. Davis (1977). A corner finding algorithm for chain–code curves. *IEEE Trans Comput.* 26:297-303.

W. Frei, C. C. Chen (1977). Fast boundary detection: a generalization and a new algorithm. *IEEE Trans. Comput.* C–26:988–998.

B. R. Frieden (1988). A comparison of maximum entropy, maximum a postiori and median window restoration algorithms, in *Scanning Microscopy* (Suppl. 2) (P. Hawkes, et al., Eds.)., Scanning Microscopy International, Chicago, 107–111.

J. P. Frisby (1980). *Vision: Illusion, Brain and Mind*. Oxford Univ. Press, Oxford, U.K.

K. S. Fu (1974). *Syntactic Methods in Pattern Recognition*, Academic Press, Boston.

K. S. Fu, J. K. Mui (1981). A survey on image segmentation. *Pattern Recognition* 13:3–16.

K. S. Fu (1982). *Syntactic Pattern Recognition and Applications*, Prentice Hall, Englewood Cliffs, NJ.

H. Fuchs, S. M. Pizer, L. C. Tsai, et al. (1982). Adding a true 3–D display to a raster graphics system. *IEEE Comput. Graphics Applic.* 2:73–78.

K. Fukunaga (1990). *Statistical Pattern Recognition,* 2nd edition. Academic Press, Boston.

R. S. Gentile, J. P. Allebach, E. Walowit (1990). Quantization of color images based on uniform color spaces. *J. Imaging Technol.* 16(1):12–21.

R. C. Gonzalez, P. Wintz (1987). *Digital Image Processing*, 2nd edition. Addison-Wesley, Reading, MA.

R. C. Gonzalez, R. E. Woods (1993). *Digital Image Processing*, Addison-Wesley, Reading, MA.

R. Gordon (1974). A tutorial on ART (algebraic reconstruction techniques). *IEEE Trans.* NS-21:78–93.

Y. A. Gowayed, J. C. Russ (1991). Geometric characterization of textile composite preforms using image analysis techniques, *J. Comput.Assisted Microsc.* 3(#4):189–200.

G. H. Granlund (1972). Fourier Preprocessing for Hand Print Character Recognition, *IEEE Trans. Comput.* C21(2):195–201.

A. Grasselli (Ed.). (1969). *Automatic Interpretation and Classification of Images*. Academic Press, Boston.

C. Gratin, F. Meyer (1992). Morphological three-dimensional analysis. *Scanning Microsc. Suppl.* 6:129–135.

F. C. A. Green, I. T. Young, G. A. Lighart (1985). A comparison of different focus functions for use in autofocus algorithms. *Cytometry* 6:81091.

S. Grossberg (Ed.). (1988). *Neural Computers and Natural Intelligence*. MIT Press, Cambridge, MA.

P. Gualtieri, P. Coltelli (1992). An automated system for the analysis of moving images. *J. Comput. Assisted Microsc.* 3(#1):15–22.

H. J. G. Gundersen (1986). Stereology of arbitrary particles *J. Microsc.* 143:3–45.

H. J. G. Gundersen et al. (1988). Some new, simple and efficient stereological methods and their use in pathological research and diagnosis. *Acta Pathologica, Microbiologica et Immunologica Scandinavica* 96:857.

H. J. G. Gundersen, E. B. Jensen (1987). The efficiency of systematic sampling in stereology and its prediction. *J. Microsc.* 147:229–263.

D-P. Hader, Ed. (1992). *Image Analysis in Biology*, CRC Press, Boca Raton, FL.

K. J. Halford, K. Preston (1984). 3-D Skeletonization of Elongated Solids. *Computer Vision Graphics Image Process.* 27:78–91.

Y. S. Ham (1993). Differential absorption cone-beam microtomography, Ph.D. Thesis, North Carolina State University,

D. J. Hand (1981). *Discrimination and Classification*, John Wiley & Sons, New York, NY.

R. M. Haralick (1978). Statistical and structural approaches to texture, *Proc. 4th Intl. Joint Conf. Patt Recog.*, Kyoto, Japan, 45.

R. Haralick (1979). Statistical and textural approaches to textures. *Proc. IEEE* 67:786–804.

R. M. Haralick, I. Dinstein (1975). A spatial clustering procedure for multi-image data. *Comput. Graph. Image. Proc.* 12:60–73.

R. M. Haralick, L. G. Shapiro (1988). Segmentation and its place in machine vision. *Scanning Microscopy Supplement* 2:39–54.

R. M. Haralick, L G Shapiro (1992). *Computer and Robot Vision I*. Addison-Wesley, Reading, MA.

R. M. Haralick, K. Shanmugam, I. Dinstein (1973). Textural features for image classification. *IEEE Trans.* SMC-3:610–621.

J. A. Hartigan (1975). *Clustering Algorithms*. John Wiley & Sons, New York.

R. V. L. Hartley (1942). A more symmetrical Fourier analysis applied to transmission problems. *Proc. IRE.*

S. Haykin (1993). *Neural Networks*. MacMillan, New York.

D. Hearn, M. P. Baker (1986). *Computer Graphics.* Prentice Hall, Englewood Cliffs, NJ.

M. Heath, S. Sarkar, T. Sanocki, et al. (1997). A robust visual method for assessing the relative performance of edge-detection algorithms. *IEEE Trans. Patt. Anal. Mach. Intell.* (PAMI)19(12):1338–1359.

D. O. Hebb (1949). *The organization of behaviour.* John Wiley & Sons, New York.

P. Heckbert (1982). Color image quantization for frame buffer display. *Computer Graphics* 16(3).:297–307.

R. Hegerl (1989). Three-dimensional reconstruction from projections in electron microscopy. *European J. Cell Biol.* 48 (Suppl. 25):135–138.

H. Heijmans (1991). Theoretical aspects of grey-level morphology. *IEEE Trans. Patt. Anal. Mach. Intell.* (PAMI) 13(6):568–582.

H. Heijmans (1994). *Morphological Image Operators.* Academic Press, New York.

C. Heipke (1992). A Global Approach for Least-Squares Image Matching and Surface Reconstruction in Object Space. *Photogrammetric Eng. Remote Sensing* 58(3):317–323.

G. T. Herman (1980). *Image Reconstruction from Projections — The Fundamentals of Computerized Tomography.* Academic Press, New York.

E. C. Hildreth (1983). The detection of intensity changes by computer and biological vision systems. *Comput. Vis. Graph. Image Proc.* 22:1–27.

T. J. Holmes, S. Bhattacharyya, J. A. Cooper, et al. (1995). Light microscopic images reconstructed by maximum likelihood deconvolution, in *Handbook of Biological Confocal Microscopy* (J. Pawley, Ed.). Plenum Press, New York, 389–402.

T. J. Holmes, N. J. O'Connor (2000). Blind deconvolution of 3D transmitted light brightfield micrographs. *J. Microsc.* 200(2):114–127.

B. J. Holt, L. Hartwick (1994). Visual image retrieval for applications in art and art history. *Proc. Storage and Retrieval for Image and Video Databases II*, SPIE, San Jose.

B. K. P. Horn (1970). *Shape from Shading: A Method for Obtaining the Shape of a Smooth Opaque Object from One View* (AI Tech Report 79, Project MAC). Mass. Inst. Tech., Cambridge, MA.

B. K. P. Horn (1975). Obtaining shape from shading information, in *Psychology of Computer Vision* (P. H. Winston, Ed.). McGraw Hill New York,115–155.

P. Hough (1962). Method and means for recognizing complex patterns, U.S. Patent 3,069,654.

C. V. Howard, M. G. Reed (1998). *Unbiased Stereology, Three Dimensional Measurements in Stereology.* BIOS Scientific Publishers, Oxford, U.K.

J. Huang, S. M. Dunn, S. M. Wiener, et al. (1994). A Method for Detecting Correspondences in Stereo Pairs of Electron Micrographs of Networks. *J. Comp. Assisted Microsc.* 6(2):85–102.

T. S. Huang (1979). A fast two-dimensional median filtering algorithm. *IEEE Trans.* ASSP 27:13–18.

D. H. Hubel (1988). *Eye, Brain, and Vision,* Scientific American Library. W. H. Freeman, New York.

H. E. Hurst, R. P. Black, Y. M. Simaika (1965). *Long-Term Storage: An Experimental Study.* Constable, London.

C. Hwang, S. Venkatraman, K. R. Rao (1993). Human visual system weighted progressive image transmission using lapped orthogonal transform classified vector quantization *Optical Eng.* 32(7):1524–1530.

S. Inoue (1986). *Video Microscopy,* Plenum Press, New York.

B. Jahne (1997). *Practical Handbook on Image Processing for Scientific Applications.* CRC Press, Boca Raton, FL.

A. K. Jain (1989). *Fundamentals of Digital Image Processing.* Prentice Hall, London.

M. James (1988). *Pattern Recognition.* Blackwell Scientific, London.

J. R. Janesick (2001). *Scientific Charge-Coupled Devices.* SPIE Press, Bellingham, WA.

E. T. Jaynes (1985). Where do we go from here? in *Maximum Entropy and Bayesian Methods in Inverse Problems* (C. R. Smith, W. T. Grandy, Eds.). D. Reidel Publishing Co., Dordrecht, Holland, 21–58.

K. F. Jarausch, T .J. Stark, P. E. Russell (1996). Silicon structures for in-situ characterization of atomic force microscopy probe geometry. *J. Vac. Sci. Technol. B.* 14(6):3425.

J. P. Jernot (1982). Thése de Doctorat és Science, Université de Caen, France.

E. M. Johnson, J. J. Capowski (1985). Principles of reconstruction and three-dimensional display of serial sections using a computer, in *The Microcomputer in Cell and Neurobiology Research* (R. R. Mize, Ed.). Elsevier, New York, 249–263.

L. R. Johnson, A. K. Jain (1981). An Efficient Two-Dimensional FFT Algorithm. *IEEE Trans. PAMI* 3:698–701.

Q. C. Johnson, J. H. Kinney, U. Bonse, et al. (1986). Micro-Tomography using Synchrotron Radiation Lawrence Livermore National Laboratory Preprint UCRL-93538 A. C. Kak, M. Slaney (1988). *Principles of Computerized Tomographic Imaging.* IEEE Pub. PC–02071.

S. Joshi, M. I. Miller (1993). Maximum a posteriori estimation with good roughness for 3D optical sectioning microscopy. *Opt. Soc. Am. A.* 10:1078–1985.

M. Kaes., A. Witkin, D. Terzopoulos (1987). Snakes: active contour models, *J. Comput. Vision* 1:321–331.

A. C. Kak, M. Slaney (1987, 2001). *Principles of Computerized Tomographic Imaging.* SIAM, Philadelphia PA.

H. R. Kang (1997). *Color Technology for Electronic Imaging Devices.* SPIE Optical Engineering Press, Bellingham, WA.

H. R. Kang (1999). *Digital Color Halftoning.* SPIE Optical Engineering Press, Bellingham, WA.

J. N. Kanpur, P. K. Sahoo, A. K. C. Wong (1985). A new method for grey-level picture thresholding using the entropy of the histogram. *Comput. Vision, Graph. Image Process.* 29:273–285.

N. Karssemeijer et al. (Eds.). *Digital Mammography.* Kluwer Academic Publishers, New York.

M. Kass, A. Witkin, D. Terzopoulos (1987). Snakes: active contour models. *Int. J. Comput. Vision* 1(4):321–331.

A. E. Kayaalp, R. C. Jain (1987). Using SEM stereo to extract semiconductor wafer pattern topography. *Proc. SPIE* 775:18–26.

B. H. Kaye, J. E. LeBlanc, G. Clark (1983). A study of physical significance of three-dimensional signature waveforms. *Proc. Fineparticle Characterization Conf.*

B. H. Kaye (1986). Image analysis procedures for characterizing the fractal dimension of fineparticles. *Proc. Particle Technol. Conf.*, Nürnberg, Germany.

A. Keating (1993). Duke University, Durham, NC, private communication.

D. J. Keller (1991). Reconstruction of STM and AFM images distorted by finite-size tips. *Surf. Sci.* 253:353–364.

D. J. Keller, F. S. Franke (1993). Envelope reconstruction of probe microscope images. *Surf. Sci.* 294:409–419.

S. Kim, J. Lee, J. Kim (1988). A New Chain-Coding Algorithm for Binary Images Using Run-Length Codes. *Comput. Vision, Graph. Image Process.* 41:114–128.

J. H. Kinney, Q. C. Johnson, M. C. Nichols, et al. (1989). X-ray microtomography on beamline X at SSRL. *Rev. Sci. Instrum.* 60(7):2471–4.

J. H. Kinney, M. C. Nichols, U. Bonse, et al. (1990). Nondestructive imaging of materials microstructures using X-ray tomographic microscopy. *Proc. MRS Symp. Tomographic Imaging.* Boston, MA.

R. Kirsch (1971). Computer Determination of the Constituent Structure of Biological Images. *Comput. Biomed. Res.* 4:315–328.

J. Kittler, J. Illingworth, J. Foglein (1985). Threshold selection based on a simple image statistic. *Comput. Vision, Graph. Image Process.* 30:125–147.

V. Kober, M. Mozerov, J. Alvarez-Borrego (2001). Nonlinear filters with spatially connected neighborhood. *Opt. Eng.* 40(6):971–983.

A. Kriete, Ed. (1992). *Visualization in Biomedical Microscopies: 3D Imaging and Computer Applications,* VCH Publishers, Weinheim,

F. P. Kuhl, C. R. Giardina (1982). Elliptic Fourier features of a closed contour. *Comp. Graph. Image Process.* 18:236–258.

K. J. Kurzydlowski, B. Ralph (1995). *The Quantitative Description of the Microstructure of Materials*, CRC Press, Boca Raton, FL.

M. Kuwahara, K. Hachimura, S. Eiho, M. Kinoshita (1976). Processing of RI-angiocardiographic images, in *Digital Processing of Biomedical Images* (K. Preston, M. Onoe, Eds.)., Plenum Press, New York, 187–202.

R. L. Lagendijk, J. Biemond (1991). *Iterative identification and restoration of images.* Kluwer Academic Publishers, Boston, MA.

L. Lam, S. Lee, C. Suen (1992). Thinning methodologies — a comprehensive survey. *IEEE Trans. PAMI* 14:868–885.

C. Lantejoul, S. Beucher (1981). On the use of the geodesic metric in image analysis. *J. Microsc.* 121:39.

R. S. Ledley, M . Buas, T. J. Golab (1990). Fundamentals of true-color image processing. *Proc. Intl. Conf. Patt. Recog.* 1:791–795.

D. L. Lee, A. T. Winslow (1993). Performance of three image-quality metrics in ink-jet printing of plain papers. *J. Electron. Imaging* 2(3):174–184.

S. U. Lee, S. Y. Chung, R. H. Park (1990). A comparative performance study of several global thresholding techniques for segmentation. *Comput. Vision. Graph. Image Process.* 52:171–190.

P. E. Lestrel, Ed. (1997). *Fourier Descriptors and Their Applications in Biology*, Cambridge Univ. Press, Cambridge, MA.

J. Y. Lettvin, R. R. Maturana, W. S. McCulloch, W. H. Pitts (1959). What the frog's eye tells the frog's brain. *Proc. Inst. Rad. Eng.* 47(#11), 1940–1951.

S. Levialdi (1972). On shrinking binary picture patterns. *Commun. ACM* 15(1):7–10

H. Li, M. Novak, R. Forchheimer (1993). Fractal-based image sequence compression scheme. *Optical Eng.* 32(7):1588–1595.

B. Lichtenbelt, R. Crane, S. Naqvi (1998). *Introduction to Volume Rendering.* Prentice Hall, Saddle River, NJ.

W. Lin, T. J. Holmes, D. H. Szarowski, J. N. Turner (1994). Data corrections for three-dimensional light microscopy stereo pair reconstruction. *J.Comput. Assisted Microsc.* 6(3):113–128.

M. Lineberry (1982). Image segmentation by edge tracing. *Appl. Digital Image Process.* IV, Vol. 359.

S. Lobregt, P. W. Verbeek, F. C. A. Groen (1980). Three-dimensional skeletonization: principle and algorithm. *IEEE Trans. PAMI* 2:75–77.

E. Mach (1906). Über den Einfluss räumlich und zeitlich variierender Lichtreize auf die Gesichtswahrnehmung. *S.-B. Akad. Wiss. Wien, Math.-Nat. Kl.* 115:633–648.

J. B. MacQueen (1967). Some Methods for the Classification and Analysis of Multivariate Observations, *Proc. 5th Berkeley Symp. Mathematical Statistics Probab.*, 1, 281–297.

E. Mainsah, K. J. Stout, T. R. Thomas (2001). Surface measurement and characterization in *Metrology and Properties of Engineering Surfaces* (E. Mainsah, Ed.). Kluwer Academic Publishers, London, 1–42.

S. G. Mallat (1989). A theory for multiresolution signal decomposition: the wavelet representation. *IEEE Trans. PAMI* 11(7):674–693.

T. Malzbender, D. Gelb, D. Wolters (2001). Polynomial texture maps. *Comput. Graph., Proc. Siggraph 2001*, pp.519–528.

B. B. Mandelbrot (1967). How long is the coast of Britain? Statistical self-similarity and fractional dimension. *Science* 155:636–638.

B. B. Mandelbrot (1982). *The Fractal Geometry of Nature*. W. H. Freeman, San Francisco, CA.

B. B. Mandelbrot, D. E. Passoja, A. J. Paullay (1984). Fractal character of fracture surfaces of metals. *Nature* 308:721.

R. Mann, S. Stanley, D. Vlaev, et al. (2001). Augmented reality visualization of fluid mixing in stirred chemical reactors using electrical resistance tomography *J. Electron. Imaging* 10(3):620–629.

P. Markiewicz, M. C. Goh (1994). Atomic force microscopy probe tip visualization and improvement of images using a simple deconvolution procedure. *Langmuir* 10:5–7.

P. Markiewicz, M. C. Goh (1995). Atomic force microscope tip deconvolution using calibration arrays. *Rev. Sci. Instrum.* 66:3186–3190.

D. Marr (1982). *Vision*. W. H. Freeman, San Francisco, CA.

D. Marr, E. Hildreth (1980). Theory of edge detection. *Proc. R. Soc. Lond.* B207:187–217.

D. Marr, T. Poggio (1976). Cooperative computation of stereo disparity. *Science* 194:283–287.

G. A. Mastin (1985). Adaptive Filters for digital image noise smoothing: an evaluation. *Comput. Vis. Graph. Image Proc.* 31:102–121.

A. D. McAulay, J. Wang, J. Li (1993). Optical wavelet transform classifier with positive real Fourier transform wavelets. *Optical Eng.* 32(6):1333–1339.

W. S. McCulloch, W. Pitts (1943). A logical calculus of the ideas imminent in nervous activity. *Bull. Math. Biophys.* 5:115.

J. J. Mecholsky, D. E. Passoja (1985). Fractals and Brittle Fracture, in *Fractal Aspects of Materials Materials*. Research Society, Pittsburgh PA.

J. J. Mecholsky, T. J. Mackin, D. E. Passoja (1986). Crack propagation in brittle materials as a fractal process, in *Fractal Aspects of Materials II*. Materials Research Society, Pittsburgh, PA.

J. J. Mecholsky, D. E. Passoja, K. S. Feinberg–Ringel (1989). Quantitative analysis of brittle fracture surfaces using fractal geometry. *J. Am. Ceram. Soc.* 72:60.

G. Medioni, R. Nevatia (1985). Segment-based stereo matching. *Computer Vision, Graph. Image Process* 31:2–18.

D. L. Milgram (1975). Computer Methods for Creating Photomosaics. *IEEE Trans.* C-24:1113–1119.

D. L. Milgram, M. Herman (1979). Clustering edge values for threshold selection. *Comput. Graph. Image. Process* 10:272-280.

M. Minsky, S. Papert (1969). *Perceptrons: An Introduction to Computational Geometry*. MIT Press, Cambridge, MA.

M. W. Mitchell, D. A. Bonnell (1990). Quantitative topographic analysis of fractal surfaces by scanning tunneling microscopy. *J. Mater. Res.* 5(10):2244–2254.

J. R. Monck, A. F. Oberhauser, T. J. Keating, et al. (1992). Thin-section ratiometric Ca2+ images obtained by optical sectioning of Fura-2 loaded mast cells. *J. Cell Biol.* 116:745–759.

H. P. Moravec (1977). Towards automatic visual obstacle avoidance. *Proc. 5th IJCAI*,:584.

R. B. Mott (1995). Position-tagged spectrometry, a new approach for EDS spectrum imaging. *Proc. Microsc. Microanal.* Jones & Begall, NY, 595.

J. C. Mott-Smith (1970). Medial Axis Transformations, in *Picture Processing and Psychopictorics* (B. S. Lipkin, A. Rosenfeld, Eds.). Academic Press, New York.

H. R. Myler, A. R. Weeks (1993). *Pocket Handbook of Image Processing Algorithms in C.* Prentice Hall, Englewood Cliffs, NJ.

K. S. Nathan, J. C. Curlander (1990). Reducing speckle in one-look SAR images. *NASA Tech Briefs* Feb:70.

F. Natterer (2001). T*he Mathematics of Computerized Tomography.* SIAM, Philadelphia, PA.

F. Natterer, F. Wubbeling (2001). *Mathematical Methods in Image Reconstruction.* SIAM, Philadelphia, PA.

B. Neal, J. C. Russ, J. C. Russ (1998). A super-resolution approach to perimeter measurement. *J. Comput. Assisted Microsc.* 10(1):11–22.

C. V. Negoita, D. A. Ralescu (1987). *Simulation, Knowledge-Based Computing, and Fuzzy Statistics.* Van Nostrand Reinhold, New York. NY.

C. V. Negoita, D. A. Ralescu (1975). *Applications of Fuzzy Sets to Systems Analysis.* Halsted Press, New York, NY.

R. Nevatia, K. Babu (1980). Linear feature extraction and description. *Comput. Graph. Image Process.* Vol. 13.

W. Niblack (Ed.) (1993). Storage and Retrieval for Image and Video Databases. *SPIE Proc.* Vol. 1908.

A. Nicoulin, M. Mattavelli, W. Li, M. Kunt (1993). Subband image coding using jointly localized filter banks and entropy coding based on vector quantization. *Optical Eng.* 32(7):1430–1450.

A. Nieminen, P. Heinonen, Y. Nuevo (1987). A new class of detail-preserving filters for image processing. *IEEE Trans.* PAMI-9:74–90.

N. Nikolaidis, I. Pitas (2001). *3-D Image Processing Algorithms.* John Wiley & Sons, New York.

J. F. O'Callaghan (1974). Computing the Perceptual Boundaries of Dot Patterns. *Comp. Graph. Image Process.* 3(2):141–162.

K. Oistämö, Y. Neuvo (1990). Vector median operations for colro image processing. *Nonlinear Image Processing* (E. J. Delp, Ed.). *SPIE Proc.* 1247:2–12.

C. K. Olsson (1993). Image Processing Methods in Materials Science, Ph.D. Thesis, Technical Univ. of Denmark, Lyngby Denmark.

N. Otsu (1979). A threshold selection method from gray-level histograms. *IEEE Trans SMC* 9:62–69; 377–393.

D. P. Panda, A. Rosenfeld (1978). Image segmentation by pixel classification in (gray level, edge value) space. *IEEE Trans. Comput.* 27:875–879.

Y-H. Pao (1989). *Adaptive Pattern Recognition and Neural Networks.* Addison-Wesley, Reading, MA.

J. R. Parker (1997). *Algorithms for Image Processing and Computer Vision.* John Wiley & Sons, New York.

T. Pavlidis (1977). *Structural Pattern Recognition.* Springer Verlag, New York.

T. Pavlidis (1980). A Thinning Algorithm for Discrete Binary Images. *Comput.Graph. Image Process.* 13:142–157.

T. Pavlidis (1982). *Algorithms for Graphics and Image Processing.* Computer Science Press, Rockville, MD.

L. D. Peachey, J. P. Heath (1989). Reconstruction from stereo and multiple electron microscope images of thick sections of embedded biological specimens using computer graphics methods. *J. Microsc.* 153:193–204.

D. M. Pearsall (1978). Phytolith analysis of archaeological soils: evidence for maize cultivation in formative Ecuador. *Science* 199(4325):177–178.

S. Peleg, J. Naor, R. Hartley, et al. (1984). Multiple resolution texture analysis and classification. *IEEE Trans. PAMI* 6:518.

A. P. Pentland (1983). Fractal-based description of natural scenes IEEE Trans PAMI-6:661.

A. P. Pentland, Ed. (1986). From Pixels to Predicates, Ablex, Norwood, NJ.

A. P. Pentland, R. W. Picard, S. Sclaroff (1994). Photobook: Content-based manipulation of image databases, in *Proc. Storage Retrieval Image Video Databases II,* SPIE, San Jose, CA.

E. Persoon, K.-S. Fu (1977). Shape Descrimination Using Fourier Descriptors. *IEEE Trans. Sys. Man Cyber.* (SMC) 7:170–179.

J. L. Pfalz (1976). Surface networks. *Geographical Anal.* 8(2):77–93.

D. R. Piperno (1984). A comparison and differentiation of phytoliths from maize (Zea mays L.) and wild grasses: use of morphological criteria. *American Antiquity* 49(2).:361–383.

I. Pitas (2000). *Digital Image Processing Algorithms and Applications.* John Wiley & Sons, New York.

W. K. Pratt (1991). *Digital Image Processing,* 2nd edition. John Wiley & Sons, New York.

T. Prettyman, R. Gardner, J. Russ, et al. (1991). On the performance of a combined transmission and scattering approach to industrial computed tomography, in A*dvances in X-ray Analysis* Vol. 35. Plenum Press, New York, NY.

J. M. S. Prewitt, M. L. Mendelsohn (1966). The analysis of cell images. *Ann. N.Y. Acad. Sci.* 128:1035–1053.

L. Quam, M. J. Hannah (1974). *Stanford automated photogrammetry research AIM-254.* Stanford AI Lab, Stanford, CA.

C. F. Quate (1994). The AFM as a tool for surface imaging. *Surf. Sci. (Netherlands)* 299–300, 980–95.

J. Radon (1917). Über die Bestimmung von Funktionen durch ihre Integralwerte längs gewisser Mannigfaltigkeiten. *Berlin Sächsische Akad. Wissen.* 29:262–279.

R. Ramanath (2000). Interpolation methods for the Bayer color array, M. S. Thesis, N. C. State Univ. Dept of Electrical Eng. (www4.ncsu.edu/~rramana/Research/MastersThesis.pdf).

B. S. Reddy, B.N. Chatterji (1996). An FFT-based technique for translation, rotation, and Scale-Invariant image registration. *IEEE Trans. Image Process.* 5(8):1266–1271.

M. G. Reed, C. V. Howard, C. G. Shelton (1997). Confocal imaging and second-order stereological analysis of a liquid foam. *J. Microsc.* 185(3):313–320.

M. G. Reed, C. V. Howard (1997). Edge corrected estimates of the nearest neighbor function for three-dimensional point patterns. *J. Microsc.* (in press).

M. G. Reed, C. V. Howard (1998). *Unbiased Stereology.* Bios Scientific Publ., Oxford.

A. A. Reeves (1990). Optimized Fast Hartley Transform with Applications, in Image Processing Thesis, Dartmouth College, Hanover, NH.

R. G. Reeves, Ed. (1975). *Manual of Remote Sensing.* American Society of Photogrammetry, Falls Church, CA.

K. Rehm, S. C. Strother, J. R. Anderson, et al. (1994). Display of merged multimodality brain images using interleaved pixels with independent color scales. *J. Nucl. Med.* 35:1815–1821.

I. Rezanaka, R. Eschbach, Eds. (1996). *Recent Progress in Ink-Jet Technologies*. Soc. Imaging Science and Tech., Springfield, VA.

W. H. Richardson (1972). Bayesian-based iterative method of image restoration. *J. Opt. Soc. Am.* 62:55–59.

J. P. Rigaut (1988). Automated image segmentation by mathematical morphology and fractal geometry. *J. Microsc.* 150:21–30.

G. X. Ritter, J. N. Wilson (2001). *Handbook of Computer Vision Algorithms in Image Algebra*, 2nd edition. CRC Press, Boca Raton, FL.

L. Roberts (1982). Recognition of three-dimensional objects, in *The Handbook of Artificial Intelligence*, Vol. III (P. Cohen, E. Figenbaum, Eds.). Kaufmann, Los Gatos, CA.

L. G. Roberts (1965). Machine perception of three-dimensional solids, in *Optical and Electro-Optical Information Processing* (J. T. Tippett, Ed.) MIT Press, Cambridge, MA.

F. J. Rohlf, J.W. Archie (1984). A comparison of Fourier methods for the description of wing shape in mosquitoes (Diptera culicidae). *Syst. Zool.* 33: 302–317.

F. J. Rohlf (1990). Morphometrics. *Annu. Rev. Ecol. Syst.* 21: 299–316.

D. W. Rolston (1988). *Principles of Artificial Intelligence and Expert System Development*. McGraw-Hill, New York.

I. Rock (1984). *Perception*. W. H Freeman, New York.

B. G. Rosen, R. J. Crafoord, Eds. (1997). *Metrology and Properties of Engineering Surfaces*. Chalmers Univ., Göteborg, Sweden.

F. Rosenblatt (1958). The Perceptron: A probabilistic model for information organization and storage in the brain. *Psych. Rev.* 65:358–408.

A. Rosenfeld, A. C. Kak (1982). *Digital Picture Processing*, Vols. 1 & 2. Academic Press, New York.

I. Rovner (1971). Potential of opal phytoliths for use in paleoecological reconstruction. *Quaternary Res.* 1(#3):345–59.

Y. Rui, T. S. Huang, S-F. Chang (1999). Image Retrieval: Current techniques, promising directions and open issues, *J. Visual Commun. Image Representation* 10(1):39–62.

D. E. Rumelhart, G. E. Hinton, R. J. Williams (1986). Learning representations by back-propagating errors. *Nature* 323:533–536.

J. C. Russ (1984). Implementing a new skeletonizing method. *J. Microsc.* 136:RP7.

J. C. Russ (1986). *Practical Stereology*. Plenum Press, New York.

J. C. Russ (1988). Differential Absorption Three-Dimensional Microtomography. *Trans Amer. Nucl. Soc.* 56(3):14.

J. C. Russ (1990a). *Computer Assisted Microscopy*. Plenum Press, New York.

J. C. Russ (1990b). Surface characterization: Fractal dimensions, Hurst Coefficients and Frequency transforms. *J. Comput. Assist. Microsc.* 2(3):161–184.

J. C. Russ (1990c). Processing images with a local Hurst operator to reveal textural differences. *J. Comput. Assist. Microsc.* 2(4):249–257.

J. C. Russ (1991). Multiband thresholding of images. *J. Comput. Assist. Microsc.* 3(2):77–96.

J. C. Russ (1993). JPEG Image Compression and Image Analysis. *J. Comput. Assist. Microsc.* 5(3):237–244.

J. C. Russ (1993). Method and application for ANDing features in binary images. *J. Comput. Assist. Microsc.*, 5(4):265–272.

J. C. Russ (1994). *Fractal Surfaces*, Plenum Press, New York.

J. C. Russ (1995a). Computer-Assisted Manual Stereology. *J. Comp. Assist. Microsc.* 7(1):35–46.

J. C. Russ (1995b). Median Filtering in Color Space. *J. Comp. Assist. Microsc.* 7(2):83–90.

J. C. Russ (1995c). Thresholding Images. *J. Comp. Assist. Microsc.* 7(3):41–164.

J. C. Russ (1995d). Designing kernels for image filtering. *J. Comp. Assist. Microsc.* 7(4):179–190.

J. C. Russ (1995e). Optimal greyscale images. *J. Comp. Assist. Microsc.* 7(4):221–234.

J. C. Russ (1995f). Segmenting touching hollow features. *J. Comp. Assist. Microsc.* 7(4):253–261.

J. C. Russ (1997). Fractal dimension measurement of engineering surfaces, in *7th Intl Conf. on Metrology Properties Eng. Surf.* (B. G. Rosen, R. J. Crafoord, Eds.). Chalmers Univ., Göteborg Sweden, 170–174.

J. C. Russ (2001a). *Forensic Uses of Digital Microscopy*, CRC Press, Boca Raton, FL.

J. C. Russ (2001b). Fractal Geometry in Engineering Metrology, in *Metrology and Properties of Engineering Surfaces* (E. Mainsah et al., Eds.). Kluwer Academic Publishers, London, 43–82.

J. C. Russ, D. S. Bright, J. C. Russ, et al. (1989). Application of the Hough transform to electron diffraction patterns. *J. Comput. Assist. Microsc.* 1(1):3–77.

J. C. Russ, R. T. Dehoff (2001). *Practical Stereology,* 2nd Edition. Plenum Press, New York.

J. C. Russ, I. Rovner (1987). Stereological verification of Zea Phytolith taxonomy. *Phytolitharien Newsletter* 4(#3):10.

J. C. Russ, J. C. Russ (1988a). Automatic discrimination of features in grey scale images. *J. Microsc.* 148:263–277.

J. C. Russ, J. C. Russ (1988b). Improved implementation of a convex segmentation algorithm. *Acta Stereologica* 7:33–40.

J. C. Russ, J. C. Russ (1989a). Uses of the Euclidean Distance Map for the Measurement of Features in Images. *J. Comput. Assist. Microsc.* 1(4):343.

J. C. Russ, J. C. Russ (1989b). Topological Measurements on Skeletonized Three-Dimensional Networks. *J. Comput. Assist. Microsc.* 1:131–150.

J. C. Russ, H. Palmour, III, T. M. Hare (1989). Direct 3-D Pore Location Measurement in Alumina. *J. Microsc.* 155(2):RP1–2.

P. Russell, D. Batchelor (2001). SEM and AFM: Complementary techniques for surface investigations. *Microsc. Anal.* July 2001: 5–8.

F. F. Sabins, Jr. (1987). *Remote Sensing: Principles and Interpretation,* 2nd Edition, W. H. Freeman, New York.

K. Sahoo, S. Soltani, A. C. Wong, et al. (1988). A survey of thresholding techniques *Comput. Vision Graph. Image Process.* 41:233–260.

E. Sanchez, L. A. Zadeh, Eds. (1987). *Approximate Reasoning in Intelligent System Decision and Control.* Oxford Press, New York NY.

J. Sanchez, M. P. Canton (1999). *Space Image Processing.* CRC Press, Boca Raton, FL.

L. J. Sartor, A. R. Weeks (2001). Morphological operations on color images. *J. Elect. Imaging* 10(2):548–559.

S. Saunders (1991). Magellan: the geologic exploration of venus. *Eng. Sci.* Spring 1991:15–27.

A. Savitsky, M. J. E. Golay (1964). Smoothing and differentiation of data by simplified least squares procedures. *Anal. Chem.* 36:1627–1639.

R. J. Schalkoff (1991). *Pattern Recognition: Statistical, Syntactical and Neural Approaches.* John Wiley & Sons, New York.

D. J. Schneberk, H. E. Martz, S. G. Azavedo (1991). Multiple Energy Techniques in Industrial Computerized Tomograhy, in *Review of Progress in Quantitative Nondestructive Evaluation* (D. O. Thompson, D. E. Chimenti, Eds.)., Plenum Press, New York.

H. P. Schwartz, K. C. Shane (1969). Measurement of particle shape by Fourier analysis. *Sedimentology* 13:213–231.

H. Schwarz, H. E. Exner (1980). Implementation of the concept of fractal dimensions on a semi-automatic image analyzer. *Powder Techn.* 27:107.

H. Schwarz, H. E. Exner (1983). The characterization of the arrangement of feature centroids in planes and volumes. *J. Microsc.* 129:155.

P. J. Scott (1995). Recent advances in areal characterization. *IX Intern. Oberflächenkolloq.* Tech. Univ. Chemnitz-Zwickau, 151–158.

P. J. Scott (1997). Foundations of topological characterization of surface texture in *7th Intl Conf. on Metrology and Properties of Engineering Surfaces* (B. G. Rosen, R. J. Crafoord, Eds.)., Chalmers Univ., Göteborg, Sweden, 162–169.

J. Serra (1982). *Image Analysis and Mathematical Morphology.* Academic Press, London.

M. Seul, L. O'Gorman, M. J. Sammon (2000). *Practical Algorithms for Image Analysis.* Cambridge Univ. Press, Cambridge, MA.

L. A. Shepp, B. F. Logan (1974). The Fourier reconsruction of a head section. *IEEE Trans. NS* 21:21–43.

A. Shih, G. Wang, P. C. Cheng (2001). Fast algorithm for X-ray cone-beam microtomography. *Microsc. Microanal.* 7:13–23.

J. Skilling (1986). Theory of Maximum Entropy Image Reconstruction, in *Maximum Entropy and Bayesian Methods in Applied Statistics, Proc. 4th Max Entropy Workshop, Univ. of Calgary, 1984* (J. H. Justice, Ed.). Cambridge Univ. Press, Cambridge. MA. 156–178.

P. E. Slatter (1987). *Building Expert Systems: Cognitive Emulation.* Halsted Press, New York.

B. D. Smith (1990). Cone-beam tomography: recent advances and a tutorial review. *SPIE Optical Eng.* 29:5.

R. F. Smith (1990). *Microscopy and Photomicrography*, CRC Press, Boca Raton, FL.

B. Smolka, A. Chydzinski, K. W. Wojciechowski, et al. (2001). On the reduction of impulse noise in multichannel image processing. *Opt. Eng.* 40(6):902–908.

D. L. Snyder, T. J. Schutz, J. A. O'Sullivan (1992). Deblurring subject to nonnegative constraints. *IEEE Trans. Sig. Proc.* 40:1143–1150.

I. Sobel (1970). *Camera models and machine perception AIM-21.* Stanford Artificial Intelligence Lab, Palo Alto, CA.

P. Soille (1999). *Morphological Image Analysis*, Springer-Verlag, Berlin.

M. Sonka, V. Hlavac, R. Boyle (1999). *Image Processing, Analysis and Machine Vision*, 2nd edition, Brooks Cole, Pacific Grove, CA.

S. Srinivasan, J. C. Russ, R. O. Scattergood (1990). Fractal Analysis of Erosion Surfaces. *J. Mater. Res.* 5(11):2616–2619.

J. A. Stark, W. J. Fitzgerald (1996). An Alternative Algorithm for Adaptive Histogram Equalization. *Comput. Vis. Graph. Image Proc.* 56(2):180–185.

M. Stefik (1995). *Introduction to Knowledge Systems.* Morgan Kaufmann, San Francisco, CA.

D. C. Sterio (1984). The unbiased estimation of number and sizes of arbitrary particles using the disector. *J. Microsc.* 134:127–136.

P. L. Stewart, R. M. Burnett Seminars in Virology, cited in C. J. Mathias, Visualization Techniques Augment Lab Research into Structure of Adenovirus. *Scientific Computing Automation* 7(6).:51–56.

M. C. Stone, W. B. Cowan, J. C. Beatty (1988). Color gamut mapping and the printing of digital color images, *ACM Trans. Graphics* 7(4):249–292.

J. A. Storer (1992). *Image and Text Compression.* Kluwer Academic Publishers, New York.

K. J. Stout, P. J. Sullivan, W. P. Dong, et al. (1993). *The development of methods for the characterization of roughness in three dimensions.* Publication EUR 15178 EN of the Commission of the European Communities, Univ. of Birmingham, Edgbaston, England.

R. G. Summers, C. E. Musial, P-C. Cheng, et al. (1991). The use of confocal microscopy and stereocon reconstructions in the analysis of sea urchin emryonic cell division. *J. Electron Microscope Tech.* 18:24–30.

R. E. Swing (1997). *An Introduction to Microdensitometry.* SPIE Press, Bellingham, WA.

H. Talbot, T. Lee, D. Jeulin, et al. (2000). Image analysis of insulation mineral fibers. *J. Microsc.* 200(3):251–258.

T. R. Thomas (1999). *Rough Surfaces,* 2nd edition. Imperial College Press, London.

M. M. Thompson, Ed. (1966). *Manual of Photogrammetry,* American Society of Photogrammetry, Falls Church, VA.

J. T. Tou, R. C. Gonzalez (1981). *Pattern Recognition Principles.* Addison-Wesley, Reading, MA.

J. Trussell (1979). Comments on "Picture thresholding using an iterative selection method." *IEEE Trans SMC* 9:311.

T-M. Tu, S-C. Su, H-C. Shyu, et al. (2001). Efficient intensity-hue-saturation-based image fusion with saturation compensation. *Optical Eng.* 40(5):720–728.

J. N. Turner, D. H. Szaeowski, K. L. Smith, et al. (1991). Confocal microscopy and three-dimensional reconstruction of electrophysiologically identified neurons in thick brain slices. *J. Electron Microscope Tech.* 8:11–23.

P. C. Twiss, E. Suess and R.M. Smith (1969). Morphological classification of grass phytoliths. *Soil Science Soc. America Proc.* 33(1):109–115.

S. E. Umbaugh (1998). *Computer Vision and Image Processing.* Prentice Hall, Saddle River NJ.

E. E. Underwood (1970). Quantitative Stereology Addison-Wesley, Reading, MA.

E. E. Underwood, K. Banerji (1986). Fractals in Fractography. *Mater. Science Eng.* 80:1.

P. A. van den Elsen, J. B. A. Maintz, E-J.D. Pol, et al. (1995). Automatic Registration of CT and MR Brain Images Using Correlation of Geometrical Features. *IEEE Trans. Med. Imaging,* 14(2):384–396.

P. A. van den Elsen , E-J. D. Pol, T. S. Sumanaweera, et al.(1994). Grey value correlation techniques used for automatic matching of CT and MR brain and spine images. *SPIE Intl Conf. Visualization in Biomedical Computing* 2359:227–237.

P. A. van den Elsen, E-J. D. Pol, M.A. Viergever (1993). Medical image matching — a review with classication, *IEEE Eng. Medicine Biol.* 12(1):26–39.

J. Van Helden (1994). CrestPathway algorithm. (personal communication).

H. R. J. R. Van Helleputte, T. B. J. Haddeman, M. J. Verheijen, J-J. Baalbergen (1995). Comparative study of 3D measurement techniques (SPM, SEM, TEM) for submicron structures. *Microelectron. Eng.* 27:547.

G. M. P. Van Kempen, L. J. Van Vliet, P. J. Verveer, et al. (1997). A quantitative comparison of image restoration methods in confocal microscopy. *J. Microsc.* 185(3):354–365.

J. G. Verly, R. L. Delanoy (1993). Some principles and applications of adaptive mathematical morphology for range imagery. *Optical Eng.* 32(12):3295–3306.

H. Verschueren, B. Houben, J. De Braekeleer, et al. (1993). Methods for computer assisted analysis of lymphoid cell shape and motility, including Fourier analysis of cell outlines. *J. Immunol. Meth.* 163:99–113.

J. S. Villarrubia (1994). Morphological estimation of tip geometry for scannerd probe microscopy. *Surf. Sci.* 321:287–300.

J. S. Villarrubia (1996). Scanned probe microscope tip characterization without calibrated tip characterizers. *J. Vac. Sci. Technol.* B14:1518–1521.

J. S. Villarubbia (1997). Algorithms for scanned probe microscopy image simulation, surface reconstruction and tip estimation. *J. Res. Natl. Inst. Stand. Tech.* 102(4):425.

R. J. Wall, A. Klinger, K. R. Castleman (1974). Analysis of Image Histograms. *Proc. 2nd Joint Intl Conf. Patt. Recog. IEEE 74CH-0885-4C*, 341–344.

J. R. Walters (1988). *Crafting Knowledge-Based Systems: Expert Systems Made Easy.* John Wiley & Sons, New York.

G. Wang, T. H. Lin, P. C. Cheng, et al. (1991). Scanning cone-beam reconstruction algorithms for X-ray microtomography. *SPIE Scanning Microscope Instrumentation* 1556:99.

G. Wang, M. Vannier (2001). Micro-CT scanners for biomedical applications, *Advanced Imaging* July:18–27.

Z. Wang (1990). *Principles of Photogrammetry (with Remote Sensing).* Press of Wuhan Technical University of Surveying and Mapping, Beijing.

A. R. Weeks (1996). *Fundamentals of Electronic Image Processing,* SPIE Press, Bellingham, WA.

E. R. Weibel (1979). *Stereological Methods,* Vols. I & II. Academic Press, London.

S. Welstead (1999). *Fractal and Wavelet Image Compression Techniques.* SPIE Press, Bellingham, WA.

A. Wen, C. Lu (1993). Hybrid vector quantization *Optical Eng.* 32(7):1496–1502.

J. West, J. M. Fitzpatrick, M.Y. Wang, et al. (1997). Comparison and Evaluation of Retrospective Intermodality Registration Techniques. *J. Comput. Assist. Tomography* 21:54–566.

J. S. Weszka (1978). A survey of threshold selection techniques. *Comput. Graph. Image. Process* 7:259–265.

J. Weszka, C. Dyer, A. Rosenfeld (1976). A comparative study of texture measures for terrain classification. *IEEE Trans SMC* 6:269–285.

J. S. Weszka, A. Rosenfeld (1979). Histogram modification for threshold selection. *IEEE Trans SMC* 9:38–52.

D. J. Whitehouse (1994). *Precision — the Handbook of Surface Metrology.* Institute of Physics Publishing, Bristol.

H. K. Wickramasinghe (1991). Scanned probes old and new. *AIP Conf. Proc.* 9–22.

B. Willis, B. Roysam, J. N. Turner, et al. (1993). Iterative, constrained 3D image reconstruction of transmitted light bright field micrographs based on maximum likelihood estimation, *J. Microsc.* 169:347–361.

R. Wilson, M. Spann (1988). *Image Segmentation and Uncertainty.* John Wiley & Sons, New York.

G. Winstanley (1987). *Program Design for Knowledge-Based Systems,* Halsted Press, New York.

R. J. Woodham (1978). Photometric stereo: a reflectance map technique for determining surface orientation from image intensity. *Proc. SPIE* 155: 136–143.

G. Wolf (1991). Usage of global information and a priori knowledge for object isolation. *Proc. 8th Intl. Congr. for Stereology,* Irvine, CA., 56.

K. W. Wong (1980). Basic Mathematics of Photogrammetry, in *Manual of Photogrammetry,* 4th Edition. American Society of Photogrammetry, Falls Church, VA., 57–58.

B. P. Wrobel (1991). Least-squares methods for surface reconstruction from images. *ISPRS J. Photogrammetry Remote Sensing,* 46:67–84.

S. Wu, A. Gersho (1993). Lapped vector quantization of images. *Optical Eng.* 32(7):1489–1495.

R. R. Yager (1979). On the measures of fuzziness and negation, part 1: membership in the unit interval. *Int. J. Gen. Sys.* 5:221–229.

G. J. Yang, T. S. Huang (1981). The effect of median filtering on edge location estimation. *Comput. Graph. Image Proc.* 15:224–245.

N. Yang, J. Boselli, I. Sinclair (2001). Simulation and quantitative assessment of homogeneous and inhomogeneous particle distributions in particulate metal matrix composites. *J. Microsc.* 201(2):189–200.

Y. Yakimovsky (1976). Boundary and object detection in real world images. *J. Assoc. Comput. Mach.* 23:599–618.

R. W. Young, N. G. Kingsbury (1993). Video compression using lapped transforms for motion estimation/compensation and coding. *Optical Eng.* 32(7):1451–1463.

T. York (2001). Status of electrical tomography in industrial applications. *J. Electron. Imaging* 10(3):608–619.

A. Yoshitaka, T. Ichikawa (1999). A survey on content-based retrieval for multimedia databases. *IEEE Trans. Knowledge Data Eng.* 11(1):81–93.

L. A. Zadeh (1965). Fuzzy Sets. *Infor. Control* 8:338–353.

C. T. Zahn, R.Z. Roskies (1972). Fourier descriptors for plane closed curves. *IEEE Trans. Comput.* C-21:269–281.

X. Zhou, E. Dorrer (1994). An Automatic Image Matching Algorithm Based on Wavelet Decomposition. ISPRS *Int. Arch. of Photogrammetry Remote Sensing,* 30(3/2):951–960.

H-J. Zimmermann (1987). *Fuzzy Sets, Decision Making and Expert Systems.* Kluwer Academic Publishers, Boston, MA.

S. Zucker (1976). Region growing: childhood and adolescence. *Comput. Graph. Image Process* 5:382–399.

O. Zuniga, R. M. Haralick (1983). Corner detection using the facet model, *Comput. Vision Patt. Recog. IEEE,* 30–37.

Index

Sobel operator, 242
Venus, 632
Atomic force microscopes (AFMs)
contours, 371
distance recording, 54
image types, 54
interferometer comparison, 58–59
noncontacting measurements, 657
physical contact, 654
quantitative dimensional measurements, 656
range imaging, 55–58, 665–668
rank operations, 255
surface data analysis, 681
Atom probe ion microscope, 600
Autocorrelation process, 331–332, 685, 690–691, *see also* Correlation process; Cross-correlation process
Automated Fingerprint Identification System (AFIS), 109
Automatic scaling, 265

B

Baba studies, 591
Babu, Nevatia and, studies, 435
Background fitting, 174–179
Background subtraction, 173, *see also* Subtraction
Backprojection, 560–561, 582–584
Backup copy storage, 104
Baddeley studies, 452, 487
Baker, Hearn and, studies, 190, 606
Balasubramanian studies, 117
Ballard and Brown studies, 376, 529
Ballard studies, 491, 529
Balloons, 379
Bandwidth limitations, 18–20
Banerji, Underwood and, studies, 261
Barnard and Thompson studies, 660
Barnes studies, 570
Barnsley and Hurd studies, 126, 127
Barnsley and Sloan studies, 127
Barnsley studies, 127
Barty studies, 596
Batchelor, Russell and, studies, 654
Bayer pattern, 15
Bayes' theorem, 168, 323, 536, 567
BCC, *see* Body-centered cubic (BCC) configuration
Beam hardening, 573–578
Bertrand studies, 253
Berzins studies, 229
Besl studies, 606
Beucher, Lantejoul and, studies, 430
Beucher and Lantejoul studies, 430
Bezier curves, 508
Bially iteration, 323
Biemond, Lagendijk and, studies, 324
Binnig studies, 654
Binning, 11
Biomedical imaging, 535–536
Birmingham measurement suite, 687–693
Blackie studies, 623
Black studies, 549
"Blinking" images, *see* Astronomical imaging

Blue channel, 16
Blurring, *see also* Smoothing
deconvolution, 319, 322–324
frequency space, 324–327
horizontal line readout, 13
motion, 324–327
neighborhood averaging, 142
reconstruction, 561–562
uniformity, 321
Boddeke studies, 18, 476
Body-centered cubic (BCC) configuration, 605
Bonnell, Mitchell and, studies, 296
Boolean logic
image math, 264
images (binary), 264, 383–389
measurement templates, 396
multiple images, 59
searching databases, 105, 109
textural orientation, 353
thresholding, 337, 344, 349, 352
visualization software programs, 346
Borgefors studies, 647
Boundaries, *see also* Edges
asymmetric, 359
images (binary), processing, 439–442
line representation, 358, 367–370
pixels, 22–23
power spectrum, 295
taut-string (rubber-band), 504
Bounding box, 481
Bow studies, 547
Boyde studies, 66, 68
Bracegirdle, Bradbury and, studies, 52
Bracegirdle studies, 52
Bracewell studies, 278
Bradbury and Bracegirdle studies, 52
Bradbury studies, 52
Braudaway studies, 117
Breadth, *see* Caliper dimensions
Bresenham line drawing algorithm, 616
Briarty and Jenkins studies, 591
Bright and Steel studies, 250
Brightness
color scales substitution, 31
contrast expansion, 132–133
histogram equalization, 214
human perception, 4, 9, 23
imaging requirements, 73
large range, cameras, 26
measurements, feature specific, 475–480
pixels, 21
solid-state chip cameras, 11
surface curvature, 176
Bright studies, 669
Broadcast television, 18–19, 129, 205
Brodatz studies, 533
Brown, Ballard and, studies, 376, 529
Brown studies, 606
Browsing, 108–111
Brute-force correlation methods, 65
Bryan and Skilling studies, 170
Buckytubes, 665
Burnett, Stewart and, studies, 585

Dilation
 basics, 409–413
 Boolean operations, 425
 measurements, 417–418
 neighborhoods, 420
 noise reduction, 166
 position information, 361
 rank operations, 255
Dinstein, Haralick and, studies, 336–337
Discrete cosine transform (DCT), 118, 125–126
Display hardware, 623–624
Distance fade, 627
Distortion, 191–193, 199
Dithering, 87–88
Divijver and Kittler studies, 527
Division, 270–276, *see also* Segmentation
DOG, *see* Difference of Gaussians (DOG)
Doppler shift, 70
Dorrer, Zhou and, studies, 660
Dots in printing, 80, 83–88
Double thresholding, 405–408
Dougherty and Astola studies, 409
Dry ink printers, 95
Duda and Hart studies, 491, 527
Dust, 72
Dye-sublimation (diffusion) printers, 94–95
Dynamic ranging, 265

E

Edges, *see also* Boundaries
 enhancing operator, 242
 following, 368–369, 379
 segmentation and thresholding, 379
 Sobel and Kirsch operators, 232–248
Edwards studies, 149
Ehrlich studies, 417
Eight-connectedness, 376, 436
Electron microscopy, 192, 288, *see also* Scanning
  electron microscopes (SEMs); Transmission
  electron microscopes (TEMs) and imaging
Electrons
 diffraction patterns, 2
 noise from transfers, 13
 shifting, 8
 well capacity, 11
Elevation, 32, 59, 69
Van den Elsen studies, 606
Embossed appearance, 672
Emerging methods, 693–694
Emission tomography, 577, *see also* Positron-emission
  tomography (PET)
Engel and Massalski studies, 584
Entropy methods, 115, 362, *see also* specific type of
  entropy method
Erosion
 basics, 409–413
 Boolean operations, 425
 measurements, 417–418
 neighborhoods, 420
 noise reduction, 166
  position information, 361
Errors (dust related), 72, *see also* Defects
Euclidean distance map (EDM)

caliper dimensions, 509
edge-to-edge distances, 489
images (binary), processing, 425–444
shape, 515
standardized Euclidean distance, 539
Exner, Schwarz and, studies, 486
Expert systems, 549–550
Extremum filter, 158

F

Face-centered cubic (FCC) configuration, 605
Fahmy studies, 261
Faloutsos studies, 106
Fan-beam geometry, 578, 579
Fast Fourier transform (FFT), 278, 300, *see also* Fourier
  transforms
Feature recognition, *see also* Classification
 cross-correlation, 527–529
 decision points, 534–536
 expert systems, 549–550
 images (binary), processing, 391–405
 kNN and cluster analysis, 545–548
 learning systems, 541–545
 multidimensional classification, 536–541
 neural nets, 551–553
 parametric description, 529–534
 Sobel operator, 241
 syntactical models, 553–554
 template matching, 527–529
Feature-specific measurements, *see* Measurements,
  feature specific
Feder studies, 261, 296, 417
Feldkamp studies, 583
Feret's diameter, 484
Fern image, 126–127
FFT, *see* Fast Fourier transform (FFT)
Files, 74, 100–101
Film, 9, 11, 16
Film recorders, 98–100
Filters, *see* specific types of filters
Firestone studies, 18
Fisher studies, 127
"Fish-finder" sonar, 70
Fitzgerald, Stark and, studies, 211
Fixed pattern noise, 17–18
Fixed-point notation, 326
Fizeau optic set, 56
Flat-bed scanners, 29
Flicker, 12, 137
Flickner studies, 106
Floating-point notation, 326
Flook studies, 417
Floppy disks, 103
"Flower" image, 126–127
Fluorescence (fluorescent microscopy)
 automatic ridge-following, 369
 division, 270
 imaging requirements, 73
 noisy images, 137
 optical sectioning, 598
 voxel values, 626
Focusing, 18, 38, 292–293

Foley and Van Dam studies, 190, 606
Fourier transform infrared (FTIR) spectroscopy, 662, *see also* Infrared imaging
Fourier transforms, *see also* Frequency space
    fast Fourier transform (FFT), 278, 300
    wavelet compression, 123, 125
Fractals
    analysis, 261–263
    compression, 126–128, 130
    measurements, feature specific, 515–519
    surfaces, 694–696
Franke, Keller and, studies, 668
Frank studies, 336, 582
Frederik studies, 606
Freeman, Abbasi-Dezfouli and, studies, 660
Freeman and Davis studies, 521
Freeman studies, 374
"Freeze frame" playback, 19
Frei and Chen algorithm, 244–246, 644–645
Frequency space
    autocorrelation, 331–332
    basics, 277–278
    blurring, 324–327
    convolution, 314–317
    correlation, 328–331
    deconvolution, 322–324
    filtering, 297–314
    Fourier transform, 278–286
    frequencies and orientations, 286
    imaging system characteristics, 317–321
    masks, 303–309
    measurements, 286–297
    motion blur, 324–327
    orientation and spacing, 286–290
    periodic information selection, 309–314
    periodic noise isolation, 297–303
    template matching, 328–331
    texture and fractals, 295–297
Frieden studies, 168
Frisby studies, 5
FTIR spectroscopy, *see* Fourier transform infrared (FTIR) spectroscopy
Fu and Mui studies, 380
Fuchs studies, 623
Fudge, 556
Fukunaga studies, 380, 547
Functional parameters, 687, 691–692
Fusion, *see* Stereology (stereoscopy)
Fu studies, 553
Future trends, 649–650
Fuzzy classification, 380, *see also* Classification
Fuzzy logic, 107, 542, 550

G

Gamut (color range), 88, 96–97
Gaussian properties
    Difference of Gaussian (DOG), 243, 247
    Laplacian method, 228
    neighborhood averaging, 142–149
    noise reduction, 165
    periodic noise isolation, 243
Gauss-Jordan elimination, 567

Gentile studies, 117
Geographical information system (GIS), 100–101, 108, 606, 610
Geometrical distortion, 191–193
Gersho, Wu and, studies, 130
Gestalt theory, 4–5
Gibbs studies, 567
Global image measurements, *see* Measurements, global (scene-based)
Global Positioning System (GPS), 108
Global uniformity, 71
Goh, Markiewicz and, studies, 668
Golay, Savitsky and, studies, 148, 231
Gonzalez, Tou and, studies, 553
Gonzalez and Wintz studies, 277, 380
Gonzalez and Woods studies, 73
Gordon studies, 563
Gouraud shading, 636, 676
Gowayed studies, 643
Gradient measurements, 466–469
Graphs, human reliance on, 2
Grasselli studies, 539
Gratin and Meyer studies, 647
Gravity waves, 1
Green studies, 18
Grey-scale, *see also* Halftoning
    basics, 23–24, 208
    brightness measurements, 476
    converting color images, 46
    Euclidean distance map (EDM), 427
    histogram equalization, 214
    images (binary), 172, 419
    masks, 391
    neighborhoods, 420
    printers, 80
    subtraction effect, 181
Grigg studies, 58
Grossberg studies, 551
Grouping, 368
Gundersen and Jensen studies, 460
Gundersen studies, 400, 448
Guthrie, Arlo, 79

H

Haar functions, 123
Hader studies, 73
Halford and Preston studies, 647
Halftoning, *see also* Grey-scale
    defect removal, 170
    dot quality, 84
    printers, 80–83
Ham studies, 583, 584
Hand-held scanners, 29
Hand studies, 527
Hannah, Quam and, studies, 602
Haralick, Zuniga and, studies, 602
Haralick and Dinstein studies, 336–337
Haralick and Shapiro studies, 380, 602
Haralick studies, 259, 260, 346
Hardware, printing, 93–98
Harmonic analysis, 519–522, 649
Hart, Duda and, studies, 491, 527

Milgram studies, 194
Miller, Joshi and, studies, 324
Minkowski methods, 417, 517, 696–698
Minsky and Papert studies, 551
Mirau optic set, 56
Mirrors (prisms), 658, 659
Mitchell and Bonnell studies, 296
Mode filter, 157
Moiré patterns, 308
Monck studies, 324
Monitors (computer), 15–16, 50–52
Moravec studies, 602
Morphology (morphing), 202–205, 409, 420–425
Morse code, 113
Motif approach, 685
Motion, *see* Sequential images
Motion blur, 324–327, *see also* Blurring
Motion flow technique, 60, 65
Mott-Smith studies, 436
Mott studies, 669
Movies, digital, 128–130, 160, 205
Moving Pictures Expert Group (MPEG) standard, 129–130, 605–606
MP3 format, 129
MRIs, *see* Magnetic resonance images (MRIs)
Mui, Fu and, studies, 380
Multiband images, 336–338
Multiband thresholding, 341–346
Multidimensional classification, 536–541
Multiple images, 59–64
Multiplication, 270–276
Muybridge, Eadweard, 609
Myler and Weeks studies, 73

N

Nathan and Curlander studies, 165
National Television Systems Committee (NTSC), 28, 33–35
Natterer and Wubbeling studies, 558
Natterer studies, 558
Natural language rules, 109
Navatia and Medoni and, studies, 601
Neal studies, 510
Negoita and Ralescu studies, 542
Neighborhood techniques
    defects, correcting, 140–167
    fractal analysis, 261–262
    histogram equalization, 217–219
    isotropy, 413–416
    measurements, 358, 491–496
    method implementation, 263–265
    morphology, 420–425
    nearest neighbor measurements, 140–167
    rank operations, 249
    shape of edge-finding operations, 247
    time requirements, 646
Neural networks, 551–553
Nevatia and Babu studies, 435
Niblack studies, 106
Nieminen studies, 157
Nikolaidis and Pitas studies, 73, 644
Nobel prize, 559

Noise
    basics, 24–26
    complementary metal oxide semiconductor (CMOS) cameras, 17–18
    defects, correcting, 137–140
    electron transfers, 13
    filtering images, 297–303
    fixed pattern noise (FPN), 17–18
    position information, 360
    scanners, 29
    spikes, 298, 303, 305
    Weiner deconvolution, 322–324
Noncontacting measurements, 657–659
Non-planar view defects, 188–189
Nonuniform illumination, 171–174
NTSC, *see* National Television Systems Committee (NTSC)
Nuts learning systems example, 542–544
Nyquist frequency, 279

O

Object motion measurement, 268
O'Callaghan studies, 360
Oistämö and Neuvo studies, 154
Oldham studies, 585
Olsson studies, 247, 407
Olympic filter, 162
Opal phytoliths, 544–545
Opaque properties, 465–466, 556, 598–600
Opening (erosion/dilation), 410–413
Optical character recognition (OCR), 527–528
Optical density, 476
Optical sectioning, 61, 596–598
Orientation, 286–290, 484–486
Otsu studies, 335, 364
Outlining of regions, 167
Out-of-focus, *see* Blurring
Overshooting, 225–226

P

Palettes, reduced color, 117–118
PAL (European) television, 18
Pancorbo studies, 58
Panda and Rosenfeld studies, 349
Pao studies, 527
Pap smears, 535–536
Parallax (vergence), 65
Parametric description, features, 529–534
Parker studies, 73, 364
Parzen window function, 299
Passoja, Mecholsky and, studies, 261
Pavlidis studies, 73, 435, 553
Pearsall studies, 545
Peleg studies, 261
Pentland studies, 105, 261, 547, 600, 659
Perimeter, features, 509–512
Periodic information selection, 309–314
Periodic noise isolation, 297–303
PET, *see* Positron-emission tomography (PET)
Pfalz graph, 693

Phong shading, 673, 676
Photo-CD (Kodak)
file storage, 101
JPEG comparison, 119, 120
multiple resolution versions, 109
Physical sectioning, 596
Phytoliths, 544–545
PICT standard format, 110, 116
Piezo device, 16
Piperno studies, 545
Pitas, Nikolaidis and, studies, 73, 644
Pitas studies, 73
Pixels, *see also* Resolution
basics, 20–23
calibration, 481
cameras, 8, 10, 15
compression, 112
direction information, 239–240
fractal analysis, 261
grouping, 391–397, 392
HDTV, 28
histograms, 217, 366
image enhancement, 74
imaging systems, 375, 505
neighborhood ranking, 152
printing, 79
rounded address values, 199
shuttering problems, 12
speckle (random noise), 320, 355
two-dimensional images, 207
voxels comparison, 62
Plane photography, *see* Aerial photography
Point operations, 134
Point spread function (PSF), 318, 321–322
Poisson distribution, 487
Polarized light microscopy, 272
Polaroid instant prints, 82
Polynominal curves, 508
Population classes, 537–541
"Portrait of a Lady," 186
Position information, 359–366
Positron-emission tomography (PET), 579–580, 606,
    see also Emission tomography
Posterization, 216
PostScript language, 79, 86
Power spectrum (spectral density), 279, *see also*
    Frequency space
Pratt studies, 73, 277, 380
Predictive vector quantization, 130
Preferred orientation, 290–295
Presentation, surfaces, 669–674
Preston, Halford and, studies, 647
Prettyman studies, 573
Prewitt and Mendelsohn studies, 335
Printers, 79–83, 93–98
Printing
basics, 79–83
color, 88–93
dots, 83–88
hardware, 93–98
Processing images, *see* Images, processing
Profile measurements, surfaces, 683–686
Profilometers

physical contact, 654–655
range imaging, 54–55, 665
technology comparison, 28
Progressive scans, 16, 28
PSD standard format, 110
Pseudo-color
grey-scale value, 54
lookup tables, 211
multiply connected surfaces, 642–643
pixel value changes, 31–32
three-dimensional images, 615
PSF, *see* Point spread function (PSF)
Pythagorean distance, 427–428, 510

Q

QBIC, *see* Query by image content (QBIC)
Quality control applications, 75, 268, 660
Quam and Hannah studies, 602
Quate studies, 654
Query by image content (QBIC), 105–106
Quicktime movies, 128, 609

R

Radar imaging, *see* Synthetic aperture radar (SAR)
RAID, *see* Redundant hard disks (RAID)
Ralescu, Negoita and, studies, 542
Ralph, Kurzydlowski and, studies, 445
Ramanesh studies, 15
Random pixel noise (speckle), 320, 355
Range imaging, 54–59, 664–668
Rank leveling, 179–181
Rank operations, 248–257, 258, 646
Ray tracing, 624–628, 673
Readout noise reduction, 13
"Real time" imaging, 25
Reconnaissance photos, *see* Aerial photography
Reconstruction, three-dimensional images, 558–567, 589
Red, green, blue (RGB) signals
color median filters, 134
color printing, 88–90
color space, 40–46
contrast expansion, 133
histogram equalization, 212
ink-jet printers, 96
reduced color palettes, 117
thresholding, 337–338
two-dimensional thresholds, 338–343
Reddy and Chatterji studies, 606
Reduced color palettes, 117–118
Redundant hard disks (RAID), 104
Reed, Howard and, studies, 445
Reed and Howard studies, 486
Reed studies, 487
Reeves studies, 278, 379
Reflection, 628–633
Region-growing method, 378–379
Reiss studies, 58
Remote sensing, 534, 539, 668
Rendering surfaces, 674–677
Reproducibility, 357–359

Rescaled range analysis, 261
Resolution, 15–16, 99, *see also* High-depth (resolution) images; Pixels
RGB signals, *see* Red, green, blue (RGB) signals
Rhines, Dehoff and, studies, 445
Richardson studies and methods, 324, 516, 517, 694, 697
Ridge-finding algorithm, 253
Rigaut studies, 335
Ringing reduction, 300
Ritter and Wilson studies, 73, 435
Ritter studies, 392
Roberts' Cross operator
    derivatives, 231–232
    neighborhood implementation, 264
    Sobel and Kirsch operators, 235, 247
Roberts studies, 529, 600
Robinson studies, 55
Rock studies, 5
Rolling ball filter, 166–167, 252, 255
Rolston studies, 549
Rosen and Crafoord studies, 685
Rosenblatt studies, 551
Rosenfeld, Panda and, studies, 349
Rosenfeld, Weszka and, studies, 366
Rosenfeld and Kak studies, 73, 380, 427
Rotini noodles, 556
Rovner, Russ and, studies, 544
Rovner studies, 545
Rubber-band boundary, 504, *see also* Boundaries
Rubber-sheeting, *see* Warping
Rui studies, 105
Rumelhart studies, 552
Run-length encoding (RLE)
    lossless coding, 116
    storage, 110, 373–374
    touching of pixels, 392
    two-dimensional images, 605
Russ and Dehoff studies, 445
Russ and Rovner studies, 544
Russ and Russ studies
    perimeter length change, 363
    Pythagorean distances, 428
    segmentation, 430
    threshold settings, 335
    topological properties, 649
Russell and Batchelor studies, 654
Russ studies
    asbestos fiber identification, 495
    boundary as fractal, 417
    color median filter, 154
    cone-beam geometry, 587
    digital imaging processing, 73
    erosion, 435
    Euclidean distance map (EDM), 434
    forgery detection, 391
    fractal dimensions, 296, 695
    grey scale values, 46
    grid superimposition, 397
    hole filling, 433
    Hough transform, 495
    nearest-neighbor distance method, 487
    rescaled range analysis, 261
    segmentation, 380

stereological methods, 445
surfaces, 659, 698
threshold settings, 335
weight values, 142

S

Sabins studies, 77, 271, 539
Sahoo studies, 335
Sampling strategies, 459–461
Sanchez and Canton studies, 73
Sanchez and Zadeh studies, 542
SAR, *see* Synthetic aperture radar (SAR)
Sartor and Weeks studies, 154
Satellite imaging, *see also* Aerial photography; Astronomical imaging; Landsat images; Weather imaging
    alignment, 195
    Boolean operations, 387
    classification, 379–380
    color shading, 181, 184
    geographical information system (GIS), 100
    geometrical distortion, 191
    GOES satellite, 188
    ice floe tracking, 268
    multiple images, 60
    remote sensing classification, 534
    subtraction, 268
    texture, 259
    two-dimensional thresholding, 340
Savitsky and Golay studies, 148–149, 231
Scanners, 29
Scanning electron microscopes (SEMs)
    Boolean operations, 387
    brightness measurements, 479
    color imaging, 30
    distortion, 191, 201
    filling holes, 393
    fractal surface dimensions, 296
    grey-scale images, 24
    image types, 53
    imaging requirements, 73
    multiband thresholding, 344
    multiple images, 59
    noisy images, 139–140
    nonuniform illumination, 173
    particle selection, 400
    physical contact, 654
    Polaroid instant prints, 82
    profile measurements, 683
    range imaging, 54
    rank leveling, 179
    stereoscopy, 66, 69, 600, 661
    surfaces, 660, 681–683
    technology comparison, 28
    voxel values, 626
Scanning tunneling microscopes (STMs)
    contours, 371
    high-resolution limit, 58
    image types, 54
    operational mode, 656
    physical contact, 654
    technology comparison, 28–29
Schalkoff studies, 527, 553

three-dimensional images, 524, 525, 604–605
three-dimensional transforms, 278

W

Van der Waals forces, 655
Wall studies, 362
Walters studies, 549
Wang and Vannier studies, 587
Wang studies, 581, 660
Warping
    alignment, 194
    imaging requirements, 73
    interpolation, 200
    morphing, 202
    square pixels, 505
    subtraction, 268
Watershed segmentation, 429–433, 500
Wavelet compression, 123–126
Weather imaging, *see also* Satellite imaging
    data sets, 609
    maps, 2
    multiple images, 60
    nonuniform illumination, 172
Weeks, Myler and, studies, 73
Weeks, Sartor and, studies, 154
Weeks studies, 73
Weibel studies, 445, 471
Welch and Hanning window functions, 299
Welstead studies, 123
Wen and Lu studies, 130
West studies, 606
Weszka and Rosenfeld studies, 366
Weszka studies, 259, 335, 362
Whitehouse studies, 685
Wickramasinghe studies, 56, 654
Wiener methods, 322–324, 620
Wilson, Ritter and, studies, 73, 435

Wilson and Spann studies, 376
Winstanley studies, 549
Wintz, Gonzalez and, studies, 277, 380
Wolf studies, 335
Wong studies, 660
Woodham studies, 600
Woods, Gonzalez and, studies, 73
Wrobel studies, 660
Wu and Gersho studies, 130
Wubbeling, Natterer and, studies, 558

X

X-ray energy spectroscopy, 668
X-rays, 573–574
X-ray tomography, 63, 558

Y

Yager studies, 364
Yakimovsky studies, 377
Yang and Huang studies, 152
Yang studies, 488
YIQ/YUV color, 40, 117, 212
York studies, 557
Yoshitaka studies, 105
Young and Kingsbury studies, 119

Z

Zadeh, Sanchez and, studies, 542
Zadeh studies, 542
Zhdan, Castle and, studies, 654
Zhou and Dorrer studies, 660
Zimmerman studies, 542
Zip disks, 103
Zucker studies, 379
Zuniga and Haralick studies, 602